AMERICA'S
TEST KITCHEN

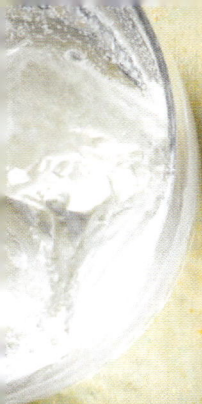

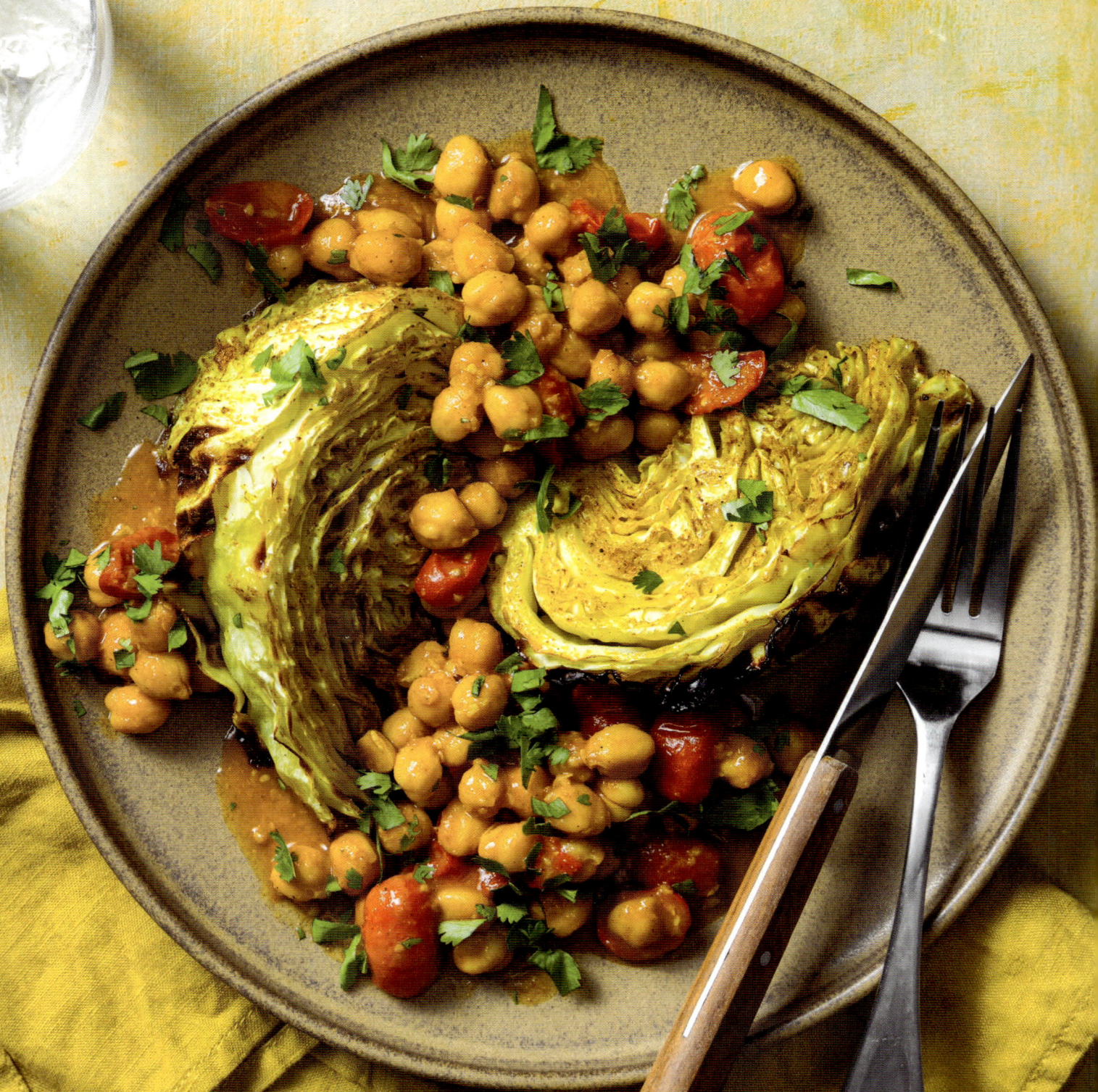

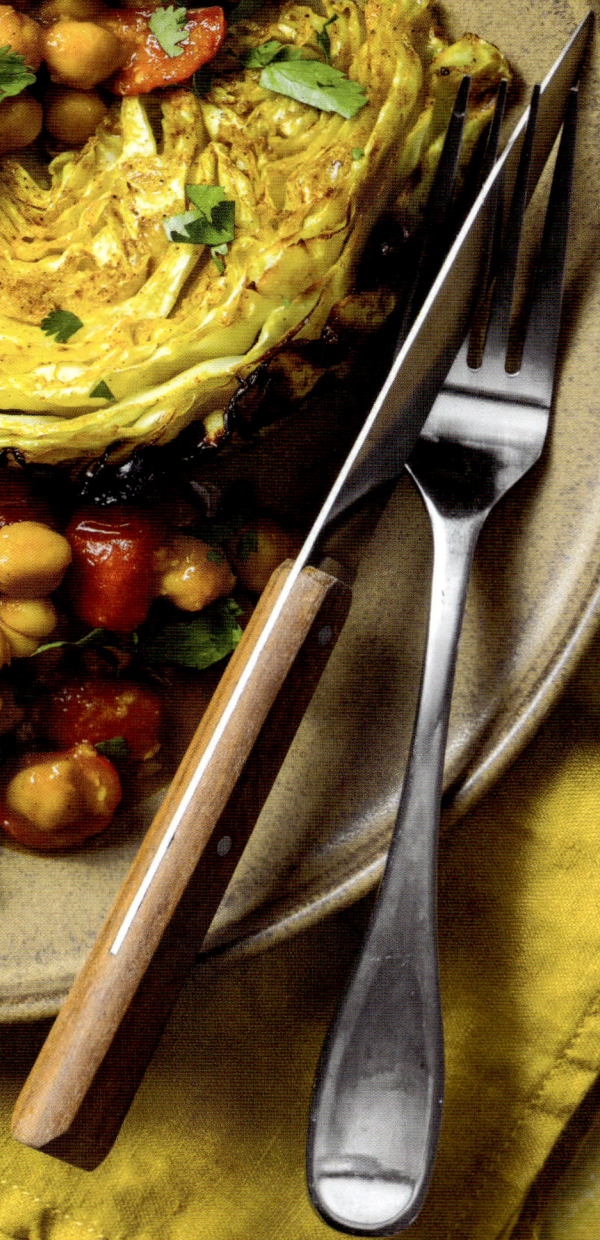

THE COMPLETE
ANTI-INFLAMMATORY
COOKBOOK

Optimize Health

Boost Your Immune System

Promote Longevity

WITH **ALICIA A. ROMANO** MS, RD, LDN

Library of Congress CIP data has been
applied for.

ISBN 978-1-954210-09-7

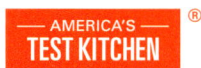

AMERICA'S
TEST KITCHEN ®

America's Test Kitchen
21 Drydock Avenue, Boston, MA 02210

Printed in Canada

10 9 8 7 6 5 4 3 2 1

Distributed by Penguin Random House
Publisher Services

Tel: 800-733-3000

Pictured on front cover: Salmon Tacos
with Super Slaw (page 246)

**Pictured on back cover (clockwise
from top):** Pressure-Cooker Chicken
with Spring Vegetables (page 310),
Kimchi Jjigae (page 79), Baked Halibut
with Cherry Tomatoes and Chickpeas
(page 243), Blueberry-Oat Smoothie
(page 47), Black-Eyed Pea Salad with
Peaches and Pecans (page 337)

Editorial Director, Books: Adam Kowit

Executive Food Editor: Dan Zuccarello

Deputy Food Editor: Stephanie Pixley

Executive Managing Editor: Debra Hudak

Project Editor: Megan Zhang

Senior Editors: Camila Chaparro, Joe Gitter, Sacha Madadian,
and Sara Mayer

Associate Editor: Claudia Catalano

Senior Photo Test Cook: José Maldonado

Test Cooks: Malcolm Jackson, Hannah Smokelin, and
Stephanie Winter

Kitchen Intern: Lillian Morrison

Assistant Editor: Julia Arwine

Consulting Nutritionist: Alicia A. Romano, MS, RD, LDN

Creative Director, Editorial: Lindsey Timko Chandler

Art Director: Nicole O'Toole

Designer: Courtney Lentz

Photography Director: Julie Bozzo Cote

Senior Photography Producer: Meredith Mulcahy

Senior Staff Photographers: Steve Klise and
Daniel J van Ackere

Staff Photographer: Kritsada Panichgul and Kevin White

Additional Photography: Beth Fuller, Nina Gallant, Joseph
Keller, and Carl Tremblay

Food Styling: Julia Heffelfinger, Joy Howard, Sheila Jarnes,
Catrine Kelty, Chantal Lambeth, Gina McCreadie,
Kendra McKnight, Ashley Moore, Christie Morrison,
Marie Piraino, Elle Simone Scott, Kendra Smith,
Sally Staub, Christine Tobin, and Janette Zepeda

Project Manager, Books: Kelly Gauthier

Senior Print Production Specialist: Lauren Robbins

Production and Imaging Coordinator: Amanda Yong

Production and Imaging Specialist: Tricia Neumyer

Production and Imaging Assistant: Chloe Petraske

Copy Editor: Elizabeth Wray Emery

Proofreader: Vicki Rowland

Indexer: Elizabeth Parson

Chief Executive Officer: Dan Suratt

Chief Content Officer: Dan Souza

Senior Content Adviser: Jack Bishop

Executive Editorial Directors: Julia Collin Davison and
Bridget Lancaster

Senior Director, Book Sales: Emily Logan

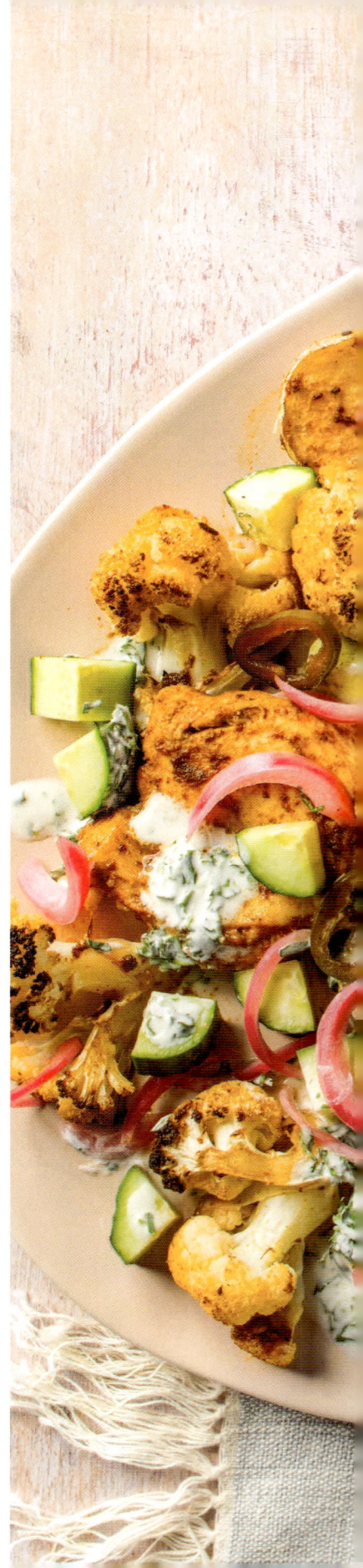

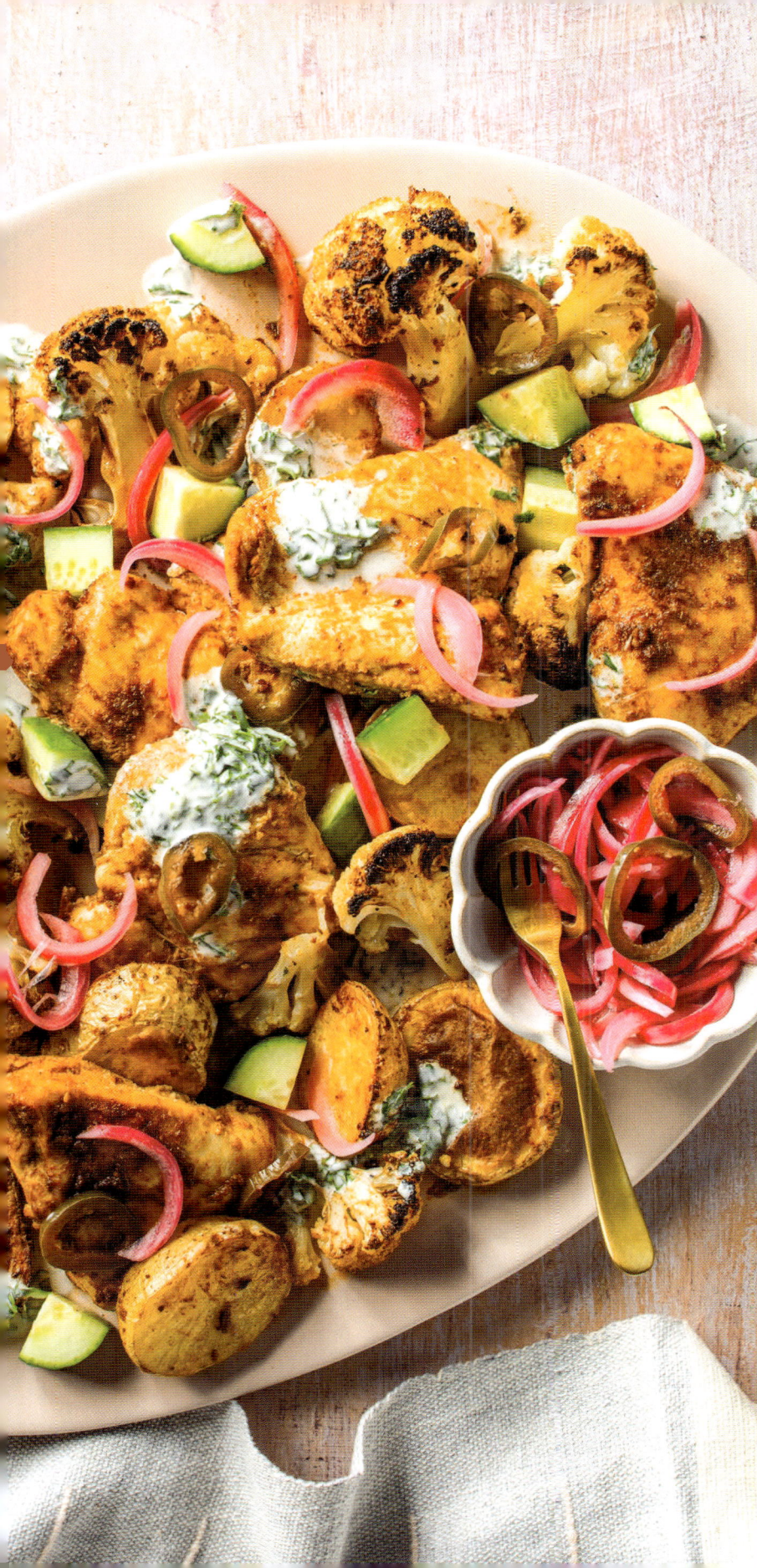

CONTENTS

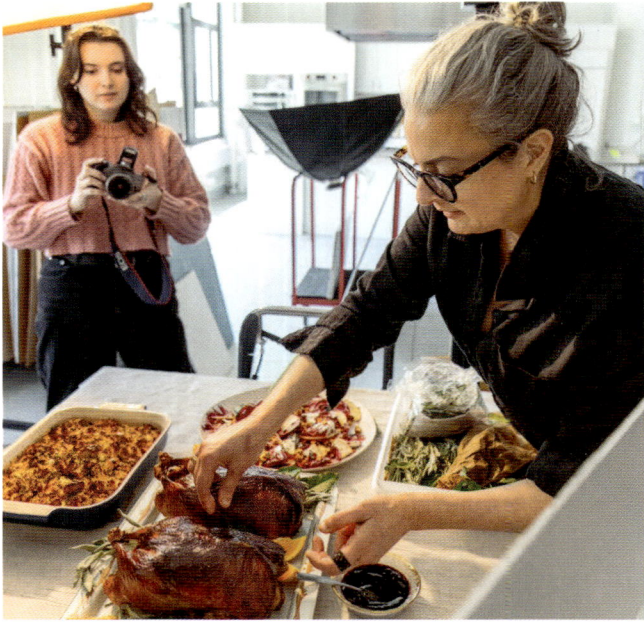
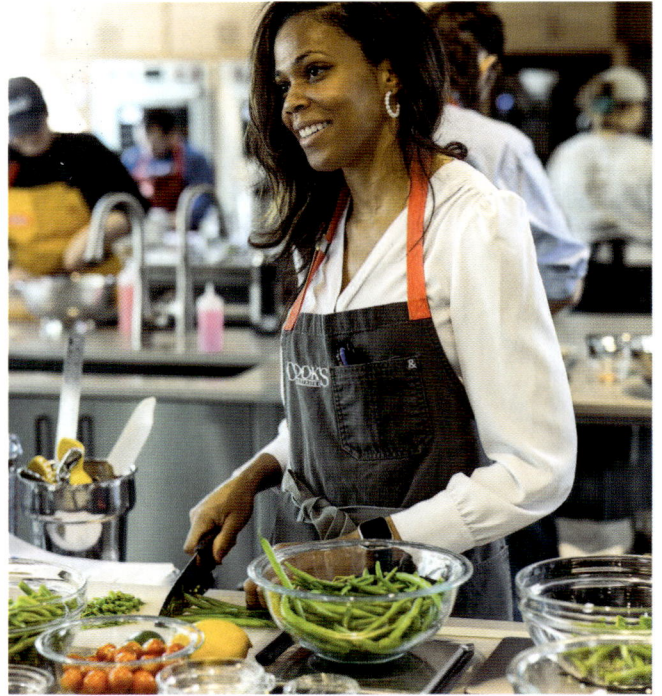
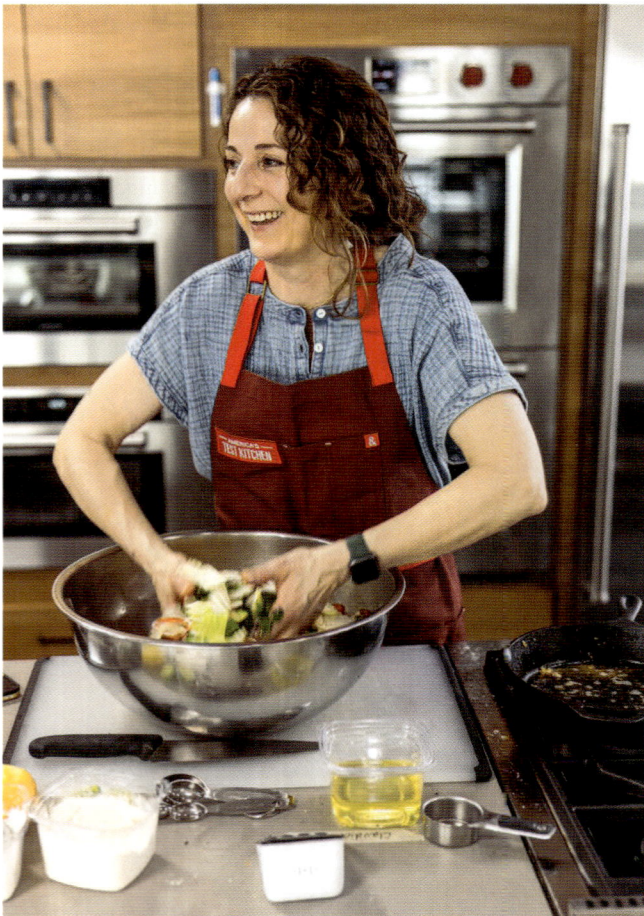
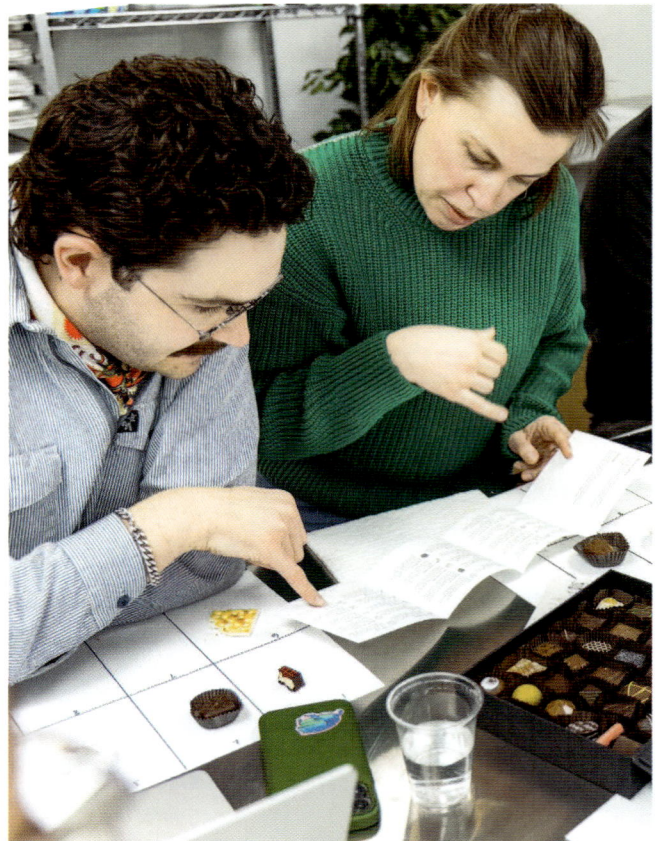

Welcome to America's Test Kitchen

This book has been tested, written, and edited by the folks at America's Test Kitchen, where curious cooks become confident cooks. Located in Boston's Seaport District in the historic Innovation and Design Building, it features 15,000 square feet of kitchen space including multiple photography and video studios. It is the home of *Cook's Illustrated* magazine and is the workday destination for more than 60 test cooks, editors, and cookware specialists. Our mission is to empower and inspire confidence, community, and creativity in the kitchen.

We start the process of testing a recipe with a complete lack of preconceptions, which means that we accept no claim, no technique, and no recipe at face value. We simply assemble as many variations as possible, test a half-dozen of the most promising, and taste the results blind. We then construct our own recipe and continue to test it, varying ingredients, techniques, and cooking times until we reach a consensus. As we like to say in the test kitchen, "We make the mistakes so you don't have to." The result, we hope, is the best version of a particular recipe, but we realize that only you can be the final judge of our success. We use the same rigorous approach when we test equipment and taste ingredients.

All of this would not be possible without a belief that good cooking, much like good music, is based on a foundation of objective technique. Some people like spicy foods and others don't, but there is a right way to sauté, there is a best way to cook a pot roast, and there are measurable scientific principles involved in producing perfectly beaten, stable egg whites. Our ultimate goal is to investigate the fundamental principles of cooking to give you the techniques, tools, and ingredients you need to become a better cook. It is as simple as that.

Find inspiration for great weeknight meals, weekend projects, holiday, and everyday cooking on our 5-star-rated app, on our social channels, and in our free email newsletters. Watch new seasons of *America's Test Kitchen* and *Cook's Country* TV shows on your public television stations and catch up with previous seasons and our original streaming series on our favorite streaming services. Start a free trial of America's Test Kitchen digital membership to access everything—including ATK Classes with focused instruction from our expert test cooks

From our kitchen to your kitchen, we welcome you into the Test Kitchen family. Please enjoy cooking with the best recipes anywhere, and follow us for daily cooking inspiration.

facebook.com/AmericasTestKitchen
instagram.com/TestKitchen
youtube.com/AmericasTestKitchen
tiktok.com/@TestKitchen
x.com/TestKitchen
pinterest.com/TestKitchen

AmericasTestKitchen.com

| JOIN OUR COMMUNITY OF RECIPE TESTERS

Our recipe testers provide valuable feedback on recipes under development by ensuring that they are foolproof in home kitchens. Help the America's Test Kitchen book team investigate the how and why behind successful recipes from your home kitchen.

Embracing an Anti-Inflammatory Way of Eating

WITH ALICIA A. ROMANO MS, RD, LDN

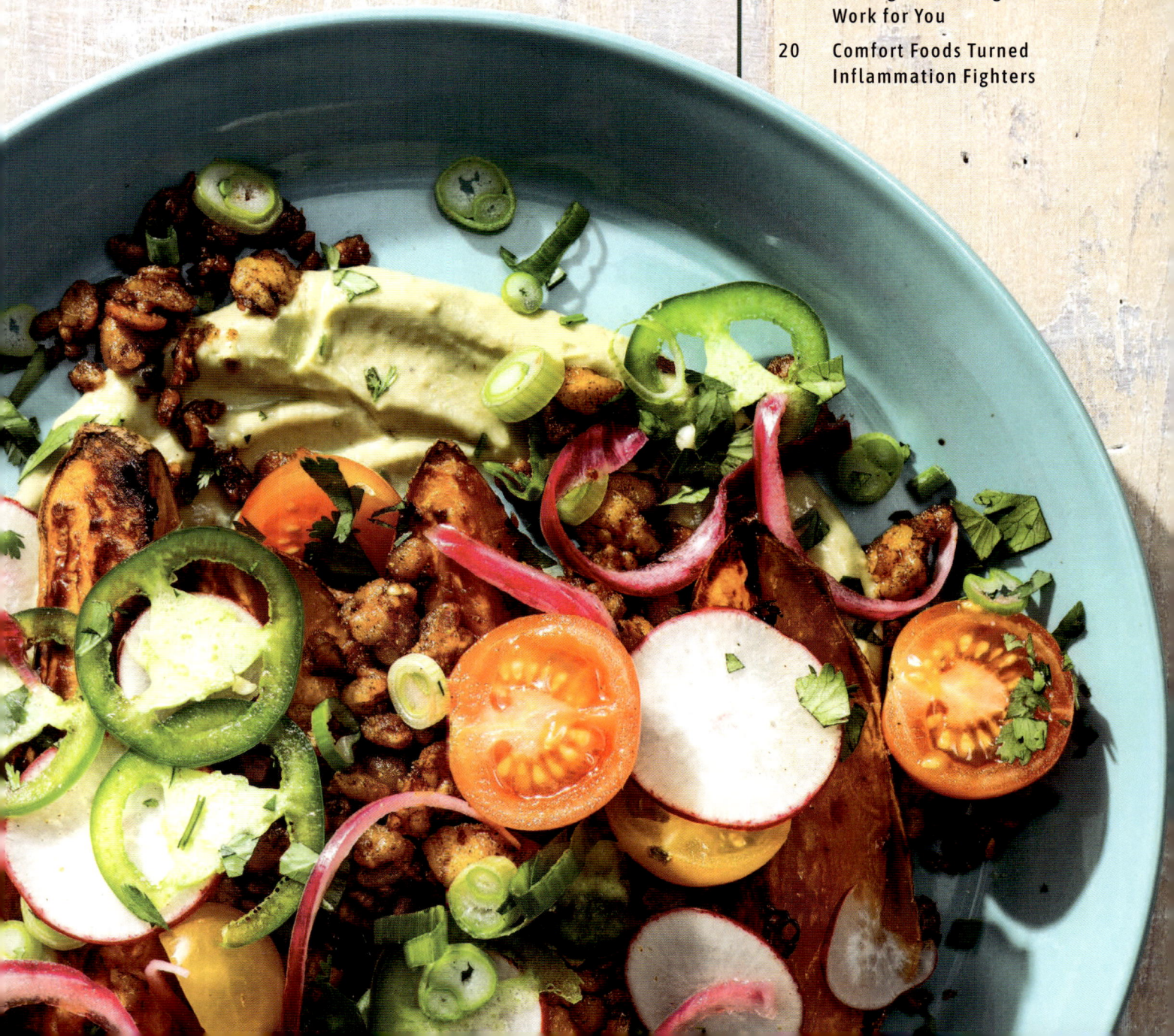

Introduction

What if we told you that the foods you eat today could have the power to shape how you feel for weeks, months, and even years to come?

The relationship between food and the way our bodies fare over time is deeply intricate, yet one topic has increasingly become a focal point for medical professionals, nutrition experts, and health-conscious eaters: chronic inflammation. This slow-burning, low-level inflammation has been linked to a staggering range of health concerns, from cardiovascular disease and type 2 diabetes to autoimmune and neurodegenerative conditions.

Unlike the body's acute inflammatory response, which plays an essential role in healing injuries and fighting infections, long-term, low-grade inflammation lingers beneath the surface, gradually damaging cells and tissues without necessarily giving noticeable warning signs. Many don't realize it's affecting them until it has taken an obvious toll on their health.

Fortunately, there's reassuring news. Research continues to reinforce that the food we put into our bodies can have a profound influence on regulating inflammation. By focusing on whole, nutrient-dense foods such as leafy greens, berries, whole grains, fatty fish, and nuts—while limiting inflammatory triggers like ultra-processed foods, refined sugars, and excessive saturated fats—we can adopt a way of eating that actively helps combat and reduce inflammation. Far from being a rigid set of restrictions, an anti-inflammatory eating pattern embraces abundance: filling your plate with more of the foods that nourish and protect, while naturally crowding out those that could drive inflammation. Small, satisfying choices made consistently over the long term can have a powerful and lasting impact on managing and lowering inflammation.

As with any healthful approach to eating, the key to long-term success is enjoyment and sustainability. That's where we, and this book, come in. If you have ever felt overwhelmed by or unsure about the convoluted nutrition advice out there, you're certainly not alone—the wellness industry can be rife with conflicting information and pseudoscience.

That's why we at America's Test Kitchen have teamed up with our longtime collaborator Alicia Romano, MS, RD, LDN, to give you expert nutritional insight alongside our trusted approach to recipe development. In a world where diet trends and alleged quick fixes come and go, the principles of anti-inflammatory eating are rooted in a solid foundation of science and balance.

With over 400 meticulously tested, dietitian-approved recipes, this comprehensive book offers everything you need to eat well for years to come. To set you up for success, we worked with Romano to clearly break down the essential dos and don'ts of anti-inflammatory eating, including which foods actively fight inflammation and which may contribute to it. We arm you with simple ingredient swaps, such as gluten-free and dairy-free tweaks, so you can adapt recipes based on dietary needs. We offer make-ahead strategies, so you can fit these recipes seamlessly into your routine, no matter how busy life may get. After all, in order for dietary adjustments to stick, meals need to be practical, satiating, and full of flavor. Whether it's a vibrant, fiberful grain bowl with roasted vegetables; a hearty fish stew rich in omega-3s; or a simple and delicious on-the-go snack, these recipes are designed to work for real life. From energizing breakfasts to filling dinners, plus drinks and snacks in between, this book covers you for every meal of the day, so you always have an anti-inflammatory bite at your fingertips.

> **FAR FROM BEING A RIGID SET OF RESTRICTIONS, AN ANTI-INFLAMMATORY EATING PATTERN EMBRACES ABUNDANCE: FILLING YOUR PLATE WITH MORE OF THE FOODS THAT NOURISH AND PROTECT, WHILE NATURALLY CROWDING OUT THOSE THAT COULD DRIVE INFLAMMATION.**

We created this book for anyone who wants to harness the power of food to reduce inflammation and bolster overall well-being. The reality is that inflammation could affect us all: Some of you may already feel its impact in symptoms like joint pain, digestive trouble, or autoimmune issues. Others may not have an immediate reason to worry about inflammation but still want to develop eating habits that lower the risk of chronic diseases. Whether you are dealing with existing inflammation, or simply wish to proactively keep issues at bay, following an anti-inflammatory eating pattern will support your body now and for many years to come.

At its core, this book is an invitation to take an empowered role in caring for your long-term health while continuing to partake in the pleasures of enjoying great food. We're excited to support and guide you on this delicious journey—and can't wait for you to cook and eat your way to better health.

A Close-Up Look at Inflammation

Inflammation is the body's natural defense mechanism that protects against injury, infection, and other environmental factors that may cause damage—while also promoting healing. It is a complex reaction involving the immune system, blood vessels, and various cellular actions in the body. Inflammation may be acute (short term) or chronic (long term) in nature.

THE BODY INITIATES INFLAMMATION AS A PROTECTIVE MECHANISM, BUT WHEN IT FAILS TO TURN OFF PROPERLY, IT CAN BECOME HARMFUL.

Acute inflammation is the immune system's fast response to injury or infection, lasting a few hours to days, and it is essential for healing. When the body detects injury or infection, a variety of cells are released as the immune system activates. Blood vessels widen (sometimes triggering visible redness or warmth) and become leaky (sometimes causing swelling) to allow more immune cells to reach the area. Neutrophils arrive first to fight infection, followed by macrophages to clean up dead cells and signal for tissue repair. Platelets help repair tissue and reduce inflammation. Once the threat is gone, healing begins, and the body returns to its normal baseline.

Chronic inflammation sets in when the body's immune response stays activated for weeks, months, or years, even when there is no injury or immediate threat. Unlike acute inflammation, which is a short-term healing response, chronic inflammation is persistent and can quietly damage healthy tissues over time. This ongoing immune activity has been linked to numerous diseases and can have a negative impact on long-term health and well-being.

The body initiates inflammation as a protective mechanism, but when it fails to turn off properly, it can become harmful. Chronic inflammation may develop due to untreated infections, lingering injuries, and autoimmune disorders, where the body mistakenly attacks itself. In many cases, long-term exposure to lifestyle and environmental factors that continuously trigger the immune system may pose a risk.

Dietary Choices: Diets high in processed foods, refined sugars, and unhealthy fats and lacking in fiber, fruits, and vegetables can fuel inflammation.

Gut Imbalance: An unhealthy gut microbiome can contribute to widespread inflammation throughout the body.

Physical Inactivity: A sedentary lifestyle slows circulation and reduces the body's ability to regulate inflammation.

Chronic Stress: Prolonged stress disrupts hormonal balance and keeps the immune system on high alert.

Poor Sleep Quality: Irregular or insufficient sleep can interfere with the body's ability to repair and regulate immune function.

Smoking and Excessive Alcohol Consumption: Both introduce toxins that trigger inflammatory responses.

Environmental Exposure: Pollutants, chemicals, and other environmental toxins can overstimulate the immune system.

Social Isolation: Research suggests that lack of social connection may negatively impact immune function and inflammation.

Unlike acute inflammation, which presents with obvious symptoms such as swelling and redness, chronic inflammation develops gradually and may not always be immediately noticeable. It can cause a number of common symptoms such as:

- Digestive discomfort (bloating, diarrhea, constipation)
- Fatigue, brain fog, or difficulty concentrating
- Frequent infections or slow-healing wounds
- Mood disorders, including anxiety and depression
- Persistent joint pain or stiffness
- Skin conditions such as rashes or recurring mouth sores
- Unexplained weight fluctuations

Anti-Inflammation Outside the Kitchen

While food is a huge piece of the inflammation puzzle, it's not the only one. How we move, sleep, manage stress, and take care of our bodies all play roles in keeping inflammation in check. Small, consistent habits can make a big difference in how we feel and function every day.

Move Your Body
Regular exercise helps lower inflammation by improving circulation, balancing blood sugar, and reducing stress hormones. It doesn't have to be intense—strength training, yoga, walking, or anything that gets you moving can help

Prioritize Sleep
Poor sleep throws off the body's natural repair processes, making it harder to regulate inflammation. Aim for 7–9 hours of quality sleep and keep a consistent routine to support overall health.

Manage Stress
Chronic stress keeps the body in a constant state of inflammation. Finding ways to reset—whether it's deep breathing, meditation, journaling, or just getting outside—can help calm the nervous system and reduce that inflammatory load.

Protect Your Skin
Too much sun exposure can lead to oxidative stress and inflammation. Daily SPF, shade, and smart sun habits go a long way in protecting your skin and overall health.

Stay Hydrated
Hydration is key for digestion, detoxification, and cellular function—all of which impact inflammation. Keep a water bottle handy and drink throughout the day.

Eat Mindfully
Slowing down, chewing food thoroughly, and being intentional about what you eat can improve digestion and prevent unnecessary inflammation.

Scientific research continues to explore the connection between chronic inflammation and disease. However, studies have shown that it plays a significant role in the development of many chronic conditions, including:

- Autoimmune diseases (rheumatoid arthritis, lupus, multiple sclerosis)
- Cardiovascular diseases (heart disease, high blood pressure)
- Certain cancers
- Lung diseases (asthma, chronic obstructive pulmonary disease)
- Metabolic disorders (type 2 diabetes, obesity, non-alcoholic fatty liver disease)
- Mental health conditions (depression, anxiety)
- Neurodegenerative diseases (Alzheimer's, Parkinson's)
- Skin conditions (eczema, psoriasis)

While chronic inflammation cannot always be entirely prevented or cured, making lifestyle changes can help manage symptoms and reduce the risk of further complications. A balanced, nutrient-rich diet, regular physical activity, stress management, and quality sleep all play critical roles in managing the body's inflammatory response.

Because chronic inflammation can manifest in different ways and overlap with various conditions, self-diagnosis is not recommended. If you suspect inflammation-related health issues, consult a healthcare professional for proper evaluation and treatment.

Although lifestyle adjustments are not a cure for chronic illnesses, they can be a powerful tool in supporting healthy immune function, managing symptoms, and potentially preventing new health issues from developing. Understanding and addressing chronic inflammation is an essential step toward looking after your long-term health.

Fight Inflammation with Food

Anti-inflammatory foods can have a powerful impact on lowering the body's inflammatory response and reducing the risk of chronic conditions such as heart disease, diabetes, and arthritis. Food isn't merely fuel—it's information for your body, and every bite has the opportunity to support healing. The right nutrients help balance blood sugar, support gut health, and strengthen the immune system, all essential for reducing chronic inflammation. By making intentional food choices, you can regulate symptoms, boost energy, and protect against long-term health issues. Let's explore how food can be one of your greatest tools for fighting inflammation.

ANTIOXIDANT ALLIES

Antioxidants are powerful compounds found in many foods that play a crucial role in protecting the body from oxidative stress caused by free radicals. Free radicals are unstable molecules that can damage cells, proteins, and DNA, contributing to inflammation and increasing the risk of chronic diseases such as heart disease, diabetes, and cancer. Antioxidants work by neutralizing these free radicals: They donate electrons to stabilize the unstable molecules, preventing further damage to the body's tissues. This process supports the immune system, helps reduce inflammation, and promotes overall health.

Vitamin C

This powerhouse antioxidant helps protect your cells, support your immune system, and aid in collagen production for healthy skin and wound healing. It's a must-have for overall wellness. Find it in:

- Bell peppers
- Broccoli
- Citrus fruits like lemons, oranges, and grapefruit
- Kale
- Mango
- Papaya
- Spinach
- Strawberries

Vitamin E

Vitamin E protects against cell damage by reducing oxidative stress, thus supporting your overall immune function and regulating inflammation. Plus, it plays a particularly large role in keeping your skin and eyes in top shape. Find it in:

- Almonds, hazelnuts, and pine nuts
- Avocados
- Olive oil
- Spinach
- Sunflower seeds, pumpkin seeds, and chia seeds

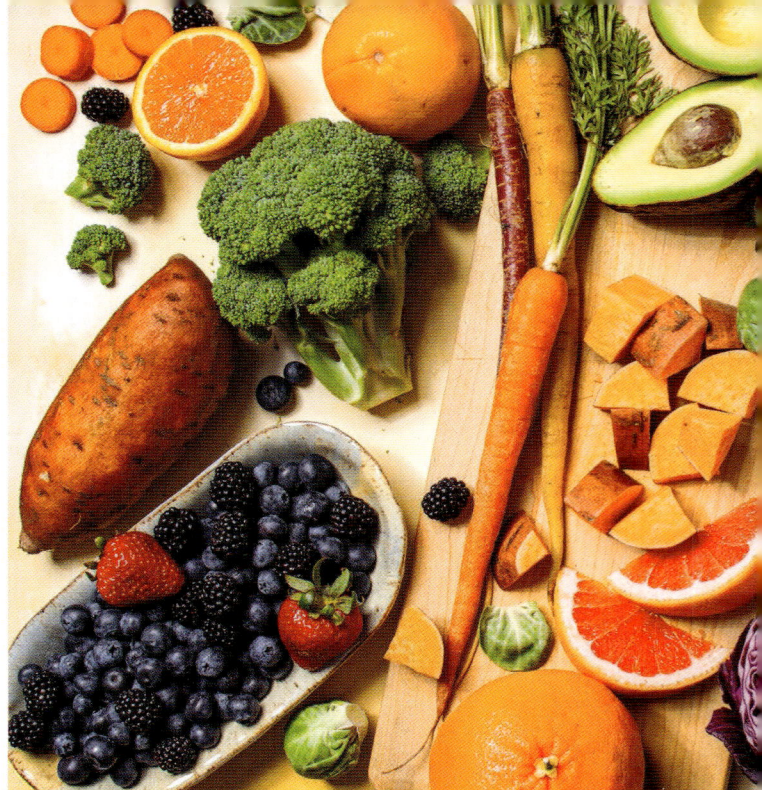

Vitamin A (Retinol & Beta-Carotene)

Vitamin A is key for your vision, immune system, and skin. Retinol, found in animal products, is the active form, while beta-carotene, found in plants, gets converted into vitamin A. Beta-carotene is particularly ample in orange and yellow vegetables. Find it in:

- Beef liver   (retinol)
- Butternut squash   (beta-carotene)
- Carrots   (beta-carotene)
- Egg yolks   (retinol)
- Fish such as salmon, mackerel, sardines, and tuna   (retinol)
- Kale   (beta-carotene)
- Spinach   (beta-carotene)
- Sweet potatoes   (beta-carotene)

Selenium

Selenium is a trace mineral that helps protect cells (particularly in the liver), supports thyroid function, and boosts your immune system. Find it in:

- Brazil nuts
- Fish such as halibut, cod, sardines, and tuna
- Lentils
- Shellfish such as shrimp, oysters, and clams
- Sunflower seeds

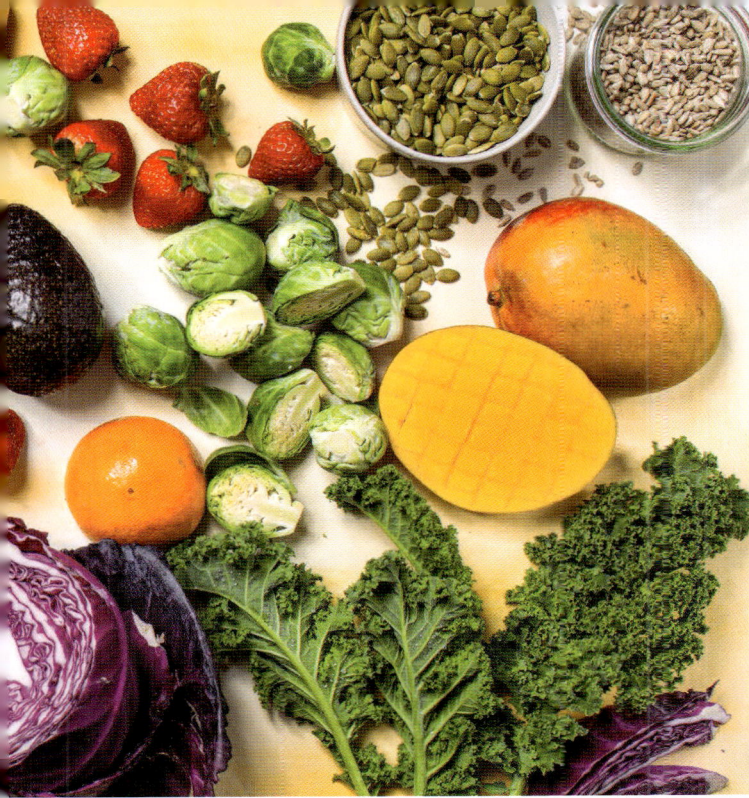

Zinc

Zinc plays a vital role in your immune health, skin, and cell repair. It's essential for overall body function and recovery. Find it in:

- Beef
- Chickpeas
- Egg yolks
- Milk
- Oysters
- Pumpkin seeds
- Sardines
- Turkey

▍ POWERFUL PHYTONUTRIENTS

Phytonutrients, also known as plant nutrients, are natural compounds found in fruits, vegetables, and other plant-based foods. These are the substances responsible for the color, flavor, and disease resistance of plants. When we eat them, they offer powerful health benefits, especially when it comes to reducing inflammation.

Many phytonutrients such as flavonoids, carotenoids, and glucosinolates have antioxidant properties, which can help neutralize the harmful free radicals that trigger inflammation. These plant compounds do more than just fight oxidative stress—they also can help regulate the immune system and decrease the production of inflammation-promoting chemicals.

Curcumin

Curcumin is the powerhouse compound in turmeric, well known for its anti-inflammatory and antioxidant properties. It's a go-to for tackling inflammation, especially for conditions like arthritis and digestive issues. It works by blocking inflammatory molecules in the body, making it a great tool for overall wellness. Find it in:

- Curry powder (often contains turmeric)
- Mustard (often has turmeric as an ingredient)
- Turmeric

Glucosinolates

These sulfur-rich compounds are found in cruciferous vegetables and help reduce inflammation in the body. They're also linked to reducing digestive inflammation and lowering the risk of certain cancers. Find them in:

- Broccoli
- Brussels sprouts
- Cauliflower
- Kale

Anthocyanins

Anthocyanins are the pigments that give fruits and vegetables their vibrant red, purple, and blue colors. Beyond looking beautiful on your plate, they are potent antioxidants that help reduce inflammation and support cardiovascular health. They are linked to balancing blood sugar and protecting cells from damage. Find them in:

- Blackberries
- Blueberries
- Cherries
- Eggplant
- Pomegranates
- Red cabbage

Lignans

Lignans are plant compounds with strong antioxidant and anti-inflammatory properties. They help regulate hormones, protect your heart, and may even reduce the risk of cancer. These compounds play a role in balancing oxidative stress in the body. Find them in:

- Beans
- Flaxseeds
- Lentils
- Sesame seeds
- Whole grains such as oats and barley

Polyphenols are a family of plant compounds known for their immune-regulating properties. While they fall under the larger umbrella of phytonutrients, their strong antioxidant and anti-inflammatory effects make them a particular standout. They interact directly with the gut microbiome, calming inflammation and enhancing the growth of beneficial bacteria. They are also particularly abundant; there are thousands of known polyphenols, and they can be found in many of our favorite foods, such as fruits, vegetables, tea, coffee, spices, and dark chocolate.

The diversity within the polyphenol family means they have wide-ranging effects; some, such as resveratrol, have been shown to offer neuroprotection, while certain flavonoids can support vascular health.

All of the polyphenols mentioned below work in different ways, but their common goal is to reduce inflammation and protect the body from damage.

Resveratrol

Resveratrol is a polyphenol known for its heart-healthy benefits and anti-inflammatory properties. It helps fight free radicals and supports immune function. Find it in:

- Blueberries
- Grapes
- Peanuts
- Red wine

Catechins

Catechins are potent antioxidants found in green tea and certain fruits. They help support cardiovascular health and combat oxidative stress. Find them in:

- Apples
- Black tea
- Grapes
- Green tea
- Pears

Flavonoids

Flavonoids are a large group of polyphenols known for their ability to reduce inflammation, protect heart health, promote circulation, and boost brain function. They help reduce inflammation by targeting specific enzymes. Find them in:

- Apples
- Blueberries
- Cherries
- Citrus fruits like lemons, oranges, and grapefruit
- Dark chocolate
- Green tea
- Kale
- Onions
- Parsley

Sulforaphane

This powerful polyphenol shows up most in cruciferous vegetables. It's known for its anti-inflammatory effects and ability to help detoxify the body. Find it in:

- Broccoli
- Brussels sprouts
- Cabbage
- Collard greens
- Kale
- Mustard greens
- Radishes
- Watercress

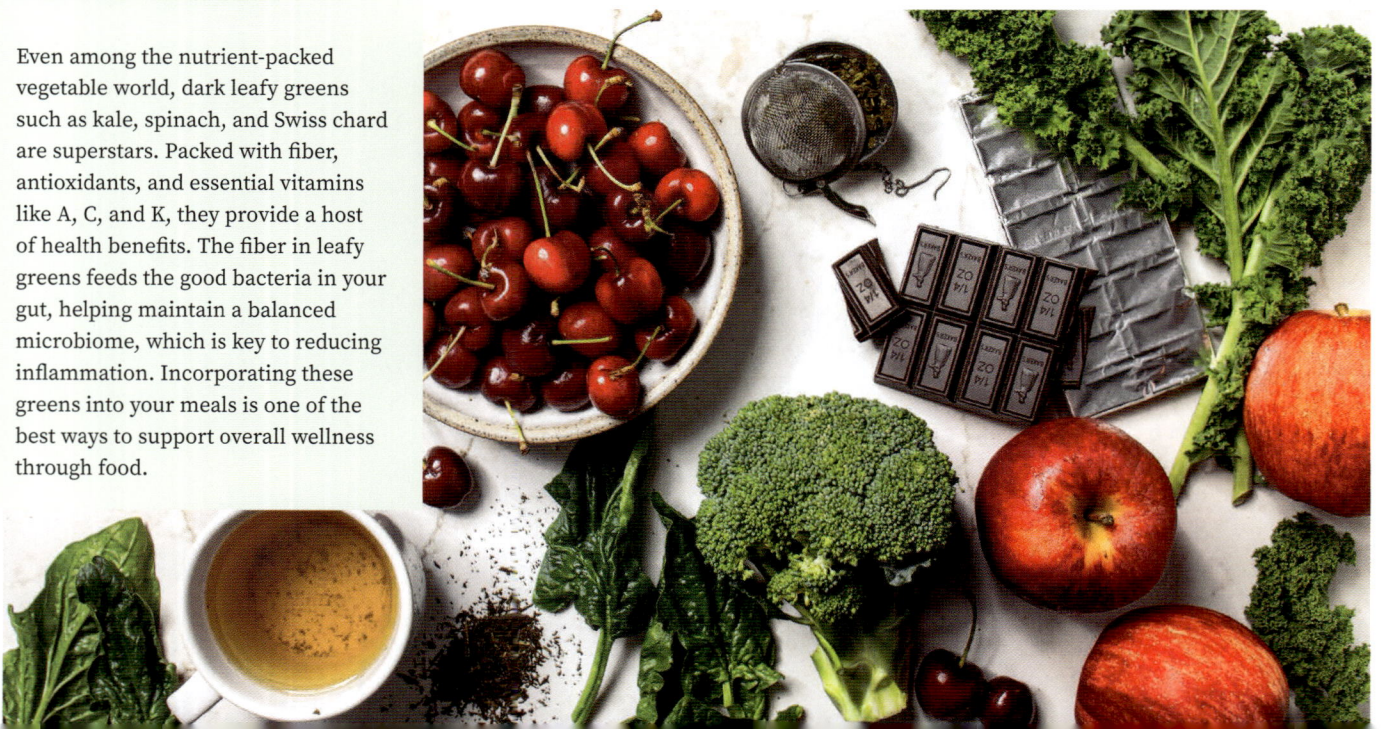

Leaf Room for Greens

Even among the nutrient-packed vegetable world, dark leafy greens such as kale, spinach, and Swiss chard are superstars. Packed with fiber, antioxidants, and essential vitamins like A, C, and K, they provide a host of health benefits. The fiber in leafy greens feeds the good bacteria in your gut, helping maintain a balanced microbiome, which is key to reducing inflammation. Incorporating these greens into your meals is one of the best ways to support overall wellness through food.

Gut-friendly fiber, prebiotics, and probiotics are all essential for managing inflammation and supporting overall gut health, which is critical for your immune system. A large portion of your immune cells are located in your gut, so a balanced microbiome plays a major role in regulating immune responses and protecting against infections.

Fiber

Fiber helps keep your digestive system running smoothly by regulating bowel movements and reducing inflammation. It also feeds the good bacteria in your gut, helping produce short-chain fatty acids (SCFAs), such as butyrate, that have anti-inflammatory benefits. Fiber comes in two forms: soluble, which dissolves in water and supports good bacteria, and insoluble, which helps eliminate waste and toxins. Both types are essential for a healthy digestive system, and eating a variety of fiber-rich foods ensures that you get enough of both kinds.

Find soluble fiber in:

- Apples
- Barley
- Chia seeds
- Citrus fruits like lemons, oranges, and grapefruit
- Flaxseeds
- Legumes such as kidney beans, black beans, and chickpeas
- Oats
- Sweet potatoes

Find insoluble fiber in:

- Cauliflower
- Celery
- Green beans
- Leafy greens such as kale, spinach, and Swiss chard
- Nuts and seeds
- Whole grains such as brown rice

Prebiotics

This special category of fiber specifically feeds your good gut bacteria. Prebiotics help your gut bacteria produce SCFAs, which further help reduce inflammation. Find them in:

- Asparagus
- Bananas
- Chicory root
- Flaxseeds
- Garlic
- Leeks
- Onions
- Seaweed
- Whole grains such as oats and barley

Probiotics

These live bacteria help balance your gut microbiome. A balanced gut means improved digestion and reduced inflammation. Together with fiber and prebiotics, probiotics work to support gut health and keep inflammation in check. Find them in:

- Kefir
- Kimchi
- Kombucha
- Natto
- Sauerkraut
- Tempeh
- Yogurt

Omega-3 fatty acids are a type of healthy fat that plays a crucial role in reducing inflammation throughout the body. When the body encounters an injury or infection, inflammation is triggered as part of the healing process. Omega-3s help regulate this inflammatory response by signaling the body to turn off inflammation once it's no longer needed. This helps prevent chronic inflammation, which can contribute to long-term damage and diseases.

Omega-3s are integral to the membranes of cells, including those in the immune system, and they influence the production of substances that control inflammation. This makes omega-3s an essential part of managing inflammation, supporting healing after immune responses, and helping prevent inflammation from becoming persistent and harmful.

Consuming foods rich in omega-3s has been linked to a reduced risk of chronic conditions such as heart disease, arthritis, and autoimmune disorders. By keeping inflammation in check, omega-3s can improve overall health. Find them in:

> **OMEGA-3S HELP REGULATE THIS INFLAMMATORY RESPONSE BY SIGNALING THE BODY TO TURN OFF INFLAMMATION ONCE IT'S NO LONGER NEEDED.**

- Chia seeds
- Fatty fish such as salmon, mackerel, and sardines
- Flaxseeds
- Grass-fed beef
- Hemp seeds
- Pasture-raised eggs
- Seaweed
- Soybeans, edamame, and tofu
- Walnuts

A Guide to an Anti-Inflammatory Diet

How can you ensure that you're eating a well-rounded diet rich in inflammation-fighting micronutrients? When it comes to embracing an anti-inflammatory way of eating, a good rule of thumb is to prioritize whole foods. Along with fruits and vegetables, it's important to include unprocessed forms of proteins, fats, and grains. Lean meats such as chicken, turkey, and tofu are packed with amino acids that support muscle and immune health. Fatty fish, rich in omega-3 fatty acids, are particularly beneficial for reducing inflammation. Healthy fats—from sources like avocados, olive oil, nuts, and seeds—are essential for managing inflammation and supporting heart health. Legumes, beans, and lentils are rich sources of plant-based protein and fiber. Whole grains such as quinoa, brown rice, and oats promote digestive health and stabilize blood sugar levels. Keep the following guidelines in mind, and you'll be well on your way to helping your body keep inflammation in check.

❙ EAT THE RAINBOW

Eating a variety of colorful fruits and vegetables is one of the simplest and most powerful ways to support your health. Each color represents a unique set of antioxidants, phytonutrients, and polyphenols—natural compounds that help reduce inflammation, support immune function, and protect your body from oxidative stress. By "eating the rainbow" you can nourish your body with a diverse range of nutrients that work together to combat inflammation and promote overall well-being.

For example, orange and yellow vegetables such as carrots and bell peppers are packed with beta-carotene, which supports immune function and eye health. Green vegetables like spinach and kale are loaded with essential vitamins such as C and K, which help manage inflammation. Purple and blue foods such as eggplant and blueberries contain anthocyanins—antioxidants that help reduce oxidative stress. Prioritizing a wide variety of colorful produce ensures that your body receives a broad spectrum of nutrients, all of which support a healthy, anti-inflammatory diet.

A Closer Look at Processed Foods

Going hand in hand with eating more whole foods is limiting ultra-processed foods, which often contain additives, preservatives, and refined sugars. These foods—think sugary snacks, fast food, pre-packaged baked goods, and sodas—are significantly altered from their natural form and can trigger inflammation in the body. Refined sugars in particular promote the production of pro-inflammatory molecules, contributing to chronic inflammation and related diseases. That's why, in developing the recipes for this book, we leaned on natural, whole-food sources for sweetness wherever possible.

Many foods you might assume are made from natural whole-food sources may actually be highly processed. Flavored yogurts usually contain thickeners and artificial flavors, plant-based meats typically include stabilizers and preservatives, and salad dressings often have flavor enhancers and emulsifiers. Condiments can be especially sneaky—ketchup, barbecue sauce, and relishes frequently contain added sugar and a host of other additives.

While it's crucial to limit processed foods, not all processed foods are created equal. Many minimally processed foods—think natural nut butters, store-bought hummus, whole-grain bread, canned beans, and smoked fish—provide essential nutrients and can be integrated into a balanced anti-inflammatory diet. Some foods are also enhanced with necessary nutrients.

Remember to read nutrition labels before jumping to conclusions about how processed a food product is. A good place to start is to flag the ingredients below, which are often used to enhance taste, texture, and shelf life but may negatively impact health when consumed in large amounts:

- Artificial sweeteners such as aspartame, sucralose, and saccharin
- Emulsifiers such as lecithin, monoglycerides, and diglycerides
- High-fructose corn syrup
- Hydrogenated oils
- Stabilizers such as pectin and carrageenan
- Texturizers such as xanthan gum and guar gum

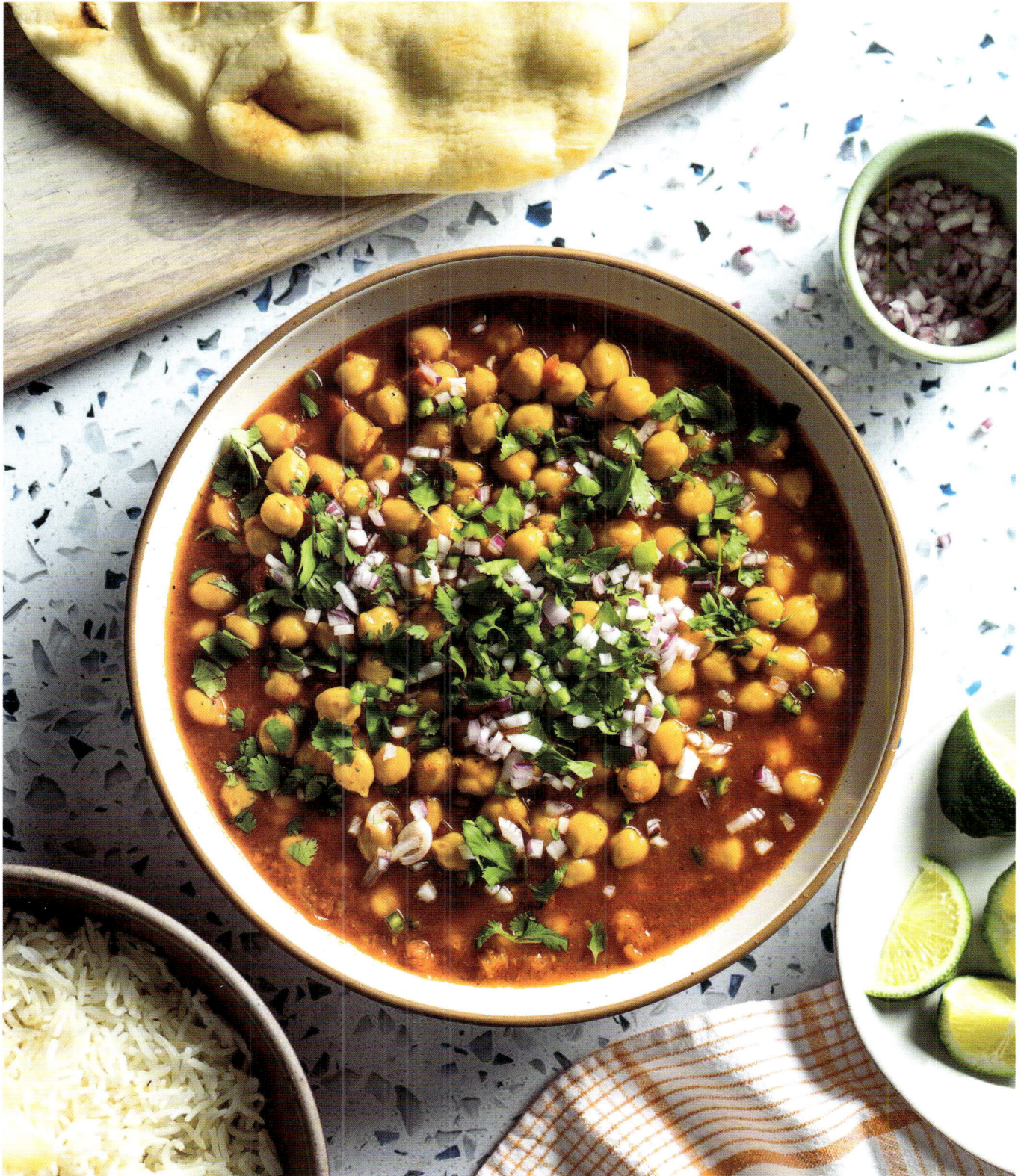

The turmeric, paprika, serrano chiles, and tomatoes in this Chana Masala (page 142) aren't just boosting flavor—their vitamins and antioxidants can help the body combat inflammation.

Choosing plant-based proteins is an effective way to reduce inflammation, support heart health, and improve overall well-being. Compared to animal meats—especially red and processed meats, which are often high in saturated fat and can trigger inflammatory responses—plant-based proteins offer numerous benefits. They are rich in antioxidants, fiber, and essential nutrients and lower in harmful inflammation-triggering compounds such as advanced glycation end-products (AGEs), which are commonly found in animal products, particularly if cooked at high temperatures (think grilling and frying). Animal products, especially meat, form more AGEs when heated due to their amino acids and fats reacting with sugars. That means that consuming too much animal protein (especially if cooked at high temperatures) can increase AGE intake, leading to inflammation, cell damage, and a higher risk of chronic diseases like heart disease and diabetes.

PLANT-BASED FOODS ARE RICH IN ANTIOXIDANTS, FIBER, AND ESSENTIAL NUTRIENTS AND LOWER IN HARMFUL INFLAMMATION-TRIGGERING COMPOUNDS.

Tofu, made from soybeans, is a great nutrient-dense option. It's low in saturated fat and rich in essential amino acids, iron, and calcium. Tofu also contains isoflavones, plant compounds that may help reduce inflammation and support hormone balance. It can be used in both savory and sweet dishes, making it a versatile choice.

Tempeh, another soy-based product, is made by fermenting cooked soybeans. It has a firmer texture and nutty flavor and is a complete protein, meaning it contains all nine essential amino acids. Tempeh is also rich in fiber, which promotes heart health and helps manage inflammation. As a fermented food, it offers probiotics that support gut health.

Legumes—a vast category that includes black beans, chickpeas, and lentils—are excellent protein sources that are also full of fiber, iron, potassium, and magnesium. They stabilize blood sugar and help reduce inflammation, thanks to their antioxidant content. The fiber in legumes also supports healthy digestion and cholesterol levels.

When it comes to fighting inflammation, the types of fats you choose can make a significant difference. Diets high in saturated fats have been linked to higher rates of inflammation. These fats, which are solid at room temperature, are typically found in animal-based products such as red meat, butter, and full-fat dairy. Unsaturated fats, on the other hand, primarily come from plant-based oils, nuts, seeds, and fatty fish. They are liquid at room temperature and fall into one of two categories: monounsaturated and polyunsaturated.

Monounsaturated fat is abundant in olive oil, avocados, and nuts (such as cashews, hazelnuts, and almonds). It enhances the function of the body's endothelial cells, which play a significant role in regulating inflammation and also support heart health. Polyunsaturated fat includes omega-3 fatty acids and omega-6 fatty acids; of these two, omega-3s are particularly revered for their anti-inflammatory benefits.

Omega-3 fatty acids are found in fatty fish—such as salmon, mackerel, and sardines—as well as in walnuts, chia seeds, and flaxseeds. Grass-fed beef and pasture-raised eggs also tend to be richer in omega-3s than their conventionally raised counterparts. Omega-3s help reduce the production of inflammatory molecules in the body; this can support heart health, promote brain function, and lower chronic inflammation. On the other hand, omega-6 fatty acids, which are common in foods such as soybean oil, corn oil, sunflower oil, and many processed food products, may fuel inflammation when consumed in large amounts. While omega-6s are essential for growth and cell repair, they're often overrepresented in the average American diet. Excess omega-6s can trigger the production of pro-inflammatory molecules, further exacerbating inflammation and contributing to an imbalance that can increase the risk of conditions such as heart disease, arthritis, and diabetes.

Ideally, the ratio of omega-6s to omega-3s in your diet should be around 4:1, but many diets today have ratios closer to 20:1, tipping the scale toward inflammation.

To keep inflammation in check, incorporate foods rich in omega-3s—fatty fish, walnuts, chia seeds, and flaxseeds—into your diet while minimizing foods high in omega-6s. When it comes to meat, choosing grass-fed over grain-fed options can help reduce omega-6 intake, as grass-fed meat tends to have a more optimal ratio of omega-3s to omega-6s.

Whole grains are an essential component of an anti-inflammatory diet. Unlike refined grains, which lose many nutrients during processing, whole grains retain their fiber, antioxidants, and essential vitamins and minerals. The high fiber content not only helps stabilize blood sugar, which can reduce spikes that contribute to inflammation, but also promotes gut health, a key factor in inflammation management—a balanced gut microbiome plays a crucial role in controlling immune responses.

Anti-inflammatory cooking doesn't need to rely strictly on whole grains, though. Flexibility is important in keeping the diet sustainable, so for instance you'll find recipes for regular pasta that incorporate fiberful vegetables, lean proteins, and healthy fats (you can also use whole-grain pasta in any of the recipes). You'll see white and brown rice in the book, as well as a variety of other whole grains, including some of our favorites listed here. And look out for the many whole-grain options available for bread, tortillas, couscous, panko, and more when shopping.

Barley : Hearty and chewy, barley offers soluble fiber and polyphenols that help regulate blood sugar and curb inflammation.

Brown and Black Rice: Both black and brown rice are loaded with fiber that helps fight inflammation (black rice also has powerful anthocyanins). They have a chewy texture and nutty flavor, making them perfect for assembling bowls or serving with stir-fries.

Fonio: This tiny West African grain is packed with iron, antioxidants, and amino acids. It cooks quickly and is easy to digest, making it a particularly gentle option for reducing inflammation.

Freekeh: Made from roasted green durum wheat, freekeh is high in fiber and antioxidants, helping to stabilize blood sugar and reduce inflammation. Its smoky flavor makes it a great side dish.

Quinoa: A gluten-free, protein-rich grain that contains all nine essential amino acids, quinoa is high in fiber and antioxidants, cooks quickly, and is a versatile option for any meal.

Teff: This tiny, nutrient-dense grain is rich in calcium and iron. It's a great gluten-free option for porridge or baked goods.

Wheat Berries: Packed with fiber, protein, and antioxidants, wheat berries support digestive health and help reduce inflammation. They have a nutty flavor and chewy texture.

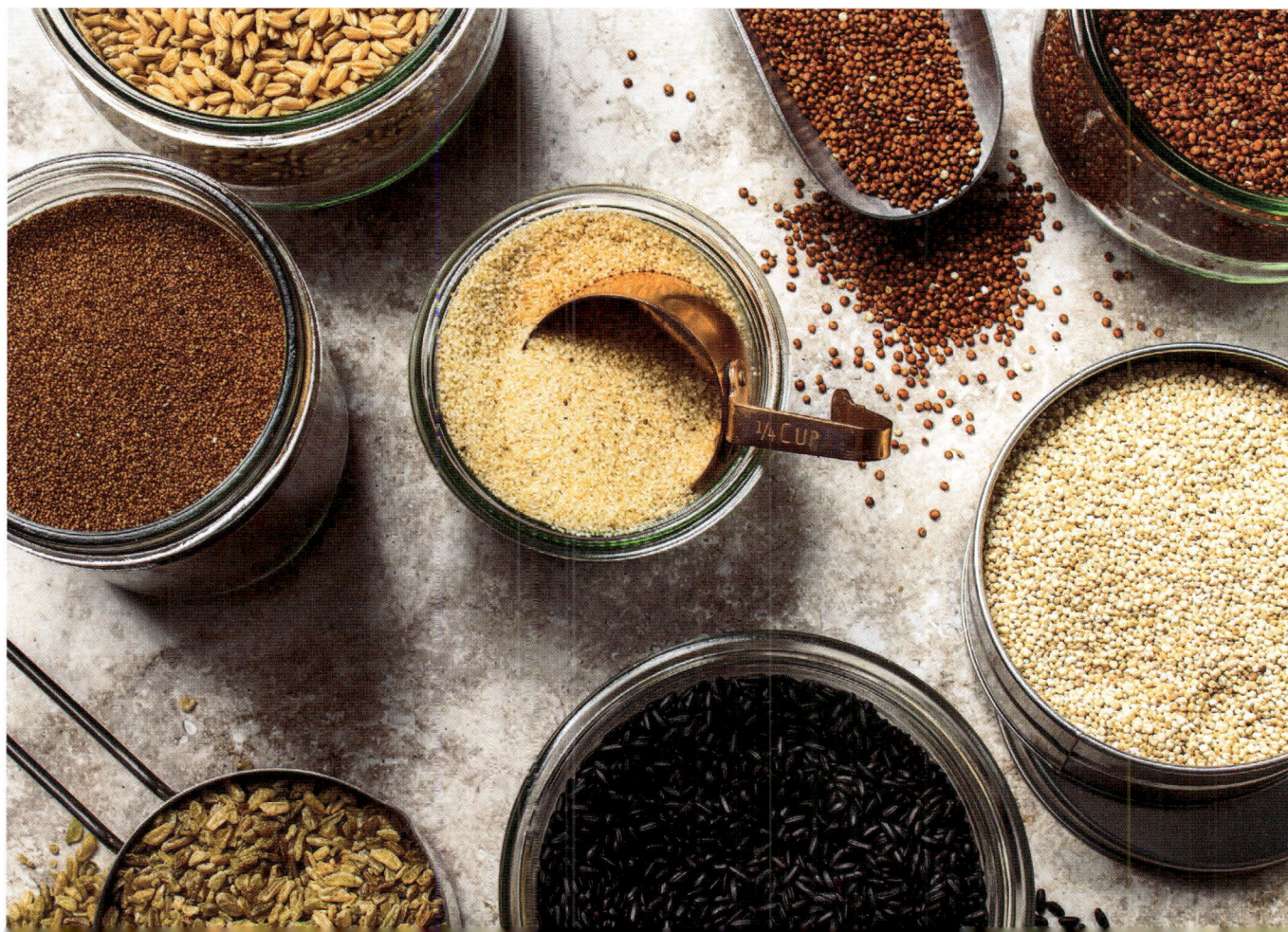

Spices and herbs don't just make food taste better—they're packed with antioxidants and compounds that help fight inflammation. Adding a variety to your meals is an easy (and delicious) way to support your health while keeping things exciting in the kitchen.

Here are some of the most potently anti-inflammatory spices and herbs from around the world that we love to reach for:

Basil: Naturally antibacterial and anti-inflammatory, basil makes a fresh, earthy addition to pestos, salads, and noodle dishes. Experiment with different varieties, from Thai basil to holy basil.

Chile Peppers: If you like a little heat, cayenne, ancho chile powder, gochugaru, and other spices and condiments made from spicy chiles are a great way to get a dose of capsaicin, which helps reduce inflammation. Different cuisines have different star chiles with varying levels of heat—keep a handful of varieties in your pantry to spice up your meals.

Cinnamon: Loaded with antioxidants and helpful in regulating blood sugar, cinnamon adds warm, toasty flavor to oatmeal, smoothies, and baked goods.

Cloves: High in antioxidants and bold in flavor, cloves add depth to both sweet and savory dishes.

Cumin: Warm, earthy, and packed with flavor, cumin helps with digestion and is a mainstay in cuisines around the world, including Indian, Mexican, Chinese, and Levantine cooking.

Garlic: Garlic is chock-full of sulfur compounds that support the immune system and reduce inflammation—and it happens to be one of the most used seasonings all over the world.

Ginger: Fresh or ground, this root should be a mainstay in your kitchen. The inflammation fighter and digestion aid adds warmth to stir-fries, teas, and marinades.

Oregano: Toss this polyphenol-packed herb into pasta sauces, dressings, and roasted veggies for its ability to fight oxidative stress.

Star Anise: Bold and aromatic, star anise comes with a dose of antibacterial and anti-inflammatory benefits. It makes a warming addition to teas, broths, and spice blends.

Sumac: This tangy, citrusy spice, rich in vitamin C and anti-inflammatory compounds, is a pantry staple in North African, Levantine, and Kurdish cuisines, among others. It adds lovely brightness to salads, roasted veggies, stews, and more.

Thyme: This slightly citrusy herb with strong anti-inflammatory properties goes great in soups, stews, and grilled dishes.

Turmeric: Curcumin makes this one of the most powerful inflammation-fighting spices on the planet. Best absorbed by the body when it's consumed with black pepper, turmeric is an excellent addition to curries, soups, and smoothies.

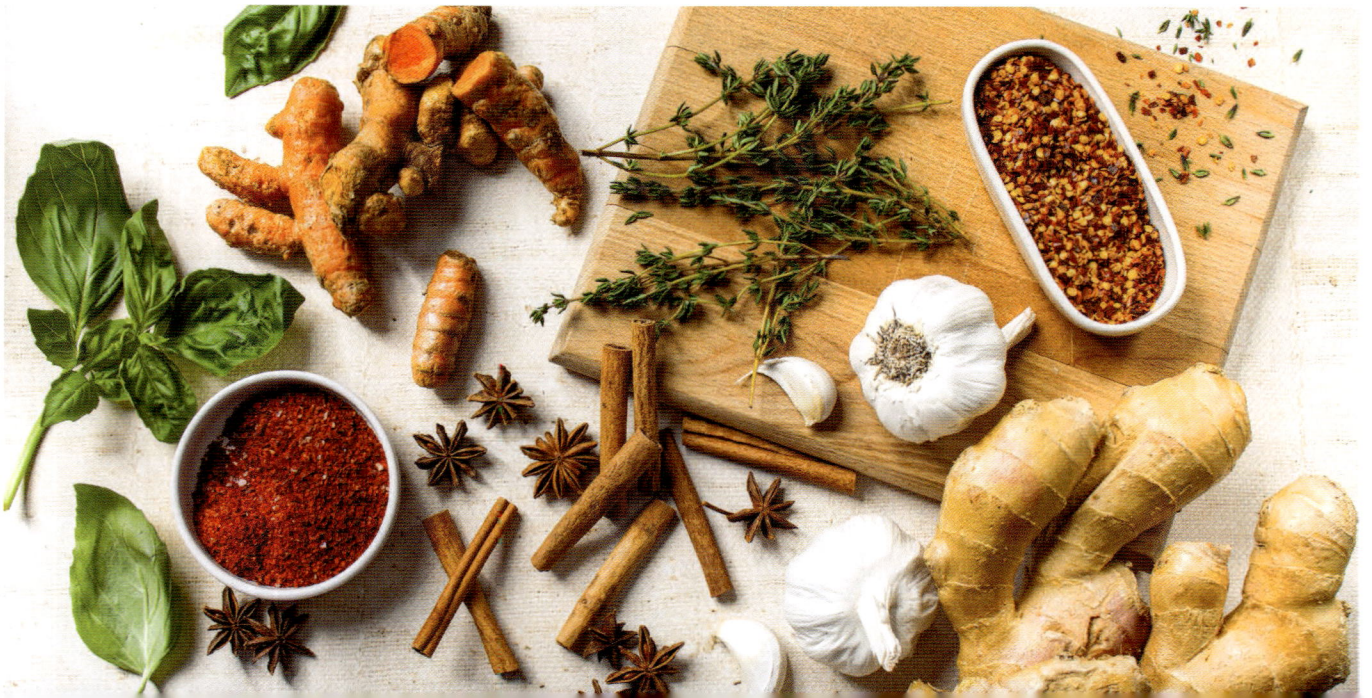

Smart Choices for Every Day

Now that you know what kinds of ingredients support an anti-inflammatory way of eating, the next step is putting that knowledge into action. This section gives you practical tips for grocery shopping and cooking, helping you stock your pantry mindfully and create nourishing meals that naturally fight inflammation. From label reading to seamless swaps, these strategies are designed to make it simpler—and more delicious—to eat in a way that supports long-term wellness.

AT THE STORE

Smart shopping lays the foundation for anti-inflammatory eating. Learn to navigate labels, choose optimal pantry staples, and make strategic swaps that support your health without sacrificing flavor.

USE THE RIGHT OILS

Not all oils are created equal: Some support health with their nutrient profiles, while others may contribute to inflammation due to processing and high omega-6 content. The key is choosing oils rich in monounsaturated fats and beneficial compounds, such as avocado oil and olive oil, which we use throughout our recipes for both flavor and health benefits. Extra-virgin olive oil (EVOO) is rich in monounsaturated fats and polyphenols, which help reduce inflammation and support heart health. Avocado oil contains high levels of oleic acid and vitamin E, promoting cardiovascular function and enhancing the absorption of fat-soluble nutrients.

Incorporating a variety of oils ensures a broader range of anti-inflammatory benefits. Other good options include flaxseed and walnut oils, which provide omega-3s to fight inflammation. Pumpkin seed and sesame oils offer additional vitamins and minerals. Try using flaxseed, walnut, pumpkin seed, and sesame oils to make dressings and sauces, or drizzle over finished salads and bowls before serving.

Limit highly processed oils such as corn, soybean, and sunflower oils, which are high in omega-6 fatty acids and can promote inflammation when consumed in excess.

Understanding smoke point is also important when choosing oils for cooking. This refers to the temperature at which an oil begins to break down and release harmful compounds. Oils with higher smoke points are optimal for cooking over high heat for prolonged periods, common in methods such as grilling or stir-frying. Avocado oil has one of the highest smoke points (up to 520°F), making it ideal for these methods. Extra-virgin olive oil, which has a lower smoke point (375–410°F), is best used in low-to-medium-high heat cooking. It also makes a flavorful finishing oil.

CHOOSE THE RIGHT MILK (FOR YOU)

The choice between plant-based milk and dairy is highly personal and should be guided by individual health needs and preferences. While plant milks, such as almond, oat, or soy milk, can be a great alternative for those avoiding dairy, they often undergo processing, which may include the addition of sugars, emulsifiers, and other additives. Emulsifiers such as guar gum, xanthan gum, and lecithin are commonly used in processed plant milks to improve texture and shelf life; these ingredients can sometimes contribute to inflammation, especially when consumed in excess. In sensitive individuals, they can potentially impact gut health by affecting the gut microbiome and contribute to digestive issues or inflammation. If inflammation or gut health is a concern, it's important to choose plant milks with minimal to zero added sugars and fewer emulsifiers, which can help reduce the risk of inflammatory response.

On the other hand, dairy offers essential nutrients such as calcium and vitamin D, but contains proteins like casein and whey, which can be inflammatory for those with sensitivities or intolerances.

Ultimately, whether you choose plant-based milk or dairy depends on your personal health, how your body responds, and what feels best for you. If inflammation is a concern, it's worth experimenting with different options and reading labels carefully—choosing products with fewer additives and more natural ingredients to reduce potential triggers. It's about finding the balance that works for your body while supporting your health goals.

MINIMIZE RED MEAT

Red meat, while rich in essential nutrients such as protein, iron, and zinc, should be consumed in moderation on an anti-inflammatory diet. Red meat is often high in saturated fats, which, when consumed in excess, may contribute to inflammation and increase the risk of chronic conditions like heart disease, type 2 diabetes, and even certain cancers. Additionally, processed red meats—such as bacon, sausages, and deli meats—are especially concerning due to their high levels of sodium, preservatives, and saturated fats, which can further promote inflammation and other health issues.

To reap the nutritional benefits of red meat while minimizing its potential inflammatory impact, enjoy it occasionally while incorporating a variety of other protein sources into your regular diet. The recipes in this book demonstrate how to enjoy red meat in dishes that limit saturated fat and also incorporate an array of anti-inflammatory ingredients such as vegetables, spices and herbs, and more.

Throughout this book, we mostly use leaner cuts such as filet mignon and pork tenderloin, which are lower in fat than options like rib eye or T-bone steaks. But fattier cuts aren't off the table: Our recipes show how a smaller amount of these can pack a great deal of meaty flavor. A little usually goes a long way, imbuing vegetables with intense savoriness and depth while keeping saturated fat in check. If available and within your budget, grass-fed or pasture-raised beef is a great choice. These options typically have a more favorable nutrient profile, including higher levels of omega-3 fatty acids. While grass-fed may not always be accessible, opting for leaner cuts and reducing red meat intake overall remains a good strategy for managing inflammation.

Processed red meats such as sausages, hot dogs, and deli meats should be avoided whenever possible. These types of meats are linked to higher levels of inflammation, and their long-term consumption has been associated with an increased risk of cardiovascular diseases and cancer.

By comparison, poultry—especially chicken and turkey—offers a lean source of protein that fits well into an anti-inflammatory diet. It's generally considered a neutral ingredient: lower in saturated fat than red meat but without the beneficial anti-inflammatory omega-3s found in fatty fish.

▮ FILL UP ON FISH

Fish is a powerful ally to an anti-inflammatory diet, primarily because of its rich content of omega-3 fatty acids. These healthy fats, particularly EPA and DHA, help reduce inflammation and support overall health. Omega-3s are known to have a calming effect on the body's inflammatory processes, which is crucial for preventing chronic conditions such as heart disease, arthritis, and autoimmune diseases. Plus, fish is packed with high-quality protein, vitamins like D and B_{12}, and minerals such as selenium.

While all sorts of fish can deliver anti-inflammatory benefits, wild-caught fish, when available, is often the best option for reducing inflammation. Wild fish typically have higher levels of omega-3s and lower levels of omega-6 fatty acids. Farmed fish, on the other hand, may have a less favorable fat profile and potentially higher levels of contaminants. But if wild-caught fish isn't available or within your budget, sustainably farmed options are still a good choice for incorporating fish into an anti-inflammatory diet. (Note that some wild fish, such as salmon, should be cooked to a lower temperature than their farmed counterparts, so be sure to follow the recommendations in the recipes.)

Some of the best fish for an anti-inflammatory way of eating include wild salmon, mackerel, Arctic char, sardines, anchovies, and trout. Each of these varieties offers a healthy dose of omega-3s and other nutrients; for example, mackerel and sardines are rich in vitamin D, while anchovies are packed with selenium.

When buying tinned fish, look for options packed in water or olive oil rather than vegetable oil. Check for sustainability certifications, such as Marine Stewardship Council (MSC), to ensure that the fish is wild-caught and responsibly sourced.

▮ CHOOSE LOW-SODIUM OPTIONS

Sodium is essential for bodily processes such as fluid balance and nerve function, but when we consume too much it can contribute to inflammation. High sodium intake is linked to increased blood pressure, which can elevate inflammation and stress on the cardiovascular system. For anyone managing chronic conditions like arthritis or heart disease, cutting back on sodium can help reduce inflammation and support overall health.

That's why in our recipes we use low-sodium versions of pantry staples such as chicken broth, soy sauce, tomato paste, and canned beans. By opting for these alternatives, we cut down on hidden salt. Over time, these swaps can help keep blood pressure in check and ease unnecessary stress on your body—two key steps toward keeping inflammation at bay.

While store-bought chicken and vegetable broths are convenient and efficient to keep in your pantry, we like to make them ourselves so we can better control the sodium content and flavorings.

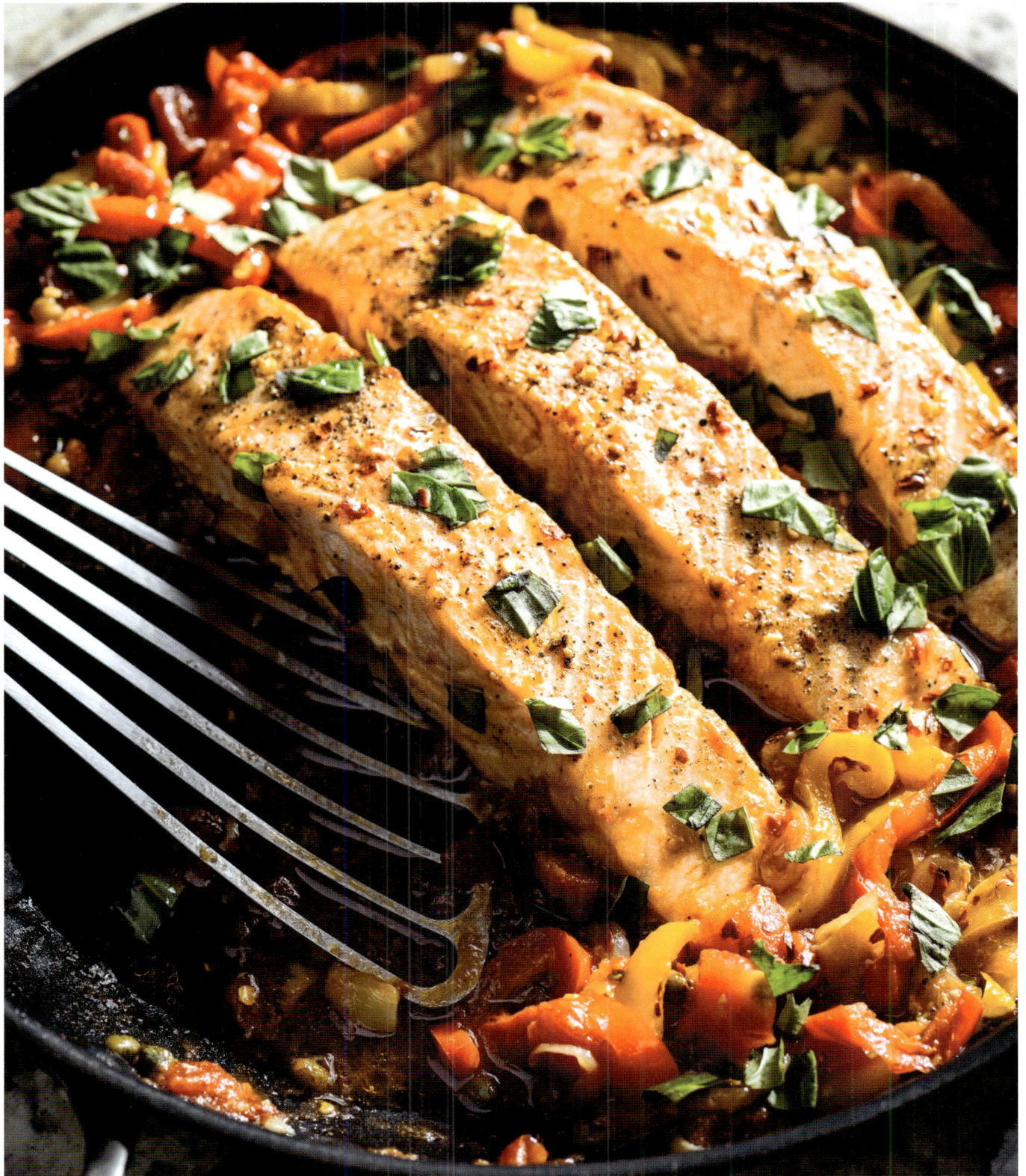

The fish in this Salmon Peperonata (page 222) is an excellent source of anti-inflammatory compounds, especially omega-3 fatty acids.

3 Stir remaining 6 cups water into pot, then return browned chicken and any accumulated juices to pot and bring to simmer. Reduce heat to low, cover, and simmer gently until broth is rich and flavorful, about 4 hours.

4 Remove large bones from pot, then strain broth through fine-mesh strainer into large container; discard solids. Let broth settle for 5 to 10 minutes, then defat using wide, shallow spoon or fat separator. (Cooled broth can be refrigerated for up to 4 days or frozen for up to 1 month.)

Vegetable Broth

makes 2 quarts · total time: 2½ hours

  3 onions, chopped
  2 celery ribs, chopped
  2 carrots, peeled and chopped
  8 scallions, chopped
 15 garlic cloves, peeled and smashed
  1 teaspoon vegetable oil
  1 teaspoon table salt
 12 cups water
  1 head cauliflower (2 pounds), cored and cut into
     1-inch florets
  1 plum tomato, cored and chopped
  8 sprigs fresh thyme
  3 bay leaves
  1 teaspoon black peppercorns

1 Combine onions, celery, carrots, scallions, garlic, oil, and salt in large Dutch oven or stockpot. Cover and cook over medium-low heat, stirring often, until golden-brown fond has formed on bottom of pot, 20 to 30 minutes.

2 Stir in water, cauliflower, tomato, thyme sprigs, bay leaves, and peppercorns, scraping up any browned bits, and bring to simmer. Partially cover pot, reduce heat to gentle simmer, and cook until stock tastes rich and flavorful, about 1½ hours.

3 Strain stock gently through fine-mesh strainer (do not press on solids). (Stock can be refrigerated for up to 4 days or frozen for up to 1 month.)

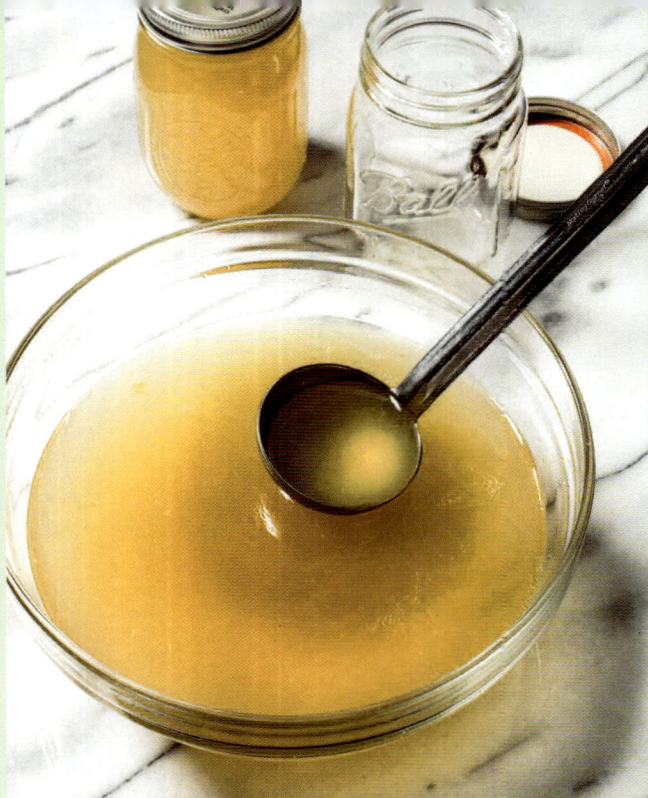

Chicken Broth

makes 2 quarts · total time: 4¾ hours

  1 tablespoon extra-virgin olive oil
  3 pounds whole chicken legs, backs, and/or wings,
     hacked into 2-inch pieces
  1 onion, chopped
  8 cups water
  3 bay leaves
  ½ teaspoon table salt

1 Heat oil in Dutch oven over medium-high heat until just smoking. Pat chicken dry with paper towels. Brown half of chicken, about 5 minutes; transfer to large bowl. Repeat with remaining chicken; transfer to bowl.

2 Add onion to fat left in pot and cook over medium heat until softened, about 5 minutes. Stir in 2 cups water, bay leaves, and salt, scraping up any browned bits.

How you cook matters just as much as what you buy. These simple techniques maximize anti-inflammation, bringing out the natural protective power of your meals while also enhancing flavor.

BLOOM SPICES IN OIL

To bring out the full potential of your spices, bloom them in a little oil before adding other ingredients. This simple technique enlivens their natural aromas, making flavors more pronounced—so you can use less salt without sacrificing taste.

BROWN, DON'T CHAR, MEAT

That blackened char on meats can contribute smoky, savory flavor, but it can also create inflammatory compounds linked to oxidative stress. Instead of grilling to a char, sauté or roast meats—these methods will still bring out rich, caramelized flavors without producing harmful byproducts in the process. Enhance the depth of flavor further with anti-inflammatory seasonings such as turmeric, ginger, and garlic to keep your meals both flavorful and nourishing. If you want to grill, choose fish or vegetables, which are less inflammatory than meat when grilled.

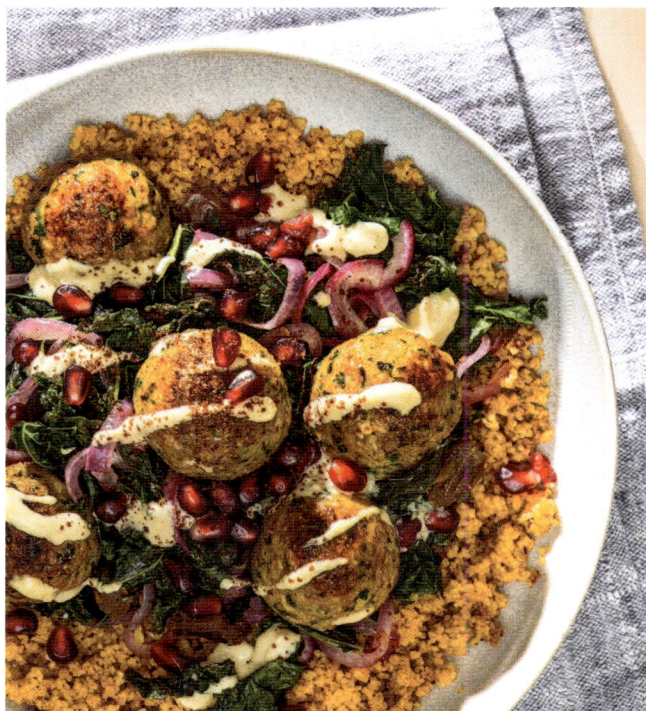

Bulgur Bowls with Chicken Meatballs and Sumac Kale, page 191

CREAM-IFY WITH WHOLESOME FOODS

You don't have to rely on heavy cream, butter, or mayonnaise to achieve silky, velvety textures. Instead, we often used naturally rich foods like Greek yogurt, blended cashews, avocado, and tahini to produce creamy satisfaction. Whether it's a luscious sauce, smooth dressing, or thick soup, a few wholesome swaps add healthy fats while keeping saturated fats in check.

COOK LOW AND SLOW

Gentle cooking preserves nutrients better than high-heat techniques. We often turned to methods such as steaming, slow-cooking, and braising to help retain water-soluble vitamins, which can be lost in frying or boiling. Gentler methods also enhance texture and flavor, resulting in tender meats and fall-apart flaky fish.

FEEL THE PRESSURE

Pressure cooking is not only a time-saver—it's also a smart way to retain nutrients. Unlike boiling or slow simmering, where vitamins and antioxidants can break down over time, pressure cooking helps lock in nutrition. It's especially useful for legumes, grains, and vegetables, making them tender and easily digestible while preserving more of their anti-inflammatory power.

Navigating the Book

To help you navigate the hundreds of recipes in this book, we created a tagging system. For quick recipes that can be cooked in 45 minutes or less, look for the **FAST** tag. These meals are ideal for busy weeknights when you want an anti-inflammatory meal with minimal time and effort. For recipes that dietitian Alicia Romano considers particularly potent sources of anti-inflammatory benefits, look for the **SUPERCHARGED** tag. These recipes are especially dense with inflammation-fighting ingredients. (Look also for the "Nutrition Knowledge" boxes from Alicia to learn more about the anti-inflammatory powerhouses in those recipes.)

Wherever possible, we also included guidance on how to make a recipe dairy-free or gluten-free. Look for that information at the bottom of recipes, along with helpful make-ahead tips so you can get a head start on cooking.

Making This Eating Pattern Work for You

Food sensitivities and allergies can play a significant role in inflammation, so it's important to understand how they impact your health. When the immune system reacts to a specific food—whether it's an allergy or a sensitivity—it sparks an inflammatory response that can range from mild discomfort like bloating or fatigue to more serious symptoms such as skin rashes, digestive problems, or joint pain.

Gluten is one of the most common culprits. For those with gluten sensitivity (not to be confused with celiac disease), gluten can trigger chronic low-grade inflammation in the gut. This ongoing inflammation can disrupt digestion and even spread throughout the body, weakening the immune system and making you more vulnerable to other health issues. Common signs of gluten sensitivity include bloating, gas, and fatigue after consuming gluten-containing foods.

Dairy is another major trigger. Whether it's due to lactose intolerance or sensitivity to casein (the protein in milk), dairy can lead to inflammation in the digestive system. This often results in symptoms such as bloating, cramps, and other gastrointestinal discomforts. For some, dairy may even trigger skin flare-ups like acne or eczema, or worsen joint pain due to inflammation. If this is the case for you, it's worth swapping in non-dairy alternatives such as oat milk, almond milk, or soy milk. While store-bought options can be great to keep on hand, you can also make them yourself to ensure that they don't contain emulsifiers and other processed additives.

If you're sensitive to any of these foods, cutting them out of your diet may help reduce inflammation and improve overall wellness. That's why we've included plenty of gluten-free and dairy-free alternatives throughout our recipes. For example, you can swap traditional noodles, pastas, and bread crumbs for their gluten-free counterparts, and use dairy-free options such as plant-based milks and dairy-free cheeses.

If you suspect you have sensitivities to dairy or gluten—or other common allergens such as nuts, eggs, or soy—it's worth getting diagnosed by a medical team. An allergist can provide food allergen testing to help identify your triggers, and a registered dietitian can work with you to create a tailored plan that supports your health while avoiding foods that cause inflammation.

Ask the Nutritionist: FAQs About Anti-Inflammatory Eating

"I heard grilled foods are inflammatory. Is that true?"
Charring meat can release compounds that contribute to inflammation if consumed in excessive amounts, especially if the protein is red meat. Avoid blackening meat, and try to grill more fish and vegetables (they produce fewer inflammatory compounds).

"Is it okay to heat extra-virgin olive oil?
Yes. Extra-virgin olive oil has a smoke point between 375 and 410 degrees Fahrenheit, so it is safe for most everyday cooking. We use it in recipes that call for medium-high heat or lower. For high-heat cooking, it's best to use another heart-healthy oil with a high smoke point, such as avocado oil.

"Do I have to avoid all sugar?"
No, but added sugar should be consumed mindfully and minimally. Excess refined sugar—think sodas, packaged sweets, and ultra-processed foods—can drive inflammation. Natural sweeteners such as honey, maple syrup, and agave nectar are less inflammatory choices, especially when consumed alongside fiber, protein, and fat to avoid a blood sugar spike.

"Should I eliminate nightshades?"
Nightshade vegetables such tomatoes, eggplants, and potatoes are dense with nutrients and not innately inflammatory. Some people with certain autoimmune or gut conditions may have sensitivities to them. Unless you've noticed that nightshades specifically trigger symptoms, there's no need to eliminate them.

"What's the connection between inflammation and gut health?"
They're closely linked. Your gut is where the majority of your immune cells live, so microbiome imbalances can trigger or worsen inflammatory symptoms. Many of the recipes in this book contain prebiotic fiber and fermented ingredients, which gently support your digestive system.

Oat Milk

serves 4 · makes about 4 cups · total time: 10 minutes, plus 1 hour chilling

    4   cups water
    ¾   cup old-fashioned rolled oats
    2   teaspoons sugar (optional)
    ¾   teaspoon avocado oil
    ½   teaspoon vanilla extract (optional)
    ⅛   teaspoon table salt

Line fine-mesh strainer with triple layer of cheesecloth overhanging edges; set aside. Process water; oats; sugar, if using; oil; vanilla, if using; and salt in blender until coarsely ground, about 10 seconds, scraping down sides of blender jar as needed. Strain blended oat mixture through prepared strainer into 4-cup liquid measuring cup or large bowl, stirring occasionally, until liquid no longer runs freely, about 5 minutes. Pull edges of cheesecloth together and squeeze pulp until liquid no longer runs freely; discard pulp. Transfer milk to airtight container and refrigerate until well chilled, about 1 hour. Serve. (Oat milk can be refrigerated for up to 4 days; stir to recombine before serving.)

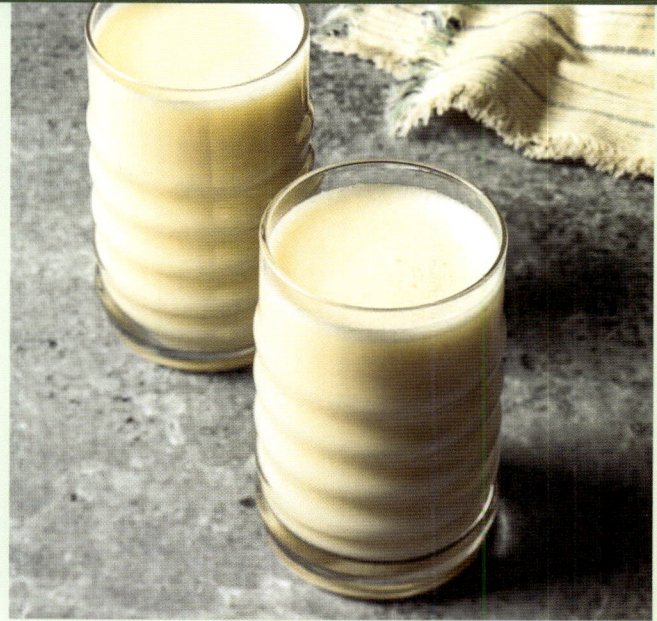

Almond Milk

serves 4 · makes about 4 cups · total time: 2 hours 10 minutes, plus 1 hour chilling

    1¼ cups whole blanched almonds
    2   tablespoons sugar (optional)
    ⅛   teaspoon table salt

1   Place almonds in large saucepan and add water to cover by 1 inch. Bring to simmer and cook until almonds are softened, 2 to 3 hours. (Alternatively, place almonds and water in slow cooker, cover, and cook on low for 2 to 3 hours.) Drain almonds and rinse well.

2   Line fine-mesh strainer with triple layer of cheesecloth overhanging edges; set aside. Process almonds and 4 cups cold water in blender until almonds are finely ground, about 2 minutes. Strain blended almond mixture through prepared strainer into 4-cup liquid measuring cup or large bowl and press to extract as much liquid as possible. Pull edges of cheesecloth together and firmly squeeze pulp until liquid no longer runs freely; discard pulp. Stir in sugar, if using, and salt until completely dissolved. Transfer milk to airtight container and refrigerate until well chilled, about 1 hour. Serve. (Almond milk can be refrigerated for up to 4 days; stir to recombine before serving.)

Soy Milk

serves 4 · makes about 4 cups · total time: 1 hour 10 minutes, plus 2 hours soaking and chilling

    ½   cup dried soybeans, picked over and rinsed
    2   teaspoons sugar (optional)
    ½   teaspoon vanilla extract (optional)
    ⅛   teaspoon table salt

1   Place soybeans in bowl and add water to cover by 2 inches. Soak soybeans at room temperature for at least 1 hour or up to 24 hours. Drain and rinse well.

2   Bring soaked soybeans and 4½ cups water to simmer in medium saucepan. Partially cover and simmer over medium-low heat until soybeans are tender, 30 to 40 minutes.

3   Line fine-mesh strainer with triple layer of cheesecloth overhanging edges; set aside. Carefully transfer soybeans and cooking liquid to blender. Add sugar, if using; vanilla, if using; and salt and process until mostly smooth, about 3 minutes. Strain blended soybean mixture through prepared strainer into 4-cup liquid measuring cup or large bowl, stirring occasionally, until liquid no longer runs freely and mixture is cool enough to touch, about 30 minutes. Pull edges of cheesecloth together and firmly squeeze pulp until liquid no longer runs freely; discard pulp. Transfer milk to airtight container and refrigerate until well chilled, about 1 hour. Serve. (Soy milk can be refrigerated for up to 4 days; stir to recombine before serving.)

Comfort Foods Turned Inflammation Fighters

Any long-term healthy eating pattern must also be satisfying. The good news is that fighting inflammation doesn't mean sacrificing the comforting flavors and hearty fare you love. Here are three examples of how our test cooks gave some of our favorite dishes an anti-inflammatory boost.

ONE BIG CAST-IRON CHICKEN AND CHARD ENCHILADA
(Page 192)

It's hard not to love enchiladas, but in order to give them an anti-inflammatory spin, we had to keep an eye on the saturated fat and fast-digesting carbohydrates. We turned to ground chicken, bulking it up with pinto beans and lots of fiberful Swiss chard. The result is a toothsome—not to mention lower-lift— one-skillet dish that is bound to satisfy.

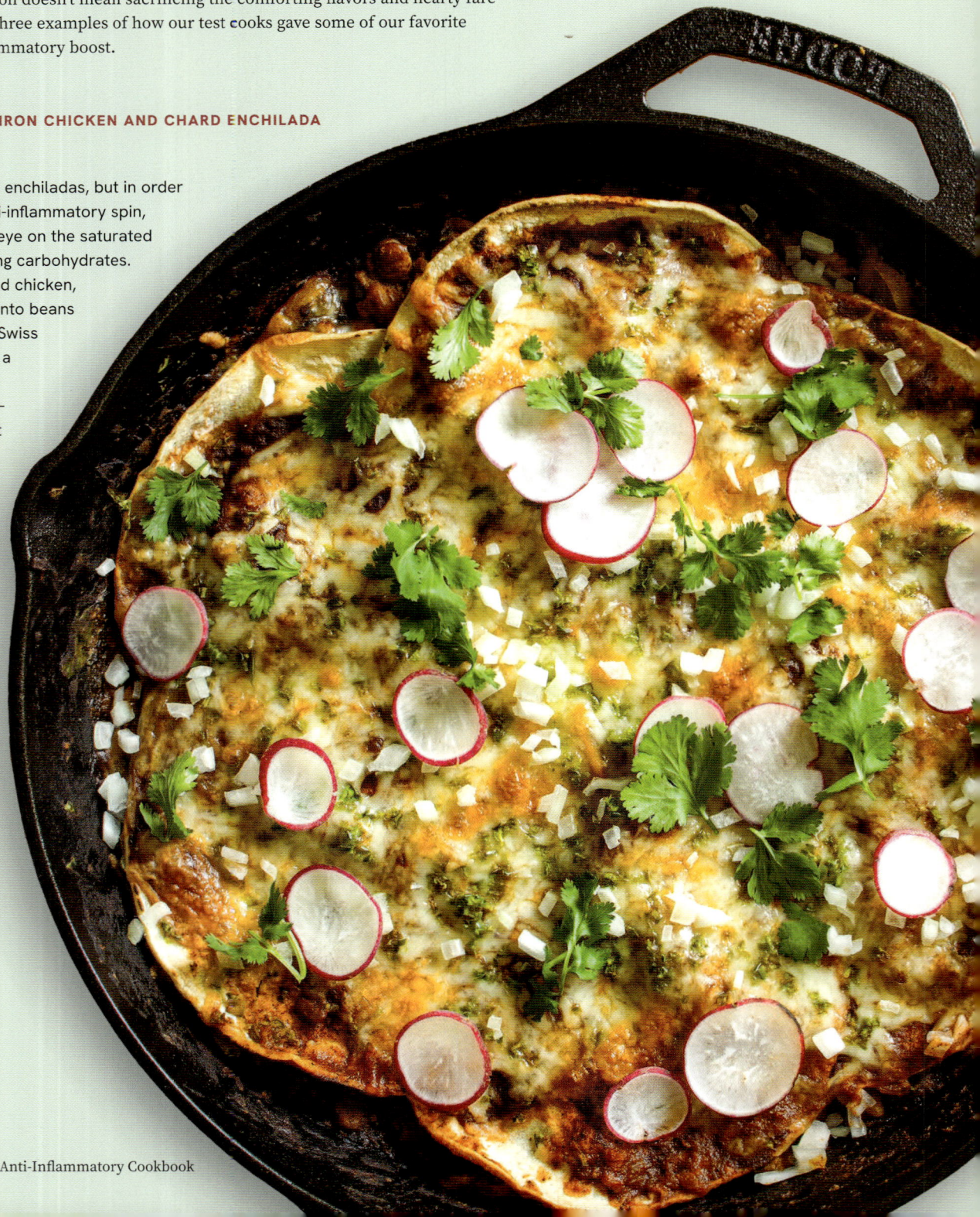

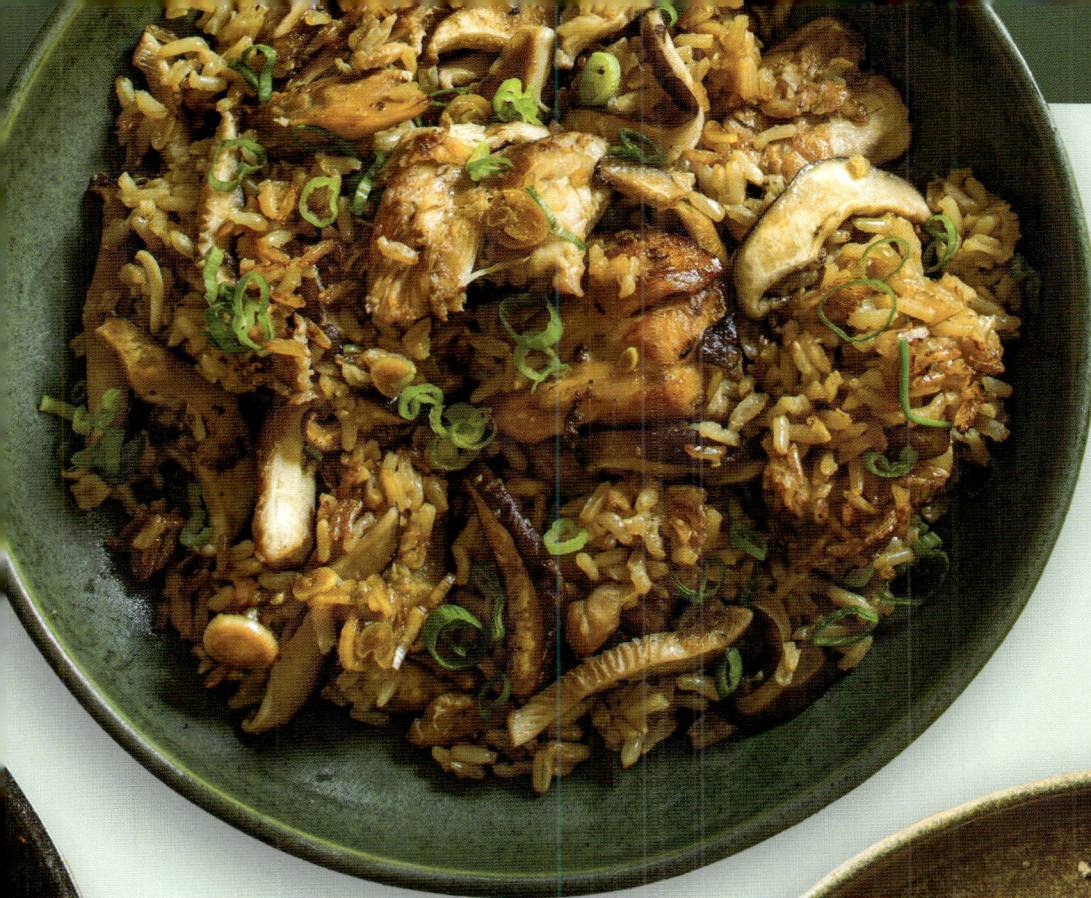

CRISPY BROWN RICE WITH SOY CHICKEN AND SHIITAKE MUSHROOMS
(Page 209)

We're big fans of Chinese clay-pot chicken rice. To enhance the dish from an inflammation-fighting perspective, we used heart-healthy avocado oil and swapped the white rice for brown—a slow-digesting alternative that keeps you full, and is satisfyingly chewy to boot.

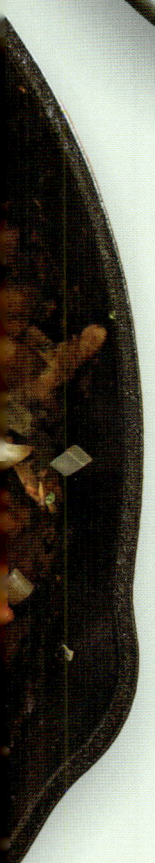

SMOKED TROUT HASH
(Page 28)

Breakfast hash is a classic. We added protein in the form of smoked trout to pack n inflammation-fighting omega-3 fatty acids, then paired it with mustard greens, a fiber-packed leafy vegetable with a horseradish-like edge. Lemon wedges and a sprinkle of dill add even more antioxidants.

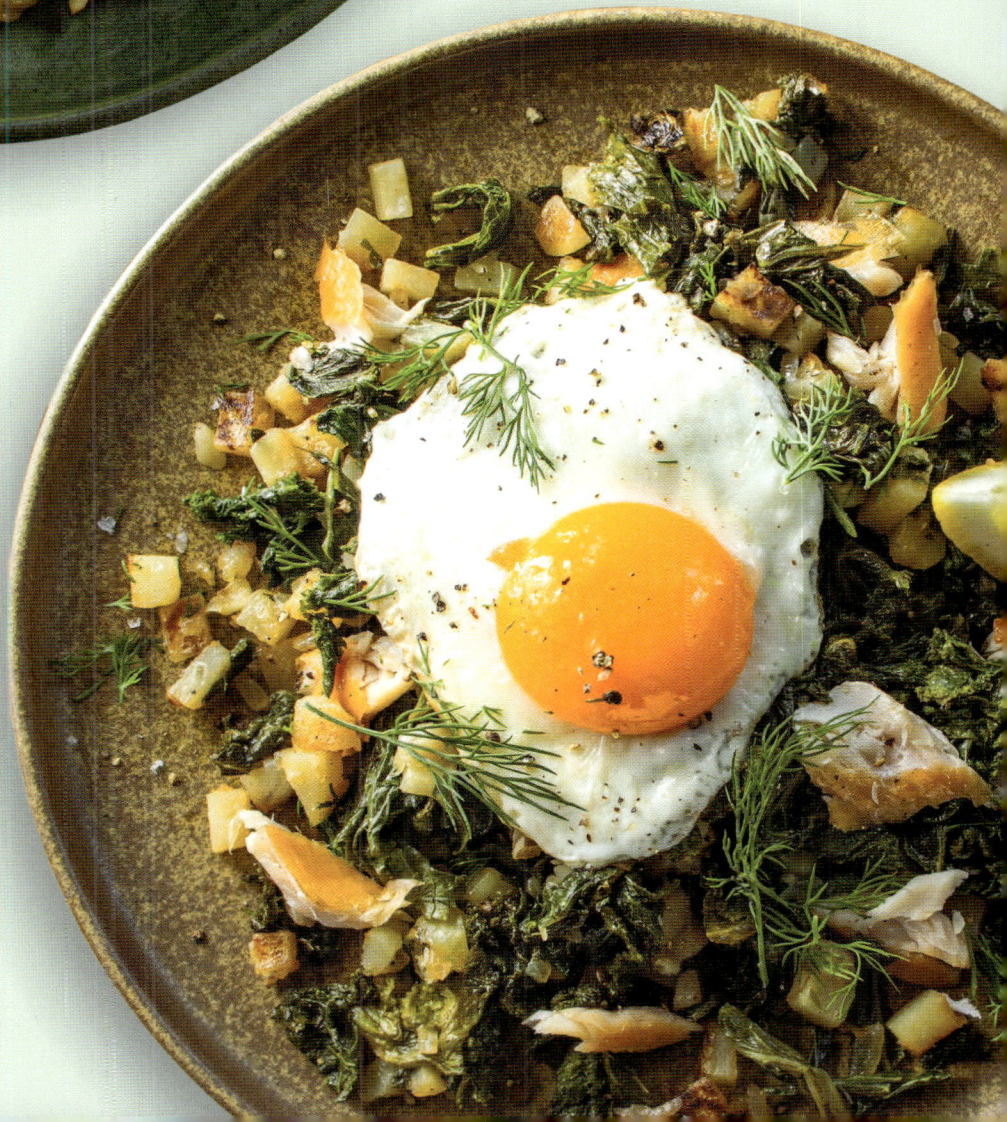

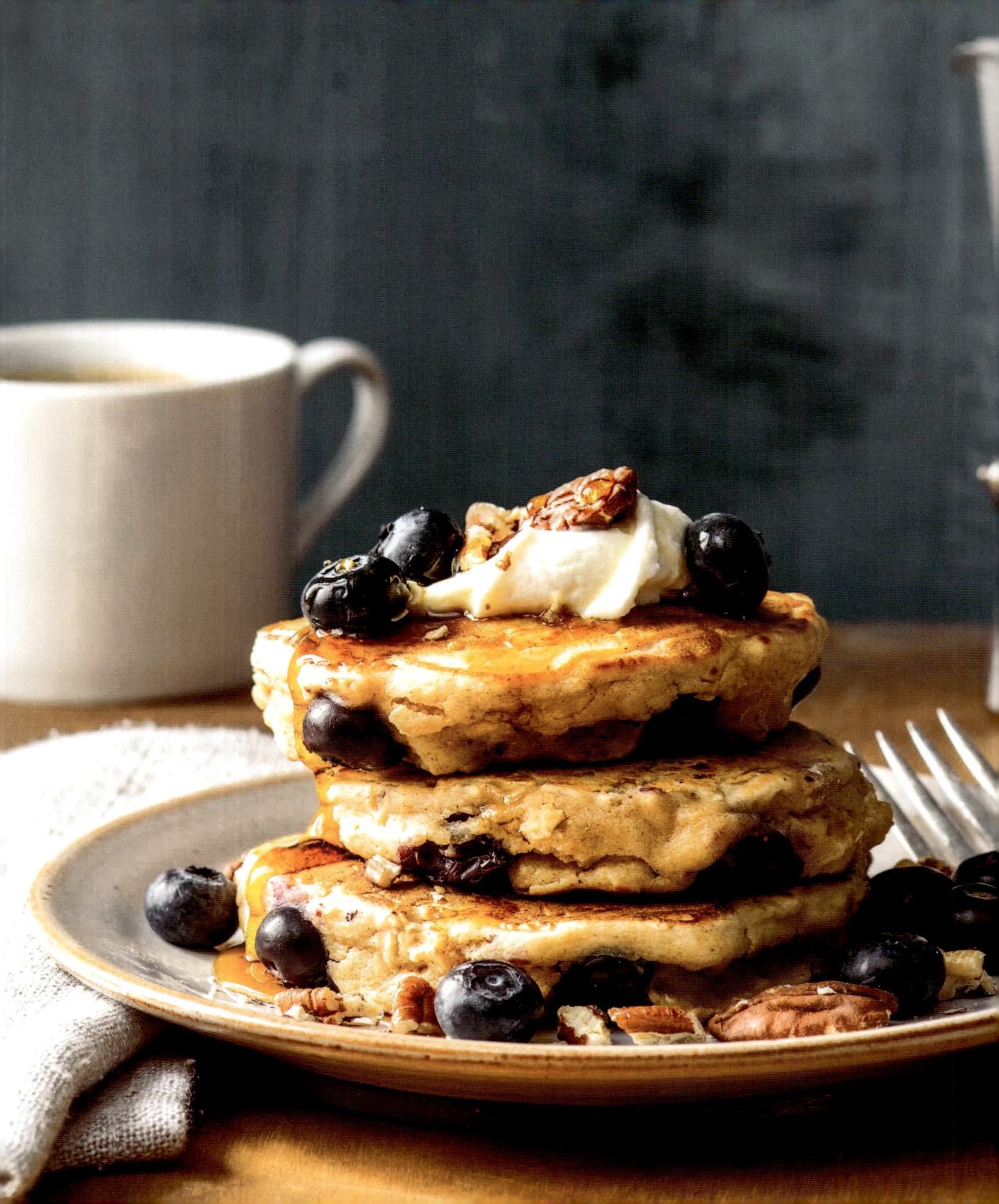

BREAKFAST

■ FAST   ■ SUPERCHARGED

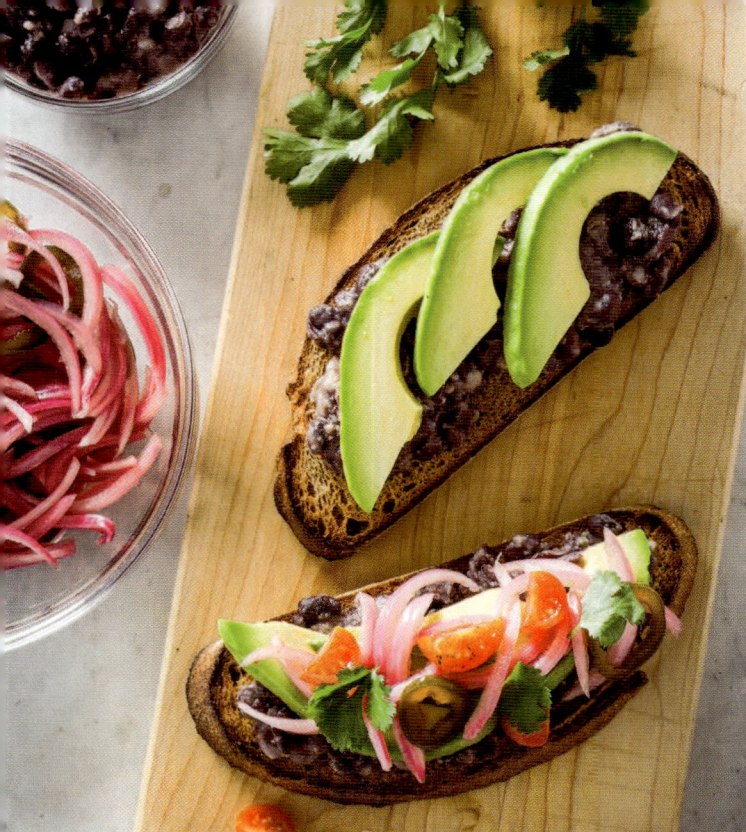

Avocado and Bean Toast

serves 4 • total time: 15 minutes **FAST**

why this recipe works • Avocado toast is one of our favorite snacks, and we wanted to add extra fiber and protein to it for a more substantial breakfast. To liven up our morning, we seasoned canned black beans with lime zest and juice and mashed them with boiling water and oil, giving us a flavorsome, well-textured base. We smeared the bread with the black bean mixture and then adorned it with heart-healthy avocado slices, lightly seasoned tomatoes, and fresh cilantro. We like to top this toast with pickled red onions, but you can use a pinch of red pepper flakes for heat if you prefer. For an accurate measure of boiling water, bring a full kettle of water to a boil and then measure out the desired amount.

    4 ounces cherry tomatoes, quartered
    4 teaspoons extra-virgin olive oil, divided
       Pinch plus ½ teaspoon table salt, divided
    ⅛ teaspoon pepper, divided
    1 (15-ounce) can no-salt-added black beans, rinsed
    ¼ cup boiling water
    ½ teaspoon grated lime zest plus 1 tablespoon juice
    4 (½-inch-thick) slices rustic bread, toasted
    1 avocado, halved, pitted, and sliced thin
    ¼ cup Quick Pickled Red Onions (recipe follows) (optional)
    ¼ cup fresh cilantro leaves

1 Combine tomatoes, 1 teaspoon oil, pinch salt, and pinch pepper in bowl; set aside. Mash beans, boiling water, lime zest and juice, remaining ½ teaspoon salt, remaining pinch pepper, and remaining 1 tablespoon oil with potato masher to coarse puree in second bowl, leaving some whole beans intact. Season with salt and pepper to taste.

2 Spread mashed bean mixture evenly over toasts, then top with avocado slices. Top with pickled onions, if using; reserved tomatoes; and cilantro. Serve.

> **MAKE AHEAD** • Mashed black beans can be refrigerated for up to 3 days; reheat in microwave before spreading over toasted bread.

> **MAKE IT GLUTEN-FREE** • Substitute gluten-free bread for the bread.

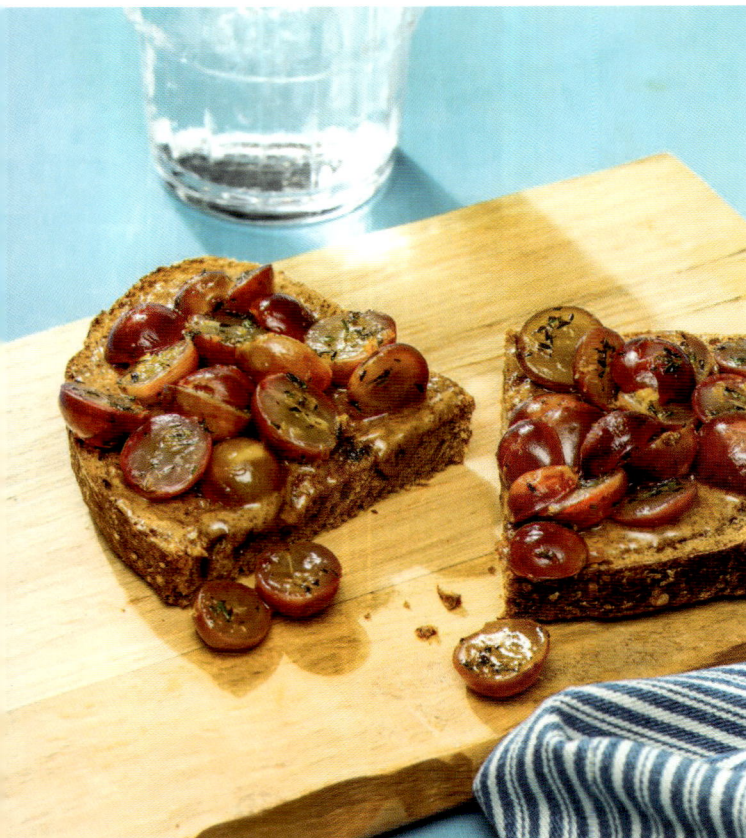

top	*Avocado and Bean Toast*
bottom	*Sautéed Grape and Almond Butter Toast*

All About Avocados

This rich fruit is an excellent source of anti-inflammatory, heart-healthy fats. We also love its buttery texture and delicate flavor. Here's how to buy and store avocados.

Buying Avocados There are many varieties of avocado, but in the United States, small, rough-skinned Hass avocados are most common, and we prefer them in the test kitchen. When ripe, their skin turns from green to dark purply black, and the fruit yields to a gentle squeeze. However, keep in mind that a soft avocado may be a bruised fruit rather than a ripe one. A good test is to try to flick the small stem off the avocado. If it comes off easily and you can see green underneath, the avocado is ripe. If you see brown underneath after prying it off, the avocado is not usable. If the stem does not come off easily, the avocado is still unripe. Because these fruits ripen off the tree, plan ahead when buying them to account for ripening time.

Ripening and Storing Avocados At room temperature, rock-hard avocados generally ripen within two days, but may do so unevenly. Once ripe, they will last two days on average if kept at room temperature. Avocados may take up to four days to ripen in the refrigerator, but will ripen more evenly. Ripe avocados last about five days when refrigerated, though some discoloration may occur. Store them toward the front of the refrigerator, on the middle to bottom shelves, where temperatures are more moderate. Avocado flesh does not freeze well; as the water in the fruit crystallizes, it destroys the avocado's creamy texture.

Keeping Leftover Avocado Green Avocado flesh turns brown very quickly once it is exposed to air. To minimize this, it's best to prepare avocados at the last moment whenever possible. However, if you need to use only half of an avocado, you can store the leftover half by rubbing 1 tablespoon of olive oil on all of the exposed flesh, allowing the excess oil to drip into a shallow bowl, then placing the avocado half cut side down in the center of the oil puddle.

Quick Pickled Red Onions

makes about 1 cup · total time: 5 minutes, plus 20 minutes pickling

- 1 red onion, halved and sliced thin through root end
- ½ cup red wine vinegar
- ½ teaspoon red pepper flakes

Combine all ingredients in bowl and let sit at room temperature for 20 minutes. (Onion can be refrigerated for up to 3 days.)

Sautéed Grape and Almond Butter Toast

serves 4 · total time: 20 minutes   **FAST**

why this recipe works · This loaded toast draws inspiration from America's most beloved sandwich but takes the simple recipe to whole new heights. Rather than smear on sugar-laden jam or jelly, we opted for something playful and unique: sautéed grapes. Not only did this swap reduce the sugar content, but the grapes were well-suited to a fun and flavorful twist. A sprinkle of thyme infused the grapes with warm and slightly peppery notes, while lemon zest and juice brought brightness and awakened the other flavors. Using a 12-inch skillet was essential, as the wide surface area allowed the mixture to reduce and thicken quickly. Peanut butter overwhelmed the lovely and delicate flavors of the sautéed grapes, but almond butter brought just the right nutty balance and allowed the topping to really shine. We finished the toast with sliced almonds for added crunch. We prefer unsweetened natural almond butter in this recipe, but you can use any kind of creamy or chunky nut or seed butter.

- 1 tablespoon extra-virgin olive oil
- 1 pound seedless red grapes, halved (2 cups)
- 1 tablespoon sugar
- 1½ teaspoons minced fresh thyme, divided
- ⅛ teaspoon table salt
- ½ teaspoon grated lemon zest plus 1 teaspoon juice
- ½ cup natural almond butter
- 4 (½-inch-thick) slices rustic bread, toasted
- ¼ cup sliced almonds, toasted

1 Heat oil in 12-inch nonstick skillet over medium-high heat until shimmering. Add grapes, sugar, 1 teaspoon thyme, and salt; cook, stirring occasionally, until grapes begin to soften and juices thicken, about 7 minutes; transfer to bowl, stir in lemon zest and juice, and set aside to cool slightly.

2 Spread almond butter evenly over toasts and, using slotted spoon, top with grapes. Drizzle with grape juice to taste and sprinkle with almonds and remaining ½ teaspoon thyme. Serve.

> **MAKE AHEAD** • Sautéed grapes can be refrigerated for up to 3 days; reheat in microwave before topping toasts.

> **MAKE IT GLUTEN-FREE** • Substitute gluten-free bread for the bread.

Fried Egg Sandwiches with Hummus and Sprouts

serves 4 • total time: 25 minutes **FAST**

why this recipe works • A hearty egg sandwich is a great way to kick-start your morning, but the typical breakfast sandwich features more saturated fat than is optimal for an anti-inflammatory way of eating. We wanted to develop a version that tasted fresher and lighter—one that you might especially crave in warmer months. We started by smearing hearty sandwich bread with creamy hummus and tart, spicy sambal oelek. The nuttiness of the hummus and heat of the sambal oelek harmonized with the richness of the oozy eggs. For a dose of fiber, not to mention some refreshing crunch, we layered the sandwiches with cucumber, red onion, tomato, and alfalfa sprouts, while a sprinkle of crumbly feta—which tends to be lower in saturated fat than many cheese varieties—injected each bite with briny tang. If you can't find sambal oelek, you can substitute chili-garlic sauce or sriracha. Store-bought garlic hummus makes for a quick and easy dose of protein on a busy morning, but you can also use our homemade Classic Hummus (page 365). This recipe can be easily halved to make 2 sandwiches rather than 4; use a 10-inch nonstick skillet for cooking the eggs.

- 2 teaspoons extra-virgin olive oil
- ½ cup garlic hummus
- 8 slices hearty sandwich bread, lightly toasted
- 2 Persian cucumbers, sliced thin on bias
- 4 teaspoons sambal oelek
- 4 large eggs
- ¼ teaspoon table salt, divided
- ¼ teaspoon pepper, divided
- 2 ounces feta cheese, crumbled (½ cup)
- 8 thin tomato slices
- 4 thin red onion slices
- 2 ounces alfalfa sprouts (2 cups)

1 Heat oil in 12-inch nonstick skillet over low heat for 5 minutes. While pan heats, spread hummus on one side of 4 slices bread, then arrange cucumber slices on top of hummus. Spread sambal on one side of remaining 4 slices bread.

2 Crack 2 eggs into small bowl and sprinkle with ⅛ teaspoon salt and ⅛ teaspoon pepper. Repeat with remaining 2 eggs, remaining ⅛ teaspoon salt, and remaining ⅛ teaspoon pepper in second small bowl.

3 Increase heat to medium-high and heat until oil shimmers. Working quickly, pour 1 bowl of eggs on one side of pan and second bowl of eggs on other side. Cover and cook for 1 minute. Remove skillet from burner and let stand, covered, 15 to 45 seconds for runny yolks (white around edge of yolk will be barely opaque), 45 to 60 seconds for soft but set yolks, and about 2 minutes for medium-set yolks.

4 Using spatula, place eggs on top of cucumbers. Top each egg with feta, tomato slices, onion slices, and sprouts. Top with remaining bread slices and serve.

> **MAKE IT GLUTEN-FREE** • Substitute gluten-free bread for the bread.

> **MAKE IT DAIRY-FREE** • Substitute plant-based feta cheese for the dairy feta cheese or omit the cheese.

Kale and Black Bean Breakfast Burritos

serves 4 • total time: 45 minutes **FAST**

why this recipe works • We love the handheld convenience and heartiness of breakfast burritos, but many versions are quite heavy. We wanted a burrito that would be just as portable and satisfying yet keep saturated fat to a minimum and nourish you with anti-inflammatory nutrients. To build a flavorful base, we sautéed onion and poblano with garlic and cumin before adding filling black beans, mashing half to create a creamier consistency while retaining the legumes' hearty bite. To work in some dark leafy greens, we quickly braised kale until tender and then used the same skillet to scramble a few eggs—a breakfast burrito staple, plus a great source of protein—before folding in the kale. We spread the bean mixture onto tortillas, added the fluffy egg-kale scramble, and finished with chopped tomato for a dose of freshness. Softening the tortillas in the microwave makes them easier to roll.

- 5 teaspoons extra-virgin olive oil, divided, plus extra for drizzling
- 1 small onion, chopped fine
- 1 poblano, stemmed, seeded, and chopped fine
- ¼ teaspoon, plus ⅛ teaspoon, plus pinch table salt, divided
- 2 garlic cloves, minced
- ½ teaspoon ground cumin
- 1 cup canned no-salt-added black beans, rinsed
- ½ cup water
- 5 ounces baby kale, roughly chopped
- 4 large eggs
- 1 tablespoon milk
  Pinch pepper
- 4 (10-inch) flour tortillas
- 1 plum tomato, cored and chopped fine
  Hot sauce

1 Heat 2 teaspoons oil in 12-inch nonstick skillet over medium-high heat until shimmering. Add onion, poblano, and ¼ teaspoon salt and cook until softened, about 5 minutes. Stir in garlic and cumin and cook until fragrant, about 30 seconds. Stir in beans and water and cook until beans are warmed through, 3 to 4 minutes. Off heat, mash half of beans to chunky paste; transfer to bowl, season with salt and pepper to taste, and cover to keep warm. Wipe out skillet with paper towels.

2 In now-empty skillet, heat 2 teaspoons oil over medium-high heat until shimmering. Add kale and ⅛ teaspoon salt, and cook until kale wilts, 3 to 4 minutes; transfer to second bowl. Wipe out skillet with paper towels.

3 Beat eggs, milk, remaining pinch salt, and pepper with fork in bowl until eggs are thoroughly combined and color is pure yellow.

4 Heat remaining 1 teaspoon oil in again-empty skillet over medium-high heat until shimmering. Add egg mixture and, using silicone spatula, constantly and firmly scrape along bottom and sides of skillet until eggs begin to clump and spatula leaves trail on bottom of pan, 1½ to 2½ minutes. Off heat, gently stir in kale and constantly fold eggs and kale until eggs have finished cooking, 30 to 60 seconds. Cover to keep warm.

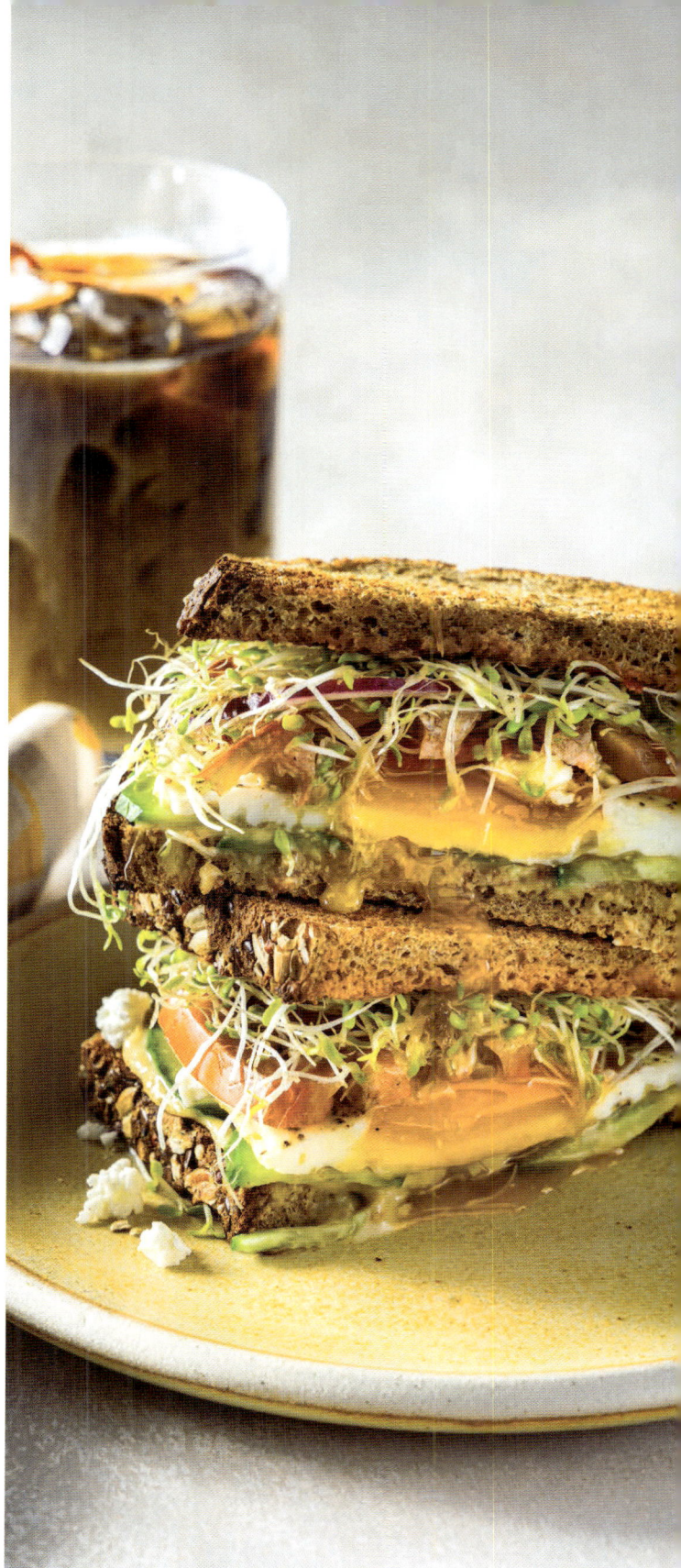

Fried Egg Sandwiches with Hummus and Sprouts

5 Wrap tortillas in damp dish towel and microwave until warm and pliable, about 1 minute. Lay warm tortillas on counter and spread bean mixture evenly across center of each tortilla, close to bottom edge. Top with kale-egg mixture, then sprinkle with tomato and drizzle with extra oil to taste. Working with 1 tortilla at a time, fold sides then bottom of tortilla over filling, then continue to roll tightly into wrap. Serve with hot sauce.

MAKE AHEAD • Aluminum foil–wrapped burritos can be frozen for up to 2 months. To serve, bake frozen foil-wrapped burritos in 325 degree oven, air fryer, or toaster oven until warmed through, about 30 minutes. Let sit for 5 minutes before serving. Alternatively, thaw burritos overnight in refrigerator, then bake for 15 minutes.

MAKE IT GLUTEN-FREE • Substitute gluten-free tortillas for the flour tortillas.

MAKE IT DAIRY-FREE • Substitute plant-based milk or water for the dairy milk.

Smoked Trout Hash

serves 4 • total time: 45 minutes   **FAST**

why this recipe works • We give breakfast hash a protein boost and a dose of omega-3 fatty acids by choosing an unusual star ingredient: smoked trout. Since this rich fish is often paired with mustard or horseradish, we partnered the trout with mustard greens, an antioxidant-packed leafy vegetable with a horseradish-like edge. Their spice stood up perfectly to the fish, and they provided leafy chew and pleasantly crisp, lacy edges. Before sautéing the greens with potatoes, we microwaved both to give them a head start on the cooking process. A sprinkle of grassy dill and a side of lemon wedges contributed just the dose of freshness we needed for a well-rounded flavor profile. You will need a 12-inch nonstick skillet with a tight-fitting lid for this recipe. For an even heartier breakfast, top with an egg (see pages 30–31).

  1 pound russet potatoes, peeled and cut into ¼-inch pieces
  2 tablespoons extra-virgin olive oil, divided
  ½ teaspoon table salt
  ¼ teaspoon pepper
1½ pounds mustard greens, stemmed and cut into 1-inch pieces
  1 onion, chopped fine
  1 garlic clove, minced
  4 ounces smoked trout, flaked
  1 tablespoon minced fresh dill
     Lemon wedges

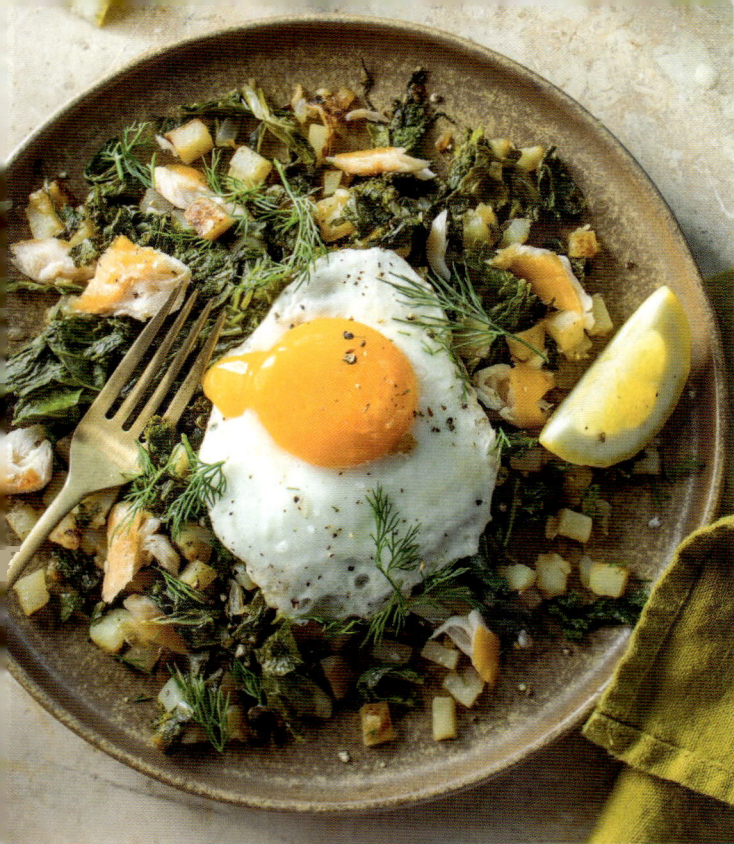
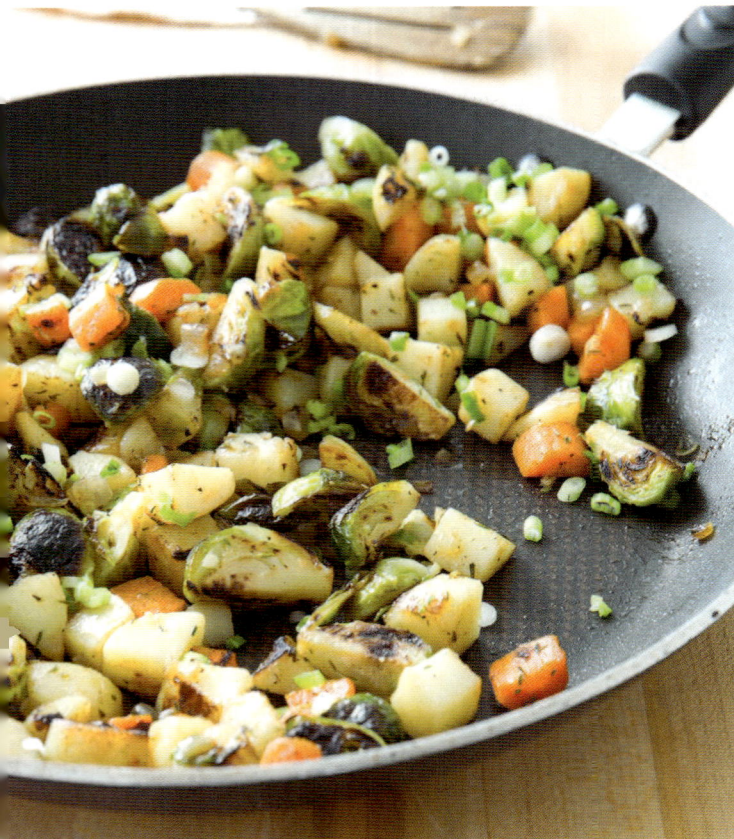

top | *Smoked Trout Hash*
bottom | *Brussels Sprout Hash*

1 Microwave potatoes, 1 tablespoon oil, salt, and pepper in covered bowl until potatoes are translucent around edges, 5 to 8 minutes, stirring halfway through microwaving.

2 Microwave mustard greens in second large covered bowl until wilted, 8 to 10 minutes, stirring halfway through microwaving. Transfer to colander, drain well, then add to bowl with potatoes; set aside.

3 Heat remaining 1 tablespoon oil in 12-inch nonstick skillet over medium-high heat until shimmering. Add onion and cook until softened and lightly browned, 5 to 7 minutes.

4 Stir in garlic and cook until fragrant, about 30 seconds. Stir in reserved potatoes and mustard greens, breaking up any clumps. Using back of spatula, firmly pack potato mixture into skillet and cook undisturbed for 2 minutes. Flip hash, one portion at a time, and repack into skillet. Repeat flipping process every few minutes until potatoes are well browned and mustard greens are tender, 6 to 8 minutes.

5 Off heat, sprinkle trout evenly over hash, then sprinkle with dill. Serve with lemon wedges.

Brussels Sprout Hash

serves 4 · total time: 25 minutes   **FAST**   **SUPERCHARGED**

why this recipe works · For a quick and hearty take on breakfast hash that makes gut-balancing vegetables the stars, we chose fiber-packed brussels sprouts and carrots, a duo of anti-inflammatory heroes that match the sturdiness of dense, filling potatoes. Brussels sprouts offer sulforaphane and other beneficial compounds, while carrots are an excellent source of beta-carotene. But hashing together different vegetables presented a challenge: The potatoes and carrots took longer than the brussels sprouts to soften. We solved this by cooking the potatoes and carrots in the microwave first, which turned them tender in only 5 minutes. Meanwhile, we cooked the brussels sprouts in a skillet to lightly caramelize their exteriors; cutting the sprouts into wedges provided nice flat surfaces that picked up flavorful browning. Finally, we added the microwaved carrots and potatoes to the skillet along with onion, garlic, and thyme, plus a little water to help the brussels sprouts finish cooking through. Look for small brussels sprouts no bigger than a golf ball, as they're likely to be sweeter and more tender than large sprouts. If you can find only large sprouts, halve them and cut each half into thirds. For an even heartier breakfast, top this hash with an egg (see pages 30–31).

1 pound red potatoes, unpeeled, cut into ½-inch pieces
2 carrots, peeled and cut into ½-inch pieces
¼ cup extra-virgin olive oil, divided
1¼ teaspoons table salt, divided
½ teaspoon pepper, divided
1 pound brussels sprouts, trimmed and quartered lengthwise
1 onion, chopped fine
2 tablespoons water
1 tablespoon minced fresh thyme
1 garlic clove, minced
2 scallions, sliced thin

1 Combine potatoes, carrots, 1 tablespoon oil, ½ teaspoon salt, and ¼ teaspoon pepper in large bowl. Microwave, covered, stirring occasionally, until vegetables are tender, 5 to 7 minutes.

2 Meanwhile, heat 1 tablespoon oil in 12-inch nonstick skillet over medium-high heat until shimmering. Add brussels sprouts and cook until browned, 6 to 8 minutes, stirring occasionally. Add microwaved vegetables and any accumulated juices, onion, water, thyme, garlic, 1 tablespoon oil, remaining ¾ teaspoon salt, and remaining ¼ teaspoon pepper. Reduce heat to medium, cover, and cook until brussels sprouts are just tender, 5 to 7 minutes longer, stirring halfway through cooking.

3 Off heat, stir in remaining 1 tablespoon oil and season with salt and pepper to taste. Sprinkle with scallions and serve.

QUARTERING BRUSSELS SPROUTS

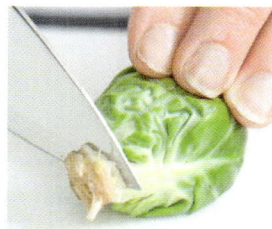

1 Use a sharp chef's knife to remove dried end where sprout was attached to stalk.

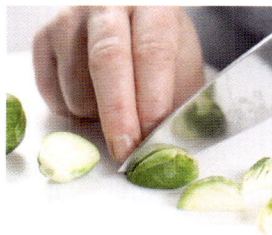

2 Slice each sprout in half through root end and then in half again to quarter it.

put an egg on it!

Adding an egg is an easy way to boost the protein and healthy fats in any meal, making it more filling and balanced. The nutrient-dense ingredient is also packed with choline and vitamin D, as well as antioxidants such as lutein and zeaxanthin. Cook up some eggs to amp up everything from sandwiches to grain bowls.

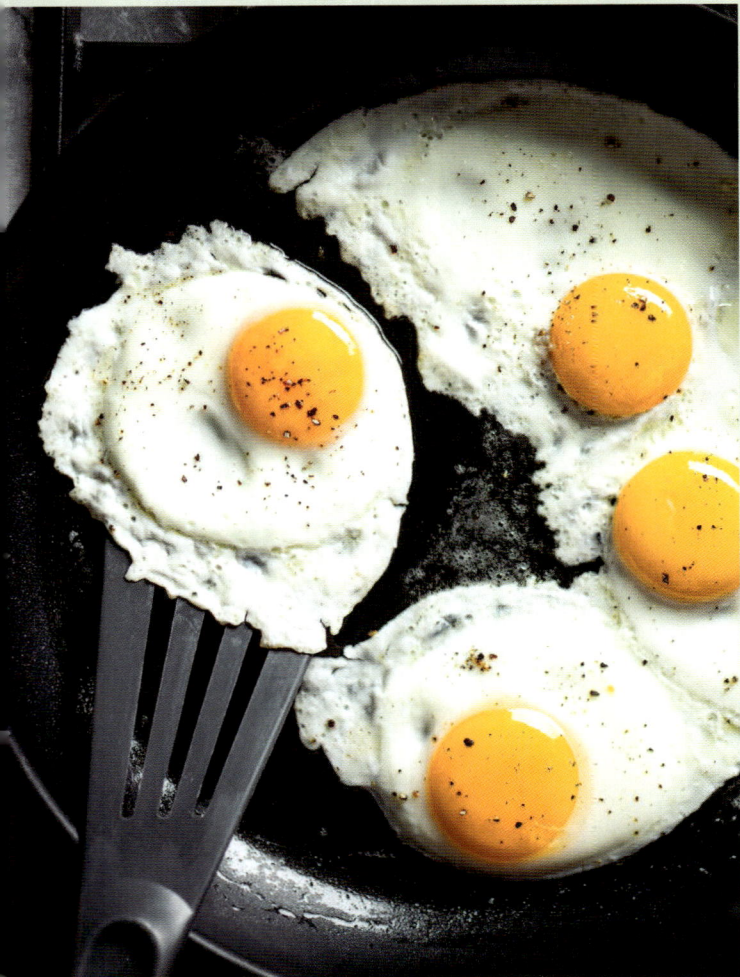

Fried Eggs

serves 2 • total time: 5 minutes

When checking for doneness, lift the lid just a crack to prevent loss of steam should they need further cooking. When cooked, the white will turn opaque, but the yolk should remain runny. You can substitute extra-large or jumbo eggs without altering the timing.

4 large eggs
2 teaspoons extra-virgin olive oil

Crack eggs into 4 small bowls. Heat oil in 12-inch nonstick skillet over medium-high heat until shimmering. Pour eggs into skillet, one at a time; cover skillet; and cook for 1 minute. Remove skillet from heat and let sit, covered, 15 to 45 seconds for runny yolks, 45 to 60 seconds for soft but set yolks, and about 2 minutes for medium-set yolks. Season with salt and pepper to taste.

Scrambled Eggs

serves 4 • total time: 10 minutes

8 large eggs
4 teaspoons water
¼ teaspoon table salt
¼ teaspoon pepper
4 teaspoons extra-virgin olive oil

Beat eggs, water, salt, and pepper together with fork in bowl until thoroughly combined and mixture is pure yellow; do not overbeat. Heat oil in 12-inch nonstick skillet over medium heat until shimmering. Add egg mixture and, using silicone spatula, constantly and firmly scrape along bottom and sides of skillet until eggs begin to clump and spatula leaves trail on bottom of skillet, 1½ to 2 minutes. Reduce heat to low and gently but constantly fold eggs until clumped and slightly wet, 30 to 60 seconds. Season with salt and pepper to taste.

Poached Eggs

makes 1 to 4 eggs • total time: 20 minutes

For the best results, be sure to use the freshest eggs possible.

1–4 large eggs
1 tablespoon distilled white vinegar
Table salt for cooking eggs

1 Bring 6 cups water to boil in Dutch oven over high heat. Meanwhile, crack eggs, one at a time, into colander set in sink or over bowl. Let stand until loose, watery whites drain away from eggs, 20 to 30 seconds. Gently transfer eggs to 2-cup liquid measuring cup.

2 Add vinegar and 1 teaspoon salt to boiling water. With lip of measuring cup just above surface of water, gently tip eggs into water, one at a time, leaving space between them. Cover pot, remove from heat, and let stand until whites closest to yolks are just set and opaque, about 3 minutes. If after 3 minutes whites are not set, let stand in water, checking every 30 seconds, until eggs reach desired doneness. (For medium-cooked yolks, let eggs sit in pot, covered, for 4 minutes, then begin checking for doneness.)

3 Using slotted spoon, carefully lift and drain each egg over Dutch oven. Season with salt and pepper to taste.

Easy-Peel Hard-Cooked Eggs

makes 1 to 6 eggs • total time: 20 minutes, plus 15 minutes chilling
Be sure to use large eggs that have no cracks and are cold from the refrigerator. If you don't have a steamer basket, use a spoon or tongs to gently place the eggs in the water. It does not matter if the eggs are above the water or partially submerged. You can double this recipe as long as you use a pot and steamer basket large enough to hold the eggs in a single layer.

1–6 large eggs

1 Bring 1 inch water to rolling boil in medium saucepan over high heat. Place eggs in steamer basket. Transfer basket to saucepan. Cover, reduce heat to medium-low, and cook eggs for 13 minutes.

2 When eggs are almost finished cooking, combine 2 cups ice cubes and 2 cups cold water in medium bowl. Using tongs or spoon, transfer eggs to ice bath; let sit for 15 minutes. Peel before using.

VARIATION

Easy-Peel Soft-Cooked Eggs
Cook eggs over medium-high heat and decrease cooking time to 6½ minutes. In step 2, submerge eggs in ice bath just until cool enough to handle, about 30 seconds.

MAKE AHEAD • Hard-cooked eggs can be refrigerated, unpeeled, for up to 1 week.

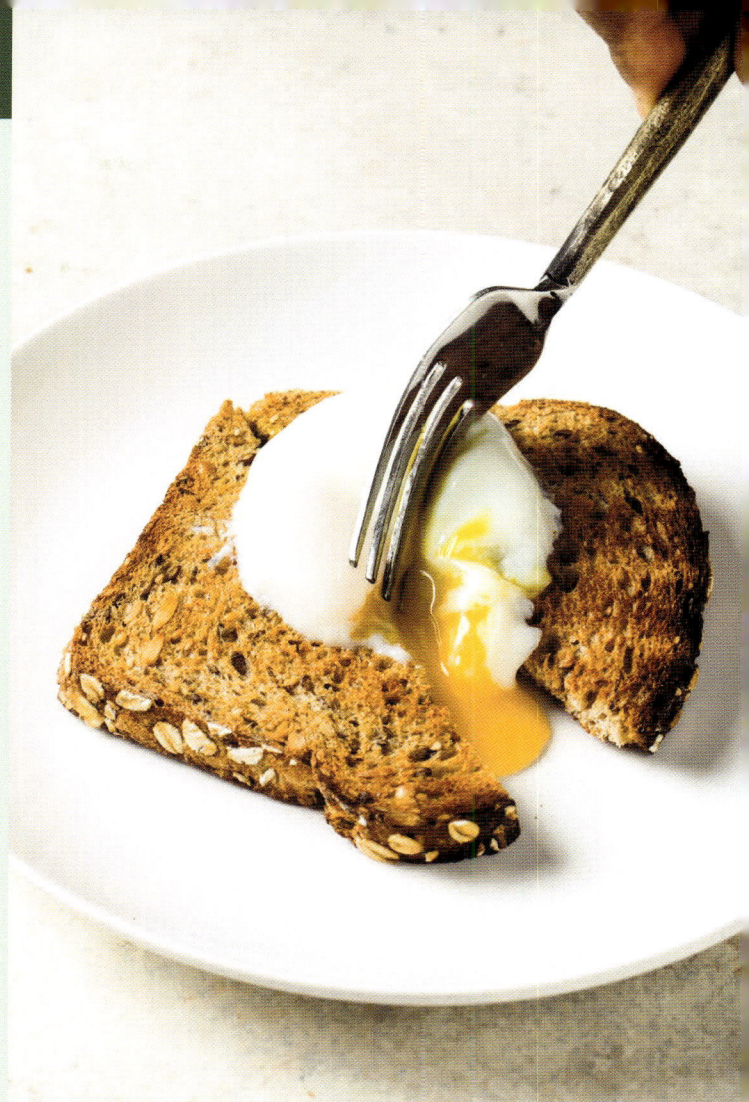

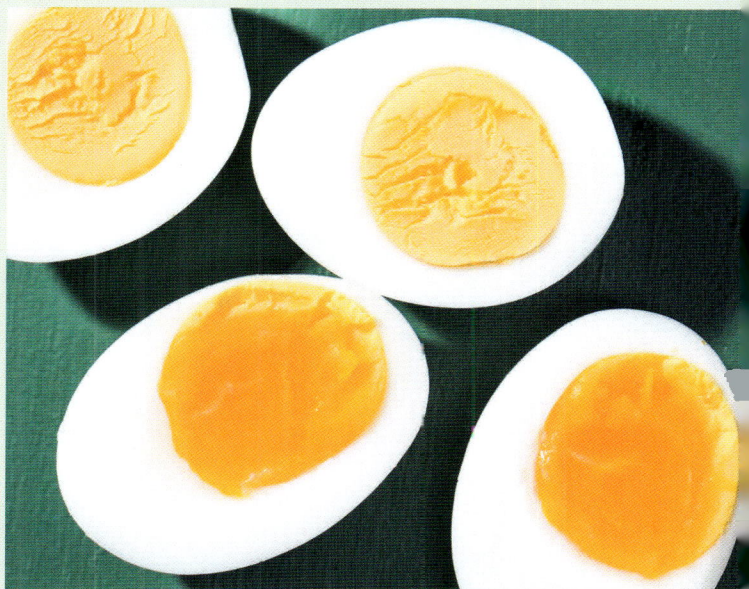

top	Poached Eggs
bottom	Easy-Peel Hard-Cooked Eggs, Easy-Feel Soft-Cooked Eggs
left	Fried Eggs

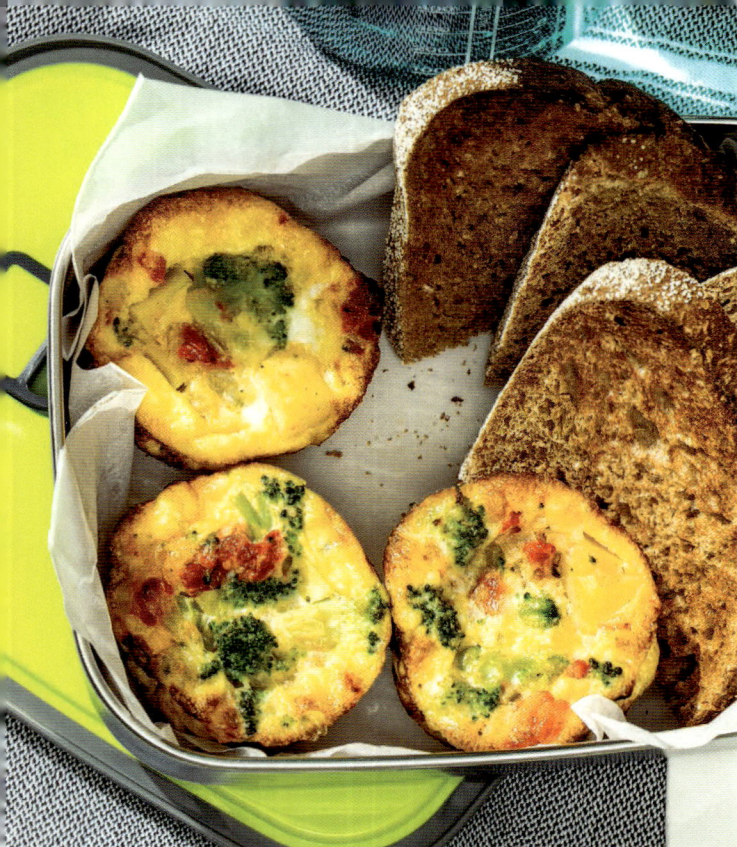

Frittata Bites with Broccoli and Sun-Dried Tomatoes

serves 4 (makes 12 frittatas) • total time: 50 minutes

why this recipe works • Once you've kick-started your morning with these vegetable-packed grab-and-go frittatas, you'll never buy the coffeehouse version again. These portable bites come together in a single bowl and are then baked in a muffin tin. After microwaving chopped potatoes—a step that ensures that they cook up nice and tender—we combined the taters with frozen broccoli and oil-packed sun-dried tomatoes, two nutrient-dense powerhouses that happen to be extra-convenient during a busy morning. A quarter cup of mozzarella was all we needed to infuse the whole batch with a little cheesy richness. After whisking in eggs and milk, we ladled the mixture into a muffin tin; it took only 15 to 20 minutes to produce beautifully puffed frittatas. Eaten with a side of hearty toasted bread, this fluffy, savory breakfast is tailor-made for enjoying on the go.

- 8 ounces Yukon Gold potatoes, peeled and cut into ½-inch pieces
- 1 onion, chopped fine
- 1 tablespoon extra-virgin olive oil
- ¼ teaspoon table salt, divided
- ⅛ teaspoon pepper
- 8 ounces frozen broccoli florets, thawed, patted dry, and cut into ½-inch pieces
- 1 ounce mozzarella cheese, shredded (¼ cup)
- ¼ cup oil-packed sun-dried tomatoes, patted dry and chopped fine
- 8 large eggs
- ¼ cup milk
- 8 (½-inch-thick) slices rustic bread, toasted

1   Adjust oven rack to lower-middle position and heat oven to 425 degrees. Toss potatoes and onion with oil, ⅛ teaspoon salt, and pepper and microwave in covered bowl until potatoes are tender and translucent around edges, 5 to 8 minutes, stirring halfway through microwaving. Remove bowl from microwave and let cool slightly, about 2 minutes. Stir in broccoli, cheese, and tomatoes.

2   Generously spray 12-cup muffin tin with avocado oil spray, then divide potato mixture evenly among cups. Whisk eggs, milk, and remaining ⅛ teaspoon salt together in large bowl until thoroughly combined and mixture is pure yellow; do not overbeat. Using ladle, evenly distribute egg mixture over filling in muffin cups.

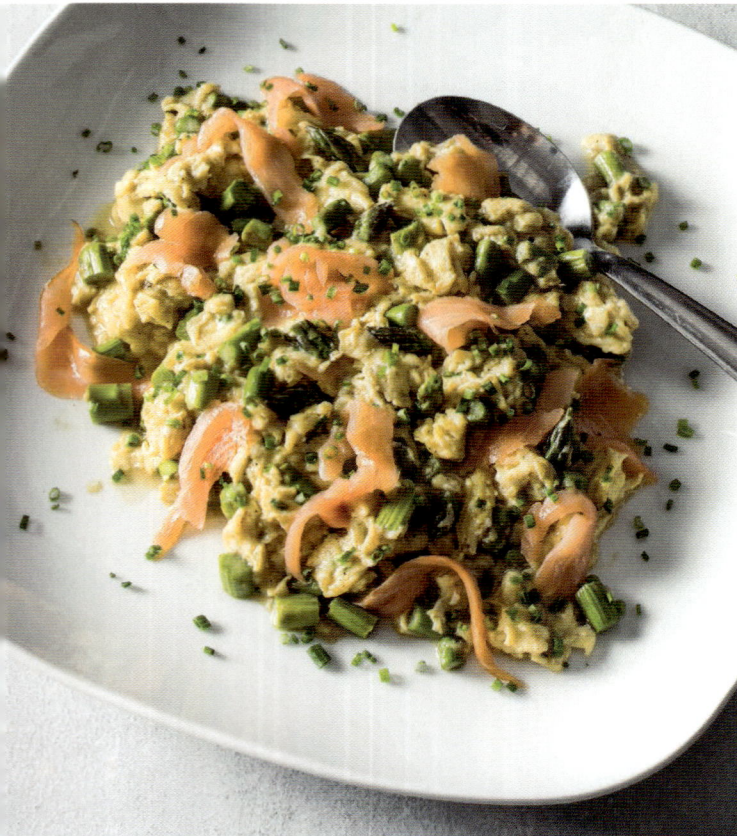

top | *Frittata Bites with Broccoli and Sun-Dried Tomatoes*
bottom | *Scrambled Eggs with Asparagus, Smoked Salmon, and Chives*

3 Bake until frittatas are lightly puffed and just set in center, 15 to 20 minutes. Transfer muffin tin to wire rack and let cool slightly, about 10 minutes. Run butter knife around edges of frittatas to loosen, then gently remove from muffin tin. Serve frittata bites with toasted bread.

MAKE AHEAD • Frittatas can be refrigerated for up to 2 days.

MAKE IT GLUTEN-FREE • Substitute gluten-free bread for the bread.

MAKE IT DAIRY-FREE • Substitute plant-based mozzarella cheese for the dairy mozzarella cheese and plant-based milk or water for the dairy milk.

Scrambled Eggs with Asparagus, Smoked Salmon, and Chives

serves 4 • total time: 20 minutes **FAST**

why this recipe works • There are countless possibilities for add-in ingredients to amp up a dish of scrambled eggs. We wanted to develop a version featuring flavorful smoked salmon for a hearty breakfast packed with omega-3 fatty acids. To tenderize and lend richness to the eggs without adding moisture, we skipped the dairy and other watery liquids and beat our eggs with extra-virgin olive oil, an excellent source of monounsaturated fats; it also added subtly fruity, grassy notes. We cooked the eggs quickly in more olive oil, stirring constantly to create large curds. Opting for a mild vegetable to counterbalance the salmon, we prepared some nutrient-packed asparagus, which we blanched in a little water before uncovering the skillet and continuing to cook until the moisture evaporated; this gave us perfectly tender asparagus that still retained a little of its satisfying snap. Once the egg curds were well established but still a little wet, we folded in the asparagus, topped the mixture with the salmon, and sprinkled over some chives for a fresh and herbaceous finish to this nutritious, well-rounded meal. If you can't find thin asparagus spears, peel the bottom halves of the spears until the white flesh is exposed, and then halve each spear lengthwise before cutting it into ½-inch pieces. You will need a 12-inch nonstick skillet with a tight-fitting lid for this recipe.

  8 large eggs
  3 tablespoons extra-virgin olive oil, divided
  2 tablespoons minced fresh chives, divided
  ¼ teaspoon table salt
  ¼ teaspoon pepper
  1 garlic clove, minced
  8 ounces thin asparagus, trimmed and cut into ½-inch pieces
  2 tablespoons water
  2 ounces smoked salmon, torn into ½-inch strips

1 Beat eggs, 2 tablespoons oil, 1 tablespoon chives, salt, and pepper together in bowl with fork until thoroughly combined and mixture is pure yellow. Heat 1 teaspoon oil and garlic in 12-inch nonstick skillet over medium heat until fragrant, about 1 minute. Add asparagus and water; cover; and cook, stirring occasionally, until asparagus is crisp-tender, 3 to 4 minutes. Uncover and continue to cook until moisture has evaporated, about 1 minute longer. Transfer asparagus mixture to small bowl and set aside. Wipe skillet clean with paper towels.

2 Heat remaining 2 teaspoons oil in now-empty skillet over medium-high heat until shimmering. Add egg mixture and, using silicone spatula, constantly and firmly scrape along bottom and sides of skillet until eggs begin to clump and spatula just leaves trail on bottom of skillet, 30 to 60 seconds. Reduce heat to low and gently but constantly fold eggs until clumped and just slightly wet, 30 to 60 seconds. Fold in asparagus mixture. Transfer to serving dish, top with salmon, and sprinkle with remaining 1 tablespoon chives. Serve.

MAKE AHEAD • Scrambled eggs can be refrigerated for up to 24 hours; serve at room temperature or reheat in microwave.

TRIMMING ASPARAGUS SPEARS

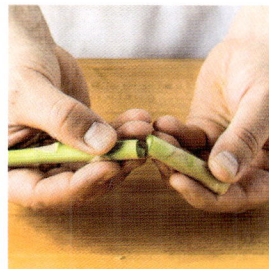

1 Remove one asparagus spear from bunch and grip stalk about halfway down; with other hand, hold stem between thumb and index finger about an inch or so from bottom and bend stalk until it snaps.

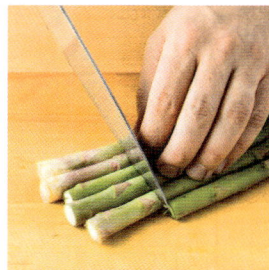

2 Using broken asparagus as guide, trim off ends of remaining spears using chef's knife.

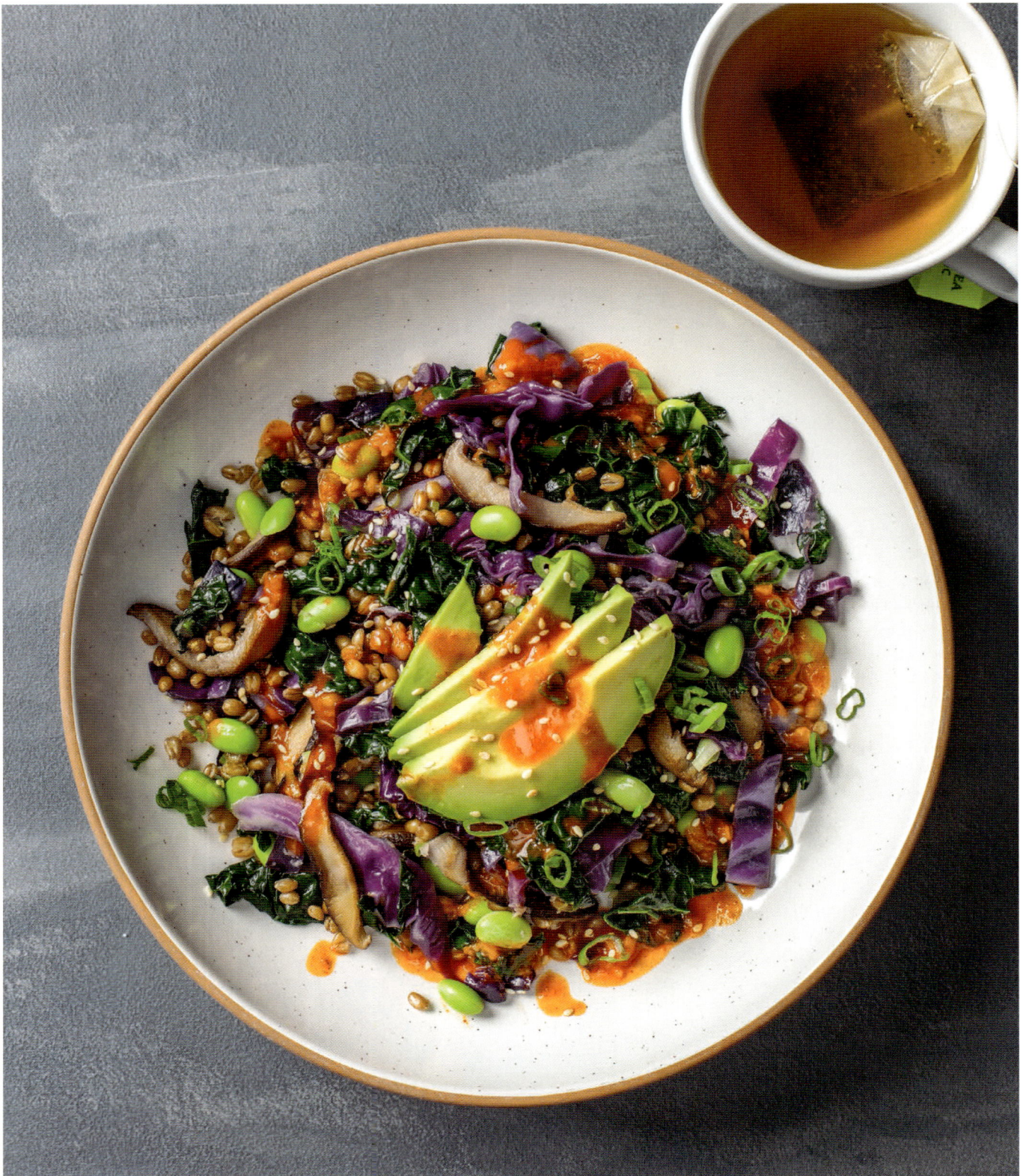

Stir Fried Breakfast Grain Bowls with Gochujang Sauce

Scrambled Eggs with Pinto Beans and Cotija Cheese

serves 4 • total time: 15 minutes **FAST**

why this recipe works • Starting the day with protein helps regulate blood sugar levels, and scrambled eggs are a great source. We upped the satiation factor even more by adding pinto beans, for a filling breakfast that comes together quickly. We started by cooking jalapeños and garlic for a bold flavor base. We then added the beans and some cilantro, letting the legumes cook just long enough to absorb the flavors before taking them out of the skillet so that they didn't soften excessively. We cooked the eggs quickly, stirring constantly to create large curds. After folding the beans back in, we sprinkled the dish with a little cotija cheese and more cilantro for a bit of fresh color and some grassy notes. If you can't find cotija cheese, you can substitute feta cheese. We like to serve these eggs with warm tortillas and hot sauce.

8	large eggs
3	tablespoons extra-virgin olive oil, divided
¼	teaspoon table salt
¼	cup jarred sliced jalapeño chiles, chopped coarse
2	garlic cloves, minced
1	(15-ounce) can no-salt-added pinto beans, rinsed
¼	cup chopped fresh cilantro, divided
1	ounce cotija cheese, crumbled (¼ cup)

1 Beat eggs, 2 tablespoons oil, and salt together in bowl with fork until thoroughly combined and mixture is pure yellow. Heat 1 teaspoon oil, jalapeños, and garlic in 12-inch nonstick skillet over medium heat until fragrant, about 1 minute. Add beans and 3 tablespoons cilantro and cook, stirring frequently, until moisture has evaporated, about 1 minute. Transfer bean mixture to small bowl and set aside. Wipe skillet clean with paper towels.

2 Heat remaining 2 teaspoons oil in now-empty skillet over medium-high heat until shimmering. Add egg mixture and, using silicone spatula, constantly and firmly scrape along bottom and sides of skillet until eggs begin to clump and spatula just leaves trail on bottom of skillet, 30 to 60 seconds. Reduce heat to low and gently but constantly fold eggs until clumped and just slightly wet, 30 to 60 seconds. Fold in bean mixture. Transfer to serving dish, sprinkle with cotija and remaining 1 tablespoon cilantro, and serve.

MAKE AHEAD • Scrambled eggs can be refrigerated for up to 24 hours; serve at room temperature or reheat in microwave.

MAKE IT DAIRY-FREE • Substitute plant-based cotija or feta cheese for the dairy cotija cheese, or omit the cheese.

Stir-Fried Breakfast Grain Bowls with Gochujang Sauce

serves 4 • total time: 35 minutes **FAST**

why this recipe works • To create this colorful breakfast, we took a cue from the one-pan simplicity of fried rice—perfect for pulling together in the morning using precooked grains. Antioxidant-dense kale joins forces with red cabbage, shiitakes, edamame, and ginger for a satisfying meal that will jump-start your day. For the grains, we chose wheat berries for their fiber and hearty chew. We topped each portion with avocado for a creamy contrast and then drizzled spicy gochujang sauce on top. Stir-frying is a fast-cooking technique, so have all your ingredients prepped before heating up the skillet. You can swap the wheat berries for other cooked whole grains such as farro, barley, or brown rice, if you prefer—just be sure they are cool or at room temperature before you start.

Gochujang Sauce

2	teaspoons toasted sesame oil
2	garlic cloves, minced
2	tablespoons gochujang
2	tablespoons water
2	teaspoons unseasoned rice vinegar

Stir-Fry

1	tablespoon toasted sesame oil
2	teaspoons grated fresh ginger
2	tablespoons avocado oil
4	ounces shiitake mushrooms, stemmed and sliced thin
¼	teaspoon table salt, divided
1½	cups thinly sliced red cabbage
6	ounces kale, stemmed and sliced thin
4	scallions, white and green parts separated and sliced thin
2	cups cooked wheat berries (page 333), room temperature
1	cup frozen shelled edamame beans, thawed and patted dry
1	avocado, halved, pitted, and sliced ¼ inch thick
1	tablespoon sesame seeds, toasted

1 For the gochujang sauce Combine oil and garlic in small bowl. Microwave until bubbly and fragrant, about 30 seconds. Stir in gochujang, water, and vinegar until combined; set aside.

2 For the stir-fry Combine sesame oil and ginger in small bowl. Heat avocado oil in 12-inch nonstick skillet over medium-high heat until shimmering. Add mushrooms and ⅛ teaspoon salt and cook, stirring frequently, until softened and lightly browned, about 3 minutes. Add cabbage, kale, and remaining ⅛ teaspoon salt and cook, stirring frequently, until kale is wilted and cabbage is slightly softened, about 2 minutes.

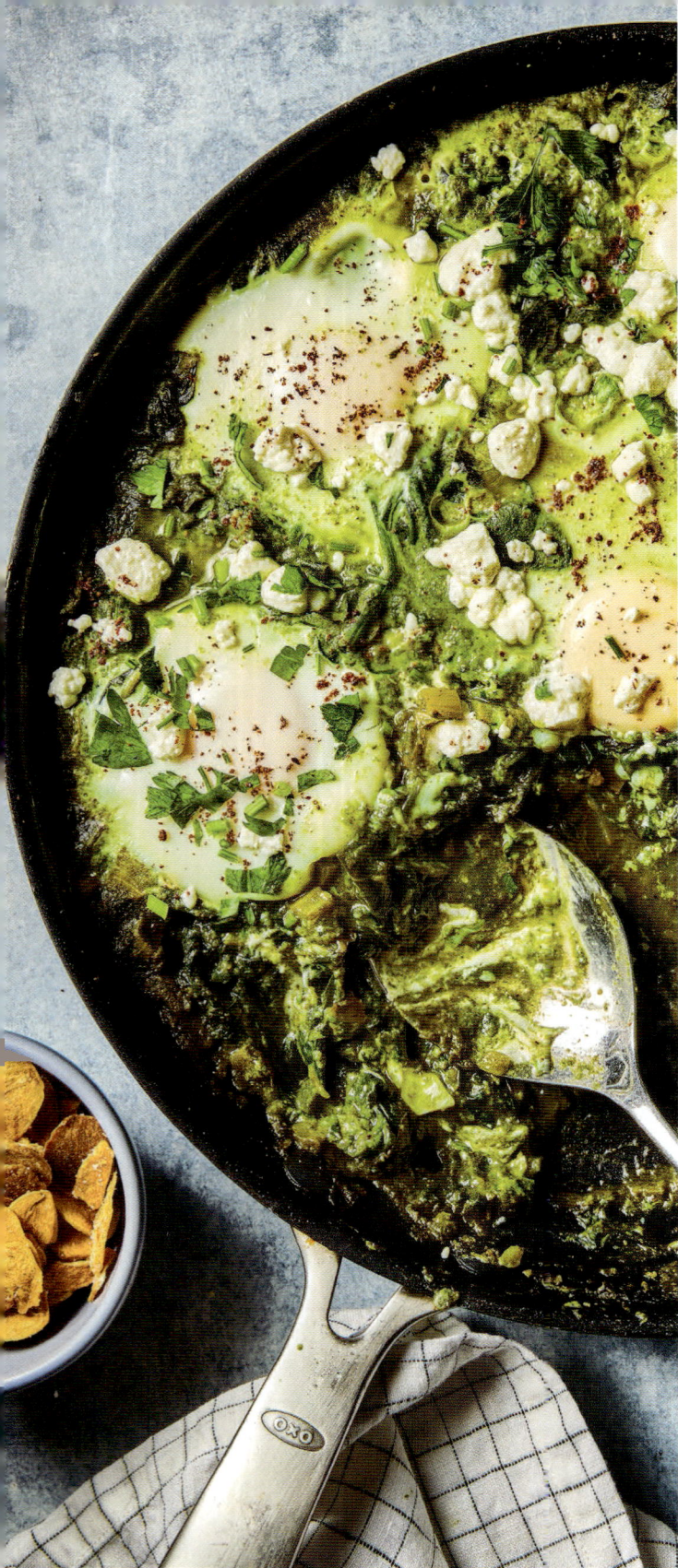

3 Push vegetables to sides of skillet to clear center; add sesame oil–ginger mixture and scallion whites to clearing and cook, mashing mixture with spoon, until fragrant, 15 to 20 seconds. Combine sesame oil–ginger-scallion mixture with vegetables. Add wheat berries and edamame and cook, stirring frequently, until warmed through, about 2 minutes.

4 Divide mixture evenly among serving bowls. Top with avocado, drizzle with sauce, and sprinkle with scallion greens and sesame seeds. Serve.

MAKE AHEAD • Gochujang sauce can be refrigerated for up to 2 days.

MAKE IT GLUTEN-FREE • Substitute oat berries, quinoa, or brown rice for the wheat berries. Be sure to use gluten-free gochujang.

Green Shakshuka

serves 4 • total time: 45 minutes FAST SUPERCHARGED

why this recipe works • For a nutritionally supercharged take on shakshuka, we replaced the robust tomato-pepper sauce from the red version of the dish with a cornucopia of digestion-enhancing leafy greens: mineral-y Swiss chard, tender baby spinach, and a bunch of fresh parsley. We started by softening the fiberful chard stems with onion and garlic in extra-virgin olive oil, which infused the vegetables with nuttiness. We pureed a portion of the cooked greens with water and bread, giving us a perfectly thick, homogeneous puree. The smooth mixture was just the right vehicle for evenly transferring heat to several eggs, which we cracked directly into the puree. A sprinkle of sumac brought its signature brightness, while a little crumbled goat cheese offered milky tang. If you can't find sumac, omit it and serve with lemon wedges (lemon juice may dull the color of the greens). Use a glass lid if you have one. If not, peek at the eggs frequently as they cook. Serve with hot sauce and garnish with Microwave-Fried Garlic Chips (recipe follows). You will need a 12-inch nonstick skillet with a tight-fitting lid for this recipe.

  6 tablespoons extra-virgin olive oil
  1 pound Swiss chard, stems sliced ¼ inch thick (2 cups), leaves cut into 1½- to 2-inch pieces (8 cups)
  1 onion, chopped fine
  8 garlic cloves, sliced thin
  ¾ teaspoon table salt, divided
  2 teaspoons ground coriander
  2 teaspoons ground cumin

2   cups plus 2 tablespoons chopped fresh parsley leaves
    and stems, divided
1   pound (16 cups) baby spinach
1   ounce rustic bread, cut into ½-inch pieces (½ cup)
1¼ cups water
1½ teaspoons ground sumac, divided
8   large eggs
1   ounce goat cheese or feta cheese, crumbled (¼ cup)
    (optional)

1 Heat oil in 12-inch nonstick skillet over medium heat until shimmering. Add chard stems, onion, garlic, and ¼ teaspoon salt. Cook, stirring occasionally, until vegetables are soft and lightly browned, 8 to 10 minutes.

2 Add coriander and cumin and cook until fragrant, about 1 minute. Add chard leaves and 2 cups parsley. Reduce heat to medium-low and cook, covered, stirring occasionally, until greens are just wilted but still bright green, 2 to 3 minutes.

3 Add half of spinach, cover, and cook until just wilted. Add remaining spinach and cook, covered, stirring occasionally, until all spinach is wilted but still bright green, 3 to 5 minutes. Off heat, transfer 1½ cups greens mixture to blender. Add bread, water, 1 teaspoon sumac, and remaining ½ teaspoon salt. Process until smooth puree forms, about 1 minute, scraping sides of blender jar as needed. Stir puree into remaining greens in skillet and smooth into even layer.

4 Using back of spoon, make 8 shallow indentations (about 1 inch wide) in surface of greens (seven around perimeter and one in center). Crack 1 egg into each indentation (which will hold yolk in place but not fully contain egg). Spoon greens over edges of egg whites so whites are partially covered and yolks are exposed.

5 Bring to simmer over medium heat. Cover and cook until yolks film over, 3 to 5 minutes, adjusting heat to maintain gentle simmer. Continue to cook, covered, until whites are softly but uniformly set (if skillet is shaken lightly, each egg should jiggle as single unit), 1 to 2 minutes longer. Off heat, sprinkle with goat cheese, if using; remaining 2 tablespoons parsley; and remaining ½ teaspoon sumac. Season with salt to taste, and serve.

| **MAKE IT GLUTEN-FREE** • Substitute gluten-free bread for the bread.

Microwave-Fried Garlic Chips

makes ½ cup • total time: 15 minutes
The confectioners' sugar helps to offset any bitterness; taste your garlic chips and decide for yourself if they need it.

½   cup thinly sliced garlic
½   cup avocado oil
1   teaspoon confectioners' sugar (optional)

Combine garlic and oil in medium bowl, stirring to separate any stuck-together cloves. Microwave for 3 minutes. If the garlic hasn't begun to brown, stir and microwave 90 seconds longer. Repeat stirring and microwaving in 30-second increments until deep golden brown (30 seconds to 2 minutes). Using slotted spoon, transfer garlic to paper towel–lined plate; dust with confectioners' sugar, if using; and season with salt to taste. Let drain and crisp for about 5 minutes. (Fried garlic can be stored in airtight container at room temperature for up to 2 days.)

Blueberry and Almond Oatmeal

serves 4 • total time: 35 minutes FAST

why this recipe works • Too often, speed trumps quality when it comes to cooking steel-cut oatmeal. You deserve to enjoy this satiating, slow-digesting breakfast at its best: pleasantly chewy and ultracreamy. But the reality is that steel-cut oats typically require a long simmering time in order to break down sufficiently; we needed to come up with a cooking method that would speed up the process yet still produce satisfying oats. For a lighter lift in the morning, we found a simple solution: toasting the raw oats in a little avocado oil. Not only did this step build flavor by drawing out the oats' inherent nuttiness, it also jump-started the cooking process. Once we added water and simmered the mixture, it took only 20 minutes for the oats to reach a state of toothsome perfection. For fresh stir-ins and minimal fuss, we chose almond butter, sliced almonds, and blueberries—an antioxidant-rich take on the flavors of a classic PB&J. If you want a less-sweet oatmeal, use just 1 tablespoon of the brown sugar, or skip it.

1 tablespoon avocado oil
1 cup steel-cut oats
4 cups water
¼ teaspoon table salt
2½ ounces (½ cup) blueberries
½ cup whole almonds, toasted and chopped
1–3 tablespoons packed light brown sugar (optional)
2 tablespoons natural almond butter

1 Heat oil in large saucepan over medium heat until shimmering. Add oats and toast, stirring constantly, until fragrant and golden, about 2 minutes.

2 Add water and bring to boil over high heat. Reduce heat to medium-low and simmer gently, stirring occasionally to avoid scorching, until mixture is creamy and oats are tender but chewy, about 20 minutes.

3 Off heat, stir in salt, cover, and let stand for 5 minutes. Stir in blueberries; almonds; sugar, if using; and almond butter. Season with salt to taste. Serve immediately.

MAKE AHEAD • Oats can be prepared through step 2 and refrigerated for up to 4 days. Reheat in microwave or saucepan and thin with water if needed before topping with blueberries, almonds, sugar, and almond butter.

Savory Oatmeal with Tex-Mex Flavors

serves 4 • **total time: 10 minutes, plus overnight soaking**

FAST

why this recipe works • What would we get if we combined filling, fiber-rich oatmeal with the bold, craveable flavors of nachos? That's the question we asked ourselves in order to come up with this glorious meal that will make savory breakfast lovers eager to climb out of bed in the morning. Most oatmeal fans agree that the steel-cut version of the grain offers the best texture, but many balk at the cooking time. In this recipe, we decreased the cooking time to only 5 minutes by stirring steel-cut oats into boiling water the night before, a trick that allowed the grains to hydrate and soften overnight. In the morning, we added vegetable broth and chili powder for a boost of savory flavor, then simmered the mixture briefly until it turned thick and creamy. Taking a page from the nacho playbook, we stirred in some cotija for a rich, cheesy backbone; sautéed corn and shallots for pops of savory sweetness; and pickled jalapeños for a dose of tangy heat. Crowned with spicy salsa, cooling avocado, and grassy cilantro, this nutritious, well-rounded meal isn't your typical bowl of breakfast oats. If you can't find cotija cheese, you can substitute feta cheese. For an even heartier breakfast, top with an egg (see pages 30–31).

3 cups water
1 cup steel-cut oats
¼ teaspoon table salt
1 cup unsalted vegetable or chicken broth
2 teaspoons chili powder
2 teaspoons extra-virgin olive oil
1 cup frozen corn
1 shallot, chopped fine
3 ounces cotija cheese, crumbled (¾ cup), divided
1 tablespoon chopped jarred jalapeño chiles, plus 1 teaspoon brine
½ avocado, sliced thin
¼ cup jarred salsa
¼ cup fresh cilantro leaves

1 Bring water to boil in large saucepan over high heat. Off heat, stir in oats and salt. Cover saucepan and let stand for at least 2 hours or up to 10 hours.

2 Stir broth and chili powder into oats and bring to boil over medium-high heat. Reduce heat to medium and cook, stirring occasionally, until oats are softened but still retain some chew and mixture thickens and resembles warm pudding, 4 to 6 minutes.

3 While oats cook, heat oil in 10-inch nonstick skillet over medium-high heat until shimmering. Add corn and cook, stirring frequently, until starting to brown and pop, about 4 minutes. Reduce heat to low; add shallot; and cook, stirring constantly, until shallot is slightly softened, about 1 minute.

4 Stir corn mixture, ½ cup cotija, jalapeños, and brine into oats. Let stand for 5 minutes. Season with salt and pepper to taste. Serve, topping each portion with avocado, salsa, cilantro, and remaining ¼ cup cotija.

MAKE AHEAD • Oats can be prepared through step 2 and refrigerated for up to 4 days. Reheat in microwave or saucepan and thin with water if needed before adding corn, jalapeños and brine, avocado, salsa, cilantro, and cotija.

MAKE IT DAIRY-FREE • Substitute plant-based cotija cheese for the dairy cotija cheese.

Baked Oatmeal with Apple and Pecans

serves 4 • total time: 1 hour

why this recipe works • Thanks to hearty whole grains and protein-packed pecans, this baked oatmeal will give you the sustained energy you need to take on the day. We stirred old-fashioned rolled oats together with shredded apples, apple cider, toasted pecans, vanilla, and cinnamon and then baked the mixture. The cider pulled double duty, lending sweetness—without introducing as much sugar as the same amount of granulated sugar would—and also amping up the apple flavor. We liked the hands-off approach of baking the oatmeal, which gave us a crisp top and tender interior. For an even more efficient morning, we suggest stirring the oat mixture together the night before—that way, the baking time is the only wait you'll have to endure come morning. For wholesome topping ideas, see pages 44–45.

- 2 cups apple cider
- 2 tablespoons extra-virgin olive oil
- 1 tablespoon ground cinnamon
- 2 teaspoons vanilla extract
- ½ teaspoon table salt
- 2 cups (6 ounces) old-fashioned rolled oats
- 1 cup pecans, toasted and chopped
- 2 apples, shredded (2 cups)

1 Adjust oven rack to middle position and heat oven to 375 degrees. Grease 8-inch square baking pan.

2 Whisk apple cider, oil, cinnamon, vanilla, and salt together in large bowl. Stir in oats and pecans until well combined, then fold in apples until just combined. Transfer oat mixture to prepared pan and spread into even layer.

3 Bake until top of oatmeal is golden brown and edges are deep golden brown, 30 to 40 minutes. Let oatmeal cool in pan on wire rack for 10 minutes before serving.

VARIATION
Baked Oatmeal with Banana and Cacao
Substitute milk for the apple cider and cacao nibs for the pecans. Substitute 2 cups chopped banana for the apple.

MAKE AHEAD • Oatmeal can be prepared through step 2 and refrigerated for up to 24 hours. Alternatively, baked oatmeal can be refrigerated for up to 3 days.

MAKE IT DAIRY-FREE • In the variation, substitute plant-based milk or water for the dairy milk.

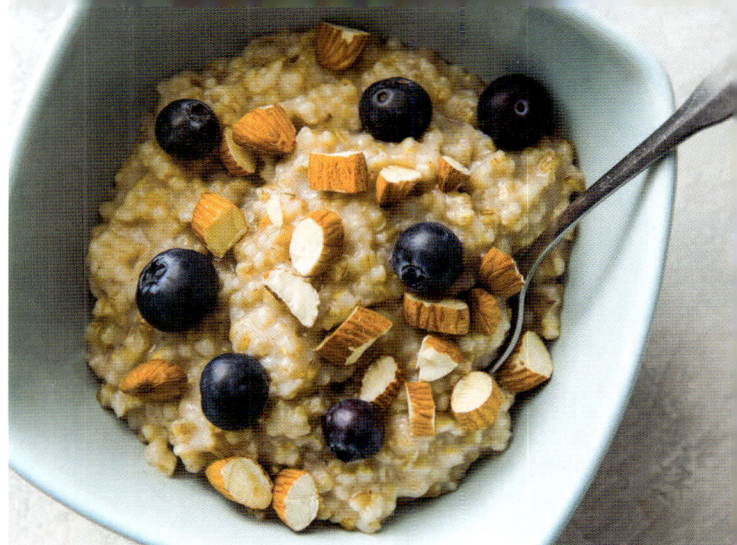

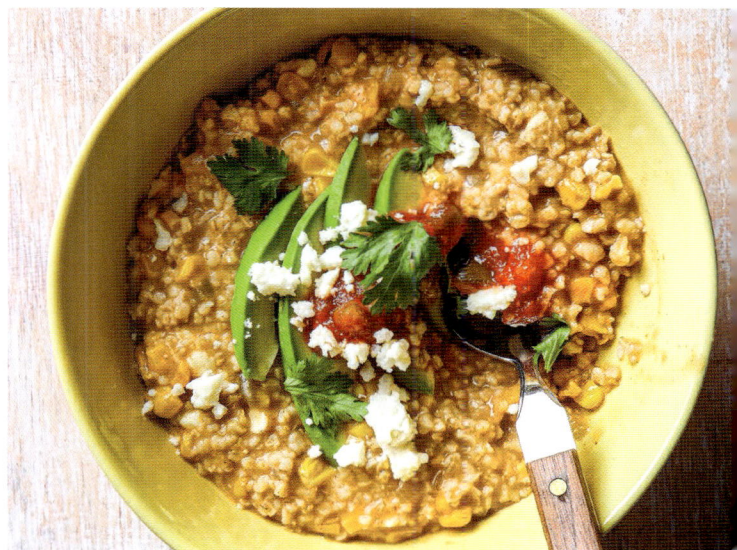

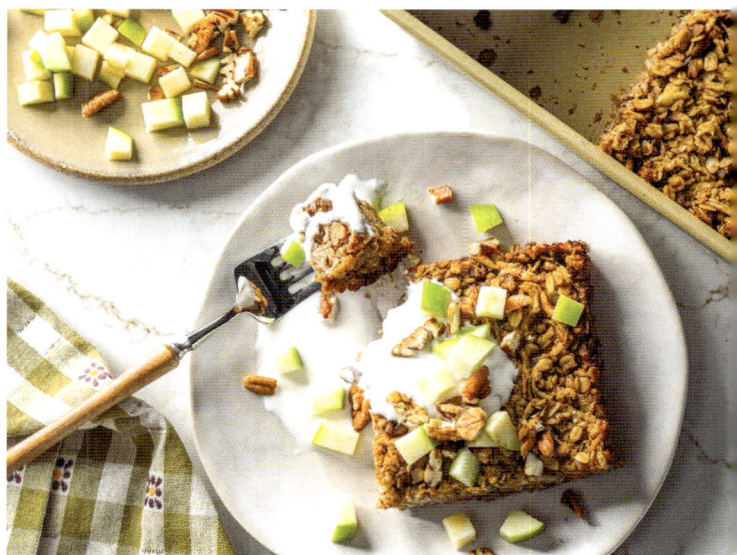

top	*Blueberry and Almond Oatmeal*
middle	*Savory Oatmeal with Tex-Mex Flavors*
bottom	*Baked Oatmeal with Apple and Pecans*

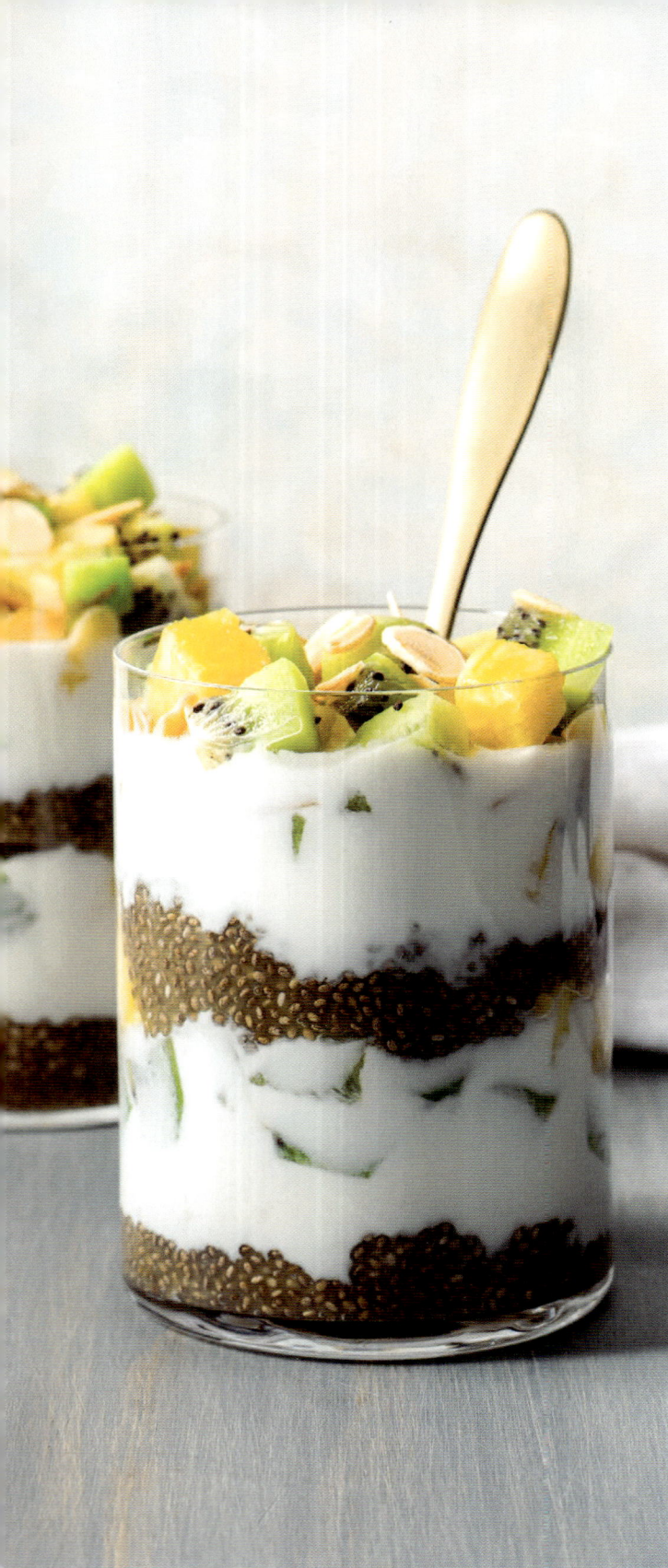

Chia Pudding Parfaits with Pineapple and Kiwi

serves 4 · total time: 30 minutes, plus 8 hours chilling

SUPERCHARGED

why this recipe works · Chia pudding, the tapioca-like result of soaking chia seeds in liquid, is a breakfast staple for many, but if that's as far as your chia adventures have taken you, it's time to explore a new horizon: chia pudding parfaits. The tiny seeds boast impressive anti-inflammatory benefits—including fiber and omega-3 fatty acids—and they possess the unique ability to gel liquid into a pudding-like consistency. To pack tropical flavor into these nourishing parfaits, we soaked the seeds in unsweetened pineapple juice. Once the pudding thickened (an overnight rest did the trick), we layered it with yogurt for creaminess and the added benefit of probiotics and with fresh pineapple and kiwi for sweetness and fiber. The result was a nutrient-rich, impressive-looking parfait that belied the ease with which it came together. Fresh, canned, or thawed frozen pineapple will work here; if using canned, look for pineapple chunks, rings, or tidbits canned in natural pineapple juice and use the fruit and the juice in the recipe. For a portable breakfast, use 2-cup jars with tight-fitting lids to store the parfaits.

  2½ cups no-sugar-added pineapple juice
  ⅔ cup chia seeds
  ¼ teaspoon table salt
  1 cup pineapple, cut into ½-inch pieces
  4 kiwis, peeled and cut into ½-inch pieces
  2 cups plain yogurt
  ¼ cup sliced almonds, toasted

1 Whisk pineapple juice, chia seeds, and salt together in bowl. Let mixture sit for 15 minutes, then whisk again to break up any clumps. Cover bowl with plastic wrap and refrigerate for at least 8 hours.

2 Combine pineapple and kiwi in bowl. Scoop ⅓ cup chia pudding into each of 4 jars or parfait glasses. Top each layer of chia pudding with ¼ cup yogurt and ¼ cup fruit mixture. Repeat layering process with remaining chia pudding, remaining yogurt, and remaining fruit. Sprinkle each parfait with 1 tablespoon almonds just before serving.

MAKE AHEAD · Chia pudding can be prepared through step 1 and refrigerated for up to 1 week. Assemble parfaits just before serving.

MAKE IT DAIRY-FREE · Substitute plant-based yogurt for the dairy yogurt.

Pepita, Almond, and Goji Berry Muesli

serves 4 • **total time: 10 minutes, plus 8 hours chilling**

SUPERCHARGED

why this recipe works • Muesli, a nutrient-packed breakfast created by a Swiss physician for his patients, started as a combination of rolled oats, nuts, seeds, and dried fruit that was soaked overnight in milk or water for improved texture and digestibility. Today's mueslis include all manner of ingredients, so we wanted to take a particularly gut-fortifying, nutrient-dense approach. An oat-forward mixture of 3 parts oats to 2 parts add-ins—a nut, a seed, and two dried fruits—gave us an ideal balance of flavor, texture, and nutrients. While traditional methods leave everything raw, we found that toasted nuts and seeds brought greater depth of flavor to this simple dish. For the nuts we opted for sliced almonds, which require almost no prep work. We chose roasted pepitas for our star seed because we loved their nutty flavor. To round out our muesli, we brought in an antioxidant-rich superfood: goji berries. A treasure trove of nutrients, the fruit is native to China and used commonly in Chinese dietary therapy. During the overnight soak, the berries softened and plumped to a lovely chewy consistency. You can also serve muesli like cereal by skipping the overnight soak if you prefer. This recipe can easily be doubled. To make a single serving, combine ½ cup muesli with ⅔ cup milk in bowl, cover, and refrigerate overnight. We like raisins and goji berries here, but you can substitute other dried fruit, if you prefer.

- 1½ cups (4½ ounces) old-fashioned rolled oats
- ¼ cup raisins
- ¼ cup goji berries
- ¼ cup sliced almonds, toasted and chopped
- ¼ cup roasted pepitas
- 1⅔ cups milk
- 5 ounces (1 cup) blueberries, raspberries, and/or blackberries

1 Combine oats, raisins, goji berries, almonds, and pepitas in bowl.

2 Stir milk into muesli until combined. Cover bowl with plastic wrap and refrigerate for 8 to 12 hours.

3 Sprinkle with berries and serve.

MAKE AHEAD • Oat mixture in step 1 can be stored at room temperature for up to 2 weeks.

MAKE IT DAIRY-FREE • Substitute plant-based milk for the dairy milk.

Nutrition Knowledge Goji berries, packed with antioxidants such as zeaxanthin, are a star in this anti-inflammatory muesli. Zeaxanthin is a carotenoid that supports eye health, while the berries' polyphenols help combat oxidative stress and inflammation in the body. Almonds and pepitas add vitamin E and magnesium, both of which are vital for cellular health and reducing inflammation. Raisins and fresh berries contribute additional antioxidants, making this a powerhouse breakfast for overall wellness. —*Alicia*

NOTES FROM THE TEST KITCHEN

Dried Fruit

Want to add other dried fruits to your muesli? Their concentrated sweet-tart flavor can be a delicious complement to sweet dishes—and savory ones as well. Here's a quick rundown of our favorites.

Apricots Apricots treated with sulfur dioxide keep longer and have a sunny orange color; untreated apricots are much darker. They taste the same, however.

Blueberries The dried variety are typically wild blueberries, which are small and fleshy, with a highly concentrated blueberry flavor.

Cherries Ninety percent of dried cherries are made from sour cherries. Often the dried sour cherries are sweetened, but not always.

Cranberries Fresh cranberries are usually infused with sweetened cranberry juice in the process of being dried.

Currants Currants are made from black Corinth grapes (not currant berries). Often called Zante currants, these fruits are smaller than raisins.

Goji Berries Goji berries are small, nutrient-dense red berries prized for their antioxidants. They are traditionally used in Chinese medicine for their many health benefits.

Green Granola

serves 24 (makes 12 cups) • **total time: 1 hour, plus 1 hour cooling**

why this recipe works • Granola gets a green makeover and a surge of antioxidants in this nutrient-packed version. For layers of crunch and plant-powered protein, we mixed in pepitas, quinoa, millet, hemp hearts, and chia seeds. A touch of ginger brought warmth that married well with the earthiness of the nuts and seeds. Extra-virgin olive oil infused the mix with healthy fats and depth of flavor, while maple syrup and brown sugar contributed just enough sweetness. Think of this mix as endlessly adaptable— toss in your favorite toasted nuts or dried fruit for extra nutrients and flavor. Whether sprinkled over yogurt, served with milk, or eaten by the handful, every bite is wholesome and satisfying. We like the convenience of prewashed quinoa (washing removes the quinoa's bitter protective coating, called saponin). You can use 1⅓ cups prewashed white quinoa if you prefer to omit the millet.

- ¼ cup maple syrup
- ¼ cup packed (1¾ ounces) light brown sugar
- 2 teaspoons vanilla extract
- ½ teaspoon table salt
- ½ cup extra-virgin olive oil
- 5 cups (15 ounces) old-fashioned rolled oats
- 1½ cups unsalted, raw pepitas
- ⅔ cup millet
- ⅔ cup prewashed white quinoa
- ½ cup hemp hearts
- 2 tablespoons chia seeds
- 1½ teaspoons ground ginger
- 2 cups dried fruit and/or toasted nuts, chopped (optional)

1 Adjust oven rack to upper-middle position and heat oven to 325 degrees. Line rimmed baking sheet with parchment paper.

2 Whisk maple syrup, sugar, vanilla, and salt together in large bowl. Whisk in oil until fully emulsified. Fold in oats, pepitas, millet, quinoa, hemp hearts, chia seeds, and ginger until thoroughly coated.

3 Transfer oat mixture to prepared sheet and spread into even layer. Using back of spatula, evenly compress mixture until very compact. Bake until lightly browned, about 45 minutes, rotating pan halfway through baking. Remove granola from oven and cool to room temperature on wire rack, about 1 hour. Break cooled granola into pieces of desired size. Fold in dried fruit and/or nuts, if using, and serve.

MAKE AHEAD • Granola can be stored in airtight container at room temperature for up to 2 weeks.

NOTES FROM THE TEST KITCHEN

All About Nuts and Seeds

Tiny but mighty, nuts and seeds are indispensable ingredients in any anti-inflammatory pantry. They are high in healthy fats, vitamins, and minerals, plus they have great texture and rich flavor. Their convenience and versatility make them a supersimple way to amp up the nutritional profile of virtually any dish, from breakfast to main courses to sides to desserts. Here's what you need to know to make the most of these powerhouses.

Storing Nuts and Seeds All nuts and seeds are high in oil and will become rancid fairly quickly if left at room temperature. In the test kitchen, we store all nuts and seeds in the freezer in freezer-safe zipper-lock bags. They will keep for months stored this way, and there's no need to defrost before using or toasting them.

Toasting Nuts Toasting nuts deepens their flavors and gives them a satisfying crunchy texture. To toast a small amount (less than 1 cup), put the nuts in a dry 12-inch skillet over medium heat. Shake the skillet occasionally to prevent scorching and toast until they are lightly browned and fragrant, 3 to 8 minutes. To toast more than 1 cup, spread the nuts in a single layer on a rimmed baking sheet and toast in a 350-degree oven. To promote even toasting, shake the baking sheet every few minutes, and toast until the nuts are lightly browned and fragrant, 5 to 10 minutes. To prevent burning, remove them from the skillet or baking sheet immediately after toasting.

Toasting Seeds Toast seeds in a dry 12-inch non-stick skillet over medium heat until the seeds turn golden and fragrant, about 5 minutes. To prevent burning, remove them from the skillet after toasting.

Skinning Toasted Nuts The skins from some nuts, such as hazelnuts and walnuts, can impart a bitter flavor and an undesirable texture in some dishes. To remove the skins from toasted nuts, simply rub the hot toasted nuts inside a clean dish towel.

100 Percent Whole-Wheat Pancakes

serves 4 to 6 (makes 18 pancakes) · total time 45 minutes **FAST**

why this recipe works · Most pancake recipes shy away from using only whole-wheat flour, often cutting it with white. But these 100 percent whole-wheat pancakes are far from dense—rather, they're fluffy and ultratender. That's because the bran in whole-wheat flour—the same stuff that contributes fiber—cuts through gluten strands that form, preventing the batter from getting tough. In fact, while many recipes advise undermixing to avoid tough pancakes, here whole-wheat flour produced soft, nutty cakes even as we whisked the batter to a smooth consistency. You can use an electric griddle set at 350 degrees instead of a skillet. For wholesome topping ideas, see pages 44–45.

  2   cups (11 ounces) whole-wheat flour
  2   tablespoons sugar
1½   teaspoons baking powder
  ½   teaspoon baking soda
  ¾   teaspoon table salt
2¼   cups buttermilk
  5   tablespoons plus 2 teaspoons avocado oil, divided
  2   large eggs

1   Adjust oven rack to middle position and heat oven to 200 degrees. Set wire rack in rimmed baking sheet and place in oven.

2   Whisk flour, sugar, baking powder, baking soda, and salt together in large bowl. In separate bowl, whisk buttermilk, 5 tablespoons oil, and eggs together until combined. Whisk buttermilk mixture into flour mixture until smooth. (Mixture will be thick; do not add more buttermilk.)

3   Heat 1 teaspoon oil in 12-inch nonstick skillet over medium heat until shimmering, 3 to 5 minutes. Using paper towels, wipe out oil, leaving thin film in pan. Using ¼-cup measure, portion batter into pan, spreading each into 4-inch round using back of spoon. Cook until edges are set, first side is golden, and bubbles on surface are just beginning to break, 2 to 3 minutes.

4   Flip pancakes and cook until second side is golden, 1 to 2 minutes longer. Serve or transfer to wire rack in oven. Repeat with remaining batter, adding remaining oil to pan as necessary.

MAKE AHEAD · Pancakes can be wrapped in plastic wrap in bundles of 2 or 3, sealed in zipper-lock bags, and frozen for up to 1 month. To reheat, microwave frozen pancakes in single layer until hot, about 2 minutes, flipping halfway through.

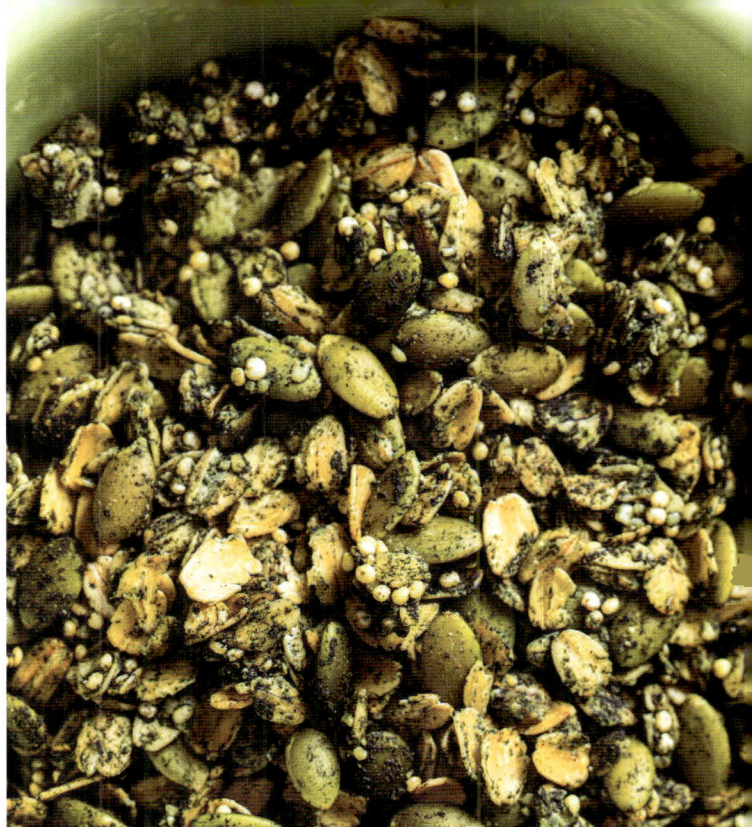

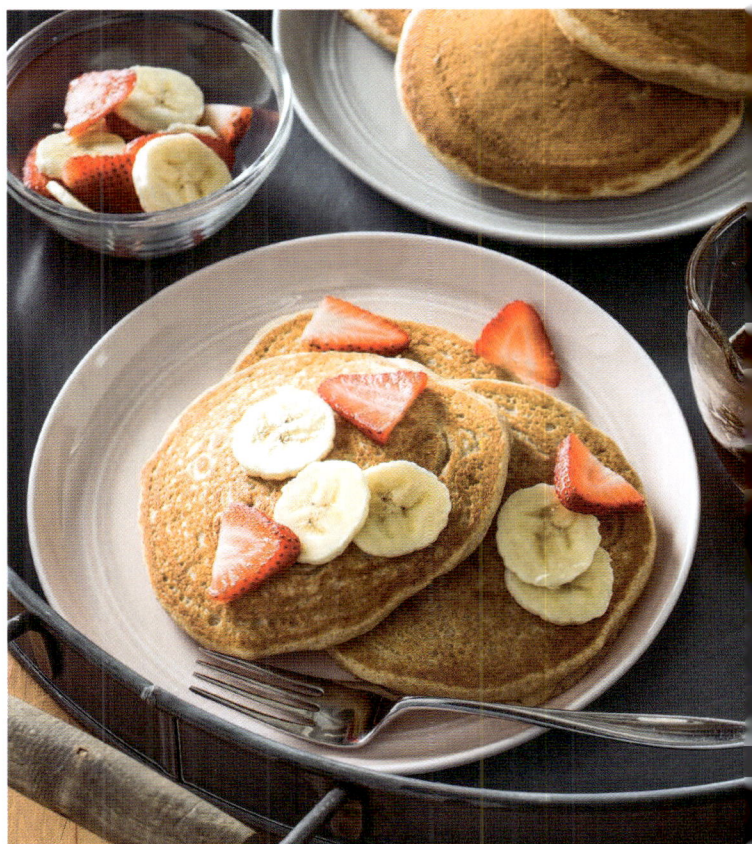

top │ *Green Granola*
middle │ *100 Percent Whole-Wheat Pancakes*

top it off

These nourishing toppings are an easy way to take a simple batch of pancakes to the next level. Some feature fiberful fruit, while others incorporate yogurt for a boost of probiotics, as well as small amounts of sugar for mild sweetness and aromatic spices for depth and antioxidants.

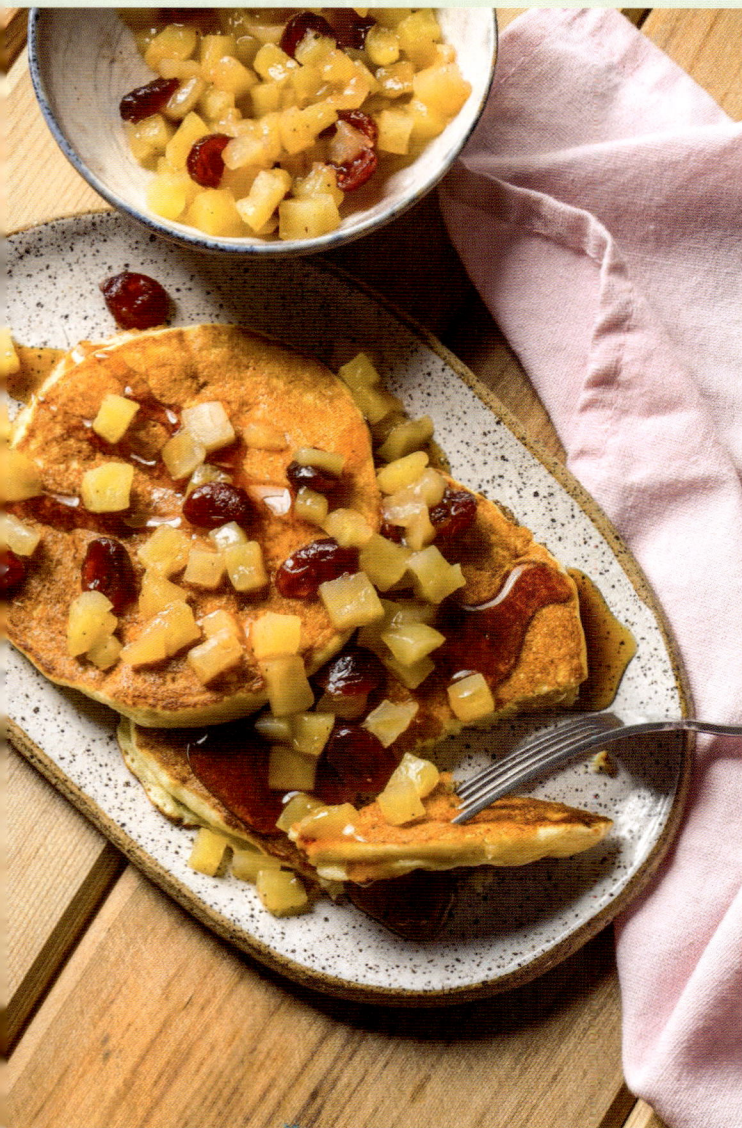

Pear-Blackberry Topping

makes 3 cups • total time: 10 minutes

- 3 ripe pears, peeled, halved, cored, and cut into ¼-inch pieces
- 1 tablespoon sugar
- 1 teaspoon cornstarch
  Pinch table salt
  Pinch ground cardamom
- 5 ounces (1 cup) blackberries

Combine pears, sugar, cornstarch, salt, and cardamom in bowl and microwave, covered, until pears are softened but not mushy and juices are slightly thickened, 4 to 6 minutes, stirring once halfway through microwaving. Stir in blackberries.

Apple-Cranberry Topping

makes 2½ cups • total time: 10 minutes

- 3 Golden Delicious apples, peeled, cored, and cut into ¼-inch pieces
- ¼ cup dried cranberries
- 1 tablespoon sugar
- 1 teaspoon cornstarch
  Pinch table salt
  Pinch ground nutmeg

Combine all ingredients in bowl and microwave, covered, until apples are softened but not mushy and juices are slightly thickened, 4 to 6 minutes, stirring once halfway through microwaving. Stir before serving.

Plum-Apricot Topping

makes 2½ cups • total time: 10 minutes

- 1½ pounds plums, halved, pitted, and cut into ¼-inch pieces
- ¼ cup dried apricots, chopped coarse
- 1 tablespoon sugar
- 1 teaspoon cornstarch
  Pinch table salt
  Pinch ground cinnamon

Combine all ingredients in bowl and microwave until plums are softened but not mushy and juices are slightly thickened, 4 to 6 minutes, stirring once halfway through microwaving. Stir before serving.

Raspberry-Chia Compote

makes ¾ cup · total time: 30 minutes

- 5 ounces (1 cup) raspberries
- 1 tablespoon sugar
- 1 tablespoon water
  Pinch table salt
- 1 tablespoon chia seeds
- ¼ teaspoon vanilla extract

Cook raspberries, sugar, water, and salt in small saucepan over medium-low heat, mashing occasionally with potato masher, until bubbling and raspberries have broken down, 4 to 6 minutes. Off heat, stir in chia seeds and vanilla and let sit until thickened, about 10 minutes.

Sweet Yogurt Sauce

makes 1½ cups · total time: 5 minutes

- 1¼ cups plain yogurt
- 3 tablespoons sugar
- ½ teaspoon vanilla extract

Whisk all ingredients together in bowl.

Orange-Honey Yogurt

makes 1¼ cups · total time: 5 minutes

- 1 cup plain Greek yogurt
- 2 tablespoons honey
- ¼ teaspoon grated orange zest plus 2 tablespoons juice

Whisk all ingredients together in bowl.

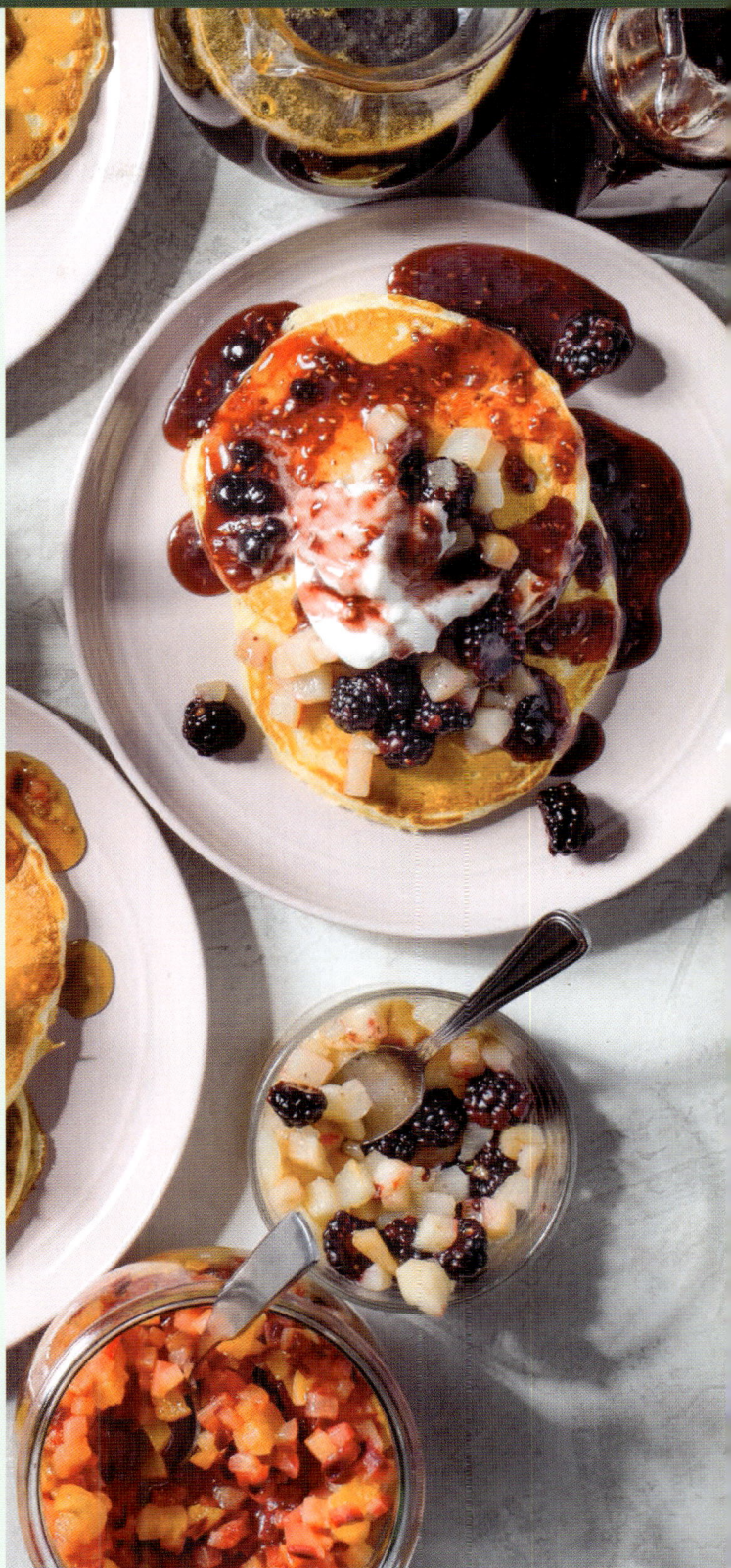

Pear-Blackberry Topping and Plum-Apricot Topping

Blueberry-Oat Pancakes

serves 4 to 6 (makes 18 pancakes)
total time: 50 minutes, plus 15 minutes resting

why this recipe works • To give classic blueberry pancakes a nutrient boost, we turned to oats. Not only is the whole grain high in gut-balancing fiber, but it also offers lovely nutty flavor and a hearty bite. We were able to create a smooth base for our batter using a combination of oat flour and a little all-purpose flour, with the latter providing structure and lift. We stirred whole rolled oats into our batter as well; presoaked until just softened, they gave our pancakes a wonderfully satisfying chew. Blueberries offered the perfect fresh counterpart to the toasty oats, while cinnamon and nutmeg infused the pancakes with comforting warmth. Switching from whole milk to buttermilk not only helped us manage the saturated fat content in this recipe but also went a long way in keeping our pancakes light and fluffy. We prefer using store-bought oat flour, as it has a very fine grind and creates the fluffiest pancakes, but you can make your own in a pinch: Grind 1½ cups (4½ ounces) old-fashioned rolled oats in a food processor to a fine meal, about 2 minutes; note, pancakes will be denser if using ground oats. Do not use toasted oat flour or quick, instant, or thick-cut oats in this recipe. You can use an electric griddle set at 350 degrees instead of a skillet. For wholesome topping ideas, see pages 44–45.

    2   cups buttermilk, divided, plus extra as needed
    1   cup (3 ounces) old-fashioned rolled oats
1½   cups (4½ ounces) oat flour
    ½   cup (2½ ounces) all-purpose flour
2½   teaspoons baking powder
    1   teaspoon ground cinnamon
    ¼   teaspoon table salt
    ⅛   teaspoon ground nutmeg
    2   large eggs
    3   tablespoons plus 2 teaspoons avocado oil, divided
    3   tablespoons sugar
    2   teaspoons vanilla extract
7½   ounces (1½ cups) blueberries, divided

1   Adjust oven rack to middle position and heat oven to 200 degrees. Set wire rack in rimmed baking sheet and place in oven. Combine 1 cup buttermilk and oats in bowl and let sit at room temperature until softened, about 15 minutes.

2   Whisk oat flour, all-purpose flour, baking powder, cinnamon, salt, and nutmeg together in large bowl. In separate bowl, whisk remaining 1 cup buttermilk, eggs, 3 tablespoons oil, sugar, and vanilla together until frothy, about 1 minute. Whisk buttermilk mixture into flour mixture until smooth. Using silicone spatula, fold in soaked oat-buttermilk mixture.

3   Heat 1 teaspoon oil in 12-inch nonstick skillet over medium heat until shimmering, 3 to 5 minutes. Using paper towels, wipe out oil, leaving thin film in pan. Using ¼-cup measuring cup, portion batter into pan, spreading each into 4-inch round using back of spoon. Sprinkle each pancake with 1 tablespoon blueberries. Cook until edges are set and first side is golden, 2 to 3 minutes.

4   Flip pancakes and cook until second side is golden, 2 to 3 minutes. Serve or transfer to wire rack in oven. Repeat with remaining batter, whisking additional buttermilk into batter as needed to loosen, and adding remaining oil to pan as necessary.

MAKE AHEAD • Pancakes can be wrapped in plastic wrap in bundles of 2 or 3, sealed in zipper-lock bags, and frozen for up to 1 month. To reheat, microwave frozen pancakes in single layer until hot, about 2 minutes, flipping halfway through.

Berry-Oat Smoothie

serves 2 • total time: 10 minutes   FAST   SUPERCHARGED

why this recipe works • This health-fortifying smoothie is deceptive because it tastes like a treat: It evokes the indulgent flavors of berry cobbler yet contains no added sugar, leaning entirely on the natural sweetness of the fruit and some choice spices. To ensure an ideal blend of tart and sweet, we used antioxidant-rich mixed berries. But despite the berries' star billing, it was the old-fashioned rolled oats we added that turned out to be the cornerstone of this smoothie: The fiber-loaded oats thickened the texture and gave us a particularly creamy drink. Though it may seem counterintuitive to toast the oats before blending them into a drink, this step contributed a nuttiness to our smoothie that amplified the cobbler flavor profile. Adding yogurt to the mix made the smoothie creamier and brought in some gut-healthy probiotics, while cinnamon, ginger, and lemon zest further echoed the baked-dessert flavor that we aspired to. This recipe is flexible, so if you have a favorite cobbler, you can swap in whatever frozen berry you like best. Toast the oats in a dry skillet over medium heat until fragrant, about 2 minutes, and then remove the skillet from the heat so the oats won't scorch.

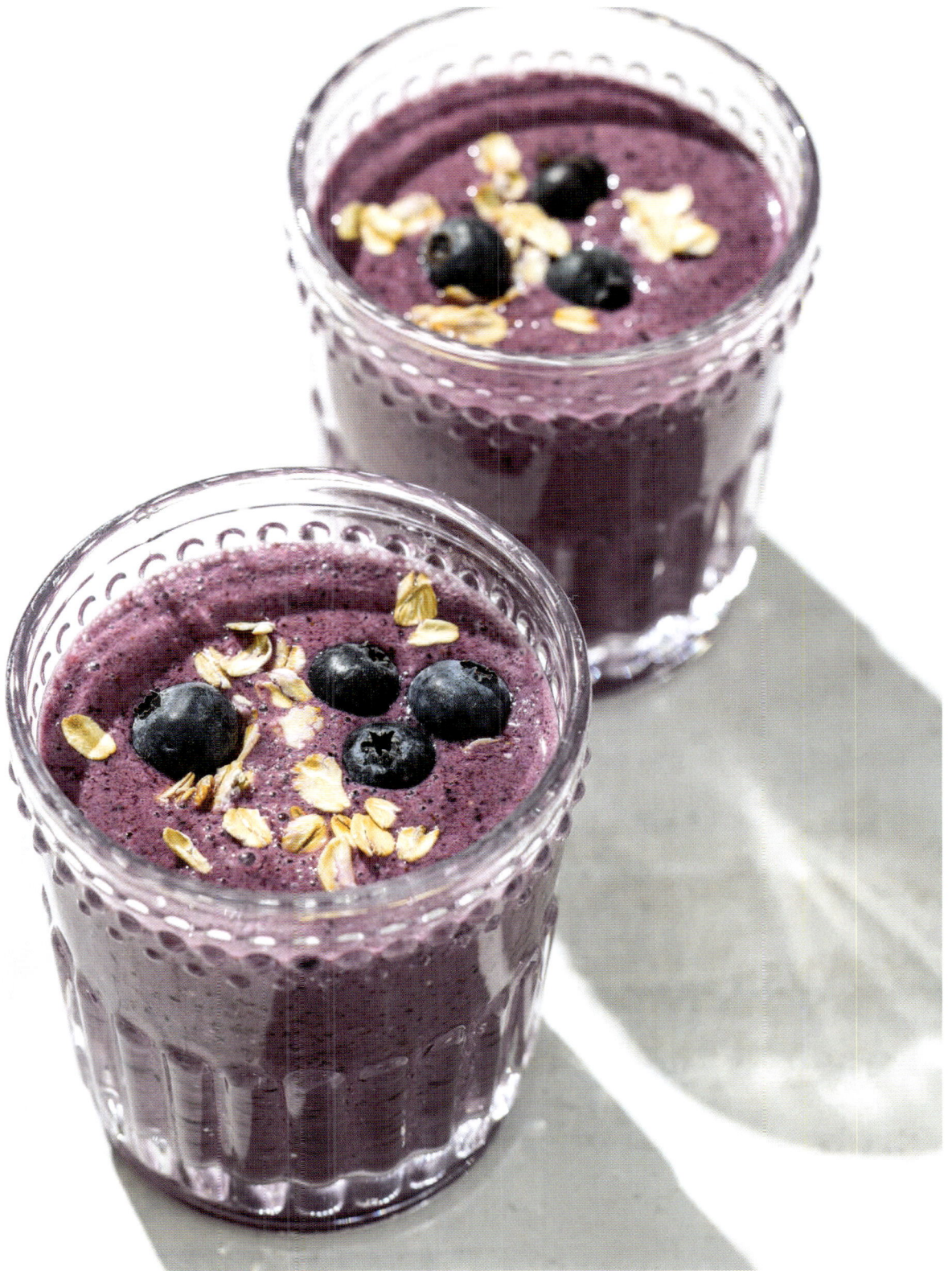

½ cup old-fashioned rolled oats, toasted

1¾ cups frozen mixed berries

½ teaspoon grated lemon zest

¼ teaspoon ground cinnamon

⅛ teaspoon ground ginger

½ cup plain yogurt

1 cup water, plus extra as needed

In order listed, add all ingredients to blender and process on low speed until mixture is combined but still coarse in texture, about 10 seconds, scraping down sides of blender jar as needed. Gradually increase speed to high and process until completely smooth, about 1 minute. Adjust consistency with water as needed. Serve.

MAKE AHEAD • Smoothie can be refrigerated for up to 24 hours; stir vigorously and thin with additional water before serving if needed.

MAKE IT DAIRY-FREE • Substitute plant-based yogurt for the dairy yogurt.

Super Greens Smoothie

serves 2 • total time: 10 minutes `FAST` `SUPERCHARGED`

why this recipe works • For many nutrition-minded eaters, a smoothie made from an assortment of greens is the epitome of wholesomeness. To make sure our recipe offered peak nutrient density, we loaded it with six phytonutrient-rich greens, choosing them with care to ensure a pleasantly vegetal beverage. Spinach and parsley brought mild grassiness, broccoli unexpectedly offered subtle sweetness, cucumber contributed a refreshing note, and avocado acted as an emulsifier and thickener that held the mixture together. Our final "green" came from the superfood spirulina, a plant-based algae high in antioxidants. Because all those greens can taste intense, we incorporated unsweetened apple juice, which balanced out the bitterness of the greens and rounded out the drink's flavor profile. Blending the ingredients with 2 cups of ice added light aeration and broke up all the fibrous greens for a smooth texture. You can use either blue or green spirulina in this recipe, but blue spirulina will affect the color of your smoothie.

NOTES FROM THE TEST KITCHEN

Measuring Frozen Fruit

Though we usually reserve liquid measuring cups for liquids, we find it easier to measure chunky frozen fruit for smoothies and other recipes in a 2-cup glass measure instead of traditional dry measuring cups. To measure 2 cups of frozen fruit, fill the cup to the top with fruit and then gently press down so that it spreads somewhat to the edges of the glass. Once pressed, the top of the fruit should sit just slightly above the 2-cup mark.

1 cup baby spinach

2 cups ice

4 ounces cucumber, cut into 2-inch pieces (1 cup)

3 ounces broccoli florets, cut into 1-inch pieces (1 cup)

½ ripe avocado

¼ cup fresh parsley leaves

2 teaspoons spirulina

1 cup unsweetened apple juice, plus extra as needed

In order listed, add all ingredients to blender and process on low speed until mixture is combined but still coarse in texture, about 10 seconds, scraping down sides of blender jar as needed. Gradually increase speed to high and process until completely smooth, about 2 minutes. Adjust consistency with extra apple juice as needed. Serve.

MAKE AHEAD • Smoothie can be refrigerated for up to 24 hours; stir vigorously before serving.

Nutrition Knowledge   In this powerhouse of a green smoothie, spinach, parsley, and broccoli provide antioxidants such as lutein and quercetin, while avocado offers healthy monounsaturated fats that support anti-inflammation. I love that the drink also features spirulina, a plant-based algae rich in phycocyanin, a powerful anti-inflammatory compound.   —*Alicia*

Passionate Dragon Smoothie

serves 2 · total time: 5 minutes   **FAST**

why this recipe works · We wanted to develop a smoothie that stars dragon fruit, a dramatic-looking fruit that comes in a variety of colors and has a light, mild flavor. That delicate flavor proved to be a perfect partner for the assertive taste of tart, tangy passion fruit. Blending in banana gave an almost buttery quality to the smoothie, and its mild sweetness helped balance the tartness of the passion fruit. For a creamy emulsifier that disappeared into the drink, we added protein-dense silken tofu and blended everything for a full minute to achieve our desired smooth texture. This combination of tropical fruit in a smoothie is irresistible, and it's as visually inviting as it is delicious. Passion fruit pulp is often sold in the freezer section with other fruits. Do not substitute soft or firm tofu.

2½ cups frozen dragon fruit chunks
 4 ounces frozen passion fruit pulp, broken into 2-inch pieces
 4 ounces silken tofu
 ½ ripe banana, peeled
 1 cup water, plus extra as needed

In order listed, add all ingredients to blender and process on low speed until mixture is combined but still coarse in texture, about 10 seconds, scraping down sides of blender jar as needed. Gradually increase speed to high and process until completely smooth, about 1 minute. Adjust consistency with extra water as needed. Serve.

MAKE AHEAD · Smoothie can be refrigerated for up to 24 hours; stir vigorously before serving.

Matcha Fauxba

serves 2 · total time: 10 minutes   **FAST**   **SUPERCHARGED**

why this recipe works · We love boba tea with its tapioca pearls and wanted to develop a morning smoothie that evokes the fun of slurping those chewy pearls through a wide straw. So we came up with this nutrient-loaded "fauxba," which uses antioxidant-packed blueberries to channel boba's signature pearls. Boba is often made with tea, so we played with that expectation by adding a couple teaspoons of antioxidant-rich matcha powder. Matcha has a subtly tannic flavor and offers a striking green hue in addition to some energizing caffeine. Fiberful baby spinach offered a dose of leafy greens, while a juicy orange and ripe pear provided additional

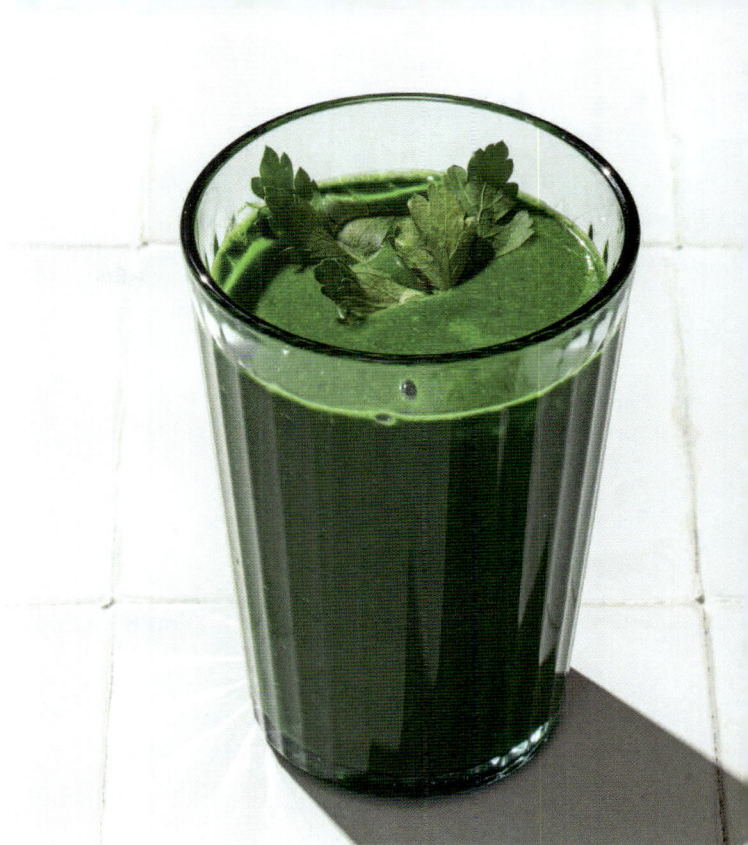

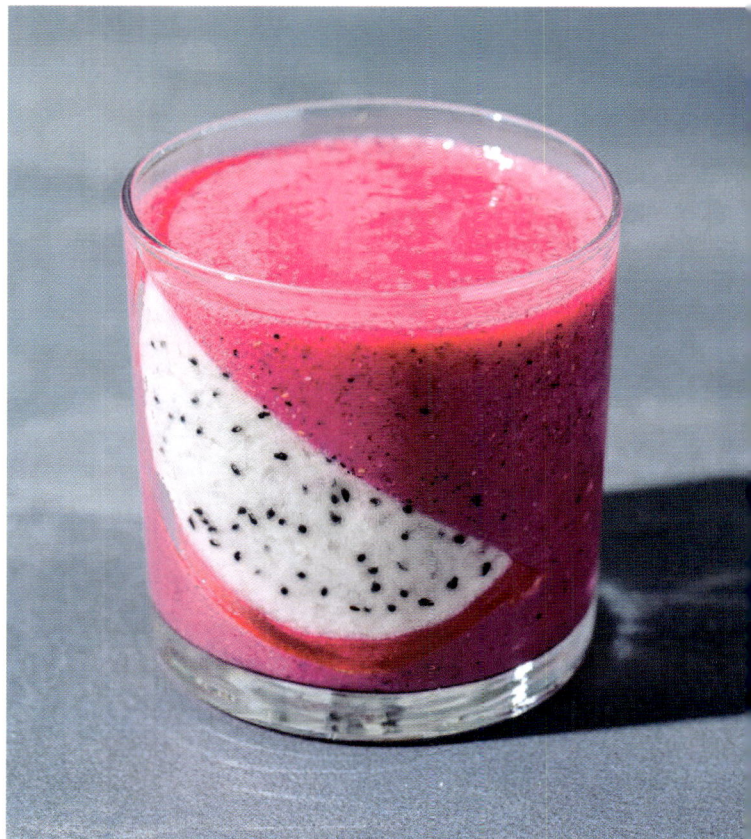

top | *Super Greens Smoothie*
bottom | *Passionate Dragon Smoothie*

fiber. Most boba drinks are loaded with added sugar, but our fauxba derives its sweetness exclusively from natural sources. For creaminess, we used silken tofu, which had the added bonus of boosting the protein content. Placing the blueberries in the bottom of the glass before pouring the smoothie on top helped us recreate the boba-drinking experience, so this smoothie is best enjoyed with a wide straw. Do not substitute soft or firm tofu.

- 1½ ounces (1½ cups) baby spinach
- 1 cup ice
- 1 orange, peeled and quartered
- 1 very ripe Asian pear, peeled, quartered, and cored
- 4 ounces silken tofu
- 2 teaspoons matcha powder
- ¼ cup water, plus extra as needed
- ½ cup fresh or thawed frozen blueberries

1 In order listed, add spinach, ice, orange, pear, tofu, matcha, and water to blender and process on low speed until mixture is combined but still coarse in texture, about 10 seconds, scraping down sides of blender jar as needed. Gradually increase speed to high and process until completely smooth, about 90 seconds. Adjust consistency with extra water as needed.

2 Divide blueberries between 2 glasses and top with smoothie. Serve.

> **MAKE AHEAD** • Smoothie can be refrigerated for up to 24 hours; stir vigorously and add blueberries to glasses just before serving.

Nutrition Knowledge   The matcha in this "fauxba" is a rich source of anti-inflammatory compounds, particularly EGCG (epigallocatechin gallate), which helps combat oxidative stress and inflammation. Its catechins support immune function and may reduce markers of chronic inflammation. Combined with vitamin C-rich orange and fiber-packed spinach, this smoothie is fun way to kick-start your morning on an anti-inflammatory note. —*Alicia*

Green Apple Pie Smoothie

serves 2 • **total time: 10 minutes** `FAST`

why this recipe works • We approached this recipe with one goal in mind: Produce a spinach smoothie that makes you want to drink your greens because it tastes like a classic baked-apple dessert. For our apple element, we chose fresh apple for its nutrients and sweet-tart flavor; peeling it first eliminated any mealy texture. We also added walnuts, an excellent source of healthy fats, which did double duty: Not only did their nuttiness evoke the toasty warmth of a well-baked crust, but they also helped thicken our smoothie to a rich, creamy consistency. During testing, we found that blending the walnuts and milk first on high—with some baby spinach for extra fiber—gave us a smooth paste to work with while creating room in the blender jar for more ingredients. To enhance that familiar autumnal pie flavor, we seasoned the smoothie with lemon zest, vanilla extract, and a touch of cinnamon. We had the best success using McIntosh and Golden Delicious apples, as they blend well, but you can use any variety.

- 2½ ounces (2½ cups) baby spinach
- 1¼ cups milk, plus extra as needed
- ⅓ cup walnuts, toasted and chopped
- ½ cup ice
- 1 apple, peeled, cored, and cut into 1-inch pieces
- ½ teaspoon grated lemon zest
- ¼ teaspoon vanilla extract
- ⅛ teaspoon ground cinnamon

1 Add spinach, milk, and walnuts to blender and process on high speed until smooth, about 1 minute.

2 In order listed, add ice, apple, lemon zest, vanilla, and cinnamon and blend on low speed until mixture is combined but still coarse in texture, about 10 seconds, scraping down sides of blender jar as needed. Gradually increase speed to high and process until completely smooth, about 90 seconds. Adjust consistency with extra milk as needed. Serve.

> **MAKE AHEAD** • Smoothie can be refrigerated for up to 24 hours; stir vigorously before serving.

> **MAKE IT DAIRY-FREE** • Substitute plant-based milk for the dairy milk.

Ruby Red Smoothie

serves 2 · **total time: 15 minutes** `FAST`

why this recipe works · Vitamin-rich, antioxidant-loaded goji berries are a nutritional powerhouse, so we wanted to develop a smoothie that made them the star. This small but mighty fruit is most readily available in its dried form, with a sweet-tart flavor reminiscent of cranberry or sour cherry. To ensure a smooth consistency when blending, we rehydrated the goji berries in warm water and reserved the soaking liquid—full of flavor and nutrients—to use in our smoothie. We paired the goji berries with frozen strawberries, which made our smoothie cold, as well as fresh grapefruit, which acted like fruit juice but offered more fiber. We then needed only a pinch of salt to heighten the fruits' natural sweetness, plus a dollop of yogurt for creaminess and some gut-friendly probiotics. The result was a refreshing and brightly colored superfood smoothie that looks as good as it will make you feel.

  2 tablespoons goji berries
  ½ cup warm water, plus extra as needed
  1 red grapefruit, peeled and quartered
  1 cup frozen strawberries
     Pinch table salt
  ½ cup plain yogurt

1   Soak goji berries in warm water in blender for at least 5 minutes or overnight.

2   In order listed, add grapefruit, strawberries, salt, and yogurt to blender and process on low speed until mixture is combined but still coarse in texture, about 10 seconds, scraping down sides of blender jar as needed. Gradually increase speed to high and process until completely smooth, about 2 minutes. Adjust consistency with extra water as needed. Serve.

MAKE AHEAD · Smoothie can be refrigerated for up to 24 hours; stir vigorously before serving.

MAKE IT DAIRY-FREE · Substitute plant-based yogurt for the dairy yogurt.

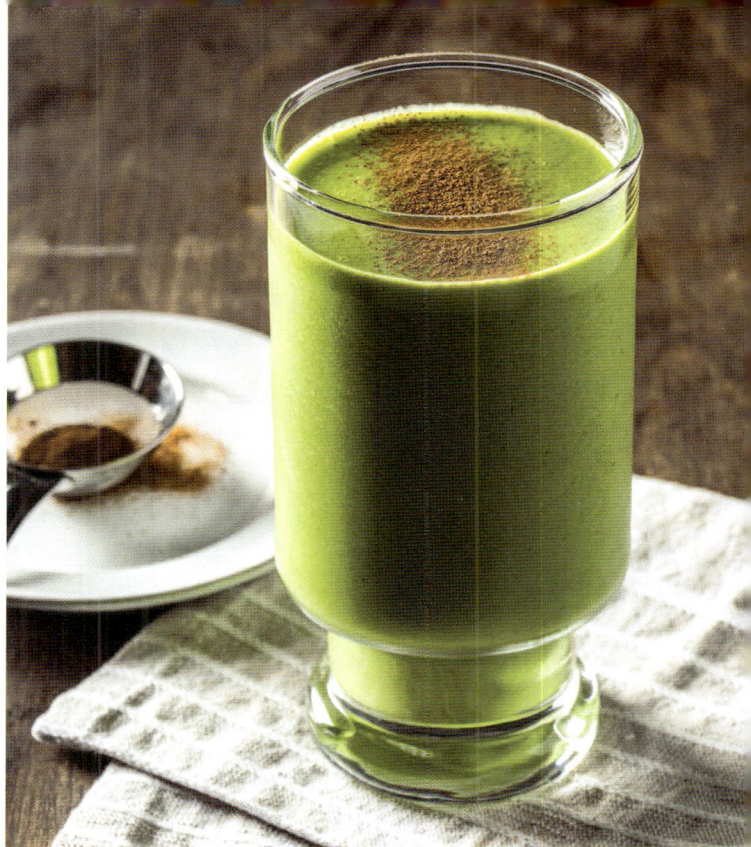

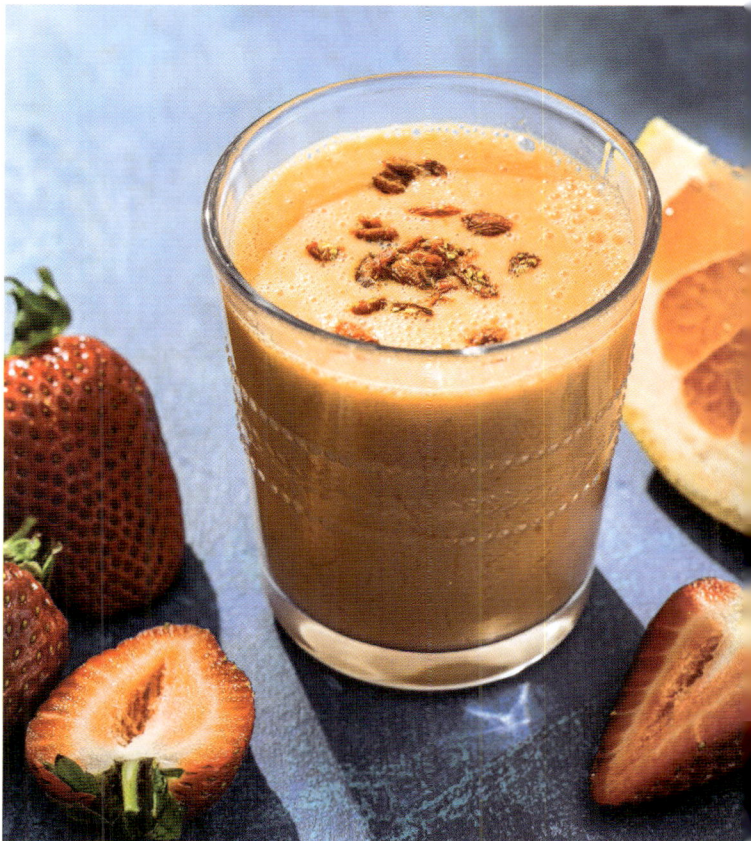

top | *Green Apple Pie Smoothie*
bottom | *Ruby Red Smoothie*

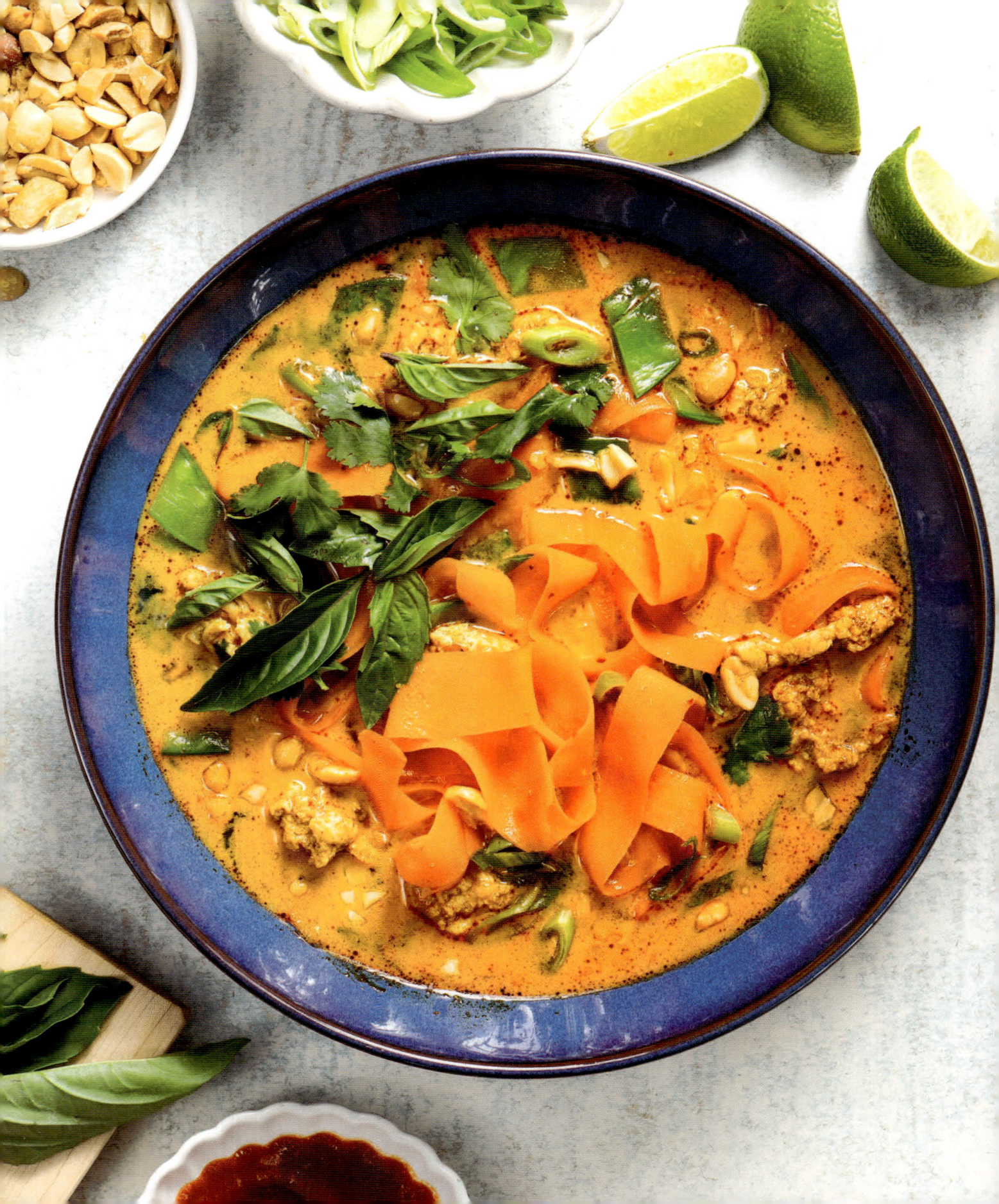

SOUPS & STEWS

■ FAST   ■ SUPERCHARGED

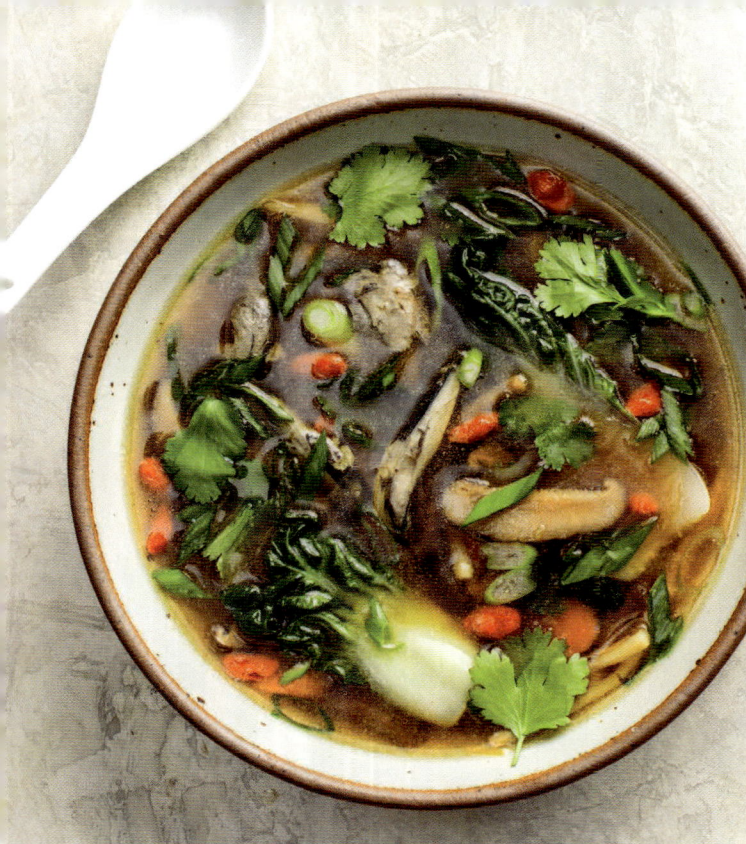

Silkie Chicken Soup with Goji Berries and Jujubes

serves 4 • total time: 1 hour 40 minutes **SUPERCHARGED**

why this recipe works • In Chinese culture, this nutrient-packed Silkie chicken soup is a dish that's widely prized for its nourishing, restorative, and anti-inflammatory properties. Believed to boost circulation and strengthen immunity, the recipe is commonly considered an example of Chinese culture's "food as medicine" philosophy and is a popular choice for illness recovery, post-partum healing, and winter wellness. Silkie chicken, also known as black-skinned chicken, is revered not only for its health benefits but also its lean, subtly sweet flavor. Traditional add-ins such as jujubes (Chinese dates), goji berries, and ginger enhance the dish's nutrient density while deepening the complexity of the broth. Straining the broth gave us a smooth, pure liquid in which to simmer lily flowers, bok choy, carrots, and more goji berries. Shaoxing wine, ginger, and soy sauce stirred in at the end rounded out the flavors of this wellness-boosting soup. Silkie chicken is traditional in this soup and is available at most Asian markets. They are commonly sold with the head and feet attached; you can ask the butcher to remove them, if desired, but we recommend leaving them intact to help enhance the flavor of the broth. If Silkie chicken is unavailable, you can substitute a 1½- to 2-pound Cornish hen. Look for jujubes and dried lily flowers at a Chinese grocer or online. Be sure to buy dried lily flowers and not dried lily bulbs, which will not soften properly in this recipe. Canned bamboo shoots, sliced into matchsticks, can be substituted for the lily flowers; there's no need to rehydrate them. The chicken skin is traditionally included in the soup with the meat, but it can be omitted, if desired.

1	(1½- to 2-pound) whole Silkie chicken, giblets discarded
12	cups water
¼	cup plus 1 tablespoon Shaoxing wine or dry sherry, divided
10	fresh cilantro stems, plus ¼ cup fresh leaves
6	scallions (4 roughly chopped, 2 sliced thin on bias)
1	(3-inch) piece ginger, peeled and sliced into ¼-inch-thick rounds, plus 1 tablespoon grated
2	ounces dried whole shiitake mushrooms
2	ounces goji berries, divided
1	ounce dried jujubes
1	ounce dried lily flowers, divided
2	star anise pods
1	teaspoon table salt
2	heads baby bok choy (4 ounces each), greens separated
2	carrots, peeled and sliced thin on bias
1½	tablespoons low-sodium soy sauce

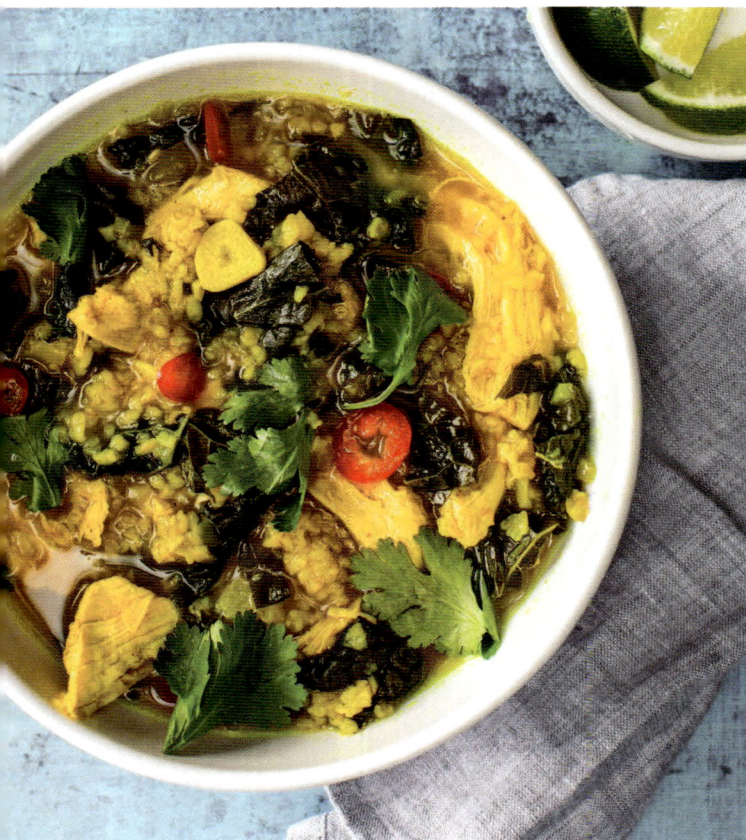

1 Place chicken in large Dutch oven or stockpot. Add water and bring to boil over high heat. Reduce to vigorous simmer and cook, turning chicken several times and skimming off any scum that rises to surface, until thighs register 175 degrees, 9 to 12 minutes. Transfer chicken to cutting board and let cool for 5 minutes. Using two forks, shred meat and skin, if using, into bite-size pieces and transfer to bowl; cover and refrigerate until ready to serve.

2 Return chicken carcass to broth along with ¼ cup Shaoxing wine, cilantro stems, chopped scallions, sliced ginger, mushrooms, 1 ounce goji berries, jujubes, ½ ounce lily flowers, star anise, and salt. Bring to boil over high heat. Reduce heat to low, cover, and simmer gently for 1 hour. Strain broth through fine-mesh strainer into large bowl, pressing on solids to extract as much liquid as possible. Reserve mushrooms; discard chicken carcass and remaining aromatics. (Broth, shredded chicken, and reserved mushrooms can be refrigerated separately for up to 3 days or frozen for up to 1 month; thaw completely before proceeding with recipe.)

3 Meanwhile, place remaining ½ ounce dried lily flowers in bowl, cover with boiling water, and let sit until tender, about 30 minutes; drain thoroughly. Stem and thinly slice reserved mushrooms.

4 Return broth to now-empty pot and bring to boil over high heat. Add lily flowers, mushrooms, bok choy, carrots, and remaining 1 ounce goji berries. Reduce to simmer and cook until vegetables are crisp-tender, about 2 minutes. Stir in chicken and cook until heated through, about 2 minutes. Stir in remaining 1 tablespoon Shaoxing wine, grated ginger, and soy sauce. Serve, garnishing individual portions with cilantro leaves and sliced scallions.

Gingery Turmeric Chicken Soup

serves 4 · total time: 1 hour

why this recipe works · This golden-hued take on classic chicken noodle soup is a bowl of warmth and comfort designed to cure what ails you. The foundation is a fragrant broth infused with turmeric, black pepper, ginger, and a whopping six cloves of garlic—ingredients known for their powerful antioxidant and immune-boosting properties. Turmeric's warm, earthy depth is enhanced by black pepper, which supports turmeric's absorption by the body, while ginger and garlic create a bold, restorative base. We also added star anise, a small but mighty pod that lends a subtle licorice-like sweetness and aids digestion. To build a broth both rich and complex, we seared the chicken for deep

umami notes and then bloomed the spices—including coriander for added warmth—to unlock their full potential. Bulgur offers hearty texture, while kale brings fiber and essential nutrients. A final addition of fresh ginger and lime zest, plus a garnish of fresh cilantro and Fresno chile, make vibrant finishing touches.

2   (10- to 12-ounce) bone-in split chicken breasts, trimmed and halved crosswise
3   tablespoons avocado oil
1   onion, chopped fine
1   teaspoon table salt
6   garlic cloves, sliced thin
2   tablespoons grated fresh ginger, divided
1   tablespoon ground turmeric
2   teaspoons ground coriander
¾   teaspoon pepper
2   star anise pods
8   cups unsalted chicken broth
2   cups water
½   cup medium-grind bulgur, rinsed
8   ounces kale, stemmed and cut into 1-inch pieces
½   teaspoon grated lime zest, plus lime wedges for serving
½   cup fresh cilantro leaves
1   Fresno chile, stemmed and sliced thin

1 Pat chicken dry with paper towels. Heat oil in Dutch oven over medium-high heat until shimmering. Place chicken skin side down in pot and cook until skin is browned, about 5 minutes; transfer to bowl. Add onion and salt to fat left in pot and cook, stirring occasionally, until onion is softened and lightly browned, 5 to 7 minutes. Add garlic, 1 tablespoon ginger, turmeric, coriander, pepper, and star anise and cook until fragrant, about 1 minute.

2 Stir in broth and water, scraping up any browned bits, and bring to boil over high heat. Add chicken and any accumulated juices, reduce heat to medium, and simmer for 10 minutes.

3 Stir in bulgur and simmer until chicken registers 160 degrees, 4 to 6 minutes. Transfer chicken to large plate, brushing any bulgur clinging to chicken back into pot, and let chicken cool slightly. Using 2 forks, shred chicken into bite-size pieces, discarding skin and bones.

4 Stir kale into soup and simmer until wilted and bulgur is tender, about 5 minutes. Stir in lime zest, shredded chicken, and remaining 1 tablespoon ginger and season with salt and pepper to taste. Sprinkle individual portions with cilantro and Fresno chile and serve with lime wedges.

Tortilla Soup with Black Beans and Spinach

serves 4 to 6 · total time: 1 hour

why this recipe works · Sopa Azteca, a tortilla soup beloved in Mexico, is light, flavorful, and full of beneficial nutrients. The broth usually gets its potency from poaching a whole chicken. To lighten our lift, we used just 12 ounces of boneless, skinless chicken thighs, but bulked up the soup with fiberful black beans and spinach. Typically, sopa Azteca calls for charring vegetables on a comal—a griddle commonly used in Mexico—before pureeing and frying them, which intensifies the ingredients' flavors. To limit the amount oil in our recipe without sacrificing flavor, we made a smoky puree of chipotles in adobo, tomatoes, onion, and garlic, then sautéed it all in a bit of extra-virgin olive oil to deepen the flavors. We also added oregano, which stood in for the more traditional but hard-to-find Mexican herb epazote. For the garnish, we oven-toasted tortilla strips—which was less inflammatory than frying, with equally crunchy results.

- 8 (6-inch) corn tortillas, cut into ½-inch-wide strips
- 3 tablespoons extra-virgin olive oil, divided
- 1 teaspoon table salt, divided
- 2 tomatoes, cored and quartered
- 1 large white onion, quartered
- 8 sprigs fresh cilantro, leaves and stems separated
- 4 garlic cloves, peeled
- 1 tablespoon minced canned chipotle chile in adobo sauce
- ¼ teaspoon dried oregano
- 4 cups unsalted chicken broth
- 2 cups water
- 1 (15-ounce) can no-salt-added black beans, rinsed
- 12 ounces boneless, skinless chicken thighs, trimmed
- 5 ounces (5 cups) baby spinach
  Lime wedges

1 Adjust oven rack to middle position and heat oven to 400 degrees. Toss tortilla strips with 1 tablespoon oil; spread over rimmed baking sheet; and bake, stirring occasionally, until golden brown and crisp, 8 to 12 minutes. Sprinkle with ¼ teaspoon salt and transfer to paper towel–lined plate.

2 Meanwhile, process tomatoes, onion, cilantro stems, garlic, chipotle, oregano, and remaining ¾ teaspoon salt in food processor until smooth, about 30 seconds, scraping down sides of bowl as needed. Heat remaining 2 tablespoons oil in Dutch oven over medium-high heat until shimmering. Add pureed tomato mixture and cook, stirring frequently, until mixture has darkened in color and liquid has evaporated, about 10 minutes.

3 Stir in broth, water, beans, and chicken, scraping up any browned bits, and bring to simmer. Cook until chicken registers 195 degrees and shreds easily with fork, 14 to 18 minutes.

4 Transfer chicken to cutting board and let cool slightly. Once cool enough to handle, shred chicken into bite-size pieces using 2 forks. Stir chicken and spinach into soup. Season with salt and pepper to taste. Place some tortilla strips in bottom of individual bowls, ladle soup over top, and sprinkle with cilantro leaves. Serve with lime wedges, passing remaining tortilla strips separately.

NOTES FROM THE TEST KITCHEN

Freezing and Reheating Soups, Stews, and Chilis

Since soup, stew, and chili recipes typically yield a generous number of servings, it is convenient to stock your freezer with leftovers for an anti-inflammatory meal on demand. To freeze them properly, first you'll need to cool them. As tempting as it might seem, don't transfer the hot soup or stew straight to the freezer or refrigerator. This can increase the fridge's internal temperature to unsafe levels for all other food. Letting the dish cool on the counter for an hour allows the temperature to drop to about 75 degrees, at which point you can transfer it safely to the freezer. For faster cooling, you can divide the pot's contents into a number of storage containers to allow the heat to dissipate more quickly or cool it rapidly by using a frozen bottle of water to stir the contents of the pot. To reheat soups, stews, and chilis, first thaw them and then simmer them gently on the stovetop in a sturdy, heavy-bottomed pot.

While most soups, stews, and chilis store just fine, those that contain pasta or dairy (plant-based or traditional) do not. The pasta turns bloated and mushy and the dairy tends to curdle as it freezes. Instead, make and freeze the dish without the pasta or dairy. When you have thawed and heated the dish through, you can stir in uncooked pasta and simmer until just tender or stir in the dairy and continue to heat gently until hot (do not boil).

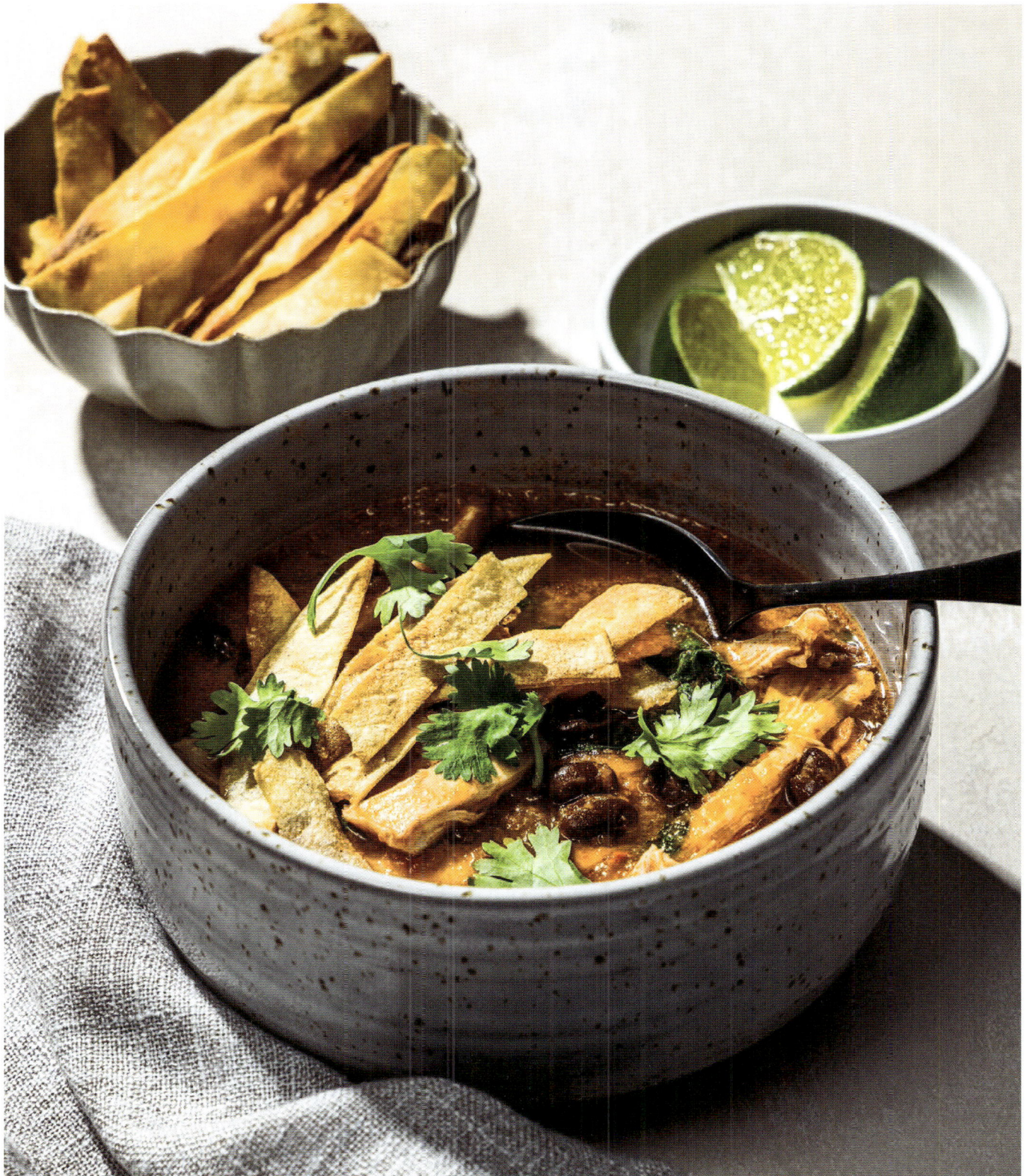

Tortilla Soup with Black Beans and Spinach

Carrot Ribbon, Chicken, and Coconut Curry Soup

serves 4 · total time: 30 minutes `FAST`

why this recipe works · We wanted to develop a wholesome, weeknight-friendly dish that drew inspiration from the many fragrant noodle soups enjoyed across Southeast Asia. For a fiberful alternative to white-rice noodles, we used a vegetable peeler to create long ribbons of carrot. Shaving the carrots thin maximized their surface area for soaking up the flavors of the soup and also made them pleasingly light and crisp. Thai curry paste, which we first bloomed in a small amount of oil so its many aromatics could thoroughly suffuse the dish, gave our soup a delectably spicy-sweet foundation. For a protein boost we added some ground chicken, which is typically lower in saturated fat than most ground meats, and simmered it in a mix of water and coconut milk; just a small amount was sufficient to make a quick, savory broth in which to cook our carrot noodles and some vitamin C–rich snow peas. We finished our soup with a mound of fresh herbs and scallions, which made for punchy final flourishes. It's worth seeking out Thai yellow curry paste for its sweet complexity; however, you can substitute red curry paste. Thai curry paste can range from mild to spicy; taste yours and, if it's very spicy, use the lower amount given. Garnish with roasted peanuts, if desired.

- 1 pound carrots, peeled
- 2 tablespoons avocado oil
- 2–4 tablespoons Thai yellow curry paste
- 12 ounces ground chicken
- 2½ cups water
- ⅓ cup canned coconut milk
- 2 tablespoons fish sauce, plus extra for serving
- 1 tablespoon sugar
- 6 ounces snow peas, trimmed and sliced ½ inch thick on bias
- 4 scallions, sliced thin on bias
- 1 cup fresh Thai basil, torn
- 1 cup fresh cilantro leaves and tender stems, torn
  Lime wedges
  Sriracha

1 Shave carrots into thin ribbons lengthwise with vegetable peeler; set aside. Combine oil and curry paste in Dutch oven and cook over medium heat until fragrant, about 3 minutes, stirring occasionally. Add chicken and cook, breaking up meat into small pieces with wooden spoon, until chicken is no longer pink, 3 to 4 minutes.

2 Add water, coconut milk, fish sauce, sugar, and reserved carrot ribbons. Bring to simmer, then add snow peas and simmer until vegetables are crisp-tender, 3 to 5 minutes.

3 Divide evenly among individual serving bowls. Sprinkle with scallions, basil, and cilantro. Serve with lime wedges, sriracha, and extra fish sauce to taste.

Chorba Frik

serves 4 to 6 · total time: 1¼ hours `SUPERCHARGED`

why this recipe works · Stews and soups are universal starters on Ramadan iftar dinner tables worldwide, as they hydrate the body and prepare it for digestion after fasting. Chorba, meaning soup, is widely consumed in different variations across Algeria, Tunisia, Morocco, and Libya and is celebrated for its nourishing qualities. Chorba frik is one version starring freekeh, a grain loaded with fiber and antioxidants; the chewy grains simmer in a tomato-based broth with cilantro, morsels of meat, and sometimes chickpeas. For our take, we kept an eye on saturated fat by making the most of just two bone-in chicken thighs. We cooked them on the stovetop to render their fat, which was a flavorful foundation on which to build the rest of our dish; we used it to cook our aromatics and bloom an assortment of inflammation-fighting spices—paprika, cumin, cayenne, and cinnamon, to name a few— before adding lycopene-rich pureed tomatoes, as well as cracked freekeh and chickpeas. We nestled the chicken into the pot with the rest of the ingredients so that the meat could stay tender while further dispersing its flavor throughout the dish. As the freekeh simmered, it retained its chew while imparting its distinctly smoky, nutty flavor. Do not use whole freekeh in this recipe.

- 1 (14.5-ounce) can no-salt-added whole peeled tomatoes
- 2 (5- to 7-ounce) bone-in chicken thighs, trimmed
- 1¼ teaspoons table salt, divided
- 2 tablespoons avocado oil
- 1 onion, chopped fine
- 1 celery rib, minced
- 1 cup minced fresh cilantro, plus ¼ cup leaves for serving
- 2 tablespoons no-salt-added tomato paste
- 3 garlic cloves, minced
- 1 tablespoon ground coriander
- 1 tablespoon paprika
- 2 teaspoons ground cumin
- ½ teaspoon pepper

¼ teaspoon ground cinnamon
¼ teaspoon cayenne pepper
6 cups water
1 (15-ounce) can no-salt-added chickpeas, undrained
½ cup cracked freekeh, rinsed
1 teaspoon dried mint
Lemon wedges

1 Process tomatoes and their juice in food processor until pureed, about 30 seconds. Pat chicken dry with paper towels and sprinkle with ¼ teaspoon salt. Heat oil in Dutch oven over medium-high heat until just smoking. Cook chicken skin side down until well browned, about 5 minutes; transfer chicken to plate. Pour off all but 2 tablespoons fat from pot.

2 Add onion, celery, and remaining 1 teaspoon salt to fat in pot and cook over medium heat until softened, about 5 minutes. Stir in minced cilantro, tomato paste, garlic, coriander, paprika, cumin, pepper, cinnamon, and cayenne and cook until fragrant, about 1 minute. Stir in pureed tomatoes, water, chickpeas and their liquid, and freekeh, scraping up any browned bits. Nestle chicken and any accumulated juices into pot and bring to simmer. Adjust heat as needed to maintain simmer and cook until freekeh is tender and chicken registers 195 degrees and shreds easily with fork, 35 to 45 minutes.

3 Transfer chicken to cutting board and let cool slightly. Once cool enough to handle, shred chicken into bite-size pieces using 2 forks, discarding skin and bones. Stir shredded chicken and any accumulated juices back into pot and season with salt and pepper to taste. Sprinkle individual portions with cilantro leaves and dried mint. Serve with lemon wedges.

MAKE IT GLUTEN-FREE • Substitute an equal amount of oat berries for the freekeh.

Nutrition Knowledge In this warming chorba frik recipe that's as nourishing as it is satisfying, coriander and paprika bring a dose of carotenoids, while cumin and cayenne add curcumin and capsaicin to help fight inflammation. Freekeh, an ancient grain rich in fiber and prebiotics, supports gut health, and chickpeas bring an extra boost of plant-based protein. —Alicia

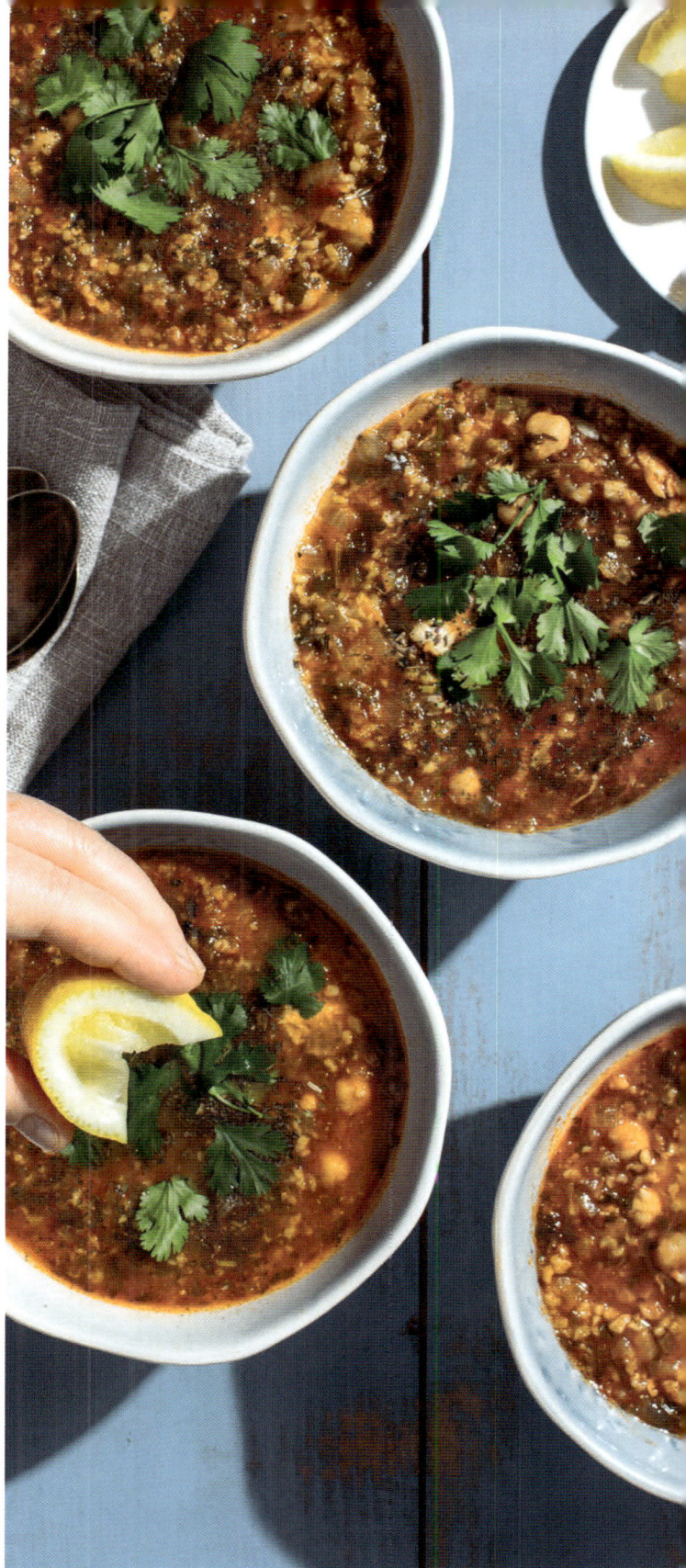

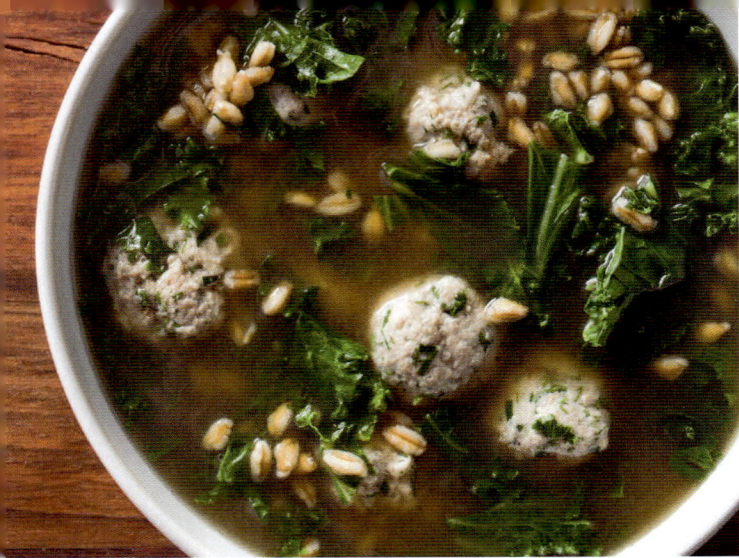

Italian Wedding Soup with Kale and Farro

serves 6 · total time: 1¾ hours

why this recipe works · Traditional Italian wedding soup is so named because of the harmonious marriage of meatballs, greens, and pasta in a savory, fortified broth. We loved the idea of a hearty, meal-in-a-bowl soup and wanted to develop a take on the dish that brings inflammation-fighting ingredients to the forefront. We replaced ditalini with hearty farro; compared with refined grains, this slow-digesting whole grain regulates blood sugar while providing lots of gut-balancing fiber. For a fast path to a complex broth, we simmered chicken broth with aromatic fennel, onion, garlic, and dried porcini mushrooms, all of which also contribute compounds that support immune function. For the meatballs, we opted to use ground turkey, which is typically lower in saturated fat than ground beef or pork. Seasoned with Parmesan, parsley, and fennel, the meatballs were deliciously herbaceous; we poached them gently in the broth, so they came out delicate and tender. Kale not only brought its characteristic assertive bite but also further upped the dish's polyphenol load and fiber content. Be sure to use 93 percent lean ground turkey, not ground turkey breast (also labeled 99 percent fat-free), in this recipe.

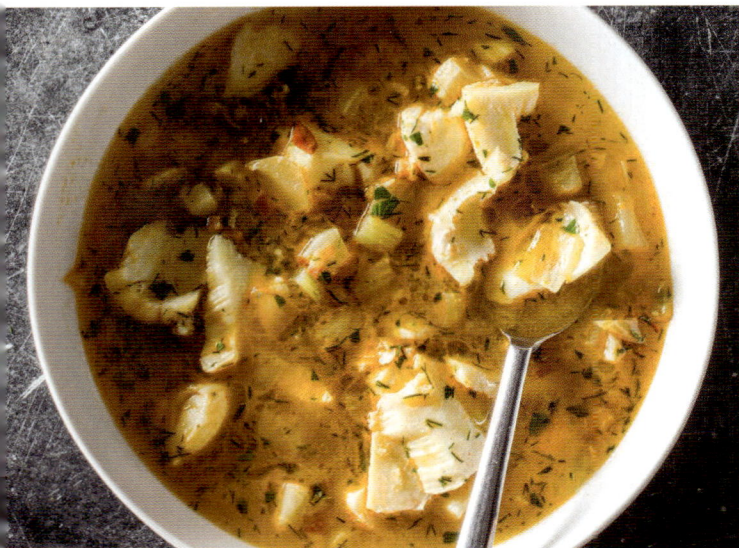

- 1 tablespoon extra-virgin olive oil
- 1 fennel bulb, ¼ cup fronds minced, stalks discarded, bulb halved, cored, and sliced thin
- 1 onion, sliced thin
- 5 garlic cloves (4 peeled and smashed, 1 minced to paste)
- ¼ ounce dried porcini mushrooms, rinsed and minced
- ½ cup dry white wine
- 1 tablespoon Worcestershire sauce
- 4 cups unsalted chicken broth
- 4 cups water
- 1 slice hearty white sandwich bread, torn into 1-inch pieces
- 5 tablespoons milk
- 12 ounces ground turkey
- ¼ cup grated Parmesan cheese
- ¼ cup minced fresh parsley
- 1 teaspoon table salt, divided
- ⅛ teaspoon pepper
- 1 cup whole farro, rinsed
- 8 ounces kale, stemmed and cut into ½-inch pieces

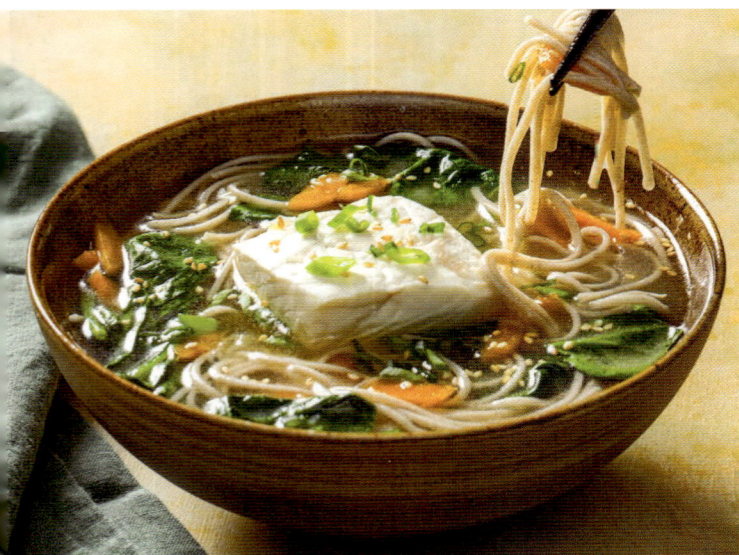

1 Heat oil in Dutch oven over medium-high heat until shimmering. Stir in fennel bulb, onion, smashed garlic, and mushrooms and cook, stirring frequently, until just softened and lightly browned, 5 to 7 minutes. Stir in wine and Worcestershire and cook for 1 minute. Stir in broth and water and bring to simmer. Reduce heat to low, cover, and simmer for 30 minutes.

2 Meanwhile, combine bread and milk in large bowl and, using fork, mash mixture to uniform paste. Add turkey, Parmesan, parsley, ½ teaspoon salt, pepper, fennel fronds, and minced garlic and knead gently with your hands until evenly combined. Using your wet hands, roll heaping teaspoon-size balls of meat mixture into meatballs and transfer to rimmed baking sheet. (You should have 35 to 40 meatballs.) Cover with greased plastic wrap and refrigerate for 30 minutes.

3 Strain broth through fine-mesh strainer set over large bowl, pressing on solids to extract as much broth as possible; discard solids. Wipe pot clean with paper towels and return strained broth to pot.

4 Bring broth to boil over medium-high heat. Add farro and remaining ½ teaspoon salt, reduce heat to medium-low, cover, and simmer until farro is just tender, about 15 minutes. Uncover, stir in meatballs and kale, and cook, stirring occasionally, until meatballs are cooked through and farro is tender, 5 to 7 minutes. Season with salt and pepper to taste, and serve.

> **MAKE AHEAD** • Shaped, uncooked meatballs can be refrigerated for up to 24 hours.

> **MAKE IT DAIRY-FREE** • Substitute plant-based milk and Parmesan cheese for the dairy milk and Parmesan cheese.

Provençal Fish Soup

serves 6 to 8 • total time: 1 hour

why this recipe works • Our Provençal-inspired fish soup makes a delicious showcase for hake, a mild white fish that's packed with omega-3 fatty acids. The fish bobs in a richly flavored broth, fragrant with digestion-supporting fennel, sweet-smoky paprika, and warm, musky saffron. To build a flavorful soup base, we cooked fennel bulb, celery, onion, and garlic before deglazing the pot with both wine and bottled clam juice, which brought oceanic flair. To ensure that the hake didn't overcook, we nestled it among the other ingredients in the pot and let it poach gently off the heat. Cod, haddock, pollock, or black sea bass can be substituted for the hake.

  1 tablespoon extra-virgin olive oil, plus extra for serving
  1 fennel bulb, 2 tablespoons fronds minced, stalks discarded, bulb halved, cored, and cut into ½-inch pieces
  1 onion, chopped
  2 celery ribs, halved lengthwise and cut into ½-inch pieces
1½ teaspoons table salt

  4 garlic cloves, minced
  1 teaspoon paprika
  ⅛ teaspoon red pepper flakes
    Pinch saffron threads, crumbled
  1 cup dry white wine
  4 cups water
  2 (8-ounce) bottles clam juice
  2 bay leaves
  2 pounds skinless hake fillets, 1 inch thick, sliced crosswise into 6 equal pieces
  2 tablespoons minced fresh parsley
  1 tablespoon grated orange zest

1 Heat oil in Dutch oven over medium heat until shimmering. Stir in fennel bulb, onion, celery, and salt and cook until vegetables are softened and lightly browned, 12 to 14 minutes. Stir in garlic, paprika, pepper flakes, and saffron and cook until fragrant, about 30 seconds.

2 Stir in wine, scraping up any browned bits. Stir in water, clam juice, and bay leaves. Bring to simmer and cook until flavors meld, 15 to 20 minutes.

3 Off heat, discard bay leaves. Nestle hake into cooking liquid, spoon some cooking liquid over top, cover, and let sit until fish flakes apart when gently prodded with paring knife and registers 135 degrees, 8 to 10 minutes. Gently stir in parsley, fennel fronds, and orange zest and break fish into large pieces. Season with salt and pepper to taste. Serve, drizzling individual portions with extra oil.

Miso Dashi Soup with Soba and Halibut

serves 4 to 6 • total time: 1¼ hours, plus 1 hour soaking

SUPERCHARGED

why this recipe works • Japanese miso soup offers a host of anti-inflammatory benefits, thanks in large part to the dashi base. Japan's versatile stock is made by extracting the umami-rich compounds in kombu (dried kelp) and katsuobushi (dried, smoked, fermented, and shaved skipjack tuna flakes); both are rich in essential minerals and omega-3 fatty acids. We steeped the kombu in cold water and then gently heated it to extract the savory compounds. After removing the kombu we added katsuobushi to give the liquid a smoky quality. Tender halibut—also a great source of omega-3 fatty acids as well as magnesium—fiberful soba noodles, carrots, and spinach further enhanced the soup's nutritional profile.

Dashi

  2 quarts cold water
1½ ounces kombu
1½ ounces katsuobushi

Soup

  8 ounces dried soba noodles
  1 tablespoon avocado oil
  3 scallions, white and green parts separated and sliced thin
  3 garlic cloves, minced
  1 tablespoon grated fresh ginger
  3 carrots, peeled, halved lengthwise, and sliced thin on bias
  1 (12-ounce) skinless halibut fillet, 1½ inches thick, cut into 2-inch pieces
  ⅓ cup white miso
  5 ounces (5 cups) baby spinach
  1 tablespoon sesame seeds, toasted

1 For the dashi Combine water and kombu in large saucepan and let sit for at least 1 hour or up to 8 hours. Meanwhile, line large fine-mesh strainer with double layer of cheesecloth, letting excess hang over sides. Set strainer over large bowl or 8-cup liquid measuring cup and set aside. After kombu has soaked, place saucepan over medium-low heat and cook until kombu-water reaches 150 degrees (water should be steaming with bubbles forming and clinging to bottom and sides of saucepan but not rising to surface), about 10 minutes. Using tongs or spider skimmer, discard kombu (or reserve for another use).

2 Increase heat to high and cook until water reaches 200 degrees (bubbles should break surface just at edges of saucepan; do not let boil), about 3 minutes. Remove saucepan from heat, add katsuobushi, and let steep for 3 minutes. Strain dashi through prepared strainer. Gather sides of cheesecloth to form bundle and lightly pinch with tongs to release any liquid into bowl. Discard bundle.

3 For the soup Bring 2 quarts water to boil in now-empty saucepan. Add noodles and cook, stirring often, until almost tender (center should still be firm with slightly opaque dot), 2 to 4 minutes (cooking times will vary). Drain noodles and set aside.

4 Wipe pot dry, then heat oil in again-empty saucepan over medium heat until shimmering. Stir in scallion whites, garlic, and ginger and cook until fragrant, about 30 seconds. Add carrots and dashi and bring to simmer. Submerge halibut in dashi and return to simmer. Reduce heat to medium-low, cover, and simmer gently until fish flakes apart when gently prodded with paring knife and registers 130 degrees, 6 to 8 minutes.

5 Stir miso into soup to dissolve. Add spinach and cook until wilted, about 30 seconds. Divide reserved noodles among bowls, then spoon soup over top. Sprinkle with scallion greens and sesame seeds and serve.

MAKE AHEAD · Dashi can be prepared through step 2 and refrigerated for up to 2 days or frozen for up to 1 month.

MAKE IT GLUTEN-FREE · For the soba noodles, look for a brand that uses 100% buckwheat flour.

NOTES FROM THE TEST KITCHEN

Getting to Know Japanese Seaweed

Seaweed, an excellent source of anti-inflammatory compounds, is a cornerstone of Japanese cuisine. It is used to flavor soups, garnish rice and noodles, and wrap maki, or rolled sushi. Here are the most common types.

Kombu Kombu is a dried kelp rich in flavor-enhancing glutamic acid. It is used extensively in Japanese cooking, one of its most popular applications being in dashi. When purchasing kombu, which is primarily sold in dried, thick sheets, take note of the chalky, white powder on the exterior. This is an indication of the glutamic acid content and translates into increased flavor.

Nori In addition to wrapping sushi, nori (Japanese for seaweed) is crumbled and garnished over soup, rice, and noodles. Nori can be plain or seasoned with soy sauce, sugar, and spices. It is often toasted before being added to a dish to release its flavor. A popular Japanese condiment, furikake, is made with nori.

Wakame Wakame is a traditional garnish in miso soup and many Japanese salads. It is available dried in thin sheets, shreds (or flakes), or fresh-salted. Dried wakame must be rehydrated in water for at least 3 to 15 minutes before using, while fresh-salted wakame should be rinsed briefly to remove the excess salt, and then soaked in water for 1 to 2 minutes.

Spring Vegetable Soup with Charred Croutons

serves 4 · total time: 1¼ hours

why this recipe works · The arrival of spring is an opportunity to show off the season's freshest vegetables, which are as visually vibrant as they are nutrient-dense. We took inspiration from this bountiful season to develop a colorful soup brimming with flavonoid-rich vegetables such as snap peas, asparagus, fennel, and leek. First, we briefly blanched the dark green part of a leek, fennel fronds, and parsley with a little baking soda—which helped retain their vibrant green color—before pureeing them with water and ice (the ice helped keep the mixture potently green, while ensuring that it didn't get too hot in the blender). For a richly flavored soup base, we cooked the white and light green parts of the leek with carrots, fennel bulb, and garlic and poured in broth. Just before serving, we added the pureed vegetables to the liquid, along with snap peas and asparagus; by only briefly cooking the latter two vegetables, we ensured that they stayed crisp-tender and maintained their bright-green hue. A touch of vinegar added welcome tang. This showstoppingly gorgeous soup is punctuated by large charred croutons, which soak up the brothy goodness. To make the croutons, we broiled them in the oven, which gave us satisfyingly crunchy results.

5 ounces rustic sourdough bread, cut into 1½-inch pieces
¾ teaspoon table salt, divided, plus salt for blanching vegetables
¼ teaspoon baking soda for blanching vegetables
2 cups fresh parsley leaves, chopped coarse
1 small leek, white and light green parts sliced into thin rounds and washed thoroughly; dark green part sliced thin and washed thoroughly
1 fennel bulb, fronds chopped coarse, stalks discarded, bulb cored and cut into ¼-inch pieces
¼ cup plus 3 tablespoons extra-virgin olive oil, divided
1½ teaspoons pepper
3 garlic cloves, sliced thin
2 carrots, peeled and cut into ¼-inch-thick rounds
4 cups unsalted vegetable or chicken broth
4 ounces thick asparagus spears, trimmed and sliced into ⅛-inch-thick rounds
4 ounces snap peas, strings removed, cut into ½-inch pieces
2 tablespoons white wine vinegar

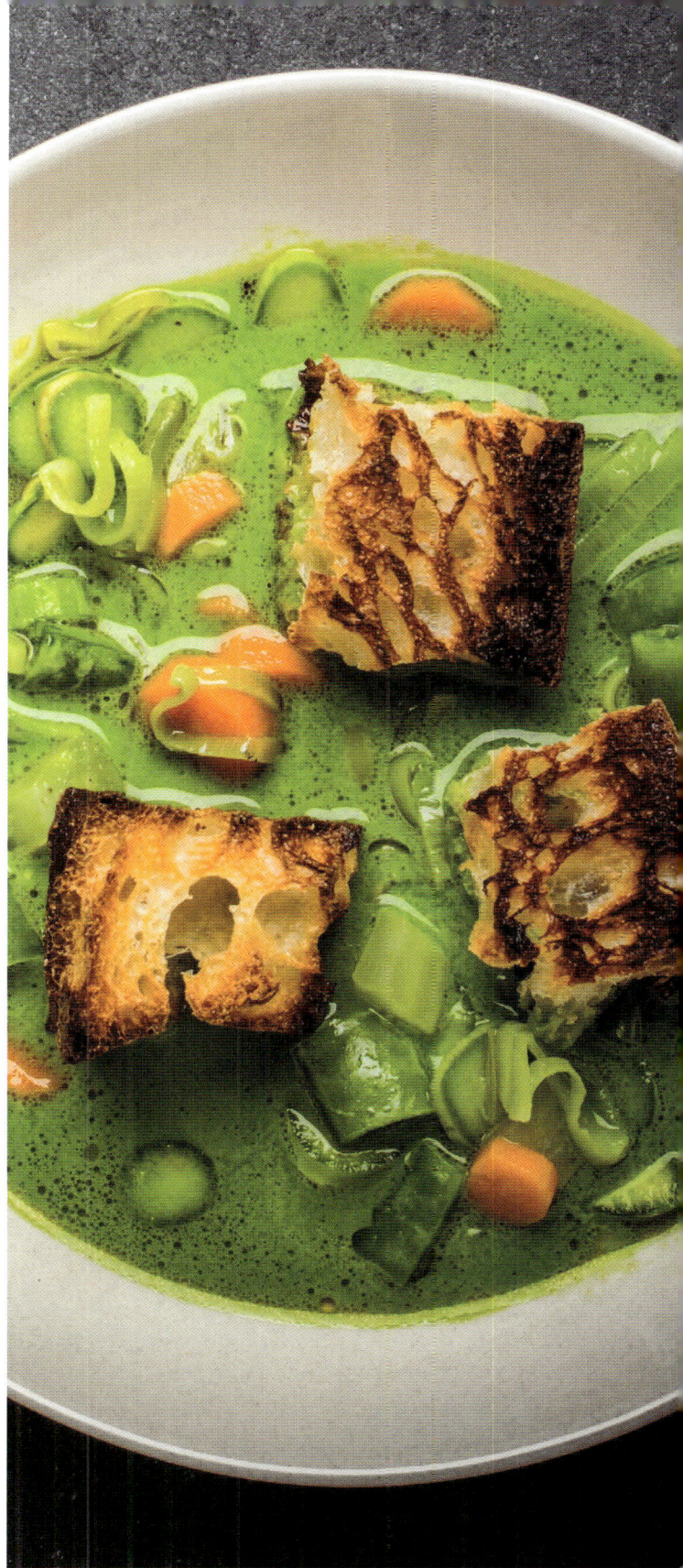

1 Adjust oven rack 8 inches from broiler element and heat broiler. Arrange bread in even layer on rimmed baking sheet. Broil until bread is charred on top, 1 to 2 minutes. Flip bread pieces and continue to broil until second side is charred, 1 to 2 minutes. Set aside.

2 Bring 10 cups water to boil in large saucepan over high heat. Meanwhile, set up ice bath by filling large bowl halfway with ice and water. Add 1½ teaspoons salt, baking soda, parsley leaves, dark green leek part, and fennel fronds to boiling water and cook for 1 minute. Drain in fine-mesh strainer or colander and immediately transfer, still in strainer, to ice bath. (Keeping the mixture in the strainer or colander makes retrieving it from the ice bath much easier.)

3 Transfer 1 cup ice and 1 cup water from ice bath to blender. Remove blanched mixture from ice bath, squeeze out excess water, and transfer to blender. Process until mostly smooth, about 1 minute. Stop blender and scrape down sides of blender jar with silicone spatula. With blender running, slowly drizzle in ¼ cup oil. Continue to process until mixture is smooth, 30 to 45 seconds. Stir in ½ teaspoon salt and set aside.

4 Heat remaining 3 tablespoons oil and pepper in Dutch oven over medium-low heat until pepper begins to sizzle, about 1 minute. Add white and light green leek parts, garlic, and remaining ¼ teaspoon salt and cook, stirring occasionally, until softened, about 3 minutes. Add carrots and fennel bulb and continue to cook, stirring occasionally, until slightly softened at edges, about 3 minutes.

5 Add broth, increase heat to medium-high, and bring to simmer, about 5 minutes. Reduce heat to medium-low and simmer gently until carrots and fennel are slightly tender but still firm, about 3 minutes.

6 Stir asparagus, snap peas, vinegar, and pureed mixture into soup. Season with salt and pepper to taste. Divide soup and charred croutons among warmed shallow bowls. Serve immediately.

NOTES FROM THE TEST KITCHEN

Pureeing Soup

The texture of a pureed soup should be as smooth and creamy as possible, so it pays to use the right appliance. With this in mind, we tried pureeing several soups with a food processor, a hand-held immersion blender, and a regular countertop blender. Here are our thoughts on each method; and because pureeing hot soup can be dangerous, we also offer some important safety tips.

Blender Is Best A standard blender turns out the smoothest pureed soups. The blade on the blender does an excellent job with soups because it pulls ingredients down from the top of the container—no stray bits go untouched by the blade. And as long as plenty of headroom is left at the top of the blender, there is no leakage.

Immersion Blender Leaves Bits Behind The immersion blender has appeal because it can be brought to the pot, eliminating the need to ladle hot ingredients from one vessel to another. However, we found that this kind of blender can leave unblended bits of food behind.

Process with Caution The food processor does a decent job of pureeing, but some small bits of vegetables can get trapped under the blade and remain unchopped. Even more troubling is the tendency of a food processor to leak hot liquid. Fill the workbowl more than halfway and you are likely to see liquid running down the side of the food processor base.

Wait Before Blending, and Blend in Batches When blending hot soup, follow a couple of precautions. Wait 5 minutes for moderate cooling, and never fill the blender jar more than halfway full; otherwise, the soup can explode out the top.

Keep the Lid Secure Don't expect the lid on a blender to stay in place. Hold the lid securely with a folded dish towel to keep it in place and to protect your hand from hot steam.

Shiitake, Tofu, and Mustard Greens Soup

serves 4 · total time: 1½ hours

why this recipe works · We wanted to develop a nourishing soup filled with anti-inflammatory vegetables swimming in a light, revitalizing broth. To build an aromatic foundation, we started by infusing broth with generous amounts of inflammation-fighting ginger and garlic. To that we added dried shiitake mushrooms, fresh shiitake stems, and just enough soy sauce to contribute savory character. Shiitakes are not only rich in glutamates but also contain anti-inflammatory compounds such as lentinans and ergothioneine. After simmering and straining the liquid, we added a splash of rice vinegar, which gave the soup subtle sweetness and tang. Sliced shiitake mushroom caps reinforced the umami-rich flavor of the broth, while a generous amount of flavonoid-rich mustard greens brought a wonderful wasabi-like kick, not to mention plenty of fiber, vitamin K, and magnesium. In lieu of refined noodles, we added tofu cubes for a satiating dose of plant-based protein. A sprinkle of sliced scallions, which contain inflammation-fighting sulfur compounds, made for the perfect fresh finish. Some tasters enjoyed a drizzle of chili oil to ramp up the spicy flavor, but it is completely optional.

- 1 tablespoon avocado oil
- 1 onion, chopped
- ¾ teaspoon table salt
- 1 (4-inch) piece ginger, peeled and sliced thin
- 5 garlic cloves, smashed
- 4 cups unsalted vegetable or chicken broth
- 4 cups water
- 8 ounces shiitake mushrooms, stemmed and sliced thin, stems reserved
- ½ ounce dried shiitake mushrooms, rinsed
- 2 tablespoons low-sodium soy sauce
- 14 ounces firm tofu, cut into ½-inch pieces
- 8 ounces mustard greens, stemmed and cut into 2-inch pieces
- 2 tablespoons unseasoned rice vinegar
- 3 scallions, sliced thin
  Chili oil (optional)

1 Heat oil in large saucepan over medium-high heat until shimmering. Stir in onion and salt and cook until softened and lightly browned, 5 to 7 minutes. Stir in ginger and garlic and cook until lightly browned, about 2 minutes.

2 Stir in broth, water, mushroom stems, dried mushrooms, and soy sauce and bring to boil. Reduce heat to low, cover, and simmer until flavors meld, about 1 hour.

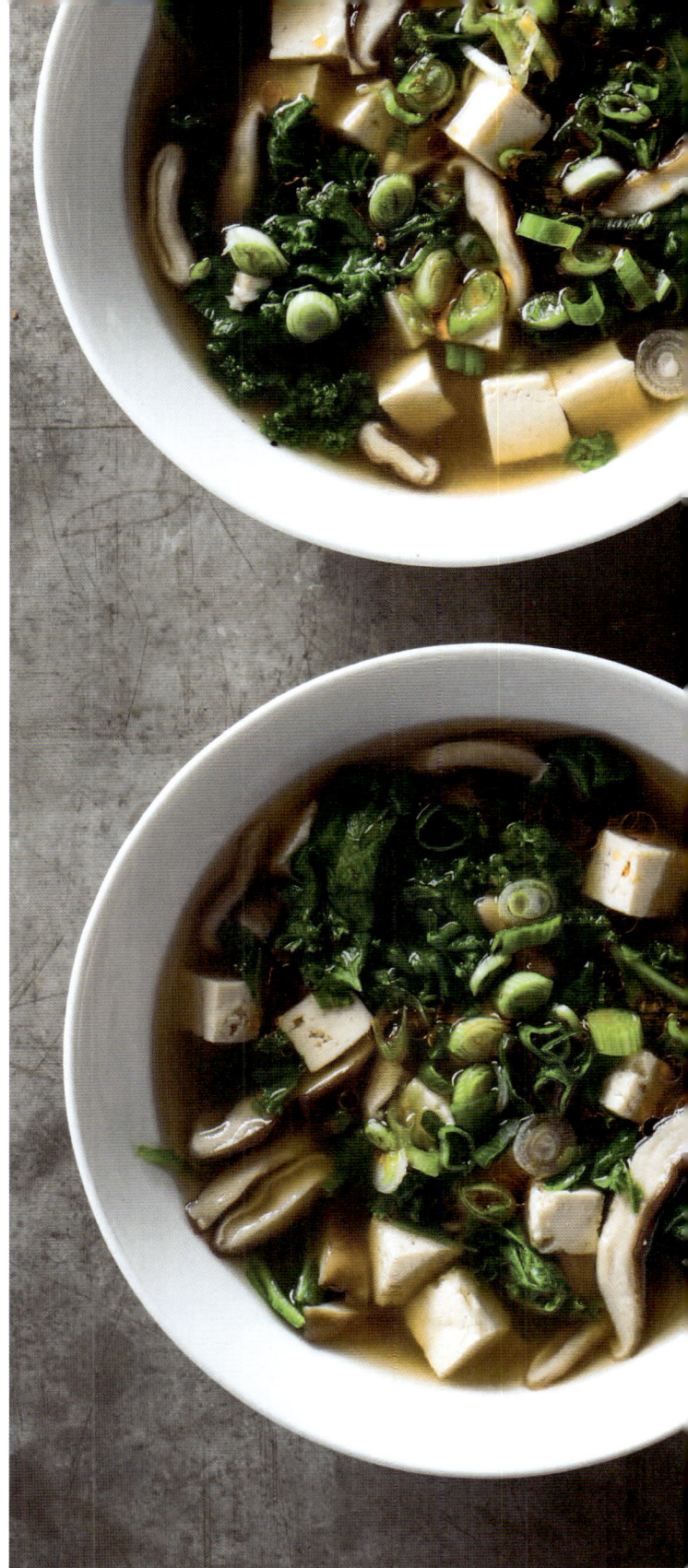

Shiitake, Tofu, and Mustard Greens Soup

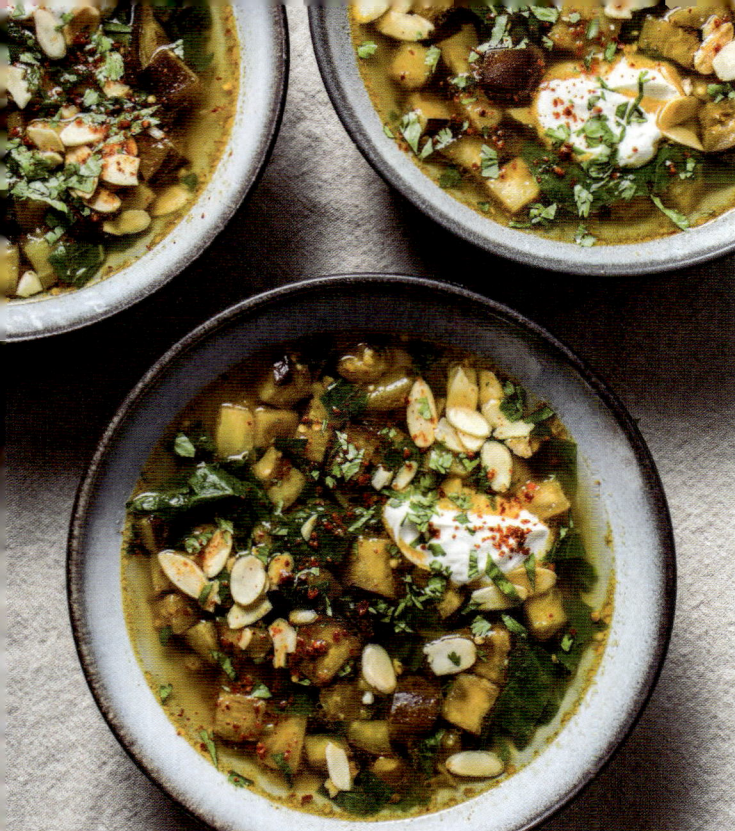

3 Strain broth through fine-mesh strainer set over large bowl, pressing on solids to extract as much liquid as possible; discard solids. Return strained broth to saucepan.

4 Stir in sliced mushrooms, tofu, mustard greens, and vinegar and cook until mushrooms and tofu are warmed through and greens are wilted, about 3 minutes. Sprinkle individual portions with scallions and drizzle with chili oil, if using. Serve.

Spiced Eggplant and Kale Soup

serves 4 • total time: 1¼ hours   **SUPERCHARGED**

why this recipe works • This fairly quick vegetarian soup featuring eggplant, kale, and ample spices is an inflammation-fighting powerhouse. We started by browning chunks of eggplant; next, we bloomed cumin, coriander, ginger, garlic, and Aleppo pepper in a bit of oil and deglazed the pot with broth and water, allowing the anti-inflammatory compounds of all our spices and aromatics to infuse the soup. Off heat, we stirred in fiberful baby kale, as well as the cooked eggplant. Diversely textured toppings took the dish to the next level: Sliced almonds brought a pleasant crunch as well as vitamin E and some monounsaturated fats; cilantro lent the soup freshness plus inflammation-reducing quercetin; and a dollop of yogurt provided rich tang coupled with gut-healthy probiotics. A final sprinkle of Aleppo pepper finished the soup with a striking pop of red.

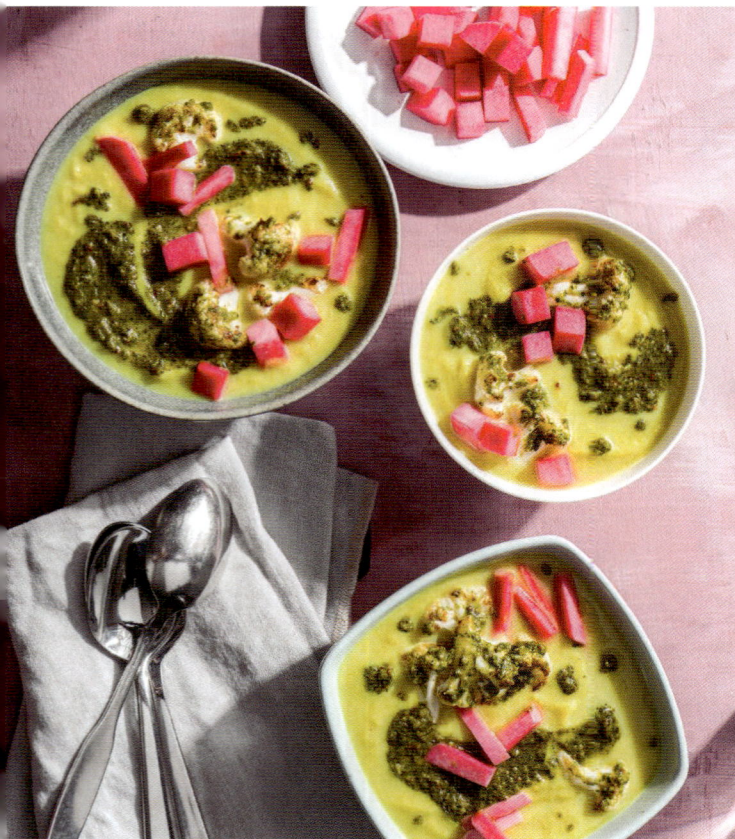

    6 tablespoons avocado oil, divided
 1¼ pounds eggplant, cut into ½-inch pieces
    2 garlic cloves, minced
 1½ teaspoons ground coriander
 1½ teaspoons ground cumin
    1 teaspoon grated fresh ginger
  ¾ teaspoon ground dried Aleppo pepper, divided
  ¼ teaspoon ground cinnamon
    1 teaspoon table salt
  ¼ teaspoon pepper
    3 cups unsalted vegetable or chicken broth
 1½ cups water
    2 ounces (2 cups) baby kale, chopped coarse
  ½ cup plain Greek yogurt
    2 tablespoons sliced almonds, toasted
    2 tablespoons minced fresh cilantro

1 Heat ¼ cup oil in Dutch oven over medium-high heat until just smoking. Add eggplant and cook, stirring occasionally, until tender and deeply browned, 6 to 8 minutes; transfer to bowl.

2   Heat remaining 2 tablespoons oil in now-empty Dutch oven over medium heat until shimmering. Stir in garlic, coriander, cumin, ginger, ½ teaspoon Aleppo pepper, cinnamon, salt, and pepper and cook until fragrant, about 30 seconds. Stir in broth and water, scraping up any browned bits, and bring to simmer. Reduce heat to medium-low, cover partially, and cook until flavors meld, about 15 minutes.

3   Off heat, stir in kale and eggplant, along with any accumulated juices. Let sit until kale is wilted and warmed through, about 2 minutes. Season with salt and pepper to taste. Dollop individual portions with yogurt and sprinkle with almonds, cilantro, and remaining ¼ teaspoon Aleppo pepper before serving.

> **MAKE IT DAIRY-FREE** • Substitute plant-based Greek yogurt for the dairy Greek yogurt.

Creamy Hawaij Cauliflower Soup with Zhoug

serves 4 to 6 • total time: 1½ hours   **SUPERCHARGED**

why this recipe works • A creamy cauliflower soup is a marvelous way to unlock the cruciferous vegetable's range of flavors—from bright and cabbage-like to nutty and even sweet—while nourishing yourself with all its nutrients, including sulforaphane, a phytonutrient known to help with detoxification. To enhance cauliflower's multiple flavor dimensions further, we turned to hawaij, the Yemeni spice blend also common in Israeli cuisine that's popularly used for soup. Thanks to turmeric, cumin, and cardamom, the seasoning mix boasts an impressive range of aromas—earthy, sweet, and distinctly savory—plus compounds that help regulate the body's inflammatory response. We cooked the cauliflower until it turned tender, adding slices of it to simmering water in two stages to infuse our soup with both the grassy flavor of just-cooked cauliflower as well as the nutty flavor of longer-cooked cauliflower. The cauliflower whipped easily into a creamy, velvety soup, no dairy required. We bloomed the hawaij with the aromatics so that the spice blend could deeply infuse the entire dish with its potent flavors. For toppings, we used a microwave and food processor to quickly make a batch of the grassy, spicy sauce known as zhoug, a flavor-packed blend of cilantro, parsley, chiles, and coriander. We also piled on browned cauliflower florets. Serve with Pink Pickled Turnips (page 68). We like to use our homemade Hawaij (page 68), but you can use store-bought if you prefer.

Zhoug
- 6 tablespoons extra-virgin olive oil
- ½ teaspoon ground coriander
- ¼ teaspoon ground cumin
- ¼ teaspoon ground cardamom
- ¼ teaspoon table salt
-   Pinch ground cloves
- ¾ cup fresh cilantro leaves
- ½ cup fresh parsley leaves
- 2 green Thai chiles, stemmed and chopped
- 2 garlic cloves, minced

Soup
- 1 head cauliflower (2 pounds)
- ¼ cup extra-virgin olive oil, divided, plus extra for serving
- 1 leek, white and light green parts only, halved lengthwise, sliced thin, and washed thoroughly
- 1 small onion, halved and sliced thin
- 1½ teaspoons table salt
- 1 tablespoon hawaij
- 4½ cups water
- 1 teaspoon white wine vinegar

1   **For the zhoug** Microwave oil, coriander, cumin, cardamom, salt, and cloves in covered bowl until fragrant, about 30 seconds; let cool completely. Pulse oil-spice mixture, cilantro, parsley, Thai chiles, and garlic in food processor until coarse paste forms, about 15 pulses, scraping down sides of bowl as needed.

2   **For the soup** Pull off outer leaves of cauliflower and trim stem. Using paring knife, cut around core to remove; slice core thin and reserve. Cut heaping 1 cup of ½-inch florets from head of cauliflower; set aside. Cut remaining cauliflower crosswise into ½-inch-thick slices.

3   Heat 3 tablespoons oil in large saucepan over medium-low heat until shimmering. Add leek, onion, and salt and cook, stirring often, until leek and onion are softened but not browned, about 7 minutes. Stir in hawaij and cook until fragrant, about 30 seconds. Stir in water, reserved sliced cauliflower core, and half of sliced cauliflower. Increase heat to medium-high and bring to simmer. Reduce heat to medium-low and simmer gently for 15 minutes. Add remaining sliced cauliflower and simmer until cauliflower is tender and crumbles easily, 15 to 20 minutes.

4 Meanwhile, heat remaining 1 tablespoon oil in 8-inch skillet over medium heat until shimmering. Add reserved florets and cook, stirring often, until golden brown, 6 to 8 minutes. Transfer to bowl, add ¼ cup zhoug, and toss until well coated. Working in batches, process soup in blender until smooth, about 45 seconds. Return pureed soup to clean pot and bring to brief simmer over medium heat. Off heat, stir in vinegar and season with salt to taste. Spoon browned florets and remaining zhoug over individual serving bowls. Serve.

MAKE AHEAD • Zhoug can be refrigerated for up to 4 days.

Nutrition Knowledge Warm, comforting, and packed with nutrients, this creamy cauliflower soup is a true anti-inflammatory delight. The spices—coriander, cumin, and cardamom—are rich in antioxidants, while garlic and Thai chiles amp up the dish's immunity-boosting power. Add in fiber-filled cauliflower, detoxifying herbs, and heart-healthy olive oil, and you've got a dish that's both tasty and nourishing. —*Alicia*

Hawaij

makes about ½ cup • total time: 15 minutes

Cloves are optional, as they're found in only some versions of hawaij, but we love the depth they add.

- 2½ tablespoons black peppercorns
- 2 tablespoons cumin seeds
- 1½ tablespoons coriander seeds
- 10 cardamom pods
- 6 whole cloves
- 1½ tablespoons ground turmeric

Process peppercorns, cumin seeds, coriander seeds, cardamom pods, and cloves in spice grinder until finely ground, about 30 seconds. Transfer to bowl and stir in turmeric. (Hawaij can be stored in airtight container at room temperature for up to 1 month.)

Pink Pickled Turnips

makes about 2 cups • total time: 45 minutes, plus 2 days pickling

- 1 cup white wine vinegar
- 1 cup water
- 1 tablespoon kosher salt
- 3 garlic cloves, smashed and peeled
- ¾ teaspoon whole allspice berries
- ¾ teaspoon black peppercorns
- 8 ounces turnips, peeled and cut into 2 by ½-inch sticks
- 1 small beet, trimmed, peeled, and cut into 1-inch pieces

1 Bring vinegar, water, salt, garlic, allspice, and peppercorns to boil in medium saucepan over medium-high heat. Cover, remove from heat, and let steep for 10 minutes. Strain brine through fine-mesh strainer, then return to saucepan.

2 Place 1-pint jar in bowl and place under hot running water until heated through, 1 to 2 minutes; shake dry. Pack turnips vertically into hot jar with beet pieces evenly distributed throughout.

3 Return brine to brief boil. Using funnel and ladle, pour hot brine over vegetables to cover. Let jar cool to room temperature, cover with lid, and refrigerate for at least 2 days before serving. (Pickled turnips can be refrigerated for up to 1 month; turnips will soften over time.)

Garlicky Wild Rice Soup with Artichokes

serves 4 • total time: 1½ hours

why this recipe works • Wild rice shines in soups, where the substantial, chewy grains bring hearty texture and filling fiber without making the dish stodgy. For this wild rice soup, we took inspiration from springtime flavors that flourish in the South of France. To get our soup off to a flavorful start, we cooked leeks, garlic, anchovies, and thyme to release their fragrance; leeks are rich in polyphenols that guard against cellular damage, while anchovies are a savory powerhouse of omega-3 fatty acids. We then deglazed the pot with a splash of wine, creating a pleasantly potent backbone for the soup. After adding broth, we simmered the rice in the liquid until the grains were almost done and then stirred in sautéed artichokes as well as asparagus, two more ingredients loaded with health benefits. Staggering the ingredients' entry into the pot ensured that everything finished cooking at the same time. Stirring in a combination of fresh tarragon, lemon zest and juice, and additional garlic off the heat rounded out the flavors of this savory, nourishing soup.

- 3 tablespoons extra-virgin olive oil, divided
- 3 cups jarred whole baby artichoke hearts packed in water, quartered, rinsed, and patted dry
- 1 leek, white and light green parts only, halved lengthwise, sliced ¼ inch thick, and washed thoroughly
- ¼ teaspoon table salt
- 8 garlic cloves, minced, divided
- 4 anchovy fillets, rinsed, patted dry, and minced
- 1 teaspoon minced fresh thyme or ¼ teaspoon dried
- ¼ cup dry white wine
- 6 cups unsalted vegetable or chicken broth
- 1 cup wild rice, rinsed
- 2 bay leaves
- 1 pound asparagus, trimmed and cut into 1-inch pieces
- 2 tablespoons minced fresh tarragon
- 1 teaspoon grated lemon zest plus 1 tablespoon juice

1 Heat 2 tablespoons oil in Dutch oven over medium heat until shimmering. Add artichokes and cook until browned, 8 to 10 minutes. Transfer to bowl and set aside.

2 Heat remaining 1 tablespoon oil in now-empty pot over medium heat until shimmering. Stir in leek and salt and cook until leek is softened and beginning to brown, 5 to 7 minutes. Stir in half of garlic, anchovies, and thyme and cook until fragrant, about 30 seconds. Stir in wine, scraping up any browned bits, and cook until nearly evaporated, about 1 minute.

3 Stir in broth, rice, and bay leaves and bring to simmer. Cover, reduce heat to medium-low, and simmer gently for 35 minutes. Stir in reserved artichokes and asparagus and cook, covered, until rice and vegetables are tender, about 10 minutes.

4 Remove pot from heat and discard bay leaves. Stir tarragon, lemon zest and juice, and remaining garlic into soup and season with salt and pepper to taste. Serve.

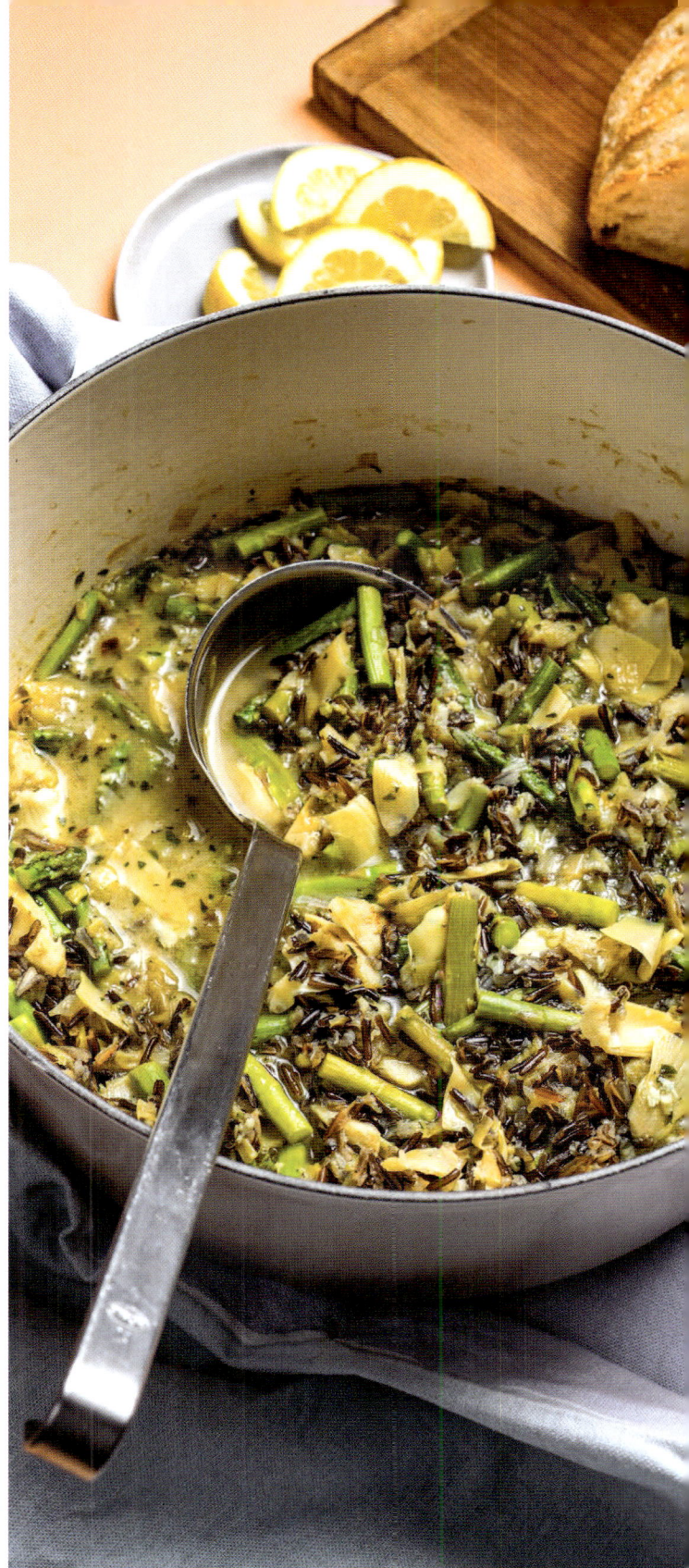

Garlicky Wild Rice Soup with Artichokes

Beet and Wheat Berry Soup with Dill Cream

serves 6 • **total time: 1¾ hours**

why this recipe works • We wanted to develop a light, fresh-tasting take on borscht that especially highlighted the flavor of the beets. Beets are an anti-inflammatory superstar, full of polyphenols, flavonoids, vitamin C, and fiber. To build a flavorful backbone for the soup, we sautéed onion, garlic, thyme, and tomato paste before stirring in the broth. Along with the beets, we also added red cabbage to the pot, further upping the gut-balancing fiber in the dish while also introducing anthocyanins, antioxidants that give the vegetable its purplish hue. Red wine vinegar and a pinch of cayenne brought a mild tartness and a bit of heat, respectively, to the dish. For even more polyphenols and fiber, we swapped out potatoes and used wheat berries, a chewy whole grain; toasting them gave the grains a rich, nutty flavor and a pleasant bite. A finishing dollop of dill-flecked sour cream brought tang and creaminess to the final dish. You can use the large holes of a box grater or a food processor fitted with a shredding disk to shred the beets and carrot. Do not use presteamed or quick-cooking wheat berries here, as they have a much shorter cooking time; read the package carefully to determine what kind of wheat berries you are using.

Dill Cream

- ½ cup sour cream
- ¼ cup minced fresh dill
- ½ teaspoon table salt

Soup

- ⅔ cup wheat berries, rinsed
- 3 tablespoons extra-virgin olive oil
- 2 onions, chopped fine
- 2 tablespoons no-salt-added tomato paste
- 4 garlic cloves, minced
- 1 teaspoon minced fresh thyme or ¼ teaspoon dried
- ¼ teaspoon cayenne pepper
- 8 cups unsalted vegetable or chicken broth
- 3 cups water
- 1½ cups thinly sliced red cabbage
- 1 pound beets, trimmed, peeled, and shredded
- 1 small carrot, peeled and shredded
- 1 bay leaf
- ¾ teaspoon pepper
- 1 tablespoon red wine vinegar
- 1 teaspoon table salt

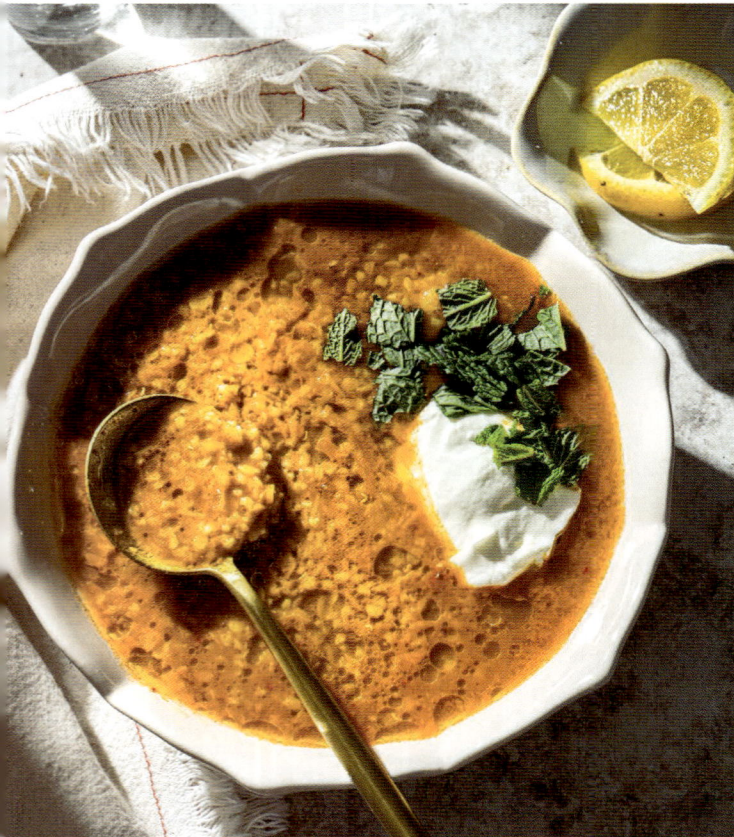

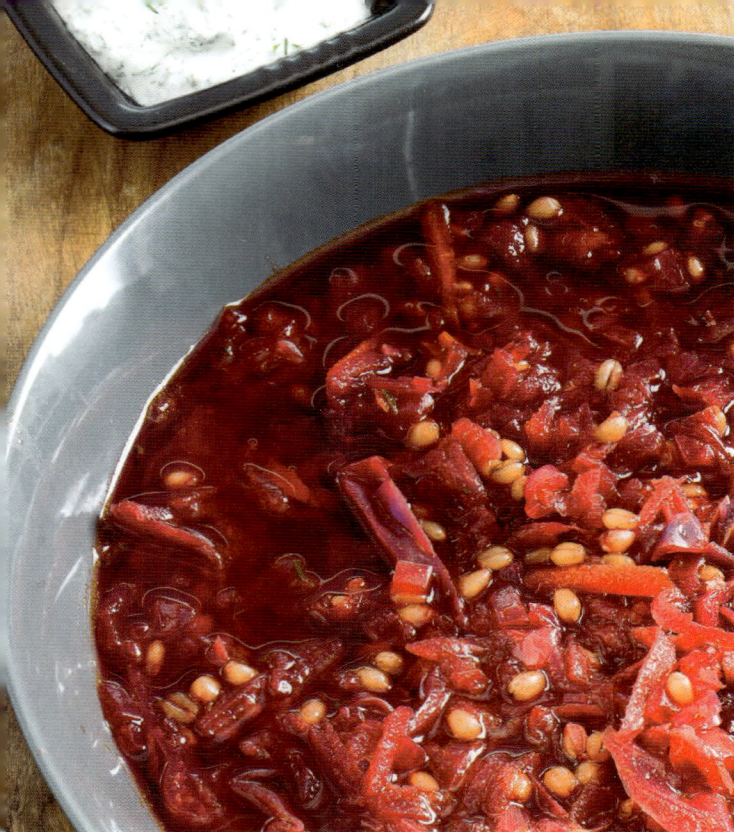

top	*Beet and Wheat Berry Soup with Dill Cream*
bottom	*Turkish Bulgur and Lentil Soup*

1   **For the dill cream** Combine all ingredients in bowl; refrigerate until ready to serve.

2   **For the soup** Toast wheat berries in Dutch oven over medium heat, stirring often, until fragrant and beginning to darken, about 5 minutes; transfer to bowl.

3   Heat oil in now-empty pot over medium heat until shimmering. Add onions and cook until softened, about 5 minutes. Stir in tomato paste, garlic, thyme, and cayenne and cook until fragrant and darkened slightly, about 2 minutes.

4   Stir in broth, water, cabbage, beets, carrot, bay leaf, pepper, and wheat berries, scraping up any browned bits, and bring to boil. Reduce heat to low and simmer until wheat berries are tender but still chewy and vegetables are tender, 45 minutes to 1¼ hours.

5   Off heat, discard bay leaf and stir in vinegar and salt. Season with additional salt and pepper to taste. Serve, passing dill cream separately.

> **MAKE IT GLUTEN-FREE** • Substitute an equal amount of oat berries for the wheat berries.

> **MAKE IT DAIRY-FREE** • Substitute plant-based sour cream for the dairy sour cream.

Turkish Bulgur and Lentil Soup

serves 4 • total time: 45 minutes   **FAST**

why this recipe works • The lore surrounding ezogelin çorbasi, a beloved Anatolian bridal soup, is that a woman created this recipe to win over her mother-in-law. Over time, the dish became associated with brides and evolved into a cultural symbol of sustenance and good fortune. But you definitely don't need to be planning a wedding to win anyone over with this one-pot dish. Heady with antioxidant-packed spices and brimming with fiber-rich lentils and bulgur, it makes a nourishing, convenient dinner for any average night. To build a flavorful base for the dish, we cooked onion and tomato paste and enhanced them with the subtle sweetness of paprika and the heat of Aleppo pepper, both of which contain immunity-boosting vitamin C. We then stirred in the lentils and bulgur so that they could toast in the saucepan, a step that drew out their nutty, earthy aroma. Vegetable or chicken broth gave the dish savory underpinnings. A shower of fresh mint and a dollop of yogurt offered a cooling contrast to the soup, while lemon wedges brought a burst of brightness.

2   tablespoons extra-virgin olive oil, plus extra for drizzling
1   small onion, chopped fine
1   teaspoon table salt
4   teaspoons paprika
1   tablespoon no-salt-added tomato paste
1   teaspoon ground dried Aleppo pepper
1   cup dried red lentils, picked over and rinsed
½   cup medium-grind bulgur, rinsed
5   cups unsalted vegetable or chicken broth
2½ cups water
¼   cup torn fresh mint
    Greek yogurt
    Lemon wedges

1   Heat oil in large saucepan over medium-high heat until shimmering. Add onion and salt and cook until softened and beginning to brown, 5 to 7 minutes. Stir in paprika, tomato paste, and Aleppo pepper and cook until fragrant, about 30 seconds.

2   Stir in lentils and bulgur and toast, stirring constantly, for 1 minute. Add broth and water and bring to boil. Reduce heat to medium-low and cook, partially covered, until lentils are broken down and bulgur is tender, 20 to 25 minutes.

3   Sprinkle individual portions with mint and drizzle with extra oil. Serve with yogurt and lemon wedges.

> **MAKE IT DAIRY-FREE** • Substitute plant-based Greek yogurt for the dairy Greek yogurt.

Lentil and Escarole Soup

serves 4 to 6 • total time: 1¾ hours

why this recipe works • This warming, main-course-worthy dish is inspired by the aromatic soups of Umbria, in which sturdy, fiber-rich lentils often play a starring role. We started by browning a medley of aromatic vegetables before stirring in broth, which gave us a savory liquid in which to cook the lentils. We opted for Umbrian lentils or lentilles du Puy, also called French green lentils, as these varieties hold their shape well during cooking; they retained their bite, while the soup stayed brothy (rather than thick and creamy). Supporting ingredients in lentil soup vary throughout Umbria, but we particularly liked escarole, a fiberful choice rich in flavonoids; adding the leafy green toward the end of cooking helped the vegetable hold on to its chewy bite and nutty taste. We also included canned diced tomatoes—a classic addition—and a couple bay leaves for warmth. A rind of Parmesan, if you have one, adds a complex note to the soup as it simmers.

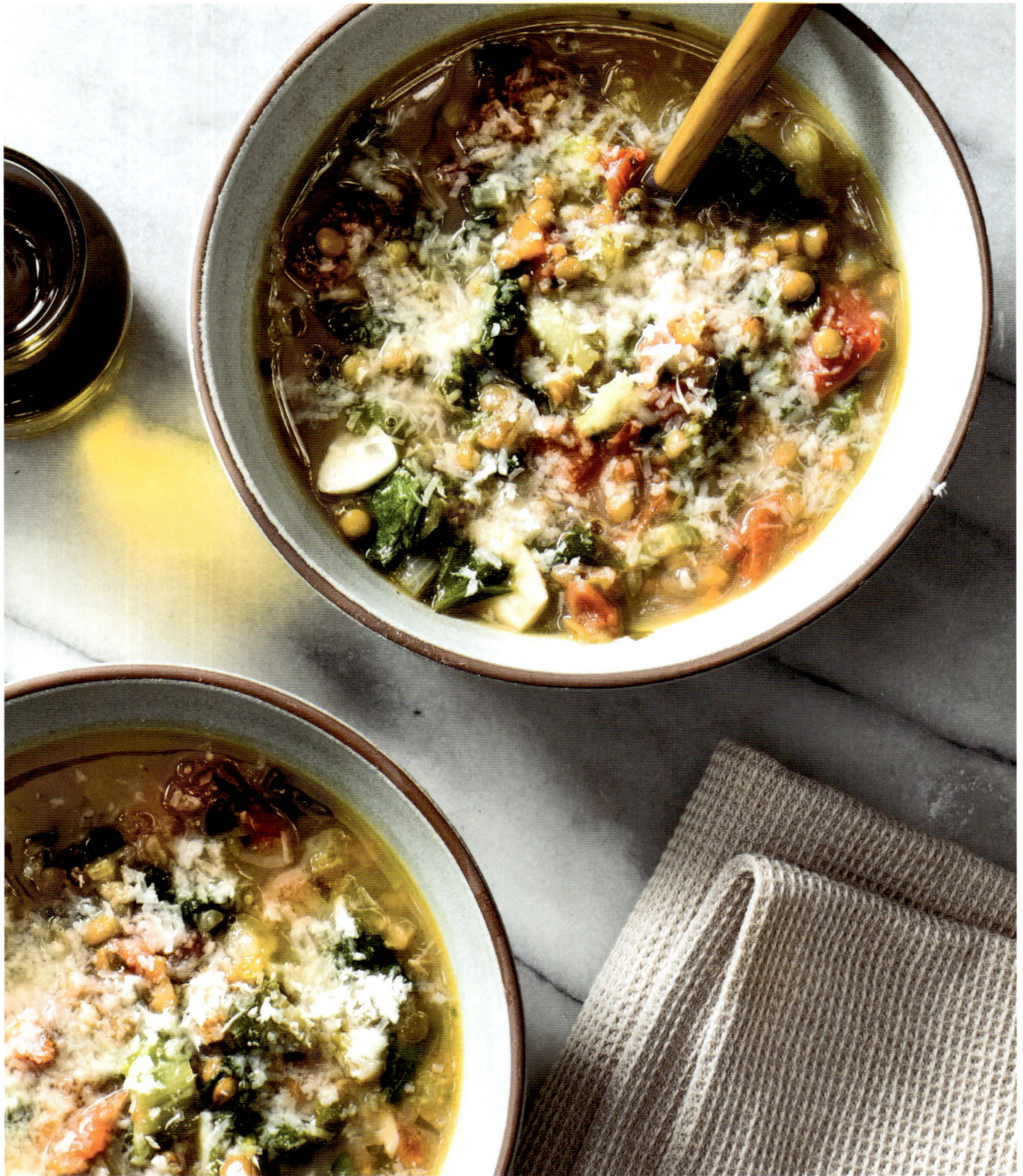

Lentil and Escarole Soup

- ¼ cup extra-virgin olive oil, plus extra for drizzling
- 1 onion, chopped fine
- 1 carrot, peeled and chopped fine
- 1 celery rib, chopped fine
- 1¼ teaspoons table salt
- 6 garlic cloves, sliced thin
- 2 tablespoons minced fresh parsley
- 4 cups unsalted vegetable or chicken broth, plus extra as needed
- 3 cups water
- 8 ounces (1¼ cups) Umbrian lentils or lentilles du Puy, picked over and rinsed
- 1 (14.5-ounce) can no-salt-added diced tomatoes
- 1 Parmesan cheese rind (optional), plus grated Parmesan for serving
- 2 bay leaves
- ½ head escarole (8 ounces), trimmed and cut into ½-inch pieces

1 Heat oil in Dutch oven over medium heat until shimmering. Add onion, carrot, celery, and salt and cook until softened and lightly browned, 8 to 10 minutes. Stir in garlic and parsley and cook until fragrant, about 30 seconds. Stir in broth; water; lentils; tomatoes and their juice; Parmesan rind, if using; and bay leaves and bring to simmer. Reduce heat to medium-low, partially cover, and simmer until lentils are tender, 1 to 1¼ hours.

2 Discard Parmesan rind, if using, and bay leaves. Stir in escarole, 1 handful at a time, and cook until wilted, about 5 minutes. Adjust consistency with extra hot broth as needed. Season with salt and pepper to taste. Drizzle individual portions with extra oil and serve, passing grated Parmesan separately.

MAKE IT DAIRY-FREE • Substitute plant-based Parmesan cheese for the dairy Parmesan cheese or omit.

Creamy White Bean Soup with Pickled Celery

serves 4 to 6 • total time: 1 hour

why this recipe works • Nutrition can come from a can, as it does in this super-creamy white bean soup with a special celery topping. To keep the promise of a smooth, velvety soup—and whipping it up quickly—we started by briefly simmering canned great Northern beans and their canning liquid with softened aromatic vegetables and herbs. Not only are great Northern beans an excellent source of plant-based protein, fiber, and magnesium,

but heating them also causes their starches to hydrate, making our soup especially creamy. Blending the beans with some liquid helped their skins break down, which also gave us an ultra-smooth puree. Broth, plus a little Parmesan cheese, boosted the soup's flavor and richness. A finishing drizzle of olive oil offered a dose of polyphenols while complementing the neutral soup base's flavor; a scattering of quick pickled celery brought welcome crunch and a tangy dimension. Use a conventional blender here; an immersion blender will not produce as smooth a soup.

Pickled Celery
- ½ cup unseasoned rice vinegar
- 1 tablespoon sugar
- ½ teaspoon table salt
- 1 celery rib, chopped fine

Soup
- ¼ cup extra-virgin olive oil, divided, plus extra for drizzling
- ½ cup chopped onion
- 1 small celery rib, chopped fine
- 1 teaspoon table salt
- 3 sprigs fresh thyme
- 2 garlic cloves, sliced thin
  Pinch cayenne pepper
- 2 (15-ounce) cans no-salt-added great Northern beans, undrained
- 2 tablespoons grated Parmesan cheese
- 2 cups unsalted vegetable or chicken broth, divided
- ½ teaspoon lemon juice, plus extra for seasoning

1 For the pickled celery Combine vinegar, sugar, and salt in medium bowl and microwave until simmering, 1 to 2 minutes. Stir in celery and let sit for 15 minutes. Drain celery, discarding liquid, and set aside until ready to serve.

2 For the soup Heat 2 tablespoons oil in large saucepan over medium heat until shimmering. Add onion, celery, and salt, and cook, stirring frequently, until softened but not browned, 6 to 8 minutes. Add thyme sprigs, garlic, and cayenne and cook, stirring constantly, until fragrant, about 1 minute. Add beans and their liquid and stir to combine. Reduce heat to medium-low, cover, and cook, stirring occasionally, until beans are heated through and just starting to break down, 6 to 8 minutes. Remove saucepan from heat and discard thyme sprigs.

3 Process bean mixture and Parmesan in blender on low speed until thick, smooth puree forms, about 2 minutes. With blender running, add 1 cup broth and remaining 2 tablespoons oil. Increase speed to high and continue to process until oil is incorporated and mixture is pourable, about 1 minute longer.

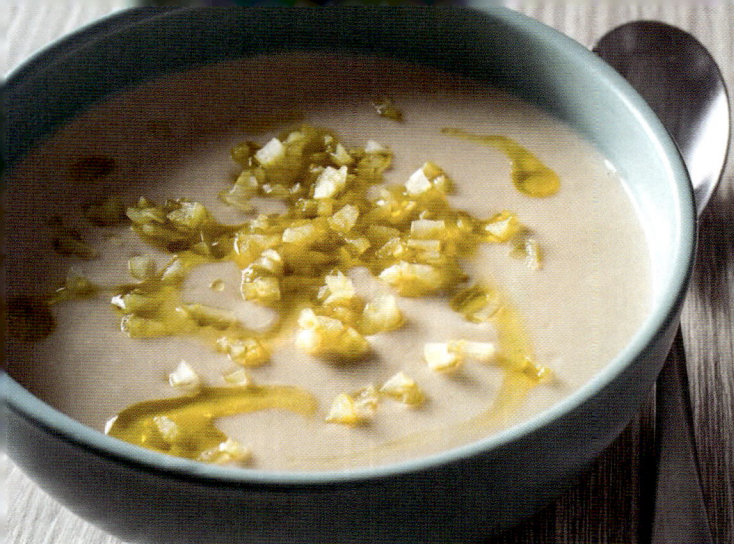

4 Return soup to clean saucepan and whisk in remaining 1 cup broth. Cover and bring to simmer over medium heat, adjusting consistency with up to 1 cup hot water as needed. Off heat, stir in lemon juice. Season with salt and extra lemon juice to taste. Drizzle each portion of soup with extra oil and sprinkle with reserved quick pickled celery.

> **MAKE IT DAIRY-FREE** • Substitute plant-based Parmesan cheese for the dairy Parmesan cheese.

Aash Reshteh

serves 6 to 8 • total time: 2¼ hours

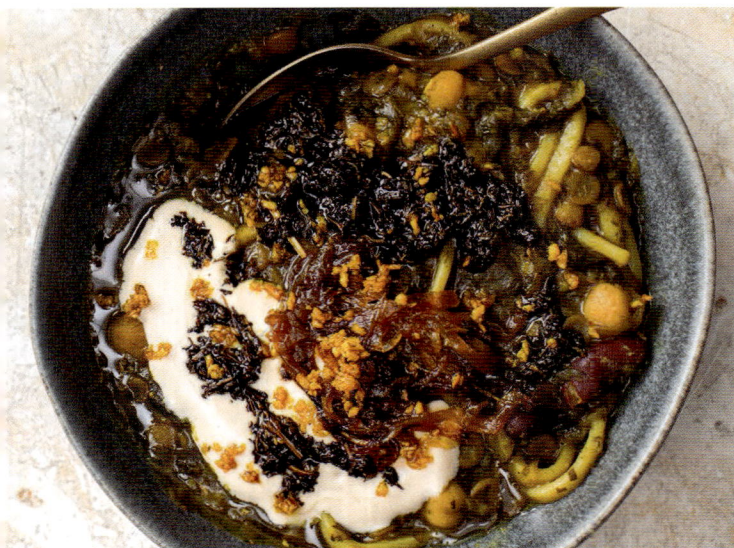

why this recipe works • Aash reshteh is a comforting and hearty Persian soup made from beans, lentils, greens, herbs, onions and noodles. The dish relies on two key ingredients unique to Persian cuisine: reshteh, the wheat noodles for which the soup is named, and kashk, a salty, tangy, fermented Iranian dairy product made from drained yogurt or whey. Another essential ingredient is time. To develop the soup's silky texture, it needs to bubble gently for some time, making this an ideal recipe for a slow, cozy afternoon. Slow-simmered lentils, chickpeas, and kidney beans gave the soup body and packed in fiber. Heaps of spinach, parsley, cilantro, and scallions contributed a hefty dose of beneficial antioxidants. Black pepper and turmeric—a powerful inflammation-fighting duo—are mellow seasonings that enhanced the flavors of the herbs. Garnishes of caramelized onions, fried garlic, mint oil, and kashk offered a final flourish that further elevated this soup. Look for reshteh and kashk in a Persian grocery, or online. We prefer jarred, refrigerated kashk rather than dehydrated because it is easier to work with. If you can't find reshteh, you can substitute linguine, which has a similar shape and mouthfeel. If you can't find kashk, you can substitute plain yogurt or sour cream, though the flavor will not be as deep or full-bodied. To prevent any bits from scorching, be sure to wipe the nonstick skillet clean in between caramelizing the onions, browning the garlic, and cooking the mint.

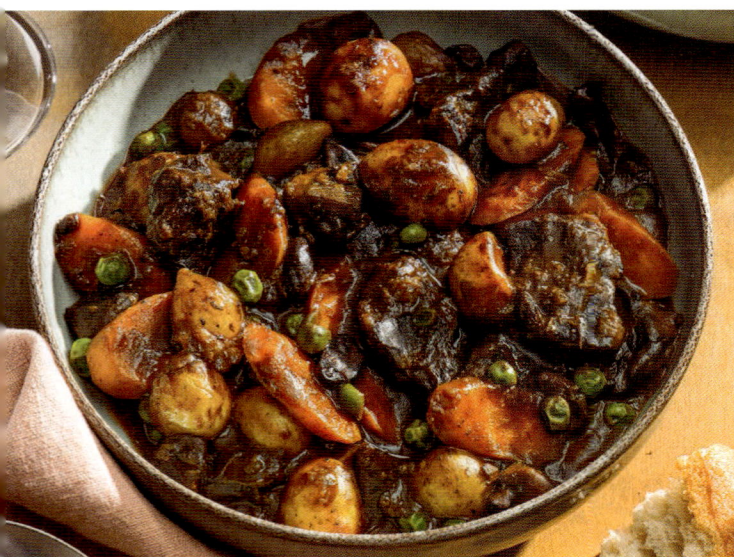

½ cup plus 2 tablespoons extra-virgin olive oil, divided
2 large onions, halved and sliced thin through root end
2¼ teaspoons table salt, divided
1 tablespoon ground turmeric, divided
8 cups unsalted vegetable or chicken broth
1 cup dried green lentils, picked over and rinsed
1 (15-ounce) can no-salt-added chickpeas, rinsed
1 (15-ounce) can no-salt-added red kidney beans, rinsed
3 tablespoons minced garlic (9 cloves)
3 tablespoons dried mint

top	*Creamy White Bean Soup with Pickled Celery*
middle	*Aash Reshteh*
bottom	*Almost Beefless Beef Stew*

12 ounces frozen chopped spinach, thawed and squeezed dry

1½ cups thinly sliced scallions (10–12 scallions)

1 cup chopped fresh parsley leaves and tender stems

1 cup chopped fresh cilantro leaves and tender stems

1 teaspoon pepper

3 ounces reshteh, broken in half

½ cup kashk

1 Heat ¼ cup oil in 12-inch nonstick skillet over medium heat until shimmering. Add onions and ¼ teaspoon salt and cook, stirring frequently, until onions are translucent, about 2 minutes. Add ¾ teaspoon turmeric and continue to cook, stirring frequently, until onions are deep golden brown and caramelized, about 25 minutes, adjusting heat as needed. Transfer to bowl and set aside. Wipe out skillet with paper towels and set skillet aside.

2 Combine broth, 2 cups water, lentils, and remaining 2 teaspoons salt in Dutch oven and bring to boil over high heat. Reduce heat to medium-low, cover, and simmer for 15 minutes, stirring occasionally and adjusting heat as needed to maintain simmer. Stir in chickpeas and kidney beans and simmer, covered, until lentils are tender, about 15 minutes, adjusting heat as needed.

3 Meanwhile, in now-empty skillet, heat 2 tablespoons oil over medium heat until shimmering. Add garlic and ¼ teaspoon turmeric and cook, stirring frequently, until garlic is just beginning to turn golden brown, about 2 minutes. Transfer garlic and oil to second bowl and set aside. Wipe out skillet with paper towels. Add remaining ¼ cup oil to again-empty skillet and heat over medium heat until shimmering. Add mint and cook, stirring frequently, until fragrant and just beginning to brown, about 1 minute. Transfer to third bowl and set aside.

4 Stir spinach, scallions, parsley, cilantro, remaining 2 teaspoons turmeric, pepper, half of reserved caramelized onions, and half of reserved browned garlic into pot with bean mixture. Cover pot and bring to boil over high heat. Reduce heat to medium-low and simmer, stirring occasionally, until greens, lentils, and beans are uniformly tender and stew has thickened, about 30 minutes.

5 Stir reshteh into pot and simmer, uncovered, until pasta is tender, about 15 minutes, stirring occasionally. Remove pot from heat and let sit until stew is thickened slightly, about 15 minutes. Season with salt to taste. Add water to kashk in bowl, 1 teaspoon at a time, until it is consistency of heavy cream. Serve soup, topping individual portions with remaining reserved caramelized onions, remaining reserved browned garlic, mint oil, and thinned kashk.

Almost Beefless Beef Stew

serves 4 to 6 · total time: 2 hours

why this recipe works · The hallmark of an excellent beef stew is exceedingly tender meat swimming in a deeply savory broth. We thought this could be achieved only by using a large cut of meat—until we tried blade steaks, which consistently turned tender and offered intense savoriness even in small amounts. We bulked up our stew with a generous amount of potatoes, carrots, peas, and pearl onions, which also made this dish much more fiberful than most beef stews. To add even more savoriness, we turned to ingredients adept at boosting flavor (while packing in more antioxidants): garlic, anchovies, and tomato paste, which combined to create a flavor-rich base for our stew. We also added a pound of cremini mushrooms, taking care to drive away moisture to concentrate their flavor. The mushrooms brought welcome umami while simultaneously affording us beneficial compounds such as selenium. Our final recipe features over 4 pounds of veggies and under a pound of beef, yet every bite brims with beefy flavor. Use extra-small Yukon Gold or red potatoes measuring less than 1 inch in diameter. You can substitute Yukon Gold or red potatoes that are 1 to 2 inches in diameter; just be sure to halve them before adding them to the stew in step 4.

2 (6- to 8-ounce) blade steaks, ¾ to 1 inch thick, trimmed and cut into 1½-inch pieces
3 tablespoons avocado oil, divided
1 pound cremini mushrooms, trimmed and halved if small or quartered if medium or large
¾ teaspoon table salt, divided
1 large onion, halved and sliced thin
6 garlic cloves, minced
2 tablespoons no-salt-added tomato paste
6 anchovy fillets, minced
¼ cup all-purpose flour
1 cup plus 2 tablespoons red wine, divided
2½ cups unsalted chicken or beef broth
1 pound extra-small potatoes, unpeeled
4 carrots, peeled and sliced ¼ inch thick on bias
1½ cups frozen pearl onions, thawed
1 cup frozen peas, thawed
¼ teaspoon pepper

1   Adjust oven rack to lower-middle position and heat oven to 325 degrees. Pat beef dry with paper towels. Heat 1 tablespoon oil in Dutch oven over medium-high heat until just smoking. Add beef and cook until well browned on all sides, 5 to 8 minutes; transfer to bowl.

2   Add mushrooms, 1 tablespoon oil, and ¼ teaspoon salt to fat left in pot and cook, covered, over medium-high heat until mushrooms have released their liquid, 3 to 5 minutes. Uncover and cook until mushrooms are well browned, 7 to 10 minutes, stirring occasionally. Transfer mushrooms to bowl with beef.

3   Add onion, remaining 1 tablespoon oil, and remaining ½ teaspoon salt to now-empty pot and cook until golden brown, 7 to 10 minutes. Add garlic, tomato paste, and anchovies and cook, stirring constantly, until tomato paste is slightly darkened, about 2 minutes. Stir in flour and cook until no dry flour remains, about 30 seconds.

4   Slowly add 1 cup wine, scraping up any browned bits. Stir in broth, potatoes, and beef-mushroom mixture and any accumulated juices. Bring to simmer, cover, and transfer to oven. Cook for 1 hour.

5   Remove pot from oven. Stir in carrots and pearl onions and bring to simmer over medium heat. Cook, stirring occasionally and scraping bottom of pot, until carrots are tender, 8 to 12 minutes.

6   Stir in peas and cook until heated through, about 2 minutes. Stir in pepper and remaining 2 tablespoons wine and season with salt and pepper to taste. Serve.

Squash, Pork, and Tamarind Curry

serves 4 · total time: 40 minutes   FAST

why this recipe works · For this simple yet highly flavorful dish, we took a cue from the curries of Myanmar (also known as Burma), which often rely on a generous amount of shallots, garlic, and ginger; a few choice spices, most commonly turmeric and chile powder; and sometimes fresh herbs, to produce an abundance of flavor in minimal time. Inspired by a tamarind and squash curry recipe in Naomi Duguid's cookbook, *Burma: Rivers of Flavor*, we made those two healthful ingredients the stars of this dish. To build a savory backbone for our curry, we browned just 8 ounces of ground pork on the stovetop to render it and made use of the flavorful fat by cooking our aromatics and spices in it. After pouring in water and scraping up the browned bits of savory goodness, we added butternut squash, which soaked up all the flavors in the pot while delivering plenty of inflammation-fighting beta-carotene, carotenoids, and potassium. Tamarind juice concentrate, a rich source of polyphenols and flavonoids, imbued the dish with a tangy, sweet, and fruity dimension that complemented the umami notes. For additional fiber and textural interest, we incorporated gai lan, also known as Chinese broccoli, a vegetable popular in Myanmar. Gai lan delivers two textures at once—tender, quick-cooking leaves and snappy, crunchy stalks—both of which contrasted deliciously with the soft, dense squash. A sprinkle of Thai basil leaves finished the curry with a dose of licorice-scented pepperiness. Look for Thai/Indonesian-style tamarind concentrate labeled "nuoc me chua"; do not use Indian-style tamarind concentrates. You can substitute kabocha squash for butternut or acorn, but you will need to extend the cooking time in step 3 to about 20 minutes. If you can't find gai lan, you can substitute broccolini, using the florets in place of the gai lan leaves. Serve with rice.

8 ounces gai lan, stalks trimmed
8 ounces ground pork
4–6 large shallots, chopped (1½ cups)
5 garlic cloves, minced
4 teaspoons grated fresh ginger
2 teaspoons paprika
1 teaspoon ground turmeric
¼ teaspoon cayenne pepper
2 cinnamon sticks
2¾ cups water
1 pound butternut or acorn squash, peeled and cut into 1-inch pieces
¼ cup tamarind juice concentrate
2 tablespoons fish sauce
½ cup fresh Thai basil leaves, torn if large

1 Remove leaves, small stems, and florets from gai lan stalks; slice leaves crosswise into 1½-inch strips (any florets and stems can go into pile with leaves); and cut stalks into ½-inch-thick pieces. Set aside.

2 Cook pork in Dutch oven over medium heat, breaking up large pieces, until golden-brown fond begins to form on bottom of pot, 5 to 8 minutes. Add shallots and cook until very soft, about 3 minutes.

3 Stir in garlic, ginger, paprika, turmeric, cayenne, and cinnamon sticks and cook until fragrant, about 30 seconds. Stir in water, scraping up any browned bits, then add squash, tamarind juice concentrate, fish sauce, and gai lan stalks. Bring to simmer, then reduce heat to medium-low; cover; and simmer until squash is tender, about 10 minutes.

4 Stir in gai lan leaves, and cook, uncovered, until leaves wilt but are still bright green, 1 to 2 minutes. Discard cinnamon sticks, sprinkle with basil, and serve.

PREPPING GAI LAN

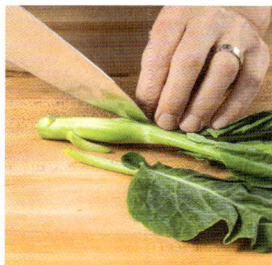

1 Cut leaves off stalks.

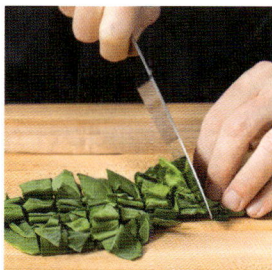

2 Slice leaves crosswise into 1½-inch strips.

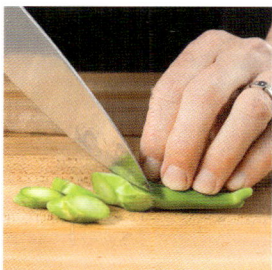

3 Cut stalks on bias into ½-inch-thick pieces.

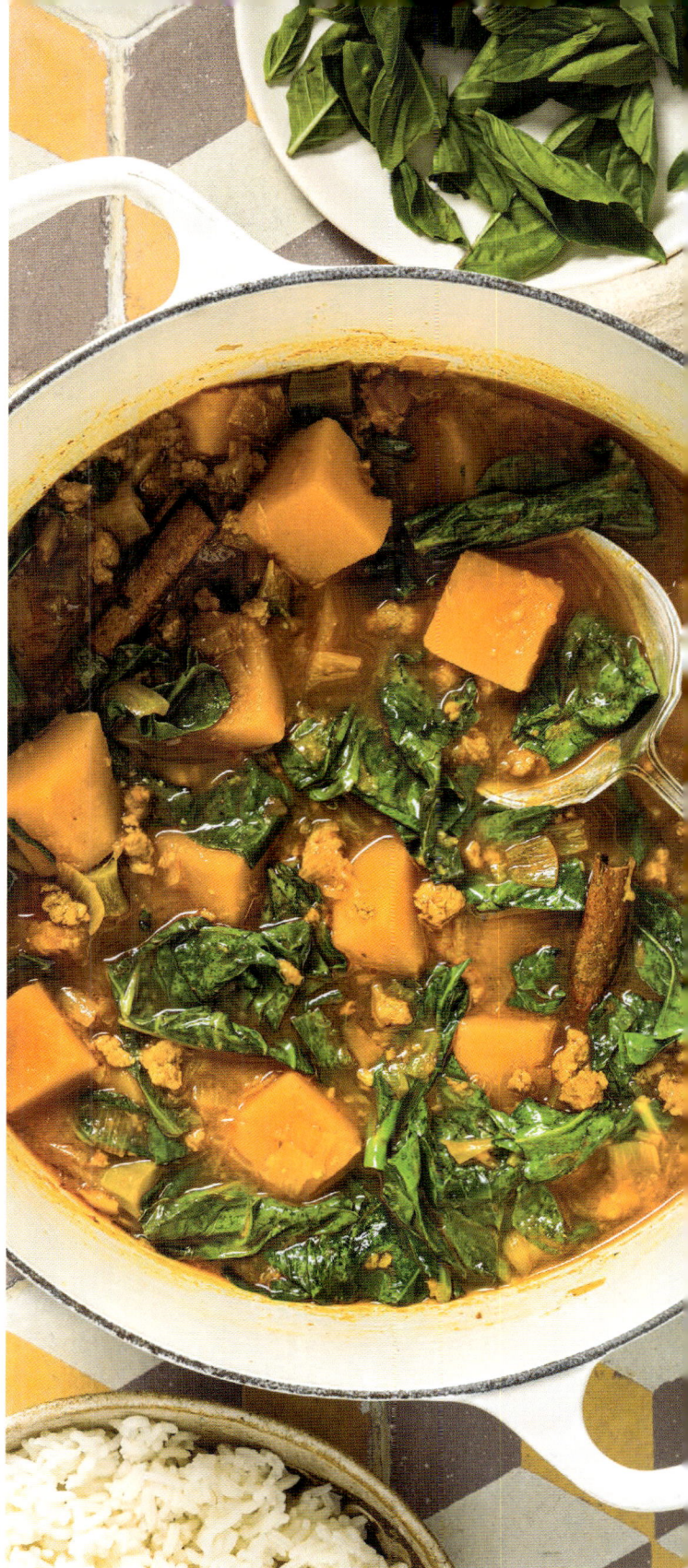

Squash, Pork, and Tamarind Curry

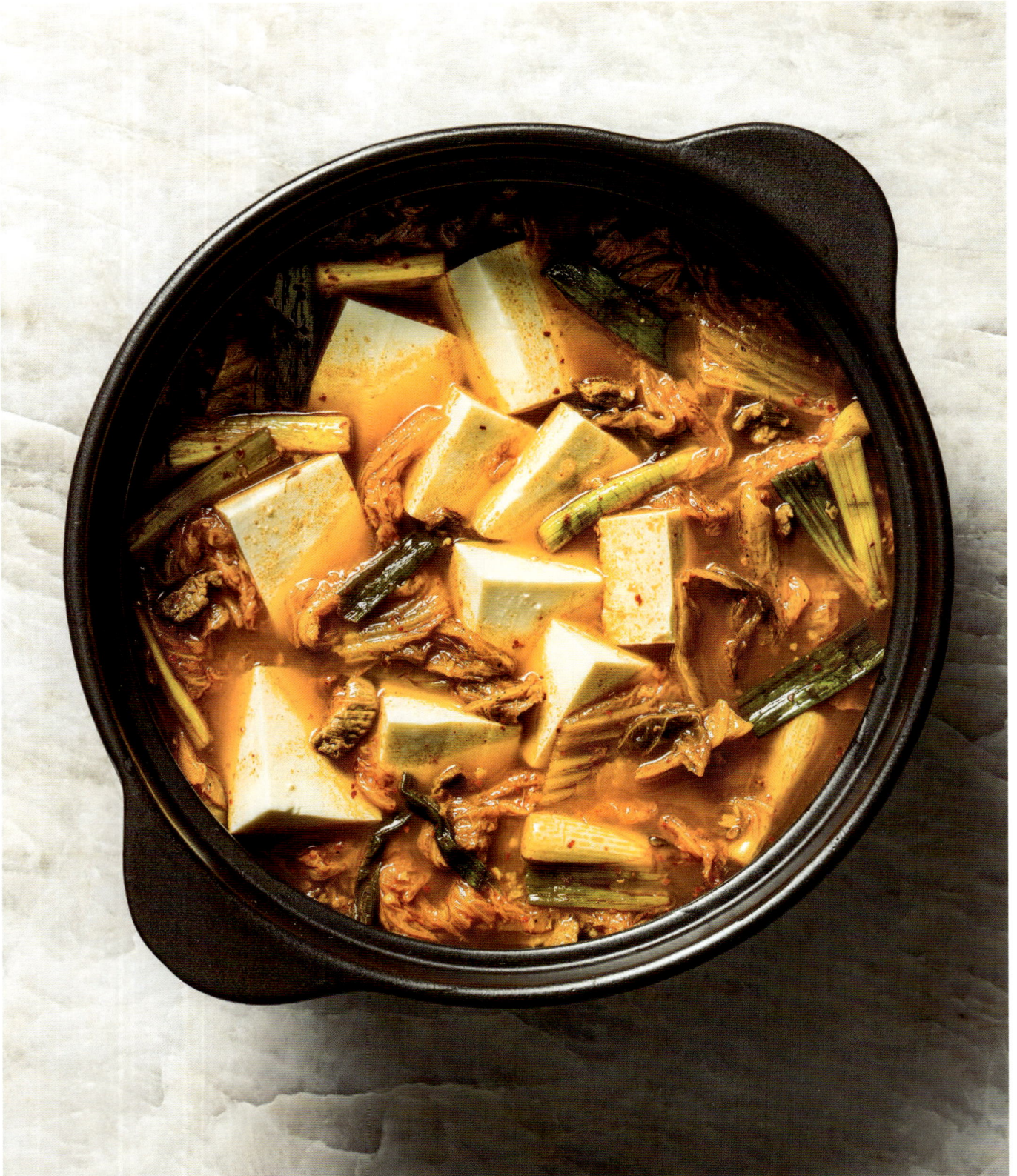

Kimchi Jjigae

Kimchi Jjigae

serves 4 · total time: 1¼ hours

why this recipe works · Korean cuisine is well celebrated for its supremely comforting stews, and kimchi jjigae may be the most famous one of all. Kimchi, the Korean dish of fermented vegetables, is packed with gut-balancing probiotics, plus antioxidants that help reduce oxidative stress. Though cooking fermented vegetables can reduce their live bacteria, some probiotics will remain, supporting a healthy gut microbiome. For the broth base, most Korean cooks use well-aged cabbage kimchi, first cooking it in oil to intensify its briny-tart fermented flavor. For the pork, we used a judicious amount of pork shoulder, a cut that is deeply flavorful and allowed us to use less while maintaining the savory essence of the dish. A dash of capsaicin-rich gochugaru, Korean chili flakes, offered mild heat and a hint of smokiness. You can substitute 8 ounces boneless pork butt roast if you prefer; pork butt roast is often labeled Boston butt in the supermarket. Serve with rice.

    2 tablespoons avocado oil, divided
    8 ounces pork shoulder steaks, trimmed, cut into 1-inch strips,
       and sliced crosswise ¼ inch thick
    ¼ teaspoon table salt
    1 pound cabbage kimchi, drained with ¼ cup juice reserved,
       cut into 2-inch pieces
    6 garlic cloves, minced
    1 tablespoon gochugaru
    2 cups unsalted chicken broth
    1 cup water
    2 teaspoons fish sauce, plus extra for seasoning
    6 scallions, cut into 2-inch lengths
   14 ounces soft or medium-firm tofu, cut into 1½-inch-wide,
       ½-inch-thick squares

1   Heat 1 tablespoon oil in Dutch oven over medium-high heat until shimmering. Add pork and salt and cook until light golden brown, 4 to 6 minutes. Add kimchi and cook until edges of white cabbage turn translucent, 5 to 7 minutes. Add garlic, gochugaru, and remaining 1 tablespoon oil and cook, stirring constantly, until fragrant, about 1 minute.

2   Stir in broth, water, fish sauce, and reserved kimchi juice. Bring to simmer; reduce heat to low; and cook, covered, until pork is tender, about 30 minutes.

3   Stir in scallions and nestle tofu into stew. Return to simmer and cook, uncovered, until scallions have softened, about 10 minutes. Season with extra fish sauce to taste. Serve.

Mapo Tofu

serves 4 to 6 · total time: 1 hour

why this recipe works · A thrilling hallmark of the Sichuan canon, mapo tofu is a fiery showcase for tofu—an excellent source of plant-based protein—as well as spices that are prominent in Sichuan cuisine. The dish uses ground pork more as a seasoning than a primary protein source; 8 ounces was enough to provide plenty of flavor without introducing a lot of saturated fat. We made the most of the fat that did render by using it to cook the bold seasonings in our sauce base. Ginger, garlic, and four Sichuan powerhouses—doubanjiang (broad bean chile paste), douchi (fermented black beans), Sichuan chili flakes, and Sichuan peppercorns—made for an immensely vibrant sauce full of antioxidants. Microwaving soft tofu in chicken broth with scallions imbued the cubes with savoriness and helped them stay intact during the braise. Stirring in cornstarch at the end created velvety thickness. If you can't find Sichuan chili flakes, you can substitute gochugaru. We developed this recipe in a 14-inch wok, but you can use a large saucepan instead. Serve with rice.

   28 ounces soft tofu, cut into ½-inch cubes
    1 cup unsalted chicken broth
    6 scallions, sliced thin
    8 ounces ground pork
    1 teaspoon avocado oil, plus extra as needed
    9 garlic cloves, minced
    ⅓ cup doubanjiang
    1 tablespoon grated fresh ginger
    1 tablespoon douchi
    1 tablespoon Sichuan chili flakes
    1 tablespoon Sichuan peppercorns, toasted and
       ground coarse
    2 tablespoons hoisin sauce
    2 teaspoons toasted sesame oil
    2 tablespoons water
    1 tablespoon cornstarch

1   Place tofu, broth, and scallions in large bowl and microwave, covered, until steaming, 5 to 7 minutes. Let stand while preparing remaining ingredients.

2   Cook pork and avocado oil in 14-inch flat-bottomed wok over medium heat, breaking up meat with wooden spoon, until meat just begins to brown, 5 to 7 minutes. Using slotted spoon, transfer pork to separate bowl. Pour off all but ¼ cup fat from wok. (If necessary, add avocado oil to equal ¼ cup.)

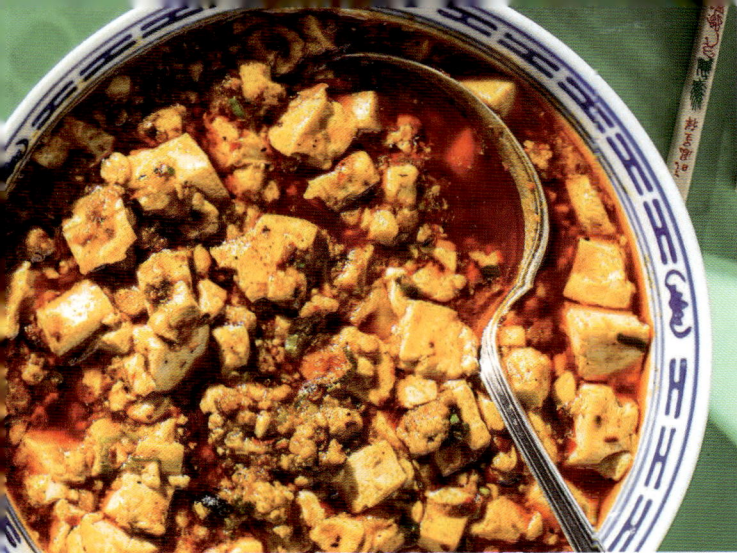

3 Add garlic, doubanjiang, ginger, douchi, chili flakes, and peppercorns to fat left in wok and cook over medium heat until spices darken and oil begins to separate from paste, 2 to 3 minutes.

4 Gently pour tofu with broth into wok, followed by hoisin, sesame oil, and cooked pork. Cook, stirring gently and frequently, until simmering, 2 to 3 minutes. Whisk water and cornstarch together in small bowl. Add cornstarch mixture to wok and continue to cook, stirring frequently, until sauce has thickened, about 3 minutes. Serve.

Maeuntang

serves 6 • total time: 35 minutes `FAST`

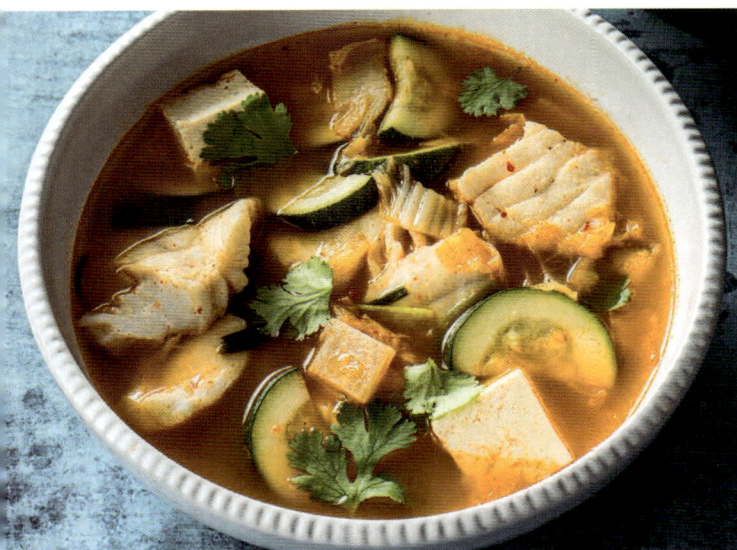

why this recipe works • Maeuntang, a traditional Korean spicy fish stew, is as flavorful as it is nourishing. Maeuntang gets its fire from both gochujang—a fermented paste made from chiles, soybeans, and rice that's funky, spicy, sweet, and salty—and the Korean red chili flakes known as gochugaru. Though the dish is traditionally made with anchovy stock, we substituted more readily available chicken broth, which gave the soup the rich body it needed. Adding ginger, garlic, and scallions to the stock brought a bevy of antioxidants, while kimchi lent the dish its gut-balancing fiber and probiotics. Simmering chunks of red snapper directly in the soup produced a rich, flavorful, and complex broth with oceanic complexity. Adding cubes of tofu and slices of zucchini—traditional mix-ins for this soup—gave us a heartier dish, and also helped counteract the heat of the fiery broth. Serve with lime wedges, if desired. Halibut, mahi-mahi, striped bass, or swordfish can be substituted for the snapper.

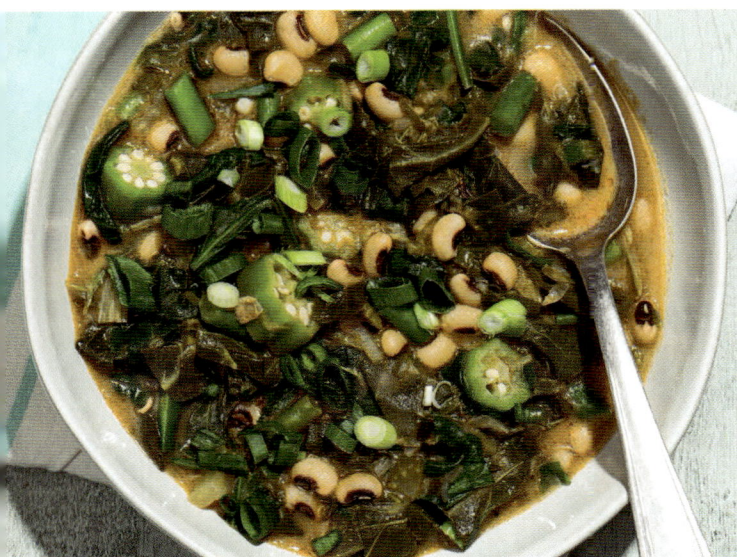

- 1 tablespoon avocado oil
- 4 garlic cloves, minced
- 1 tablespoon grated fresh ginger
- 6 cups unsalted chicken broth
- 1 cup kimchi, drained and coarsely chopped
- 1 tablespoon gochujang
- 1 tablespoon gochugaru
- ½ teaspoon pepper
- 1 (1½-pound) skinless red snapper fillet, 1 inch thick, cut into 2-inch pieces
- 7 ounces firm tofu, cut into 1-inch pieces
- 1 small zucchini, halved lengthwise and sliced ¼ inch thick
- 4 scallions, cut into 1-inch lengths
- ½ cup fresh cilantro leaves

top	*Mapo Tofu*
middle	*Maeuntang*
bottom	*Green Gumbo*

1   Heat oil in Dutch oven over medium heat until shimmering. Add garlic and ginger and cook until fragrant, about 30 seconds. Stir in broth, kimchi, gochujang, gochugaru, and pepper, then bring to simmer.

2   Stir in red snapper, tofu, zucchini, and scallions. Return to gentle simmer, then reduce heat to medium-low, cover, and cook until fish flakes apart when gently prodded with paring knife, 3 to 4 minutes. Sprinkle with cilantro and serve.

Green Gumbo

serves 6 to 8 · total time: 1 hour   **SUPERCHARGED**

why this recipe works • What sets green gumbo, or gumbo z'herbes, apart from its meatier cousins is an inflammation-fighting array of leafy green vegetables. Some versions are packed with more than a dozen kinds; to streamline, we chose one chewy variety (collards, mustard greens, or kale) and one soft one (spinach or Swiss chard) for a balance of fibrous and silky. (Do experiment with whatever greens you have on hand—they're great sources of fiber and antioxidants.) Cayenne and smoked paprika brought the benefits of capsaicin and echoed the smokiness of meaty gumbos. Though not traditional, adding other plants—okra, green beans, black-eyed peas—made an even heartier and more nutrient-rich stew. We like leaning into the green vibe with green bell pepper, but any kind will work. Don't use fresh okra here, though you can substitute frozen spinach for fresh, if you prefer. Serve over rice.

- ½   cup avocado oil
- ½   cup all-purpose flour
- 1   large onion, chopped fine
- 2   celery ribs, chopped fine
- 1   bell pepper, stemmed, seeded, and chopped fine
- 3   garlic cloves, minced
- 1   tablespoon minced fresh thyme or 1 teaspoon dried
- 2¼   teaspoons table salt, divided
- 2   teaspoons smoked paprika
- 1   teaspoon cayenne pepper
- 5   cups water
- 12   ounces collard greens, mustard greens, or kale, stemmed and cut into 1-inch pieces
- 1   cup frozen cut okra
- 1   (15-ounce) can no-salt-added black-eyed peas, rinsed
- 12   ounces curly-leaf spinach or Swiss chard, stemmed and cut into 1-inch pieces
- 6   ounces green beans, trimmed and cut into 1-inch lengths
- 1   tablespoon cider vinegar, plus extra for seasoning
- 2   scallions, sliced thin (optional)

1   Heat oil in Dutch oven over medium-high heat until just smoking. Using heat-resistant silicone spatula, stir in flour and cook, stirring constantly, until mixture is color of peanut butter, 2 to 5 minutes. Reduce heat to medium-low and continue to cook, stirring constantly, until roux has darkened to color of milk chocolate, 5 to 10 minutes longer.

2   Stir in onion, celery, bell pepper, garlic, thyme, 1 teaspoon salt, paprika, and cayenne. Cover and cook, stirring frequently, until vegetables have softened, 8 to 10 minutes.

3   Stir in water, scraping up any browned bits, and bring to boil over high heat. Stir in collard greens, 1 handful at a time; okra; and remaining 1¼ teaspoons salt. Cover, reduce heat to low, and simmer until greens are just tender, 5 to 7 minutes. Stir in black-eyed peas; spinach, 1 handful at a time; and green beans and simmer until green beans and spinach are tender, about 5 minutes. Stir in vinegar and season with salt, pepper, and extra vinegar to taste. Sprinkle with scallions, if using. Serve.

STEMMING AND SEEDING BELL PEPPERS

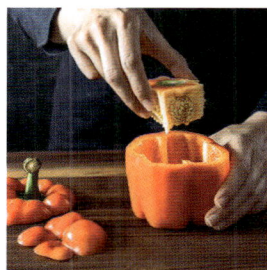

1   Slice ¼ inch from top and bottom of pepper and then gently remove stem from top lobe. Pull core out of pepper.

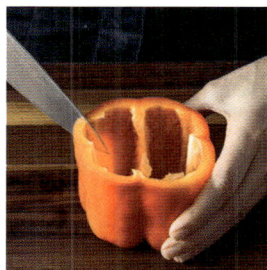

2   Make slit down one side of pepper and lay it flat, skin side down, in one long strip.

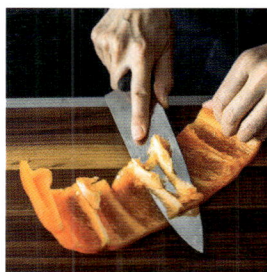

3   Slide sharp knife along inside of pepper to remove ribs and seeds.

Palak Dal

serves 4 to 6 • total time: 1¼ hours **SUPERCHARGED**

why this recipe works • In India, both raw lentils and the stews made with them are called "dal." The legumes are a staple of the vegetarian Indian meal: They're easy to prepare, affordable, and flavorful. They're also an excellent source of plant-based protein and packed with anti-inflammatory compounds. For a take on dal that's ideal for busy weeknights, we used quick-cooking red lentils. Once they had simmered to a soft texture, a vigorous whisk transformed them into a porridge-like puree, no food processor needed. We added fiber-loaded spinach, which bulked up the dish with nutrients such as carotenoids and vitamin K. Seasoning the lentils with the Indian tadka technique—frying whole spices in a few tablespoons of fat before using the mixture as a garnish—gave the dish complexity and an enticing aroma. Ghee is traditional here; you can substitute avocado oil, though the flavor will be less complex. If you can't find brown mustard seeds, you can substitute yellow. Monitor the spices and aromatics carefully during frying and reduce the heat if needed to prevent them from scorching. Serve with naan and/or rice.

4½	cups water
10½	ounces (1½ cups) dried red lentils, picked over and rinsed
1	tablespoon grated fresh ginger
¾	teaspoon ground turmeric
6	ounces (6 cups) baby spinach
1½	teaspoons table salt
3	tablespoons ghee or avocado oil
1½	teaspoons brown mustard seeds
1½	teaspoons cumin seeds
1	large onion, chopped
15	curry leaves, coarsely torn (optional)
6	garlic cloves, sliced
4	whole dried arbol chiles
1	serrano chile, halved lengthwise
1½	teaspoons lemon juice, plus extra for seasoning
⅓	cup chopped fresh cilantro

1 Bring water, lentils, ginger, and turmeric to boil in large saucepan over medium-high heat. Reduce heat to maintain vigorous simmer. Cook, uncovered, stirring occasionally, until lentils are soft and starting to break down, 18 to 20 minutes.

2 Whisk lentils vigorously until coarsely pureed, about 30 seconds. Continue to cook until lentils have consistency of loose polenta or oatmeal, up to 5 minutes. Stir in spinach and salt and continue to cook until spinach is fully wilted, 30 to 60 seconds. Cover and set aside off heat.

3 Melt ghee in 10-inch skillet over medium-high heat. Add mustard seeds and cumin seeds and cook, stirring constantly, until seeds sizzle and pop, about 30 seconds. Add onion and cook, stirring frequently, until onion is just starting to brown, about 5 minutes. Add curry leaves, if using; garlic; arbols; and serrano and cook, stirring frequently, until onion and garlic are golden brown, 3 to 4 minutes.

4 Add lemon juice to lentils and stir to incorporate. (Dal should have consistency of loose polenta. If too thick, loosen with hot water, adding 1 tablespoon at a time.) Season with salt and extra lemon juice to taste. Transfer dal to individual serving bowls and spoon onion mixture on top. Sprinkle with cilantro and serve.

Vegetable Tagine with Chickpeas and Olives

serves 4 • total time: 45 minutes **FAST**

why this recipe works • Traditional North African tagines—fragrant stews of vegetables, beans, dried fruits, and slowly braised meats—are long-simmered affairs. But making stars of the chickpeas and vegetables and skipping meat makes this tagine fast enough for a weeknight while keeping saturated fat to a minimum. We used canned chickpeas for efficiency and microwaved the potatoes and carrots before adding them to the pot to streamline the process further. For spices, we used paprika and garam masala for simplicity and lots of anti-inflammatory compounds. Oleic acid–rich green olives and vitamin C–packed lemon brought earthiness and tang, respectively, and channeled Moroccan flair. We like to use our homemade Garam Masala (page 84), but you can use store-bought if you prefer.

1	pound red potatoes, unpeeled, cut into ½-inch pieces
1	pound carrots, peeled and cut into ½-inch pieces
¼	cup extra-virgin olive oil, divided
1	teaspoon table salt
½	teaspoon pepper
1	onion, halved and sliced thin
4	(3-inch) strips lemon zest, sliced into matchsticks, plus 2 tablespoons juice
5	garlic cloves, minced
4	teaspoons paprika
2	teaspoons garam masala
3	cups unsalted vegetable or chicken broth
2	(15-ounce) cans no-salt-added chickpeas, rinsed
½	cup pitted green olives, halved
½	cup golden raisins
¼	cup minced fresh cilantro

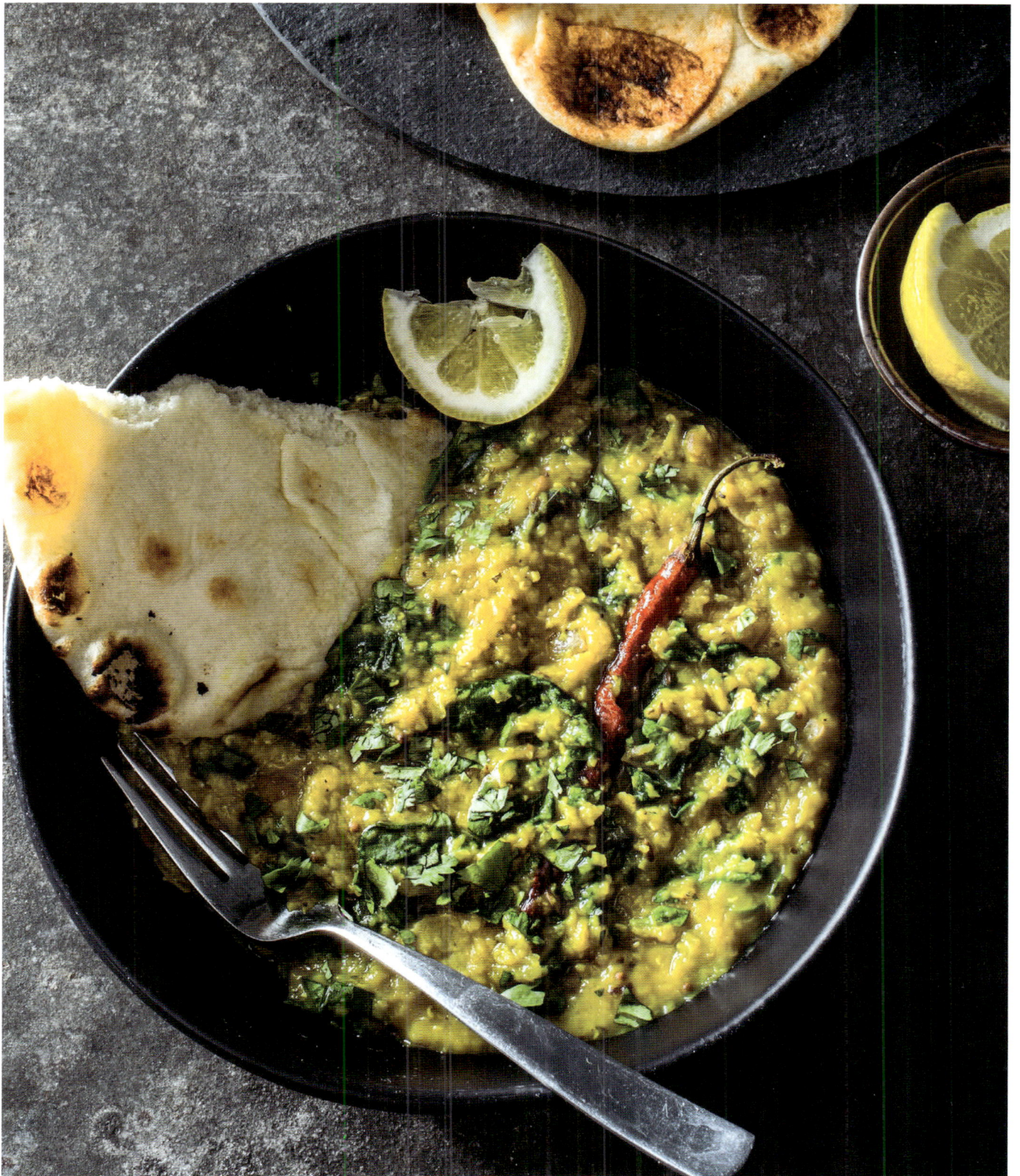

Palak Dal

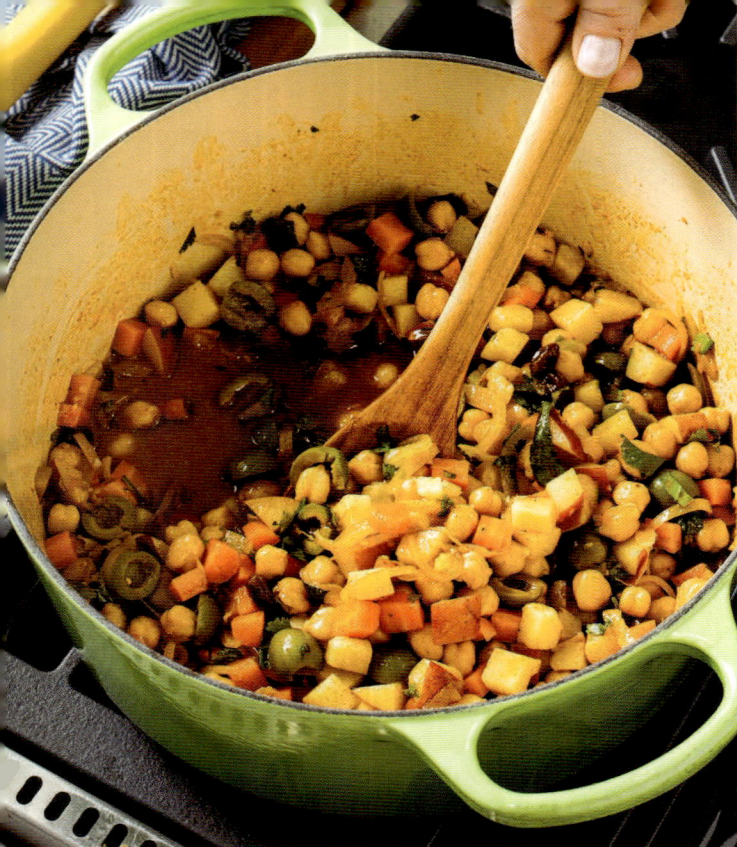

1   Microwave potatoes, carrots, 2 tablespoons oil, salt, and pepper in covered bowl until vegetables begin to soften, about 10 minutes.

2   Meanwhile, heat remaining 2 tablespoons oil in Dutch oven over medium-high heat until shimmering. Add onion and lemon zest and cook until onion begins to brown, about 8 minutes. Stir in garlic, paprika, and garam masala and cook until fragrant, about 30 seconds.

3   Add microwaved potatoes and carrots to Dutch oven and stir to coat with spices. Stir in broth, chickpeas, olives, and raisins. Cover and simmer gently until flavors blend, about 10 minutes. Uncover and simmer until vegetables are tender and sauce is slightly thickened, about 7 minutes. Stir in lemon juice and cilantro and season with salt and pepper to taste. Serve.

Garam Masala

makes ½ cup • total time: 5 minutes

      3   tablespoons black peppercorns
      8   teaspoons coriander seeds
      4   teaspoons cardamom pods
    2½   teaspoons cumin seeds
    1½   (3-inch) cinnamon sticks, broken into pieces

Process all ingredients in spice grinder until finely ground, about 30 seconds. (Garam masala can be stored in airtight container for up to 1 month.)

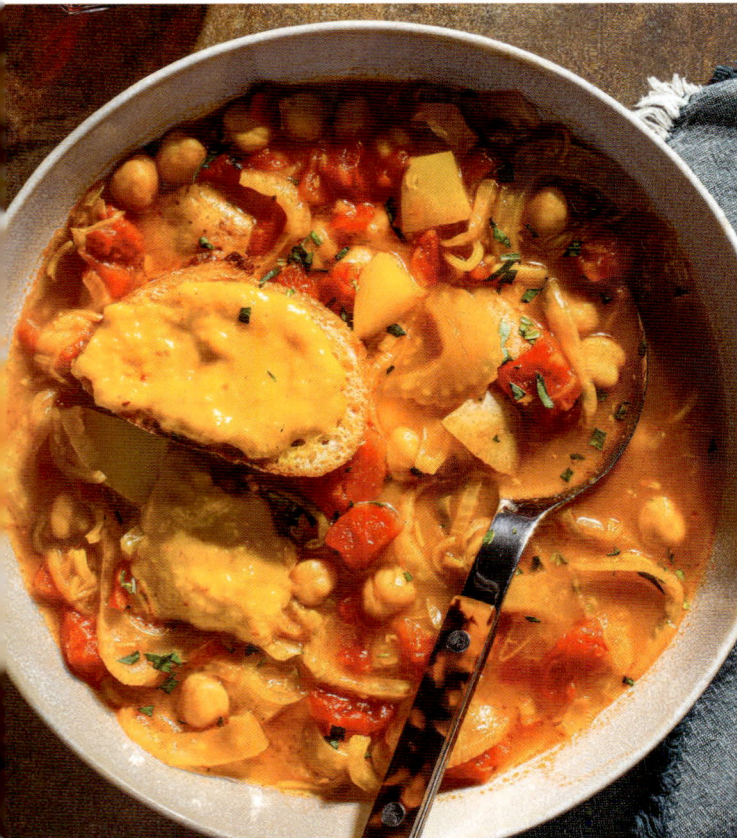

Chickpea Bouillabaisse

serves 4 to 6 • total time: 1½ hours

why this recipe works • Versatile chickpeas are at home in many cuisines. We found that the mild legumes make a protein-rich vehicle for the potent flavors of a classic bouillabaisse. To ensure a flavorful broth, we used leeks, fennel, garlic, tomato paste, and saffron. In lieu of fish stock, we opted for more readily available chicken broth plus canned chickpea liquid to create the dish's signature body. White wine, pastis, and orange zest evoked the flavors of Provence and created a more complex flavor profile. The baked croutons made for a pleasingly crunchy topping, while the rouille drizzled on top brought brightness and richness, thanks to heart-healthy extra-virgin olive oil. We prefer the robust flavor of extra-virgin olive oil in the rouille; you can use avocado oil or a combination of the two if you prefer a more neutral flavor.

Bouillabaisse

- 2 tablespoons extra-virgin olive oil
- 1 large leek, white and light green parts only, halved lengthwise, sliced thin, and washed thoroughly
- 1 fennel bulb, stalks discarded, bulb halved, cored, and sliced thin
- ¼ teaspoon table salt
- 4 garlic cloves, minced
- 1 tablespoon no-salt-added tomato paste
- 1 tablespoon all-purpose flour
- ¼ teaspoon saffron threads, crumbled
- ¼ teaspoon ground cayenne pepper
- 2 (15-ounce) cans no-salt-added chickpeas, undrained
- 3 cups unsalted chicken broth
- 1 (14.5-ounce) can no-salt-added diced tomatoes, drained
- 12 ounces Yukon Gold potatoes, unpeeled, cut into ¾-inch pieces
- ½ cup dry white wine
- ¼ cup pastis or Pernod
- 1 (3-inch) strip orange zest
- 1 tablespoon chopped fresh tarragon or parsley

Rouille and Croutons

- 3 tablespoons water
- ¼ teaspoon saffron threads, crumbled
- 1 baguette
- 4 teaspoons lemon juice
- 2 teaspoons Dijon mustard
- 1 large egg yolk
- 2 small garlic cloves, minced
- ¼ teaspoon cayenne pepper
- Pinch table salt
- ½ cup plus 2 tablespoons extra-virgin olive oil, divided

1 For the bouillabaisse Adjust oven rack to lower-middle position and heat oven to 375 degrees. Heat oil in Dutch oven over medium-high heat until shimmering. Add leek, fennel, and salt and cook, stirring often, until vegetables begin to soften, about 5 minutes. Stir in garlic, tomato paste, flour, saffron, and cayenne and cook until fragrant, about 30 seconds. Stir in chickpeas and their liquid, broth, tomatoes, potatoes, wine, pastis, and orange zest. Bring to simmer and cook over medium-low heat, partially covered, until potatoes are tender, about 20 minutes.

2 For the rouille and croutons While bouillabaisse cooks, microwave water and saffron in medium bowl until water is steaming, 15 to 30 seconds; set aside for 5 minutes. Cut 4-inch piece of baguette; remove and discard crust. Tear crustless bread into 1-inch pieces (you should have about 1 cup). Stir bread pieces and lemon juice into saffron-infused water and let sit for 5 minutes.

Using whisk, mash soaked bread mixture until uniform paste forms, 1 to 2 minutes. Whisk in mustard, egg yolk, garlic, cayenne, and salt. Whisking constantly, slowly drizzle in ¼ cup oil in steady stream until smooth mayonnaise-like consistency is reached, about 4 minutes, scraping down bowl as necessary. Slowly whisk in ¼ cup oil until smooth; set aside until ready to serve.

3 Cut remaining baguette into ¾-inch-thick slices. Toss slices with remaining 2 tablespoons oil until coated, then arrange in single layer on rimmed baking sheet. Bake until light golden brown, 10 to 15 minutes.

4 Discard orange peel from bouillabaisse. Stir in tarragon and season with salt and pepper to taste. Serve, dolloping individual serving bowls with rouille and spreading rouille over croutons.

❙ MAKE IT GLUTEN-FREE • Omit the croutons.

Roasted Poblano and White Bean Chili

serves 4 to 6 • total time: 2 hours **SUPERCHARGED**

why this recipe works • Lots of fresh chiles provide complex flavor and anti-inflammatory benefits in this chili. Processing some of the peppers with some of the beans thickened the chili. For a toasty element, plus fiber and B vitamins, we broiled fresh corn; we even simmered the cobs in the chili to extract flavor. For a spicier chili, add the seeds from the chiles. If you can't find Anaheim chiles, add two extra poblanos and one extra jalapeño. Serve with sour cream, tortilla chips, and lime wedges, if desired.

- 5 poblano chiles, halved lengthwise, stemmed, and seeded
- 3 Anaheim chiles, halved lengthwise, stemmed, and seeded
- 3 tablespoons extra-virgin olive oil, divided
- 3 ears corn, kernels cut from cobs and cobs reserved
- 2 onions, cut into large pieces
- 2 jalapeño chiles, stemmed, seeded, and chopped
- 2 (15-ounce) cans no-salt-added cannellini beans, rinsed, divided
- 4 cups unsalted vegetable or chicken broth, divided
- 6 garlic cloves, minced
- 1 tablespoon no-salt-added tomato paste
- 1 tablespoon ground cumin
- 1½ teaspoons ground coriander
- 1½ teaspoons table salt
- 1 (15-ounce) can no-salt-added pinto beans, rinsed
- 4 scallions, green parts only, sliced thin
- ¼ cup minced fresh cilantro
- 1 tablespoon lime juice

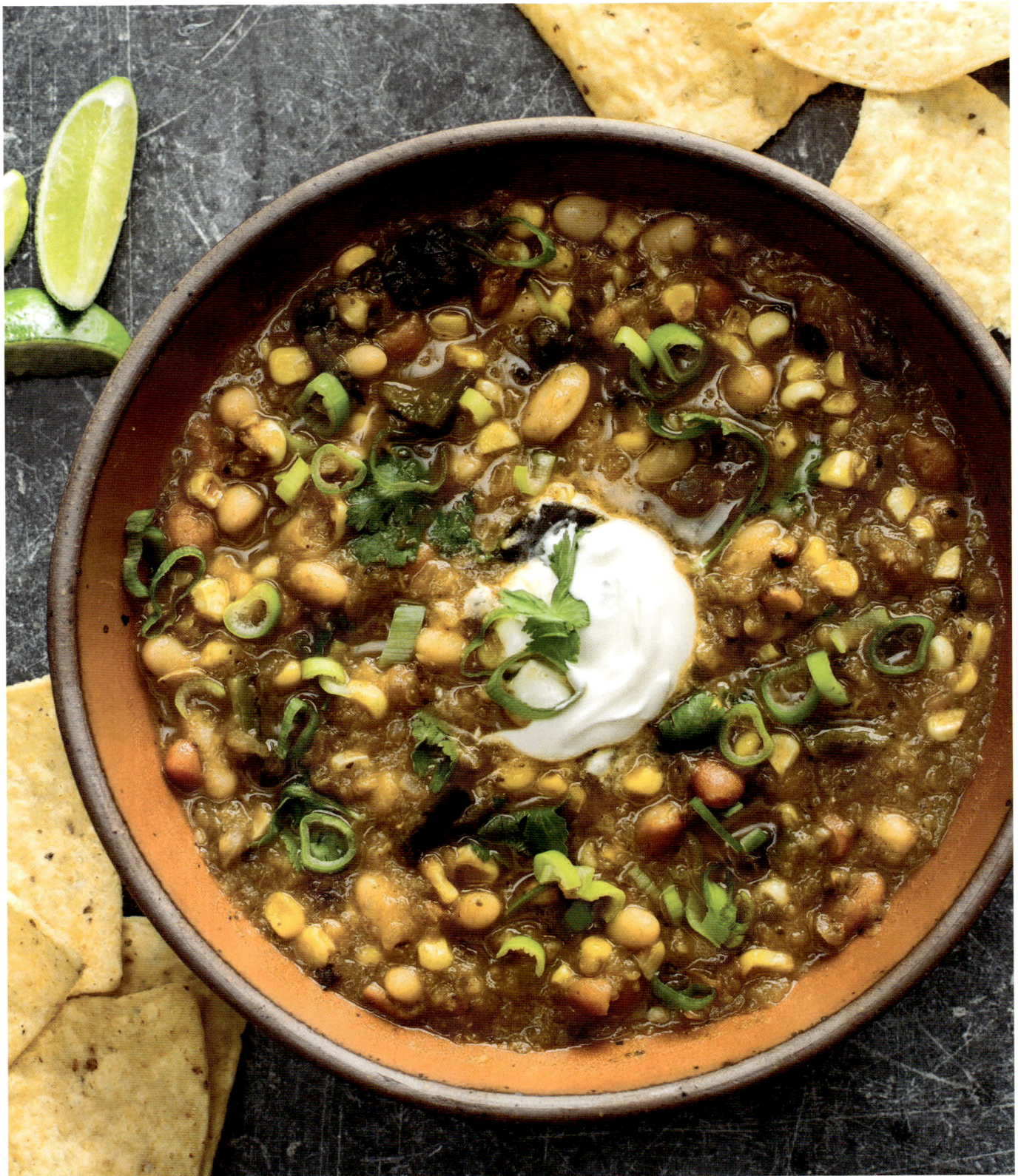

Roasted Poblano and White Bean Chili

1   Adjust oven rack 6 inches from broiler element and heat broiler. Toss poblanos and Anaheims with 1 tablespoon oil and spread, skin side up, on aluminum foil–lined rimmed baking sheet. Broil until chiles begin to blacken and soften, about 10 minutes, rotating sheet halfway through broiling. Transfer broiled chiles to bowl, cover with plastic wrap, and let steam until skins peel off easily, 10 to 15 minutes. Peel poblanos and Anaheims, then cut into ½-inch pieces, reserving any accumulated juice.

2   Meanwhile, toss corn kernels with 1 tablespoon oil, spread evenly on foil-lined baking sheet, and broil, stirring occasionally, until beginning to brown, 5 to 10 minutes; let cool on baking sheet.

3   Pulse onions and jalapeños in food processor to consistency of chunky salsa, 6 to 8 pulses; transfer to bowl. In now-empty food processor, process 1 cup cannellini beans, 1 cup broth, and ½ cup chopped roasted chiles and any accumulated juice until smooth, about 45 seconds.

4   Heat remaining 1 tablespoon oil in Dutch oven over medium heat until shimmering. Add onion-jalapeño mixture and cook until softened, 5 to 7 minutes. Stir in garlic, tomato paste, cumin, coriander, and salt and cook until tomato paste begins to darken, about 2 minutes. Stir in remaining 3 cups broth, scraping up any browned bits. Stir in pureed chile-bean mixture, remaining roasted chiles, remaining cannellini beans, pinto beans, and corn cobs. Bring to simmer, then reduce heat to low and simmer gently until thickened and flavorful, about 40 minutes.

5   Discard corn cobs. Stir in broiled corn kernels until heated through, about 1 minute. Off heat, stir in scallions, cilantro, and lime juice and season with salt and pepper to taste. Serve.

Nutrition Knowledge   Bold, spicy, and brimming with anti-inflammatory benefits, this chili is a powerhouse of flavor and wellness. Anaheim and jalapeño chiles deliver capsaicin, while cumin and coriander add antioxidants such as curcumin and quercetin to fight inflammation. The fiber from beans, garlic for immune support, and a medley of vegetables make this dish as nourishing as it is bold.

—*Alicia*

White Chicken Chili

serves 4 to 6 · **total time: 45 minutes**   **FAST**

why this recipe works · Usually chili needs to simmer for hours, but this mildly spiced, tomato-free version is ready to eat in under an hour. For a flavorful foundation, we browned chicken breasts, a lean protein source, and added poblanos and onions. For a thick consistency, we blended canned hominy, a form of corn rich in fiber and B vitamins, with broth until smooth, creating a velvety broth in which to poach the chicken. We left some of the hominy whole to stir into the chili, punctuating each bite with warm corn flavor and pleasing chew. Tomatillo salsa and cilantro brought zest and freshness. Serve with your favorite chili garnishes.

  2   (15-ounce) cans no-salt-added white or yellow hominy, rinsed, divided
  4   cups unsalted chicken broth, divided
1½   pounds boneless, skinless chicken breasts, trimmed
  ½   teaspoon table salt
  ½   teaspoon pepper
  2   tablespoons avocado oil, divided
  3   poblano chiles, stemmed, seeded, and chopped
  1   onion, chopped fine
  2   tablespoons all-purpose flour
  3   garlic cloves, minced
  1   teaspoon ground cumin
  1   teaspoon ground coriander
  ⅛   teaspoon cayenne pepper
  ½   cup jarred tomatillo salsa or salsa verde
  2   tablespoons minced fresh cilantro

1   Process 1½ cups hominy and 1 cup broth in blender until smooth, about 10 seconds; set aside.

2   Pat chicken dry with paper towels and sprinkle with salt and pepper. Heat 1 tablespoon oil in Dutch oven over medium-high heat until just smoking. Add chicken and cook until lightly browned on both sides, about 5 minutes; transfer to plate.

3   Add remaining 1 tablespoon oil, poblanos, and onion to fat left in pot and cook over medium heat until vegetables are softened, about 5 minutes. Stir in flour, garlic, cumin, coriander, and cayenne and cook until fragrant, about 1 minute. Slowly whisk in remaining 3 cups broth, scraping up any browned bits and smoothing out any lumps.

4 Stir in pureed hominy mixture and remaining hominy. Add browned chicken, along with any accumulated juices; cover; and simmer gently until chicken registers 160 degrees, about 10 minutes. Transfer chicken to cutting board; using 2 forks, shred into bite-size pieces.

5 Return chili to simmer. Stir in shredded chicken and tomatillo salsa and cook until heated through, about 1 minute. Stir in cilantro and season with salt and pepper to taste. Serve.

Simple Beef Chili with Kidney Beans

serves 6 · total time: 2½ hours

why this recipe works · Some beef chilis are all about the meat, but we wanted one that gave the same prominence to beans, an excellent source of fiber and plant-based protein. With the goal of developing a no-fuss recipe made with pantry staples, we leaned on anti-inflammatory spices such as cumin, coriander, and cayenne, which we added to the pot with the aromatics to boost their fragrance. We then added the beef, opting for a 90-percent-lean variety to keep saturated fat in check. Two forms of canned tomatoes—diced and pureed—packed the dish with lycopene, a powerful antioxidant. Cooking the chili with the lid on for half the cooking time gave it an appealingly chunky consistency. Serve with your favorite chili garnishes.

- 2 tablespoons avocado oil
- 2 onions, chopped fine
- 1 red bell pepper, stemmed, seeded, and cut into ½-inch pieces
- 6 garlic cloves, minced
- ¼ cup chili powder
- 1 tablespoon ground cumin
- 2 teaspoons ground coriander
- 1 teaspoon red pepper flakes
- 1 teaspoon dried oregano
- ½ teaspoon cayenne pepper
- 1½ pounds 90 percent lean ground beef, divided
- 2 (15-ounce) cans no-salt-added red kidney beans, rinsed
- 1 (28-ounce) can no-salt-added diced tomatoes
- 1 (28-ounce) can no-salt-added tomato puree
- ½ teaspoon table salt
  Lime wedges

1 Heat oil in Dutch oven over medium heat until shimmering. Add onions, bell pepper, garlic, chili powder, cumin, coriander, pepper flakes, oregano, and cayenne and cook, stirring occasionally, until vegetables are softened and beginning to brown, about

10 minutes. Increase heat to medium-high and add half of beef. Cook, breaking up pieces with spoon, until no longer pink and just beginning to brown, 3 to 4 minutes. Add remaining beef and cook, breaking up pieces with spoon, until no longer pink, 3 to 4 minutes.

2 Add beans, tomatoes and their juice, tomato puree, and salt; bring to boil, then reduce heat to low and simmer gently, covered, stirring occasionally, for 1 hour. Remove cover and continue to simmer 1 hour longer, stirring occasionally (if chili begins to stick to bottom of pot, stir in ½ cup water and continue to simmer), until beef is tender and chili is dark, rich, and slightly thickened. Season with salt to taste. Serve with lime wedges.

NOTES FROM THE TEST KITCHEN

All About Canned Tomatoes

Canned tomatoes are a convenient source of antioxidants. We tested a variety of canned tomato products to determine the best uses for each.

Whole Tomatoes Whole tomatoes are peeled tomatoes packed in their own juice or puree. They are quite soft and break down quickly when cooked, and are best when fresh tomato flavor is a must.

Diced Tomatoes Diced tomatoes are peeled, machine-diced, and packed in their own juice or puree. Many brands add calcium chloride, a firming agent that helps the chunks maintain their shape. These are best for chunky sauces or long-cooked stews.

Crushed Tomatoes Crushed tomatoes are whole tomatoes ground finely, then enriched with tomato puree. They work well in smooth sauces, especially when you want to make a sauce quickly.

Tomato Puree Tomato puree is made from cooked tomatoes, strained to remove their seeds and skins. Tomato puree works well in long-simmered, smooth, thick sauces with a deep, hearty flavor.

Tomato Paste Tomato paste is tomato puree that has been cooked to minimize moisture. Because it's full of glutamates, tomato paste brings out subtle depth and savory notes. It lends deep, well-rounded tomato flavor to dishes.

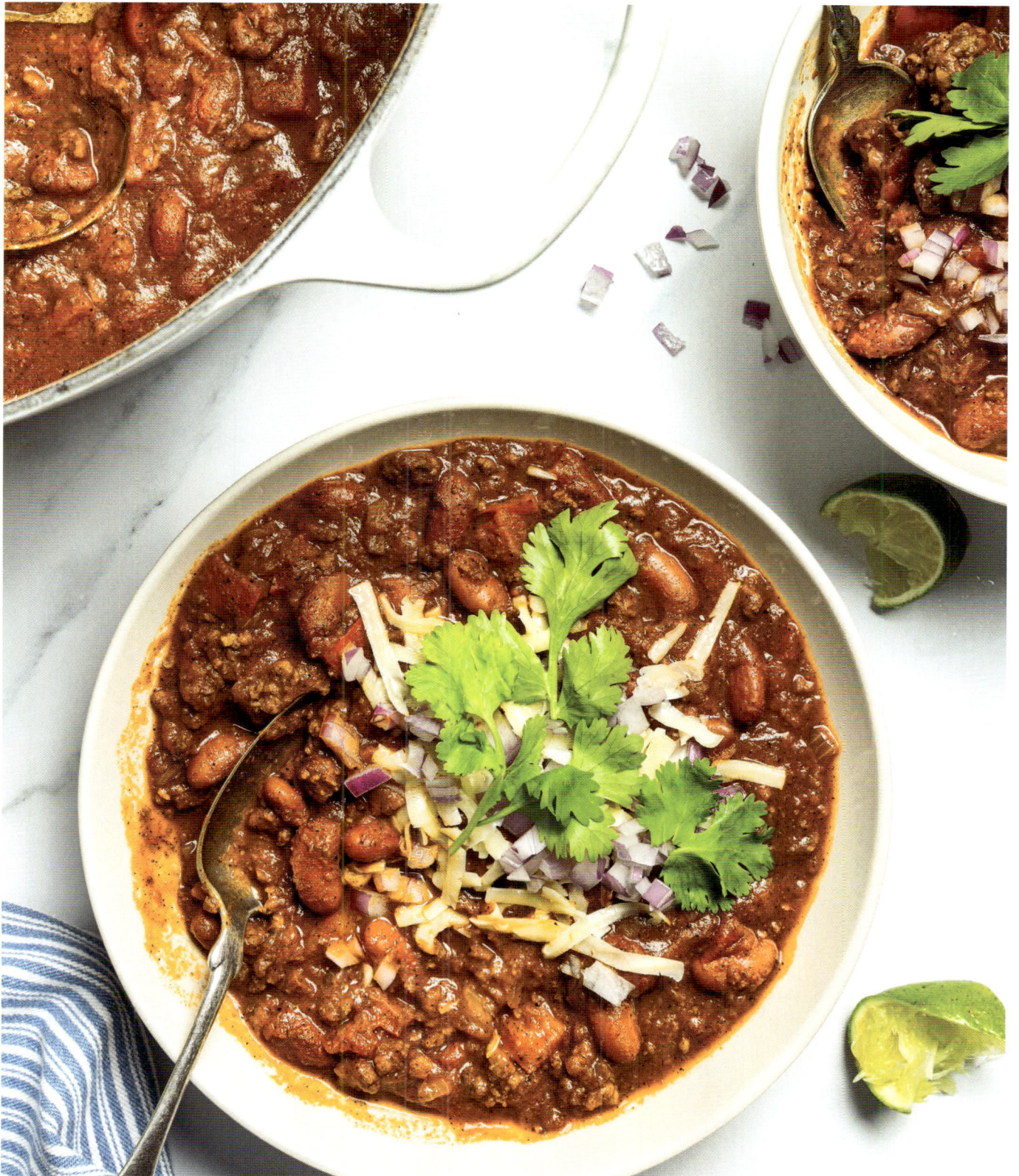

Simple Beef Chili with Kidney Beans

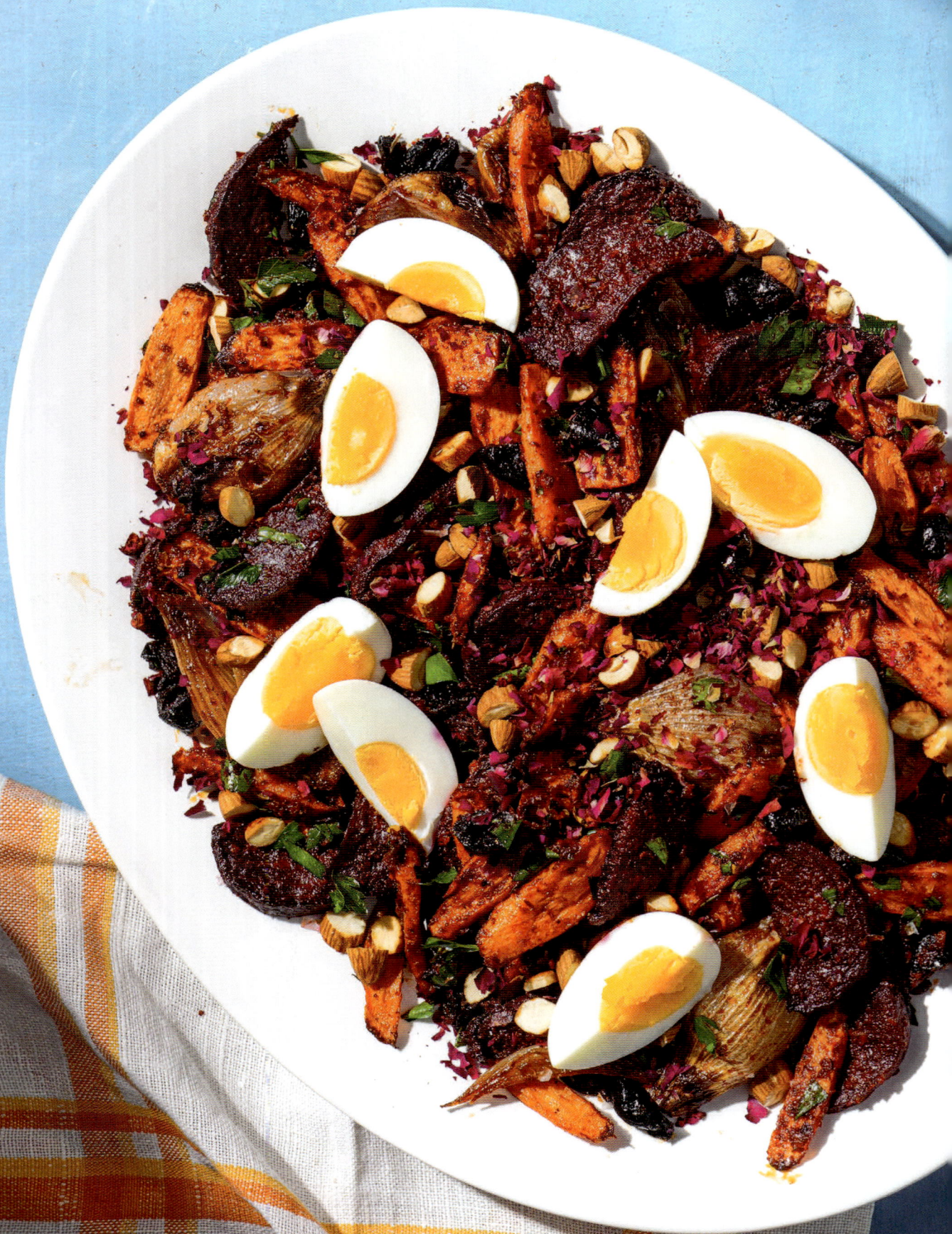

DINNER SALADS & BOWLS

■ FAST　　■ SUPERCHARGED

Chicken and Arugula Salad with Figs and Warm Spices

serves 4 • total time: 25 minutes **FAST** **SUPERCHARGED**

why this recipe works • Chicken salad provides a hearty, protein-rich base for a wide variety of anti-inflammatory mix-ins and toppings—and we added them in spades. We started with simple poached chicken, which we shredded and then jazzed up with antioxidant-rich, majestically purple figs as well as chickpeas for gut-nourishing fiber plus protein. We then dressed it all with a citrusy vinaigrette seasoned with an antioxidant-loaded trio of spices: cinnamon, coriander, and smoked paprika. To get the most out of the spices, we microwaved them with a little oil to bloom their flavor and aroma before whisking in the lemon juice. A bed of peppery, glucosinolate-rich baby arugula and a generous portion of the poached chicken soaked up our dressing. We just needed a bit of nutty crunch to play against the soft figs, and we got that from toasted chopped almonds. The result of bringing all these ingredients together is a well-rounded, anti-inflammatory powerhouse of a dish. You can substitute dried figs for the fresh figs in this recipe. We like to use our Perfect Poached Chicken (recipe follows) here, but any cooked chicken will work.

- 3 tablespoons extra-virgin olive oil, divided
- 1 teaspoon ground coriander
- ½ teaspoon smoked paprika
- ¼ teaspoon ground cinnamon
- 3 tablespoons lemon juice
- ½ teaspoon table salt
- ¼ teaspoon pepper
- 2 cups shredded cooked chicken
- 1 (15-ounce) can no-salt-added chickpeas or white beans, rinsed
- 5 ounces (5 cups) baby arugula
- ½ cup fresh parsley and/or mint leaves
- 1 shallot, sliced thin
- 8 fresh figs, stemmed and quartered
- ½ cup whole almonds, pecans, or walnuts, toasted and chopped

1 Microwave 1 tablespoon oil, coriander, paprika, and cinnamon in large bowl until fragrant, about 30 seconds. Whisk in lemon juice, salt, and pepper. Whisking constantly, slowly drizzle in remaining 2 tablespoons oil until emulsified.

2 Add chicken, chickpeas, arugula, parsley, and shallot to dressing in bowl and toss gently to combine. Season with salt and pepper to taste. Transfer salad to serving platter, arrange figs over top, and sprinkle with almonds. Serve.

Perfect Poached Chicken

makes 4 cups • total time: 50 minutes
The recipe can be easily halved; use the same amount of salt and water.

- 4 (6- to 8-ounce) boneless, skinless chicken breasts, trimmed
- Table salt for cooking chicken

1 Cover chicken breasts with plastic wrap and pound thick ends gently until ¾ inch thick. Whisk 4 quarts cool water with 2 tablespoons salt in Dutch oven.

2 Arrange chicken in steamer basket without overlapping. Submerge basket in pot. Heat over medium heat, stirring occasionally, until water registers 175 degrees, 15 to 20 minutes.

3 Turn off heat, cover pot, remove from burner, and let sit until chicken registers 160 degrees, 17 to 22 minutes. Transfer chicken to cutting board and let cool for 10 to 15 minutes. Slice, chop, or shred as desired. Serve. (Chicken can be refrigerated for up to 2 days. Let come to room temperature before using in salads.)

Dijon Chicken Salad with Raspberries and Avocado

serves 4 • total time: 45 minutes **FAST**

why this recipe works • This hearty salad will make you feel as good as it looks. Juicy, pan-seared chicken provides plenty of lean protein; we pounded down the thicker ends of the breasts to make sure that they cooked evenly and stayed tender throughout. For our greens, we used mesclun, which offers anti-inflammatory compounds and digestion-boosting fiber and delivers a mildly bitter, pleasantly peppery punch. For toppings, we leaned on sweet-tart raspberries for a dose of antioxidants, while creamy avocado contributes heart-healthy fats. For a bit of crunchy contrast, we tossed in toasted pecans, which are rich in magnesium and nutty flavor, plus a handful of refreshing basil. The dressing—made with cider vinegar, Dijon mustard, and extra-virgin olive oil—lightly coated the chicken and mesclun, offering a tangy kick that contrasted particularly well with the natural sweetness of the berries. For the best results, buy similar-size chicken breasts weighing up to 8 ounces. If using breasts that weigh 10 to 12 ounces, cook only three and increase the cooking time in step 2 to 9 to 12 minutes. We don't recommend using breasts larger than 12 ounces here as their exteriors will toughen before they cook through.

- 4 (6- to 8-ounce) boneless, skinless chicken breasts, trimmed
- ¼ cup extra-virgin olive oil, divided
- ¾ teaspoon table salt, divided
- 2 tablespoons cider vinegar
- 1 tablespoon Dijon mustard
- ¼ teaspoon pepper
- 10 ounces (10 cups) mesclun
- 5 ounces (1 cup) raspberries, halved
- 1 avocado, halved, pitted, and cut into ½-inch pieces
- ½ cup shredded fresh basil
- ½ cup pecans, toasted and chopped

1 Gently pound thicker end of each breast until ½ inch thick. Pat breasts dry with paper towels. Brush both sides of breasts with 1 tablespoon oil, then sprinkle each breast with ⅛ teaspoon salt. Place breasts, skinned side down, in 12-inch nonstick skillet, arranging narrow parts of breasts opposite wider parts. Place skillet over high heat and cook for 2 minutes. Flip breasts and cook for 2 minutes (there should be light browning).

2 Flip breasts, reduce heat to medium, and continue to cook, flipping breasts every 2 minutes, until exterior is well browned and thickest part of breast registers 155 degrees, 6 to 8 minutes. Transfer breasts to cutting board, tent with aluminum foil, and let rest for 10 minutes.

3 Slice chicken ¾ inch thick. Whisk vinegar, mustard, pepper, and remaining ¼ teaspoon salt together in large bowl. Whisking constantly, slowly drizzle in remaining 3 tablespoons oil until emulsified. Add mesclun and toss to combine. Season with salt and pepper to taste. Transfer salad to serving platter, arrange chicken, raspberries, and avocado over top, and sprinkle with basil and pecans. Serve.

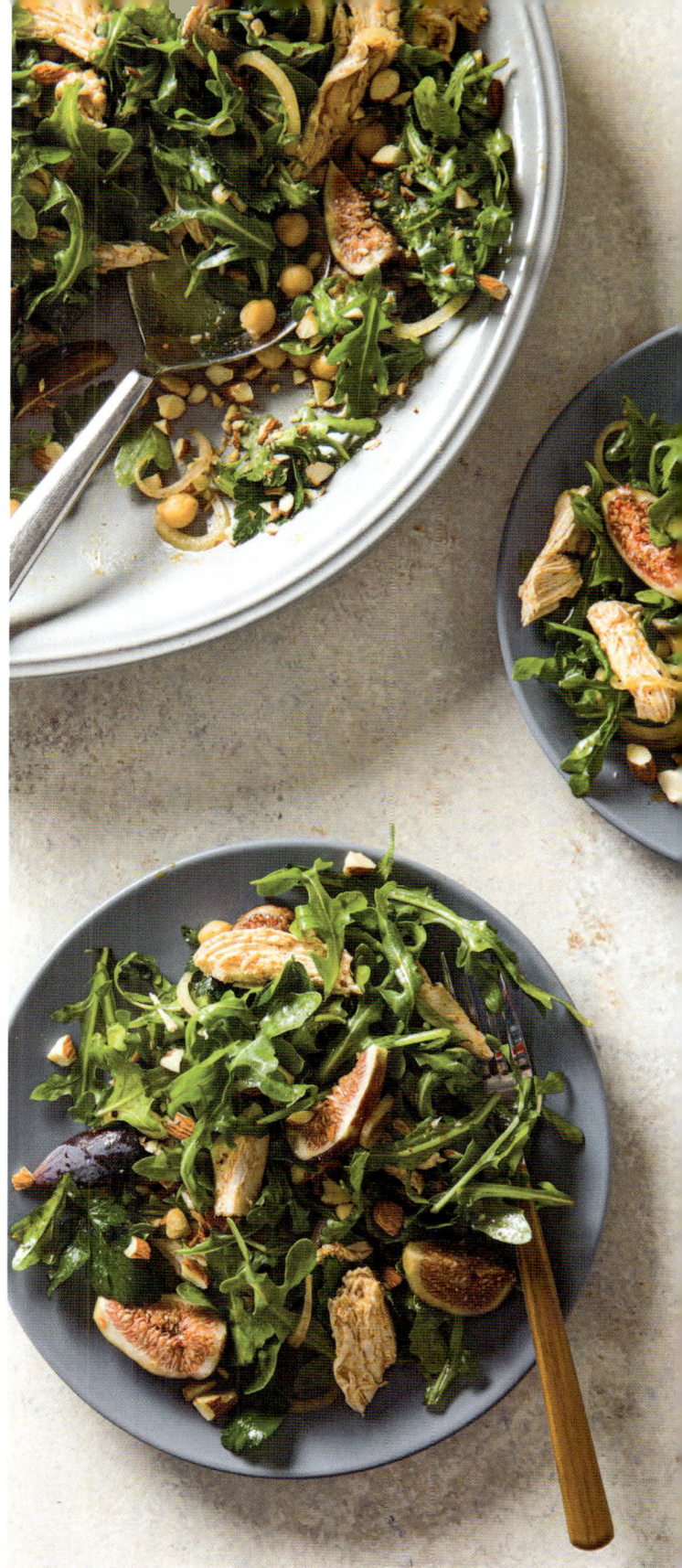

Chicken and Arugula Salad with Figs and Warm Spices

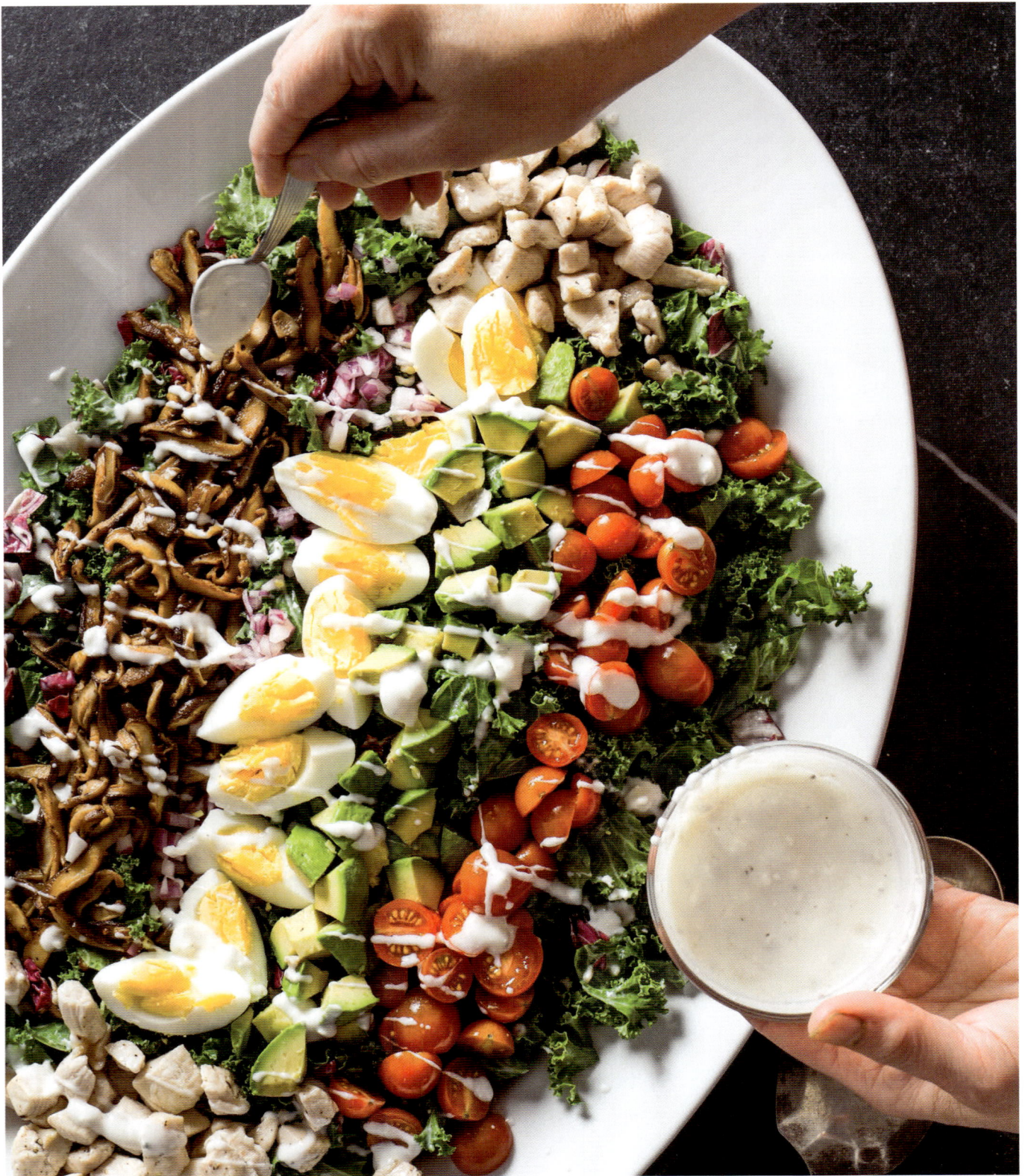

Super Cobb Salad

Super Cobb Salad

serves 4 · total time: 1 hour

why this recipe works · In addition to a stunning presentation, Cobb salad has the makings of a powerhouse meal: eggs, avocados, greens, tomatoes, and lean chicken. We just had to do something about all the bacon and cheese, which contribute more saturated fat than is optimal for an anti-inflammatory meal. We thought we'd have to sacrifice bacon's rich smoky flavor—until we tried sautéing shiitake mushrooms with smoked paprika and chili powder. Not only did this produce smokiness without the saturated fat and preservatives, but we also gained some umami meatiness. Using kale in place of romaine upped the fiber and nutritional profile, as did the radicchio, which also contributed beautiful pops of purple. For the dressing, just 3 tablespoons of blue cheese, whisked with yogurt, garlic, and lemon juice, provided the rich, tangy flavor we were after and gave us an ultracreamy salad. We tossed some with our greens and drizzled the rest over our still-classic yet mindfully updated Cobb salad.

- 8 ounces boneless, skinless chicken breasts, trimmed
- ¾ teaspoon table salt, divided
- ¼ teaspoon pepper, divided
- 2 teaspoons extra-virgin olive oil, divided
- 10 ounces shiitake mushrooms, stemmed and sliced thin
- ⅛ teaspoon smoked paprika
- ⅛ teaspoon chili powder
- 8 ounces kale, stemmed and cut into 1-inch pieces (8 cups)
- ⅓ cup finely chopped red onion
- 1 tablespoon lemon juice, divided
- ¾ cup plain yogurt
- 3 tablespoons crumbled blue cheese
- 1 garlic clove, minced
- ½ small head radicchio (3 ounces), cored and cut into ½-inch pieces
- 2 Easy-Peel Hard-Cooked Eggs (page 31), quartered
- 1 avocado, halved, pitted, and cut into ½-inch pieces
- 6 ounces cherry tomatoes, halved

1 Pat chicken dry with paper towels and cut into ½-inch pieces. Sprinkle with ⅛ teaspoon salt and ⅛ teaspoon pepper. Heat 1 teaspoon oil in 12-inch nonstick skillet over medium-high heat until shimmering. Add chicken and cook, stirring occasionally, until cooked through, 4 to 6 minutes. Transfer to plate and let cool.

2 Heat remaining 1 teaspoon oil in now-empty skillet over medium heat until shimmering. Add mushrooms and ½ teaspoon salt, cover, and cook until mushrooms have released their liquid, 4 to 6 minutes. Uncover and increase heat to medium-high. Stir in paprika, chili powder, and remaining ⅛ teaspoon pepper and cook until mushrooms are golden, 4 to 6 minutes. Transfer to second plate and let cool.

3 Place kale in large bowl and cover with warm tap water (110 to 115 degrees). Swish kale around to remove grit. Let kale sit in warm water bath for 10 minutes. Remove kale from water and spin dry in salad spinner in multiple batches. Pat leaves dry with paper towels if still wet. Toss onion with 2 teaspoons lemon juice and set aside.

4 Whisk yogurt, blue cheese, garlic, remaining 1 teaspoon lemon juice, and remaining ⅛ teaspoon salt together in bowl until well combined.

5 Toss kale and radicchio with ½ cup dressing to coat. Season with salt and pepper to taste. Transfer to serving platter and arrange in even layer. Arrange cooled mushrooms, onion, eggs, avocado, and tomatoes in single, even rows over greens, leaving space at either end. Arrange half of chicken in each open space at ends of platter. Drizzle remaining dressing over salad. Serve.

> **MAKE AHEAD** · Chicken and mushrooms can be prepared through step 2 and refrigerated separately for up to 3 days.

Sichuan-Style Chicken Salad

serves 4 to 6 · total time: 40 minutes **FAST**

why this recipe works · Sichuan's famous bang bang ji si, or bang bang chicken, is a dish composed of shredded chicken, julienned cucumber, and a spicy sauce. Taking inspiration from its satisfying, flavorful combination of textures and ingredients, we wanted to turn this dish into a main-course salad. Shredding the chicken allowed it to hold plenty of potent dressing; we made the dressing by microwaving avocado oil with garlic and ginger—to awaken the flavors of the aromatics—before straining the oil and adding umami-rich soy sauce, briny vinegar, toasty sesame oil, and pleasantly numbing Sichuan peppercorns. We tossed the dressed chicken with thinly sliced napa cabbage, cilantro, scallions, and celery for plenty of crunch and filling fiber. If you can't find Sichuan chili powder, you can swap in gochugaru—Korean red pepper flakes—for a similar flavor profile. If you prefer a less numbing dressing, use the lesser amount of Sichuan peppercorns. We like to use our Perfect Poached Chicken (page 92) in this recipe, but any cooked chicken will work.

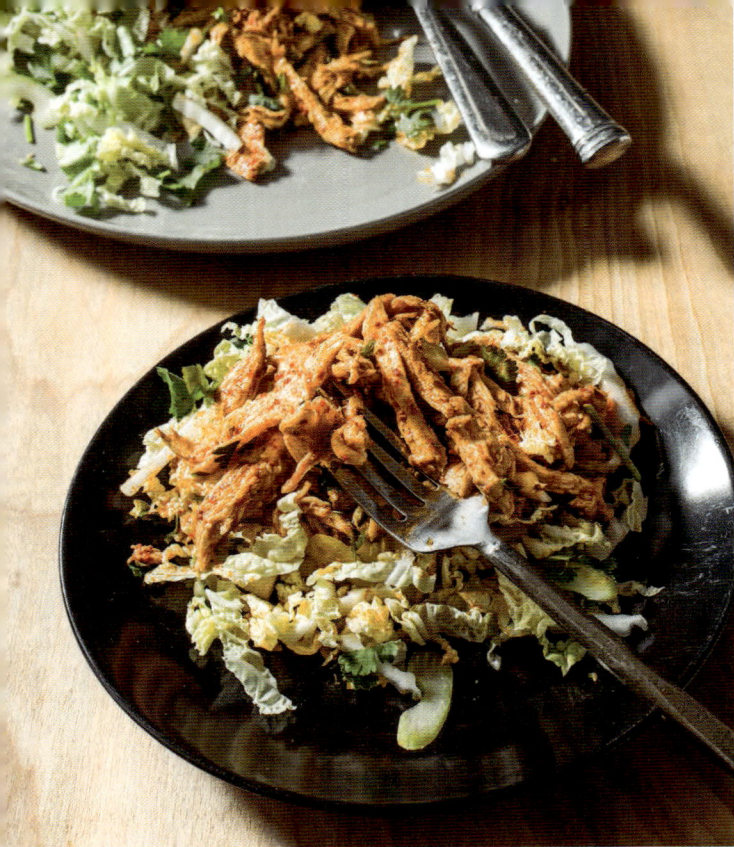

Dressing

- ¼ cup avocado oil
- 1 garlic clove, peeled and smashed
- 1 (½-inch) piece ginger, peeled and sliced in half
- 2 tablespoons Sichuan chili powder
- 2 tablespoons low-sodium soy sauce
- 1 tablespoon Chinese black vinegar or sherry vinegar
- 1 tablespoon toasted sesame oil
- 1–3 teaspoons Sichuan peppercorns, toasted and ground

Salad

- 4 cups shredded cooked chicken
- ½ head napa cabbage, sliced thin (6 cups)
- 1½ cups coarsely chopped fresh cilantro leaves and stems, divided
- 6 scallions, sliced in half lengthwise, then sliced thin on bias, divided
- 1 celery rib, sliced thin on bias
  Pinch table salt
- 2 teaspoons toasted sesame seeds (optional)

1   For the dressing Combine avocado oil, garlic, and ginger in bowl. Microwave until oil is hot and bubbling, about 2 minutes. Stir in chili powder and let cool for 10 minutes.

2   Strain oil mixture through fine-mesh strainer into large bowl; discard solids. Whisk soy sauce, vinegar, sesame oil, and 1 teaspoon peppercorns into strained oil. Add up to 2 teaspoons additional peppercorns to taste.

3   For the salad Add chicken to bowl with dressing and toss to coat. Season with salt to taste. Toss cabbage, 1 cup cilantro, two-thirds of scallions, celery, and salt in second large bowl. Season with salt and pepper to taste. Arrange cabbage mixture in even layer on serving platter. Mound chicken on top of cabbage mixture and sprinkle with remaining ½ cup cilantro; remaining scallions; and sesame seeds, if using. Serve.

MAKE IT GLUTEN-FREE • Substitute low-sodium tamari for the low-sodium soy sauce.

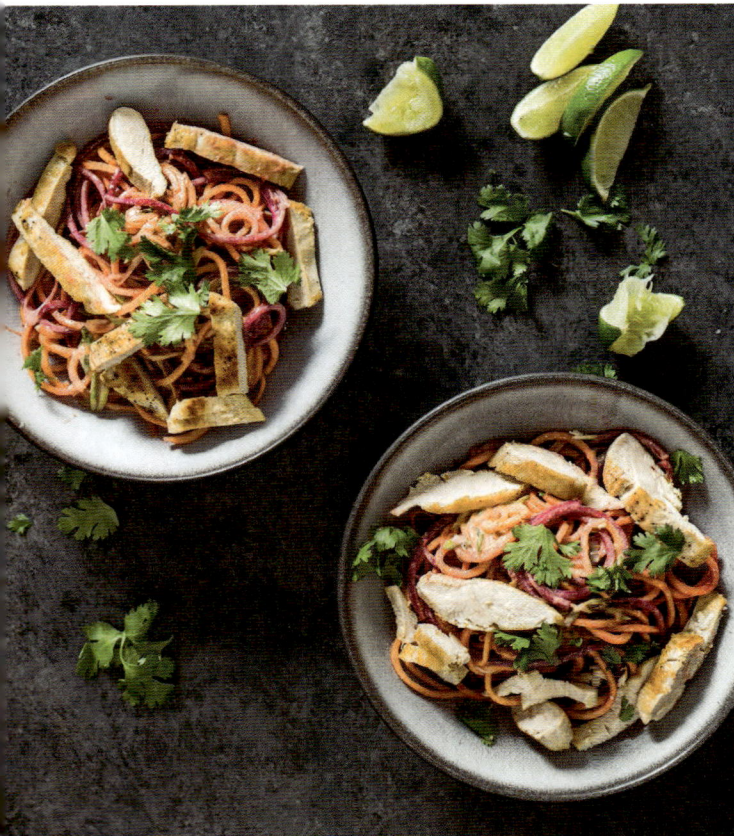

top | Sichuan-Style Chicken Salad
bottom | Beet and Carrot Noodle Salad with Chicken

Beet and Carrot Noodle Salad with Chicken

serves 4 · total time: 1 hour

why this recipe works · This colorful dish uses homemade beet and carrot noodles to marry the hearty appeal of pasta salad with the refreshing lightness of raw vegetables. With their dense texture, beets make excellent vegetable "noodles," as spiralizing renders them delicate enough to eat raw. Pairing them with carrot noodles made for a visually stunning, not to mention more nutritionally diverse, salad. The noodles' crisp-tender texture made the perfect canvas for a nutty, aromatic dressing of peanut butter, tahini, and soy sauce. Topping the salad with pan-seared chicken cutlets was a quick and fuss-free way to add protein and turn this dish into a well-rounded meal. You will need a spiralizer to make the beet and carrot noodles; if you don't have one, you can use precut store-bought vegetable noodles. You'll need about 12 ounces of each. Generously sized vegetables spiralize more easily, so use beets that are at least 1½ inches in diameter and carrots that are at least ¾ inch across at the thinnest end and 1½ inches across at the thickest end. You can use smooth or chunky peanut butter in the dressing for this recipe.

1 pound beets, trimmed and peeled
1 pound carrots, trimmed and peeled
¼ cup natural peanut butter
3 tablespoons tahini
2 tablespoons lime juice, plus lime wedges for serving
1 tablespoon low-sodium soy sauce
1 tablespoon grated fresh ginger
2 garlic cloves, minced
1 teaspoon table salt, divided
½ teaspoon toasted sesame oil
1–6 tablespoons hot tap water
5 scallions, sliced thin on bias
4 (6- to 8-ounce) boneless, skinless chicken breasts, trimmed
1 tablespoon avocado oil
½ cup fresh cilantro leaves

1 Using spiralizer, cut beets and carrots into ⅛-inch-thick noodles, cutting noodles into 6- to 8-inch lengths as you spiralize (about every 2 to 3 revolutions); set aside.

2 Whisk peanut butter, tahini, lime juice, soy sauce, ginger, garlic, ½ teaspoon salt, and sesame oil in large bowl until well combined. Whisking constantly, add hot water, 1 tablespoon at a time (up to 6 tablespoons), until dressing has consistency of heavy cream. Add beet and carrot noodles and scallions to dressing and toss to coat; set aside.

3 Gently pound thicker end of each breast until ½ inch thick. Pat breasts dry with paper towels. Brush both sides of breasts with avocado oil, then sprinkle with remaining ½ teaspoon salt. Place breasts, skinned side down, in 12-inch nonstick skillet, arranging narrow parts of breasts opposite wider parts. Place skillet over high heat and cook for 2 minutes. Flip breasts and cook for 2 minutes (there should be light browning).

4 Flip breasts, reduce heat to medium, and continue to cook, flipping breasts every 2 minutes, until exterior is well browned and thickest part of breast registers 155 degrees, 6 to 8 minutes. Transfer breasts to cutting board, tent with aluminum foil, and let rest for 10 minutes.

5 Slice chicken ¾ inch thick. Toss vegetable noodles to recoat in dressing and season with salt and pepper to taste. Transfer to serving platter and arrange chicken on top. Sprinkle with cilantro and serve with lime wedges.

MAKE IT GLUTEN-FREE · Substitute low-sodium tamari for the low-sodium soy sauce.

SPIRALIZING VEGETABLE NOODLES

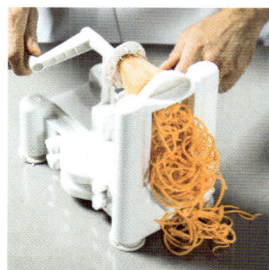

1 Trim vegetable so it will fit on prongs. Secure vegetable between prongs and blade surface. Spiralize by turning crank.

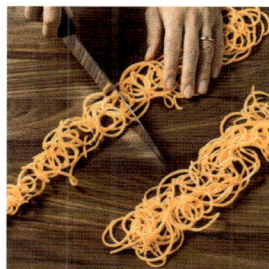

2 Pull noodles straight and cut into desired length.

Salmon and Watercress Salad with Grapefruit and Avocado

serves 4 • total time: 50 minutes **SUPERCHARGED**

why this recipe works • Seafood is an excellent way to turn a simple salad into a filling meal. Not only does it pack the protein, but it also offers additional nutrient benefits, including omega-3 fatty acids—as this simple salmon salad showcases. Add some avocado, too, and you've got a powerhouse duo that serves up an optimal dose of anti-inflammatory, heart-healthy fats. For sweet-tart contrast plus vibrant color, we added grapefruit, which also provided a welcome dose of fiber. We reserved some of the juice to use in a simple citrus vinaigrette infused with white wine vinegar and Dijon mustard. Watercress was just the right green for this salad: Its peppery punch beautifully balances the other flavorful ingredients. Finally, we added a sprinkle of crunchy toasted hazelnuts and torn mint leaves, which provided lively finishing touches. If using wild salmon, cook the fillets until they reach 120 degrees (for medium-rare) and start checking for doneness after 4 minutes.

- 2 (6- to 8-ounce) skin-on salmon fillets, 1 to 1½ inches thick
- 3 tablespoons plus 1 teaspoon extra-virgin olive oil, divided
- ¾ teaspoon table salt, divided
- ⅛ teaspoon pepper
- 2 red grapefruits
- 1 small shallot, minced
- 1 teaspoon white wine vinegar
- 1 teaspoon Dijon mustard
- 4 ounces (4 cups) watercress, torn into bite-size pieces
- 1 avocado, halved, pitted, and sliced ¼ inch thick
- ¼ cup hazelnuts, toasted, skinned, and chopped
- ¼ cup fresh mint leaves, torn

1 Adjust oven rack to lowest position, place aluminum foil–lined rimmed baking sheet on rack, and heat oven to 500 degrees. Make 4 or 5 shallow slashes, about 1 inch apart, on skin side of each fillet, being careful not to cut into flesh. Pat salmon dry with paper towels, rub with 1 teaspoon oil, and sprinkle with ¼ teaspoon salt and pepper.

2 Reduce oven temperature to 275 degrees and remove sheet from oven. Carefully place salmon skin side down on prepared sheet. Roast until center is still translucent when checked with tip of paring knife and registers 125 degrees (for medium-rare), 8 to 12 minutes. Transfer salmon to plate and let cool slightly, about 15 minutes.

3 Meanwhile, cut away peel and pith from grapefruits. Holding fruit over bowl, use paring knife to slice between membranes to release segments. Measure out 2 tablespoons grapefruit juice and transfer to separate bowl.

4 Using 2 forks, flake salmon into rough 2-inch pieces, discarding skin. Whisk shallot, vinegar, mustard, and remaining ½ teaspoon salt into bowl with grapefruit juice. Whisking constantly, slowly drizzle in remaining 3 tablespoons oil until emulsified. Season with salt and pepper to taste. Arrange watercress in even layer on serving platter. Top with salmon pieces, grapefruit segments, and avocado. Drizzle dressing over top, then sprinkle with hazelnuts and mint. Serve.

MAKE AHEAD • Roasted salmon can be refrigerated for up to 3 days.

Nutrition Knowledge This salmon and watercress salad is packed with anti-inflammatory ingredients. The omega-3s from salmon and polyphenols from grapefruit help reduce oxidative stress and support heart health. Watercress and hazelnuts provide additional antioxidants, while avocado offers gut-healthy fiber and fats. The mint and shallots, offering a nice boost of vitamin C, are the cherries on top.
—*Alicia*

Mediterranean Tuna Salad

serves 4 • total time: 30 minutes **FAST**

why this recipe works • For a tuna salad that is light and bright rather than heavy and creamy, we bypassed the mayo and instead opened a jar of oil-packed sun-dried tomatoes. Their concentrated sweet-tangy flavor was the perfect enhancement to plain canned tuna. We also didn't let the flavor-packed oil from the jar go to waste; it became an ideal base for a lemony vinaigrette that imbued every bite of our salad with warm Mediterranean flavor. Meaty cannellini beans and briny olives brought salty, savory balance to the tart dressing, while a bed of tender Bibb lettuce gave every bite a refreshing crunch. And what is tuna salad without celery providing some crunch and a mildly bitter contrast? For prominent celery flavor and even more fiber, we used both the celery ribs and the leaves, which was just the refreshing note our tuna salad needed.

2 shallots, sliced thin
3 tablespoons lemon juice
2 teaspoons Dijon mustard
1 garlic clove, minced
½ teaspoon table salt
½ teaspoon pepper
¼ cup oil-packed sun-dried tomatoes, rinsed, patted dry, and minced, plus 6 tablespoons sun-dried tomato oil
2 (6-ounce) cans solid white tuna in water, drained and flaked
1 head Bibb lettuce (8 ounces), torn into 1-inch pieces
1 cup canned no-salt-added cannellini beans, rinsed
4 celery ribs, sliced thin on bias, plus ½ cup celery leaves
½ cup pitted kalamata olives, sliced thin

1 Whisk shallots, lemon juice, mustard, garlic, salt, and pepper together in large bowl. Whisking constantly, slowly drizzle in sun-dried tomato oil until emulsified; set aside for 5 minutes.

2 Toss sun-dried tomatoes and tuna with 2 tablespoons vinaigrette. In separate bowl, toss lettuce with 2 tablespoons vinaigrette to coat. Season tomato mixture and lettuce with salt and pepper to taste. Arrange lettuce in even layer on serving platter. Top with tomato mixture, beans, celery, and olives. Drizzle with remaining vinaigrette and sprinkle with celery leaves. Serve.

Carrot and Endive Salad with Smoked Salmon

serves 4 to 6 · total time: 1¼ hours

why this recipe works · This colorful salad uses all of the carrot—greens and root!—in multiple ways. Carrots with their greens attached are sweeter than bagged carrots, and the feathery greens are fresh and slightly reminiscent of parsley. We shaved a portion of the carrots into ribbons and pickled them, which accentuated their pleasing crunch and gave them a tangy edge; we then roasted the remaining carrots to bring out their earthy sweetness. Tossing the roasted carrots with a Dijon-dill vinaigrette while they were still slightly warm allowed them to absorb even more of the dressing's citrusy flavor. Smoked salmon made a perfect addition: Not only did it add richness and brininess, but it also contributed heart-healthy protein to make this a filling, meal-worthy recipe. Finally, we incorporated raw endive for its crisp bite and color contrast, as well as grapefruit for sweet-tart flavor. Parsley can be substituted for the carrot greens. You should have about 1½ pounds of carrots after trimming the carrot greens.

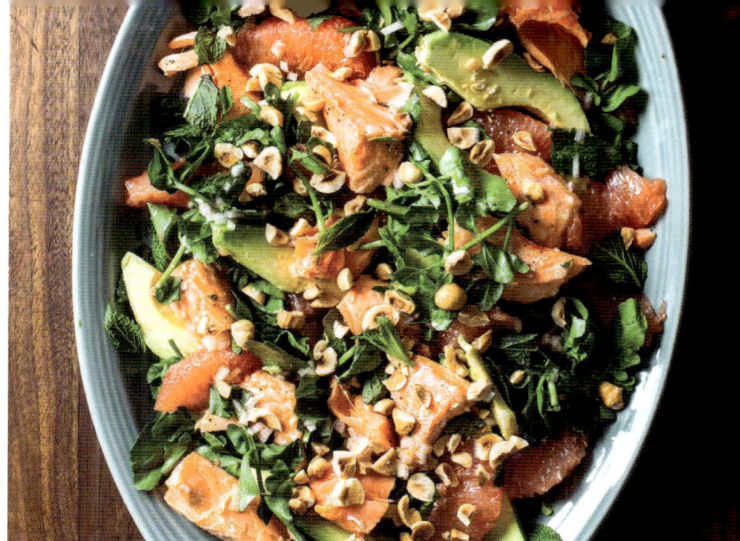

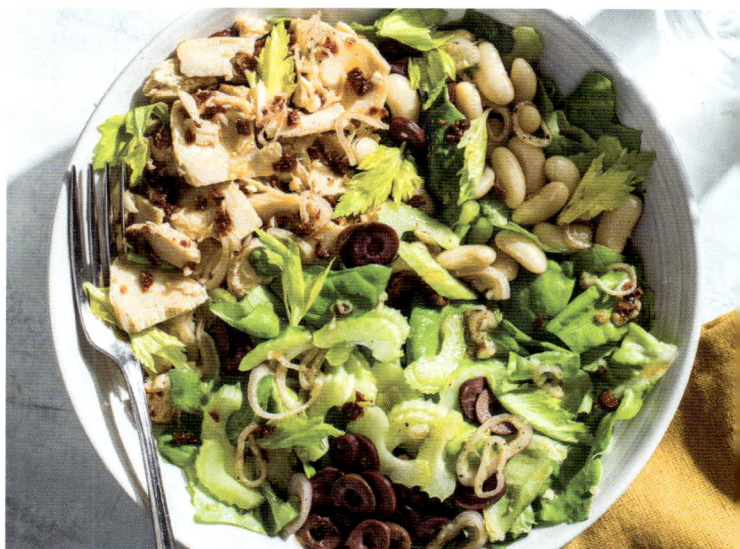

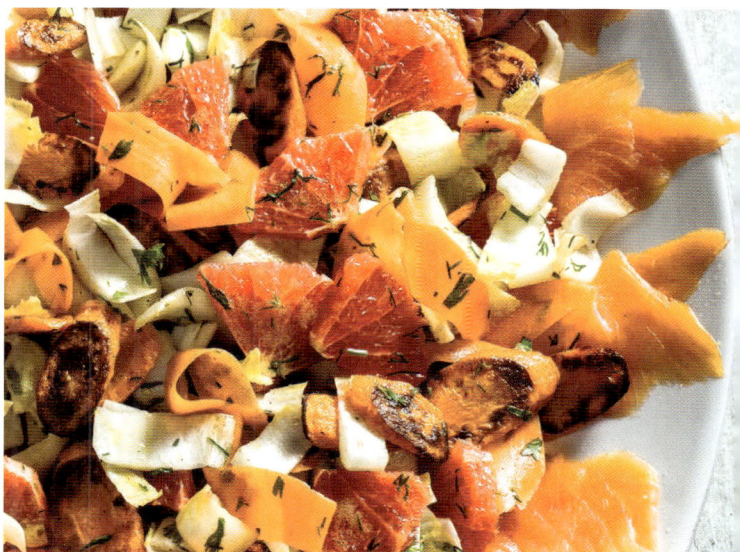

top	Salmon and Watercress Salad with Grapefruit and Avocado
middle	Mediterranean Tuna Salad
bottom	Carrot and Endive Salad with Smoked Salmon

2 pounds carrots with greens attached, divided, ¼ cup
    greens chopped
  5 tablespoons cider vinegar, divided
  ⅛ teaspoon plus ¾ teaspoon table salt, divided
  ¼ cup extra-virgin olive oil, divided
  ¼ teaspoon pepper
  1 red grapefruit
  2 tablespoons chopped fresh dill
  2 teaspoons Dijon mustard
  2 heads Belgian endive (4 ounces each), halved, cored,
    and sliced ½ inch thick
  8 ounces smoked salmon

1 Adjust oven rack to lowest position and heat oven to
450 degrees. Peel and shave 4 ounces carrots into thin ribbons
with vegetable peeler; set aside. Peel and slice remaining carrots
on bias ¼ inch thick; set aside.

2 Microwave ¼ cup vinegar and ⅛ teaspoon salt in bowl until
simmering, 1 to 2 minutes. Stir in shaved carrots and let sit,
stirring occasionally, for 45 minutes.

3 Toss sliced carrots with 1 tablespoon oil, pepper, and ½ teaspoon
salt in bowl, then spread in single layer on rimmed baking sheet,
cut side down. Roast until tender and bottoms are well browned,
15 to 25 minutes. Let cool slightly, about 15 minutes.

4 Meanwhile, cut away peel and pith from grapefruit. Quarter
grapefruit, then slice crosswise into ¼-inch-thick pieces.

5 Whisk dill, mustard, remaining 1 tablespoon vinegar, and
remaining ¼ teaspoon salt together in large bowl. Whisking
constantly, slowly drizzle in remaining 3 tablespoons oil until
emulsified. Add endive, carrot greens, roasted carrots, pickled
carrots, and grapefruit and toss to combine. Season with salt and
pepper to taste. Arrange salmon around edge of serving platter,
then transfer salad to center of platter. Serve.

MAKE AHEAD • Drained pickled carrots can be refrigerated
for up to 5 days.

Fennel and Apple Salad with Smoked Trout

serves 4 · total time: 20 minutes   FAST

why this recipe works · We enjoy a creamy seafood salad as
much as the next person, but many versions can be quite heavy
with mayonnaise. For an anti-inflammatory take on seafood
salad, we started with smoked trout, an excellent source of
unsaturated fats, vitamin D, and protein. We then deconstructed
the salad, flaking the fish atop a mix of piquant arugula and
crunchy, aromatic fennel—a wonderful but underutilized salad
candidate. Granny Smith apples contributed a little sweetness and
more crunch, and we made sure to leave the skin on to obtain all
the fruit's fiber and vitamin C. Instead of a mayo-based dressing,
we made a simple lemon and oil vinaigrette with fresh tarragon,
shallot, and tangy whole-grain mustard that brought all the
ingredients together in a much lighter way, letting the individual
elements shine through. Smoked mackerel can be substituted for
the smoked trout.

  3 tablespoons lemon juice
  1 tablespoon whole-grain mustard
  1 small shallot, minced
  2 teaspoons minced fresh tarragon, divided
  ½ teaspoon table salt
  ¼ teaspoon pepper
  ¼ cup extra-virgin olive oil
  5 ounces (5 cups) baby arugula
  2 Granny Smith apples, cored and cut into 3-inch-long
    matchsticks
  1 fennel bulb, stalks discarded, bulb halved, cored, and
    sliced thin
  8 ounces smoked trout, skin and pin bones removed, flaked

1 Whisk lemon juice, mustard, shallot, 1 teaspoon tarragon, salt,
and pepper together in large bowl. Whisking constantly, slowly
drizzle in oil until emulsified. Add arugula, apples, and fennel and
toss gently to coat. Season with salt and pepper to taste.

2 Transfer salad to serving platter, top with flaked trout, and
sprinkle with remaining 1 teaspoon tarragon. Serve.

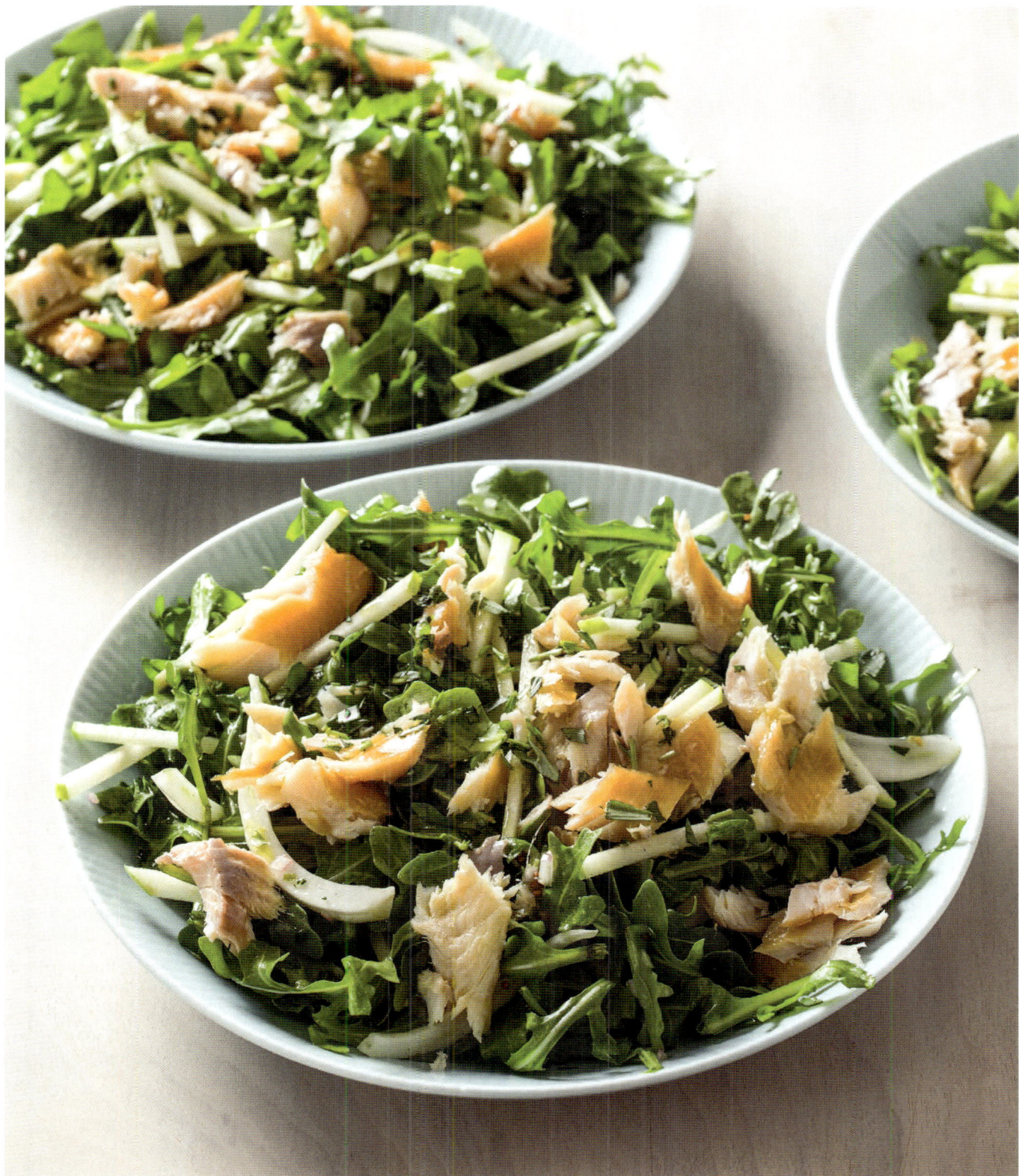

Fennel and Apple Salad with Smoked Trout

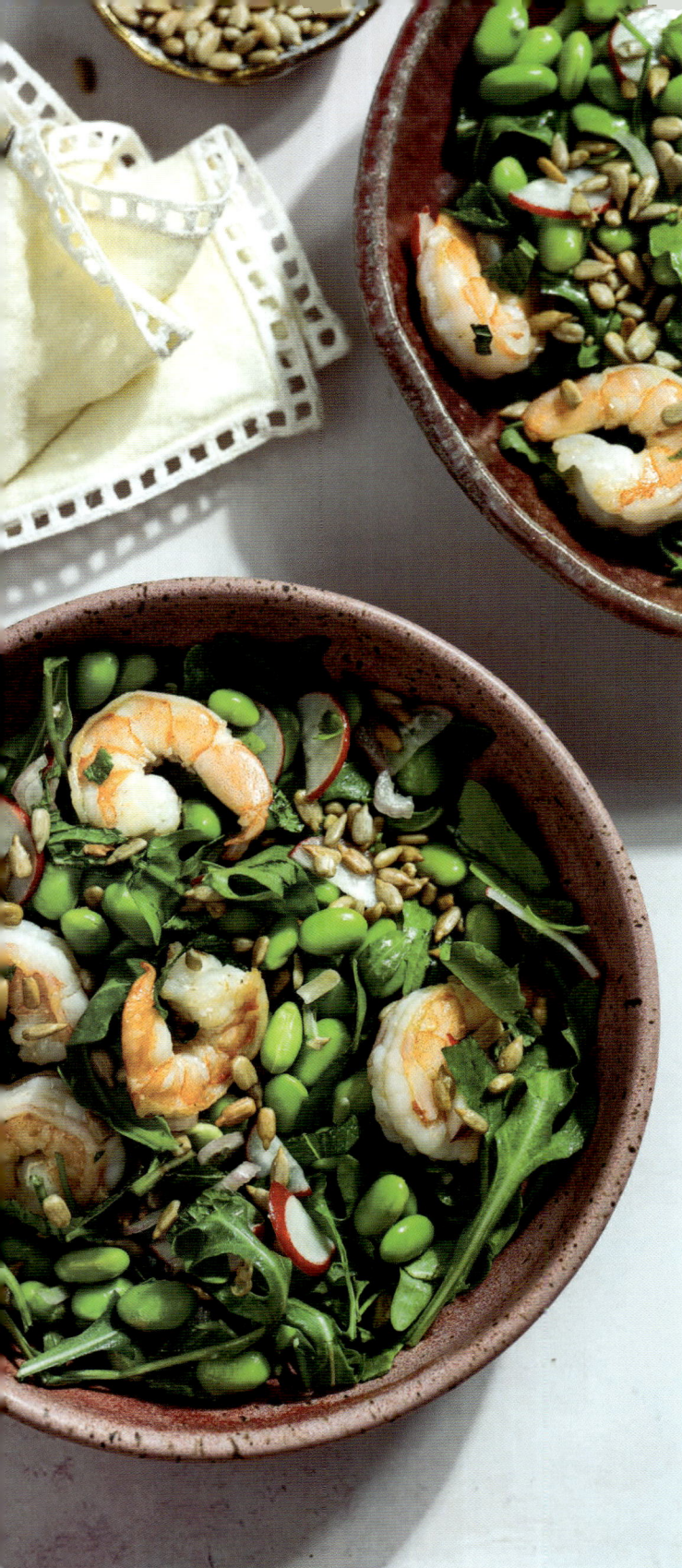

Edamame and Shrimp Salad

serves 4 • total time: 25 minutes **FAST**

why this recipe works • Edamame, which are immature soy beans, make a great addition to salads—they're ultrahigh in protein, plus their bright, fresh flavor and satisfying bite pair perfectly with leafy greens. However, their mild flavor is easily overwhelmed by tart vinaigrettes and other bold salad elements. That's why we chose to dress this salad with rice vinegar; its mild acidity allowed the flavor of the edamame to come through, and a little honey helped emulsify the dressing and added a hint of sweetness. The subtle pepperiness and delicate, tender leaves of baby arugula worked well as a flavor and texture complement, while sweet sautéed shrimp turned this bright salad into a substantial, dinner-worthy meal. Mint and basil contributed light, summery vibes, thinly sliced shallot offered mild allium notes, and radishes provided crunch and color. Garlic added aroma and flavor without overpowering the mild flavor profile, and a sprinkling of roasted sunflower seeds brought nuttiness, depth, and healthy fat.

12 ounces extra-large shrimp (21 to 25 per pound), peeled, deveined, and tails removed
1¼ teaspoons table salt, divided
¼ teaspoon pepper
1 tablespoon avocado oil
2 tablespoons unseasoned rice vinegar
1 tablespoon honey
1 small garlic clove, minced
3 tablespoons extra-virgin olive oil
3 cups frozen shelled edamame, thawed and patted dry
2 ounces (2 cups) baby arugula
½ cup shredded fresh basil
½ cup chopped fresh mint
2 radishes, trimmed, halved, and sliced thin
1 shallot, halved and sliced thin
¼ cup roasted unsalted sunflower seeds

1 Pat shrimp dry with paper towels and sprinkle with ¼ teaspoon salt and pepper. Heat avocado oil in 12-inch nonstick skillet over medium-high heat until just smoking. Add shrimp in single layer and cook, without stirring, until spotty brown and edges turn pink on bottom, about 1 minute. Flip shrimp and continue to cook until all but very center is opaque, about 30 seconds. Transfer shrimp to plate and let cool slightly, about 5 minutes.

2 Whisk vinegar, honey, garlic, and remaining 1 teaspoon salt together in large bowl. Whisking constantly, slowly drizzle in olive oil until emulsified. Add shrimp, edamame, arugula, basil, mint, radishes, and shallot and toss to combine. Season with salt and pepper to taste. Transfer salad to serving platter, sprinkle with sunflower seeds, and serve.

MAKE AHEAD • Sautéed shrimp can be refrigerated for up to 3 days.

HOW TO PEEL AND DEVEIN SHRIMP

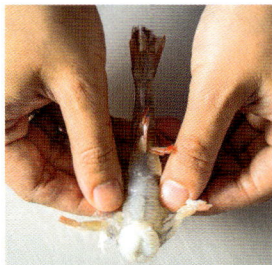

1 Break shell on underside, under swimming legs, which will come off as shell is removed.

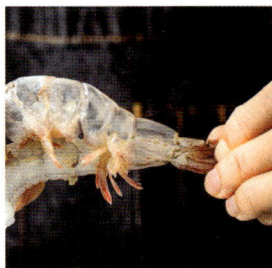

2 If recipe calls for removing tails, tug tail to remove shell. If not removing tails, pinch tail to hold in place while removing shell.

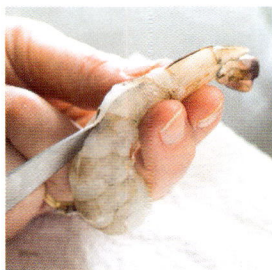

3 Using paring knife, make shallow cut along back of shrimp to expose vein-like digestive tract.

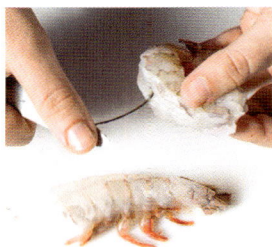

4 Using tip of knife, lift out vein. Discard vein by wiping knife blade against paper towel.

Napa Cabbage Salad with Tofu and Creamy Miso Dressing

serves 4 • total time: 45 minutes **FAST**

why this recipe works • We love the silky texture of cooked napa cabbage but find its raw flavor and texture—crisp, light, and leafy—equally delightful. This salad makes napa cabbage the star, pairing it with protein-dense tofu and a creamy cashew-based dressing for a hearty and texturally diverse meal. While tofu can be a bit bland on its own, it readily absorbed the flavor of the dressing, and pan-searing one side of the slices developed a crisp, burnished top and provided some welcome texture. Crisp snow peas and grated carrot added pops of color and also played well with this salad's light, clean flavor profile. Squeeze juice from your orange trimmings into the salad dressing, if desired.

Dressing

- ½ cup raw cashews
- ⅓ cup water, plus extra as needed
- 2 tablespoons unseasoned rice vinegar
- 2 tablespoons grated fresh ginger
- 1 tablespoons white miso
- 1 tablespoon low-sodium soy sauce
- ½ teaspoon toasted sesame oil
- ¼ teaspoon cayenne pepper

Salad

- 14 ounces firm tofu, cut crosswise into ½-inch-thick slabs
- ¼ teaspoon table salt
- 2 tablespoons avocado oil
- ¼ cup raw cashews, chopped
- 5 scallions, whites and green parts separated and sliced thin on bias
- 1 tablespoon sesame seeds
- 2 oranges
- 4 cups thinly sliced napa cabbage
- 6 ounces snow peas, strings removed, halved crosswise
- 1 cup grated carrot
- ½ cup fresh mint and/or cilantro leaves, divided

1 **For the dressing** Process cashews in blender on low speed until finely ground, about 15 seconds. Add water, vinegar, ginger, miso, soy sauce, oil, and cayenne and process on low speed until combined, about 5 seconds. Scrape down sides of blender jar and let mixture sit for 15 minutes.

2 Process cashew mixture on low speed until all ingredients are well blended, about 1 minute. Scrape down sides of blender jar, then continue to process on high speed until dressing is smooth and creamy, about 4 minutes. Adjust consistency of dressing with water as needed; set aside.

3 For the salad Spread tofu over paper towel–lined plate. Gently pat dry with paper towels and sprinkle with salt. Heat oil in 12-inch nonstick skillet over medium-high heat until just smoking. Add tofu and cook until golden brown and crisp on one side, about 5 minutes; transfer to plate browned side up.

4 Add cashews, scallion whites, and sesame seeds to fat left in skillet and cook, stirring constantly, until fragrant, about 1 minute; transfer to small bowl.

5 Cut away peel and pith from oranges. Quarter oranges, then slice crosswise into ¼-inch-thick pieces. Toss half of oranges, cabbage, snow peas, carrot, ¼ cup mint, and scallion greens together with half of dressing in large bowl. Season with salt and pepper to taste. Arrange salad on serving platter, top with tofu and remaining oranges, and sprinkle with cashew-scallion topping and remaining ¼ cup mint. Serve, passing remaining dressing separately.

MAKE AHEAD • Dressing can be prepared through step 2 and refrigerated for up to 1 week; bring it to room temperature and adjust the consistency with water before tossing it with the salad.

MAKE IT GLUTEN-FREE • Substitute low-sodium tamari for the low-sodium soy sauce.

Chopped Winter Salad with Butternut Squash and Apple

serves 4 • total time: 50 minutes

why this recipe works • The dense, satisfying texture of winter vegetables makes them perfect for starring in a filling main-course salad. That's why we decided to feature butternut squash in this salad: It's creamy and pleasantly sweet, and it readily absorbs seasonings. We deepened the squash's flavor by cutting it into pieces and tossing the pieces with balsamic vinegar and oil before roasting them. The caramelized vinegar perfectly complemented the squash's earthiness. We topped romaine and red-hued, bitter-spicy radicchio with the tender squash, plus some crunchy apple and toasted hazelnuts. Feta cheese studded the final dish with rich, creamy notes. We prefer Fuji apples, but any sweet apple will work here.

> 2 pounds butternut squash, peeled, seeded, and cut into ½-inch pieces (4½ cups)
> ¼ cup extra-virgin olive oil, divided
> 3 tablespoons balsamic vinegar, divided
> ¼ teaspoon plus ⅛ teaspoon table salt, divided
> ¼ teaspoon plus ⅛ teaspoon pepper, divided
> 1 tablespoon Dijon mustard
> 1 small head radicchio (6 ounces), trimmed, cored, and sliced ½ inch thick
> 1 romaine lettuce heart (6 ounces), cored and cut into 1-inch pieces
> 1 Fuji, Macintosh, or Red Delicious apple, unpeeled, halved, cored, and cut into ½-inch pieces
> ½ cup skinned hazelnuts, almonds, or pecans, toasted and chopped
> 2 ounces feta cheese or goat cheese (½ cup), crumbled

1 Adjust oven rack to lowest position and heat oven to 450 degrees. Toss squash with 1 tablespoon oil, 1½ teaspoons balsamic vinegar, ¼ teaspoon salt, and ¼ teaspoon pepper.

2 Spread squash in single layer on aluminum foil–lined rimmed baking sheet and roast until well browned and tender, 20 to 25 minutes, stirring halfway through roasting. Remove sheet from oven and let squash cool slightly, about 10 minutes.

3 Whisk mustard, remaining 2½ tablespoons balsamic vinegar, remaining ⅛ teaspoon salt, and remaining ⅛ teaspoon pepper together in large bowl. Whisking constantly, slowly drizzle in remaining 3 tablespoons oil until emulsified.

4 Add radicchio, romaine, and apple to bowl with dressing and toss to combine. Season with salt and pepper to taste. Transfer salad to serving platter and top with squash, hazelnuts, and feta. Serve.

MAKE AHEAD • Roasted squash can be refrigerated for up to 3 days; let it come to room temperature before assembling salad.

MAKE IT DAIRY-FREE • Omit the feta cheese or substitute plant-based feta-style cheese.

Roasted Cauliflower and Grape Salad with Chermoula

serves 4 · total time: 45 minutes   **FAST**   **SUPERCHARGED**

why this recipe works · Heady with cilantro, bright with lemon juice, and aromatic with warm spices, the North African herb sauce chermoula is often used as a marinade for meat and fish. We thought the flavorful, antioxidant-rich sauce would also be perfect for dressing up mild, nutty cauliflower—a highly nutritious vegetable rich in phytonutrients, antioxidants, and fiber—and give it a tremendous flavor boost. We started by simply cutting a head of cauliflower into florets and roasting them until caramelized. Polyphenol-rich grapes roasted alongside it for some sweet contrast. A sprinkling of fresh cilantro and crunchy walnuts provided the perfect finishing touch.

Chermoula

- 1 cup fresh cilantro or parsley leaves
- 5 tablespoons extra-virgin olive oil
- 2 tablespoons lemon juice
- 4 garlic cloves, minced
- ½ teaspoon ground cumin
- ½ teaspoon paprika
- ¼ teaspoon table salt
- ⅛ teaspoon cayenne pepper

Salad

- 1 head cauliflower (2 pounds), cored and cut into 1-inch florets
- 1 cup seedless red grapes
- ½ small red onion, sliced thin
- 2 tablespoons extra-virgin olive oil
- ½ teaspoon table salt
- ¼ teaspoon pepper
- 2 tablespoons fresh cilantro or parsley leaves
- 2 tablespoons coarsely chopped toasted walnuts or sliced almonds

1   For the chermoula Process all ingredients in food processor until smooth, about 1 minute, scraping down sides of bowl as needed; set aside.

2   For the salad Adjust oven rack to lowest position and heat oven to 475 degrees. Toss cauliflower, grapes, onion, oil, salt, and pepper together in bowl. Transfer to rimmed baking sheet and roast until vegetables are tender, florets are deep golden, and onion slices are charred at edges, 12 to 15 minutes, stirring halfway through roasting. Remove sheet from oven and let cauliflower mixture cool slightly, about 10 minutes.

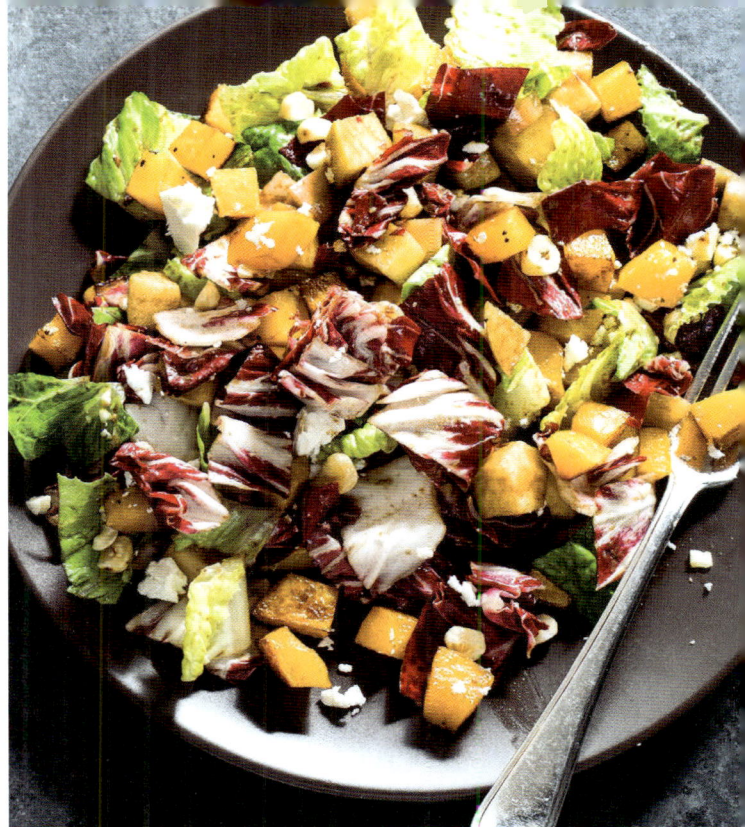

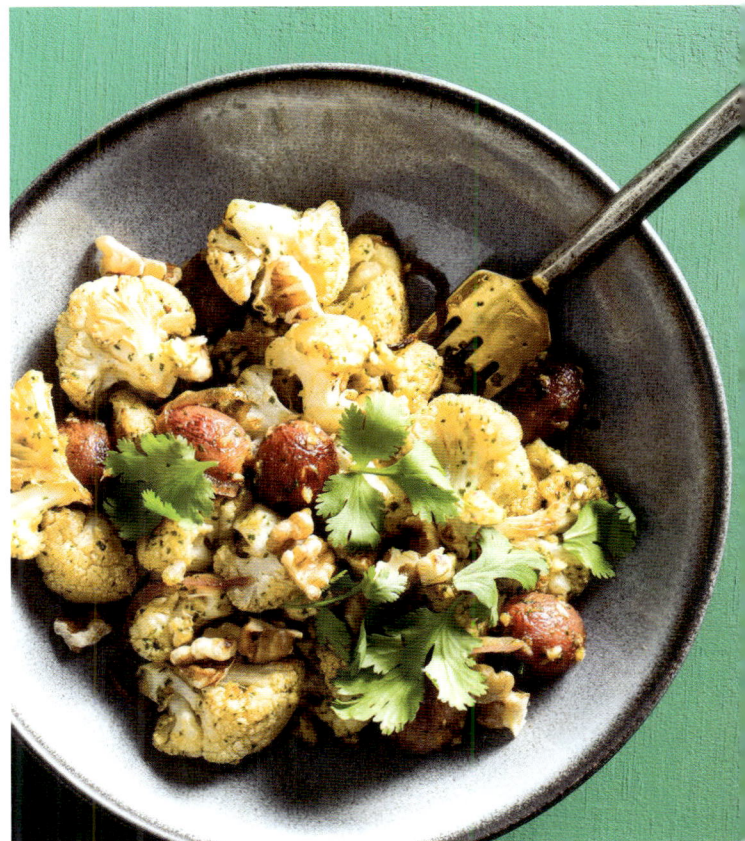

top | Chopped Winter Salad with Butternut Squash and Apple
bottom | Roasted Cauliflower and Grape Salad with Chermoula

3 Gently toss cauliflower mixture with chermoula until well coated. Season with salt and pepper to taste. Transfer cauliflower mixture to serving platter and sprinkle with cilantro and walnuts. Serve.

MAKE AHEAD • Chermoula and roasted cauliflower can be refrigerated separately for up to 3 days; let them come to room temperature before proceeding with step 3.

Roasted Carrot and Beet Salad with Harissa

serves 4 • total time: 40 minutes   **FAST**

why this recipe works • We drew inspiration from the vegetable dishes of Tunisia to develop this flavorful salad. Coating the vegetables with harissa, a spicy, aromatic chili paste, ensured bold flavor in every bite. Roasting the harissa-coated vegetables coaxed out their natural sweetness while deepening the harissa's complementary heat. Tossing the still-warm veggies with lemon juice, parsley, and a fresh hit of harissa gave us a beautifully balanced salad. Hard-cooked eggs and olives are traditional additions to many Tunisian dishes, and they make this salad substantial enough to be a light meal. Toasted almonds added a welcome crunch. We prefer our homemade Harissa (recipe follows), but you can use store-bought.

  1 pound beets, peeled and cut into ½-inch wedges
  1 pound carrots, peeled and cut ¼ inch thick on bias
  6 shallots, peeled and halved lengthwise
  3 tablespoons harissa, divided
  2 tablespoons extra-virgin olive oil
  1 tablespoon grated lemon zest plus 2 tablespoons juice
  ½ teaspoon table salt
  ¼ teaspoon pepper
  ¼ cup pitted oil-cured olives, halved
  3 tablespoons chopped fresh parsley
  3 Easy-Peel Hard-Cooked Eggs (page 31), quartered
  ¼ cup whole almonds, toasted and chopped

1 Adjust oven racks to upper-middle and lower-middle positions and heat oven to 450 degrees. Toss beets, carrots, and shallots with 1 tablespoon harissa, oil, lemon zest, salt, and pepper in large bowl. Spread in single layer over 2 rimmed baking sheets. (Do not wash bowl.) Roast until vegetables are tender and well browned on one side, 20 to 25 minutes (do not stir during roasting). Remove sheet from oven and let vegetables cool slightly, about 10 minutes.

2 Whisk lemon juice and remaining 2 tablespoons harissa in now-empty bowl. Gently toss roasted vegetables with harissa mixture until well coated. Stir in olives and parsley and season with salt and pepper to taste. Transfer vegetables to serving platter, arrange egg quarters over top, and sprinkle with almonds. Serve.

MAKE AHEAD • Roasted vegetables can be refrigerated for up to 3 days; let them come to room temperature before tossing with the harissa dressing.

Harissa

makes 1 cup • total time: 10 minutes

  ¾ cup extra-virgin olive oil
 12 garlic cloves, minced
  ¼ cup paprika
  2 tablespoons ground coriander
  2 tablespoons ground dried Aleppo pepper
  2 teaspoons ground cumin
1½ teaspoons caraway seeds
  1 teaspoon table salt

Combine all ingredients in bowl and microwave until bubbling and very fragrant, about 1 minute, stirring halfway through microwaving. Let cool completely before serving. (Harissa can be refrigerated for up to 4 days. Bring to room temperature before serving.)

Roasted Pattypan Squash Salad with Dandelion Green Pesto

serves 4 • total time: 1 hour

why this recipe works • Pattypan squash has a flavor reminiscent of zucchini, but its unique scalloped edges give it an advantage when it comes to providing texture. Pattypans come in different sizes; for this salad, we used baby green and yellow ones for their tender skin and vibrant flavor (some say the squash loses flavor as it matures). Before roasting the diminutive squashes, we cut them horizontally to make flower-shaped slabs, which we tossed, along with fresh-off-the-cob corn, in a little oil. We counter these fresh ingredients with an earthy-tasting pesto made from dandelion greens and roasted sunflower seeds. You can use baby arugula or watercress instead of dandelion greens. Use baby pattypan squashes that measure between 1½ and 2 inches in diameter. If you can't find baby pattypans, you can use zucchini or summer squash cut crosswise into 1-inch-thick rounds.

Pesto

- 1 ounce dandelion greens, trimmed and torn into bite-size pieces (1 cup)
- 3 tablespoons roasted unsalted sunflower seeds
- 3 tablespoons water
- 1 tablespoon maple syrup
- 1 tablespoon cider vinegar
- 1 garlic clove, minced
- ¼ teaspoon table salt
- ⅛ teaspoon red pepper flakes
- ¼ cup extra-virgin olive oil

Salad

- 2 tablespoons extra-virgin olive oil
- ½ teaspoon table salt
- ⅛ teaspoon pepper
- 1½ pounds baby pattypan squash, halved horizontally
- 4 ears corn, kernels cut from cobs
- 1 pound ripe tomatoes, cored, cut into ½-inch-thick wedges, and wedges halved crosswise
- 1 ounce dandelion greens, trimmed and torn into bite-size pieces (1 cup)
- 2 tablespoons roasted unsalted sunflower seeds

1   For the pesto Adjust oven rack to lowest position, place rimmed baking sheet on rack, and heat oven to 500 degrees. Process dandelion greens, sunflower seeds, water, maple syrup, vinegar, garlic, salt, and pepper flakes in food processor until finely ground, about 1 minute, scraping down sides of bowl as needed. With processor running, slowly drizzle in oil until incorporated.

2   For the salad Whisk oil, salt, and pepper together in large bowl. Add squash and corn and toss to coat. Working quickly, spread vegetables in single layer on hot sheet, arranging squash cut side down. Roast until cut side of squash is browned and tender, 15 to 18 minutes. Remove sheet from oven and let squash mixture cool slightly, about 10 minutes.

3   Gently toss roasted squash mixture, half of pesto, tomatoes, and dandelion greens together until well coated. Transfer squash mixture to serving platter, drizzle with remaining pesto, and sprinkle with sunflower seeds. Serve.

MAKE AHEAD • Pesto can be refrigerated for up to 2 days; press plastic wrap flush against surface of the pesto to minimize discoloration.

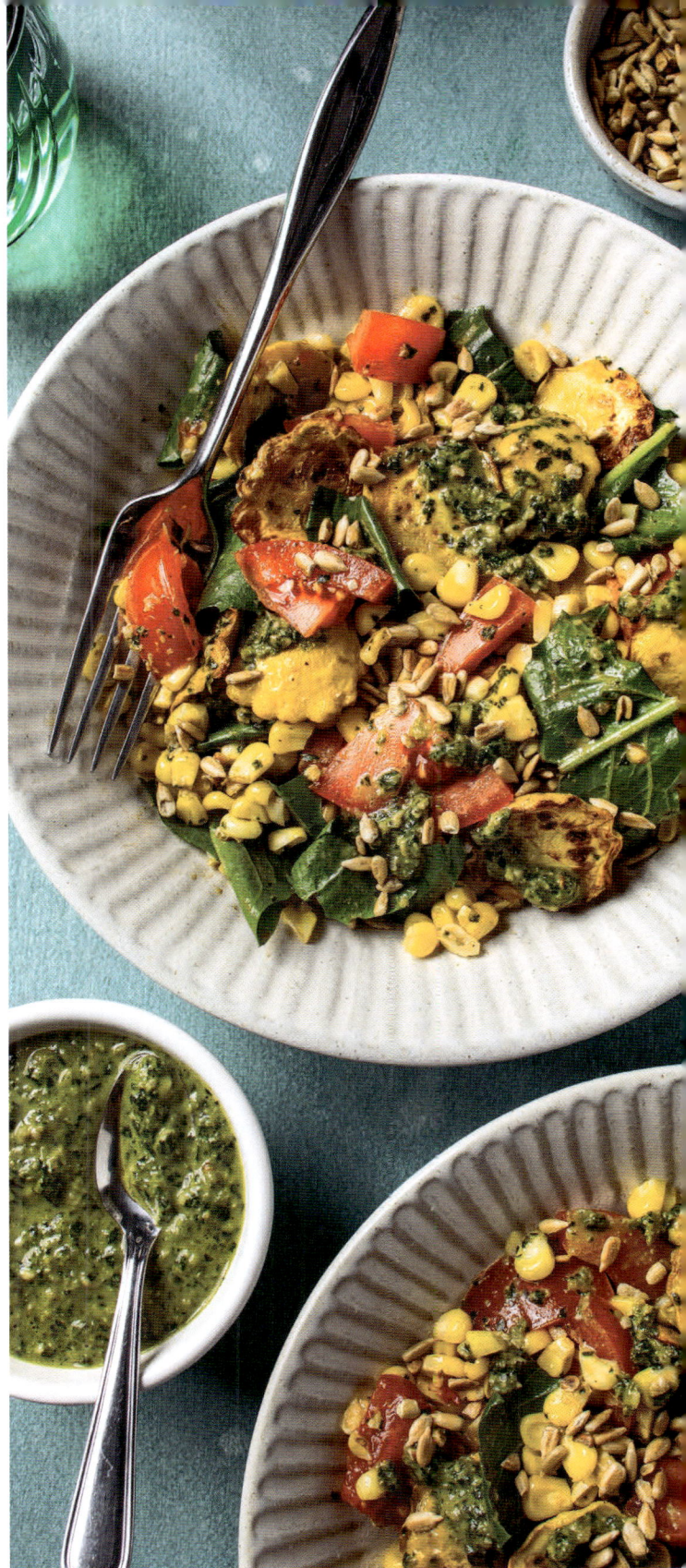

Roasted Pattypan Squash Salad with Dandelion Green Pesto

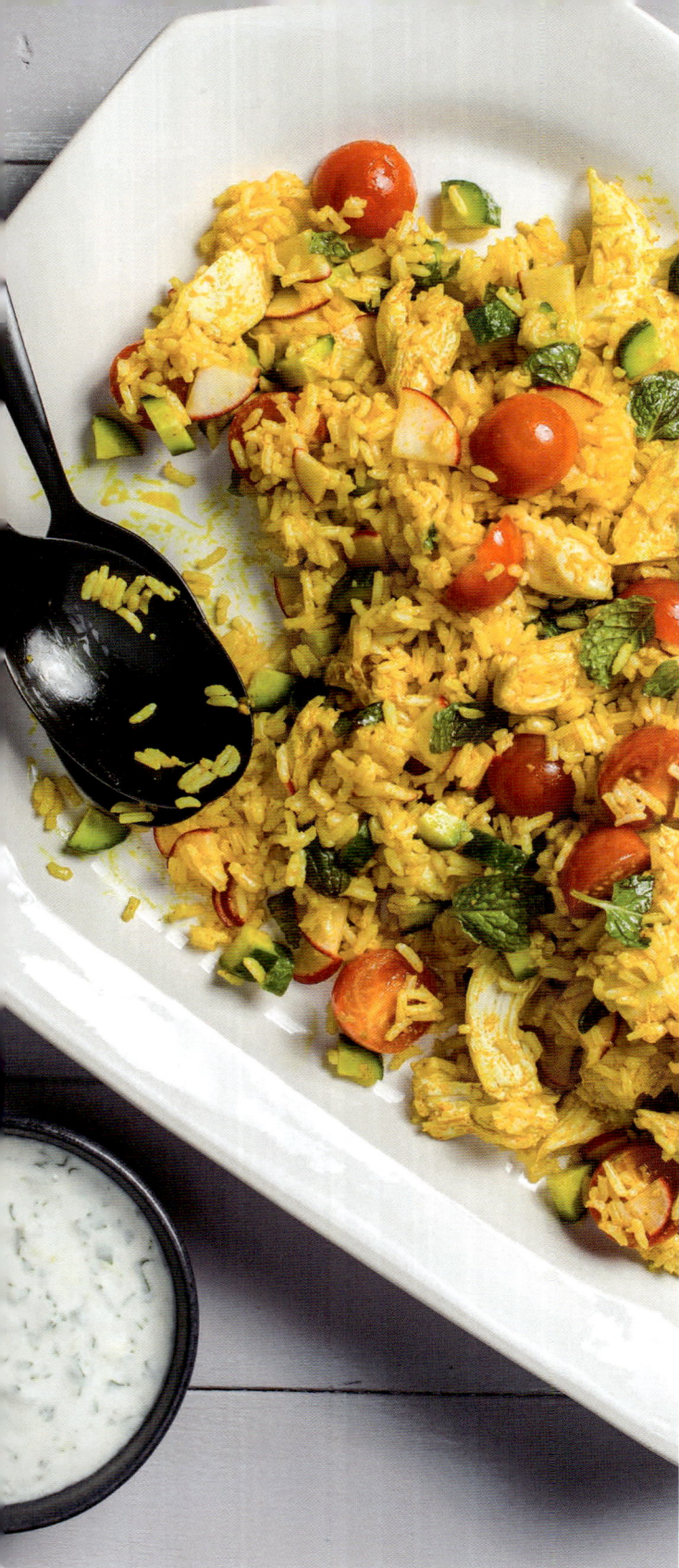

Turmeric Rice and Chicken Salad with Herbs

serves 4 · total time: 1 hour · **SUPERCHARGED**

why this recipe works · Shawarma, a street-food favorite throughout the Levant, inspired this rice and chicken salad. We started with traditional shawarma seasonings such as garlic, turmeric, paprika, cumin, and cinnamon, all of which happen to be excellent sources of inflammation-fighting antioxidants. Microwaving them with oil intensified their flavors. We love the fiber boost from brown rice, but wanted to ensure that it wouldn't stick together or get hard as it cooled; to do this, we boiled the gut-healthy grains in an abundance of salted water and then spread them on a baking sheet to prevent clumping. We added crunchy sliced cucumbers, radishes, juicy tomatoes, cilantro, and mint, which brought bursts of freshness—plus more nutrients—to every bite. A lemony herbed yogurt, drizzled over the salad, tied all the flavors together. We like using Perfect Poached Chicken (page 92) here, but any cooked chicken would work.

Herb-Yogurt Sauce

- 1 cup plain whole-milk yogurt
- 1 teaspoon grated lemon zest plus 2 tablespoons juice
- 2 tablespoons minced fresh cilantro
- 2 tablespoons minced fresh mint
- 1 garlic clove, minced

Salad

- 1 cup long-grain brown rice
- ½ teaspoon table salt, plus salt for cooking rice
- 3 tablespoons extra-virgin olive oil
- 2 garlic cloves, minced
- 1 teaspoon ground cumin
- 1 teaspoon paprika
- 1 teaspoon ground turmeric
- ⅛ teaspoon cayenne pepper
  Pinch ground cinnamon
- 3 tablespoons lemon juice
- 2 cups chopped cooked chicken
- 6 ounces cherry tomatoes, halved
- 2 Persian cucumbers, quartered lengthwise and sliced crosswise ¼ inch thick
- 3 radishes, trimmed, quartered, and sliced thin
- 1 cup torn fresh cilantro
- 1 cup torn fresh mint

1 For the herb-yogurt sauce Whisk all ingredients together in bowl. Cover and refrigerate until ready to serve.

2 For the salad Bring 4 quarts water to boil in large pot. Add rice and 2½ teaspoons salt and cook, stirring occasionally, until rice is tender, 22 to 25 minutes. Drain rice, spread onto rimmed baking sheet, and let cool for 15 minutes.

3 Microwave oil, garlic, cumin, paprika, turmeric, cayenne, and cinnamon in medium bowl until fragrant, 30 to 60 seconds. Let cool slightly, then whisk in lemon juice and salt

4 Combine rice, dressing, chicken, tomatoes, cucumbers, radishes, cilantro, and mint in large bowl and toss to combine. Season with salt and pepper to taste. Serve with herb-yogurt sauce.

MAKE AHEAD • Yogurt sauce can be refrigerated for up to 4 days.

MAKE IT DAIRY-FREE • Substitute plant-based yogurt for the dairy yogurt.

Nutrition Knowledge I love that the sauce in this rice and chicken salad gets its creaminess from probiotic-rich yogurt, blending in mint and cilantro for antioxidants and punchy flavor. The choice of brown rice is great for digestive function, while turmeric (hello, curcumin!), cumin, and paprika make a delicious case for spicing your grains with antioxidant-rich seasonings. The lean chicken is a great protein source, plus a superb vehicle for all that flavor.   —*Alicia*

Harvest Salad with Wild Rice and Sweet Potatoes

serves 4 to 6 • total time: 1¾ hours

why this recipe works • When the chill of autumn is in the air, fall food calls to us. Hearty wild rice, caramelized roasted sweet potatoes, leafy green kale, and tart apples make for a seasonal salad that packs in fiber and tastes delicious to boot. A cider and caraway vinaigrette fit the autumnal theme; we toasted and cracked the caraway seeds but left them whole for texture. Feta cheese added briny contrast, while dried cranberries contributed sweet tang for the perfect finishing touches to this harvest meal. To crack the caraway seeds, rock the bottom edge of a skillet over the toasted seeds on a cutting board until they crack. You can substitute brown rice for the wild rice but will need to adjust the cooking time.

- ½ cup wild rice
- ½ teaspoon table salt, divided, plus salt for cooking rice
- 1 pound sweet potatoes, unpeeled, halved lengthwise and sliced crosswise ¼ inch thick
- 5 tablespoons extra-virgin olive oil, divided
- 2 tablespoons plus 2 teaspoons cider vinegar
- 4 teaspoons Dijon mustard
- 2 teaspoons caraway seeds, toasted and cracked
- ¼ teaspoon pepper
- 8 ounces (8 cups) baby kale
- 1 Granny Smith apple, cored and cut into ½-inch pieces
- 4 ounces feta cheese, crumbled (1 cup)
- ¼ cup dried cranberries

1 Bring 2 quarts water to boil in large saucepan. Add rice and ½ teaspoon salt and cook until rice is tender, 35 to 40 minutes. Drain rice, spread onto rimmed baking sheet, and let cool for 15 minutes.

2 Meanwhile, adjust oven rack to middle position and heat oven to 400 degrees. Toss potatoes, 1 tablespoon oil, and ¼ teaspoon salt together in bowl, then spread in even layer on aluminum foil–lined rimmed baking sheet. Roast until potatoes are beginning to brown, 15 to 20 minutes, flipping slices halfway through roasting. Let potatoes cool for 5 minutes.

3 Whisk vinegar, 2 tablespoons water, mustard, caraway seeds, pepper, and remaining ¼ teaspoon salt together in bowl. Whisking constantly, slowly drizzle in remaining ¼ cup oil until emulsified. Toss kale with half of vinaigrette in large bowl to coat, then season with salt and pepper to taste. Transfer to serving platter and top with cooled rice, cooled sweet potatoes, apple, feta, and cranberries. Drizzle with remaining vinaigrette and serve.

MAKE AHEAD • The rice and potatoes can be prepared through step 2 and refrigerated separately for up to 3 days; let them come to room temperature before assembling the salad.

MAKE IT DAIRY-FREE • Omit the feta cheese or substitute plant-based feta-style cheese.

Bulgur Salad with Curry Roasted Sweet Potatoes and Chickpeas

serves 4 to 6 • total time: 1¼ hours

why this recipe works • Bulgur is made from wheat berries that have been steamed or boiled and ground into fine, medium, coarse, or very coarse grains. Because it is parcooked, bulgur takes very little time to simmer and becomes somewhat tender while retaining its satisfying chew. Tabbouleh may be the most globally iconic bulgur dish; however, bulgur's potential for amping up salads shouldn't end there. For a satisfying dinner salad with layers of flavor, we combined bulgur with kale and topped it with protein-rich chickpeas and sweet potatoes spiced with curry powder. Tossing the chopped kale with the warm bulgur softened the sturdy leaves. We finished our salad with crumbles of creamy goat cheese, crunchy walnuts, and sweet-tart dried cranberries for a pop of color. Look for small sweet potatoes that weigh about 8 ounces each. Don't confuse bulgur with cracked wheat, which has a much longer cooking time and will not work in this recipe.

- 1 pound sweet potatoes, unpeeled, cut lengthwise into 1-inch-thick wedges
- 1 (15-ounce) can no-salt-added chickpeas, rinsed
- ½ cup extra-virgin olive oil, divided, plus extra for drizzling
- 1 tablespoon curry powder
- 1½ teaspoons table salt, divided, plus salt for cooking bulgur
- 1¼ cups medium-grind bulgur
- 5 tablespoons cider vinegar
- 6 ounces kale, stemmed and chopped
- 4 ounces goat cheese, crumbled (1 cup)
- ½ cup walnuts, toasted and chopped
- ⅓ cup dried cranberries

1 Adjust oven rack to middle position and heat oven to 450 degrees. Line rimmed baking sheet with parchment paper. Toss sweet potatoes, chickpeas, 1 tablespoon oil, curry powder, and ½ teaspoon salt together in large bowl. Arrange in single layer on prepared sheet. Roast until sweet potatoes are lightly browned and tender, about 20 minutes.

2 Meanwhile, bring 2 quarts water to boil in large saucepan. Add bulgur and 1 teaspoon salt, reduce heat to medium-low, and simmer until grains are tender, 5 to 8 minutes. Drain bulgur.

3 Whisk vinegar, remaining 7 tablespoons oil, and remaining 1 teaspoon salt together in now-empty bowl. Add drained bulgur and kale and toss to combine. Season with salt and pepper to taste. Transfer bulgur mixture to serving platter; top with sweet potatoes and chickpeas; and sprinkle with goat cheese, walnuts, and cranberries. Drizzle with extra oil and serve.

MAKE AHEAD • Roasted potatoes can be refrigerated for up to 3 days; let them come to room temperature before assembling salad.

MAKE IT DAIRY-FREE • Omit the goat cheese or substitute plant-based goat cheese–style cheese.

NOTES FROM THE TEST KITCHEN

Big and Little Bulgur

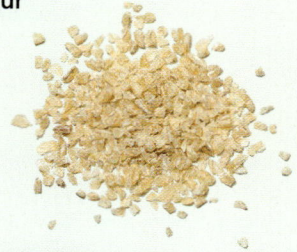

Bulgur has been a source of nutrition across the Mediterranean for roughly 4,000 years. It's made from par-boiled or steamed wheat kernels/berries that are then dried, partially stripped of their outer bran layer, and ground. The result is a fast-cooking, highly nutritious grain. Chewy-firm coarse-grind bulgur, which requires simmering, is our choice for pilaf; we like medium-grind bulgur best in salads in which it's soaked or simmered until tender; fine-grind bulgur rehydrates into a seamless binder for dishes such as baked kibbeh. Fine granules are similar in size to raw sugar, medium granules are similar to mustard seeds, and coarse granules are about the size of sesame seeds. Cracked wheat, sold alongside bulgur, is not precooked and cannot be substituted.

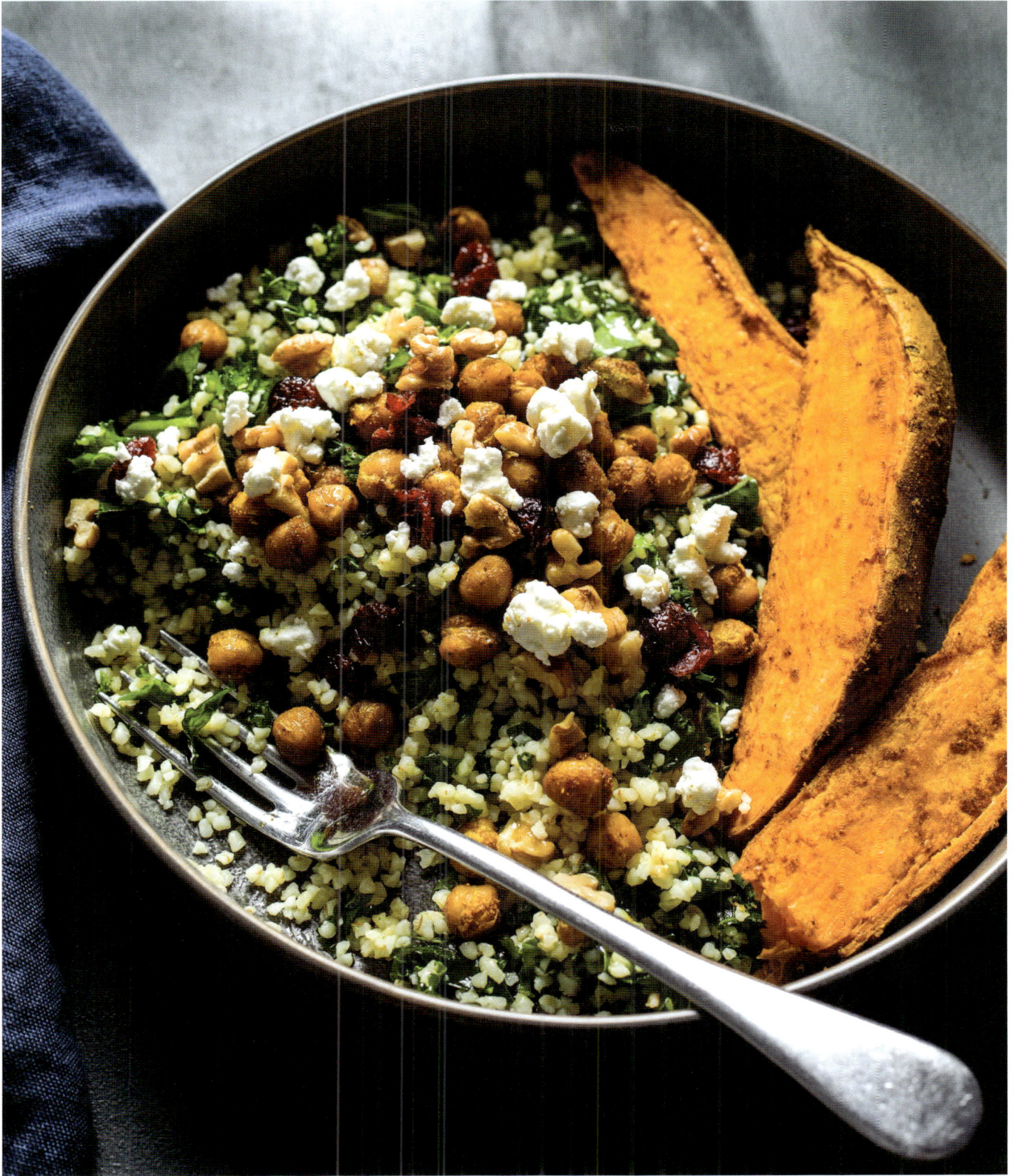

Bulgur Salad with Curry Roasted Sweet Potatoes and Chickpeas

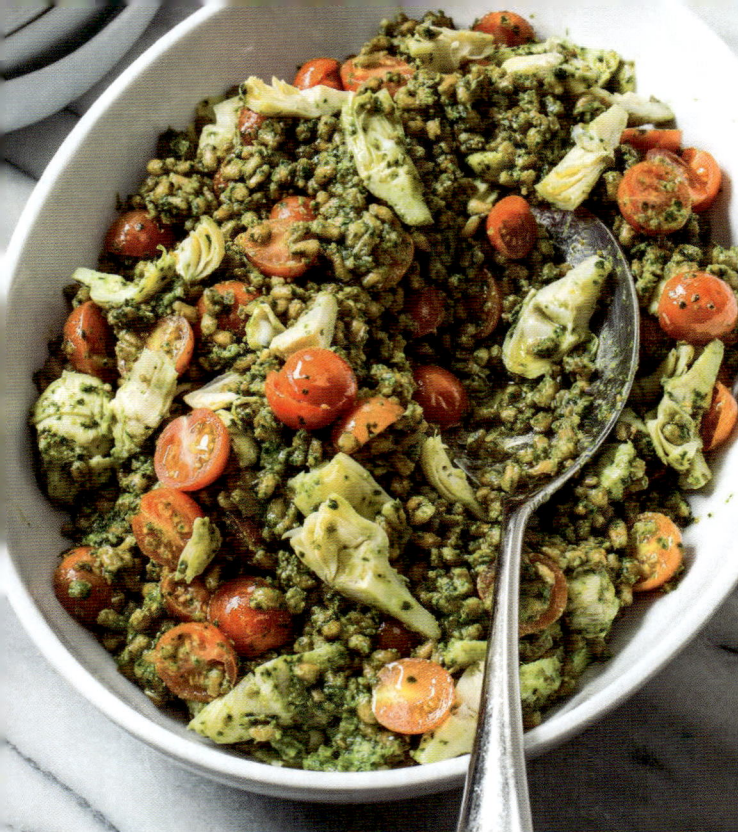

Pesto Farro Salad with Cherry Tomatoes and Artichokes

serves 4 to 6 • total time: 1 hour

why this recipe works • Farro's distinct, chewy-tender texture and earthy flavor make it perfect for a nourishing update on pesto pasta salad. We amped up the nutrients in the pesto by adding spinach, which gave us a dose of leafy greens and kept the sauce vividly green. We also incorporated sunflower seeds and cut the oil with yogurt, creating a nice creamy texture. Cherry tomatoes brightened the whole dish, while jarred artichoke hearts made a flavorful and meaty addition, with plenty of vitamins to boot.

- 1½   cups whole farro
- ½   teaspoon table salt, plus salt for cooking farro
- 2   cups fresh basil leaves
- 1½   ounces (1½ cups) baby spinach
- ½   cup roasted unsalted sunflower seeds
- 1   ounce Parmesan cheese, grated (½ cup)
- 2   garlic cloves, minced
- ¼   teaspoon pepper
- ½   cup extra-virgin olive oil
- ⅓   cup plain yogurt
- 12   ounces cherry tomatoes, halved
- 2   cups jarred whole baby artichoke hearts packed in water, rinsed, patted dry, and quartered

1   Bring 4 quarts water to boil in large pot. Stir in farro and 1 tablespoon salt, return to boil, and cook until grains are tender with slight chew, 15 to 30 minutes. Drain farro, spread onto rimmed baking sheet, and let cool for about 15 minutes.

2   Meanwhile, pulse basil, spinach, sunflower seeds, Parmesan, garlic, pepper, and salt in food processor until finely ground, 20 to 30 pulses, scraping down sides of bowl as needed. With processor running, slowly add oil until incorporated. Add yogurt and pulse to incorporate, about 5 pulses; transfer pesto to large bowl.

3   Toss cooled farro with pesto until combined. Gently stir in tomatoes and artichoke hearts and season with salt and pepper to taste. Stir in warm water as needed, 1 tablespoon at a time, to adjust consistency. Serve.

MAKE AHEAD • Cooked farro can be refrigerated for up to 3 days; let it come to room temperature before tossing with pesto.

MAKE IT DAIRY-FREE • Substitute plant-based Parmesan cheese and yogurt for the dairy Parmesan cheese and yogurt.

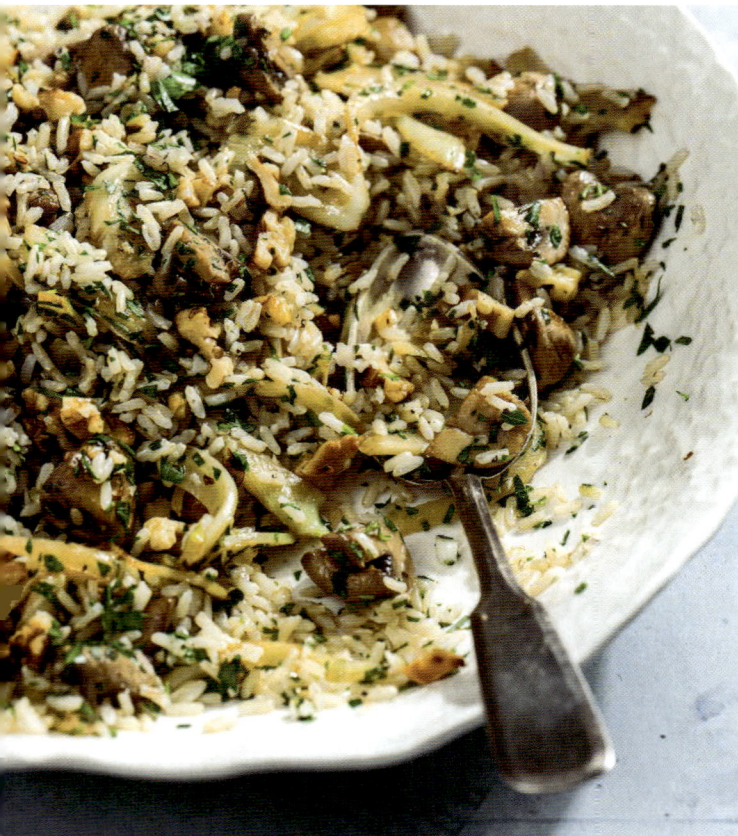

top | *Pesto Farro Salad with Cherry Tomatoes and Artichokes*
bottom | *Lentil and Brown Rice Salad with Fennel, Mushrooms, and Walnuts*

Quinoa, Black Bean, and Mango Salad with Lime Dressing

serves 4 to 6 · total time: 1 hour

why this recipe works · The quinoa seed is often called a "super-grain" because it's a nutritionally complete protein. To feature its delicate texture and nuttiness in a salad that could hold its own as a main course, we toasted the quinoa to bring out its flavor before adding liquid to the pan and then simmered the grains until they were nearly tender. Then, as we do with other grains, we spread the quinoa on a rimmed baking sheet to cool, which prevented clumping. The residual heat finished cooking the grains, giving us lovely, fluffy kernels. Black beans, mango, and bell pepper added fiber, flavor, and color to the salad, while our blended dressing made from jalapeño, cilantro, and lime juice offered freshness and zesty flavor. If you buy unwashed quinoa (or if you are unsure whether it's been washed), be sure to rinse it before cooking to remove its bitter protective coating (called saponin).

1½ cups prewashed white quinoa
2¼ cups water
1½ teaspoons table salt, divided
5 tablespoons lime juice (3 limes)
½ jalapeño chile, seeded and chopped
¾ teaspoon ground cumin
½ cup extra-virgin olive oil
⅓ cup fresh cilantro leaves
1 red bell pepper, stemmed, seeded, and chopped
1 mango, peeled, pitted, and cut into ¼-inch pieces
1 (15-ounce) can no-salt-added black beans, rinsed
1 avocado, halved, pitted, and cut into 1-inch pieces
2 scallions, sliced thin

1 Toast quinoa in large saucepan over medium-high heat, stirring often, until very fragrant and quinoa makes continuous popping sound, 5 to 7 minutes. Stir in water and ½ teaspoon salt and bring to simmer. Cover, reduce heat to low, and simmer gently until most of water has been absorbed and quinoa is nearly tender, about 15 minutes. Let sit off heat, covered, for 10 minutes. Spread quinoa onto rimmed baking sheet and let cool for 15 minutes.

2 Meanwhile, process lime juice, jalapeño, cumin, and remaining 1 teaspoon salt in blender until jalapeño is finely chopped, about 15 seconds. With blender running, add oil and cilantro and process until smooth and emulsified, about 20 seconds.

3 Toss cooled quinoa, bell pepper, mango, beans, avocado, and scallions with dressing in large bowl until well combined. Season with salt and pepper to taste. Serve.

MAKE AHEAD · Cooked quinoa can be refrigerated for up to 3 days; let it come to room temperature before tossing with dressing.

Lentil and Brown Rice Salad with Fennel, Mushrooms, and Walnuts

serves 4 · total time: 1¼ hours **SUPERCHARGED**

why this recipe works · Rice salads are a great way to enliven the flavor of hearty, earthy brown rice. Dressing the anti-inflammatory grain with bright flavors, adding lots of fresh vegetables, and pairing it with a powerhouse plant-based protein source turns brown rice into a filling, nutrient-dense meal. To ensure that the rice wouldn't clump or turn gummy, we cooked it like pasta, boiling it in a large pot of water, a method that washes away the rice's excess starches. We spread the cooked rice on a baking sheet to cool rapidly, preventing it from overcooking as it sat. To give every grain a flavor infusion, we drizzled the rice with white wine vinegar while still warm. Lentils added a satisfying, hearty chew and made the dish even more filling. Sautéed mushrooms, browned fennel, a generous amount of fresh herbs, and a sprinkling of toasted walnuts loaded the salad with fresh flavors, contrasting textures, and a more diverse array of inflammation-fighting compounds. You can substitute cremini mushrooms for the white mushrooms. Any variety of canned lentils will work in this recipe. We prefer a combination of herbs in this salad, but a single variety will also work. If your fennel bulb comes with fronds, consider including them with the other fresh herbs.

1½ cups long-grain brown rice
1¼ teaspoons table salt, divided, plus salt for cooking rice
3 tablespoons white wine vinegar, divided
¼ cup extra-virgin olive oil, divided
1 pound white mushrooms, trimmed and quartered
1 large fennel bulb, stalks discarded, bulb halved, cored, and sliced thin
1 shallot, minced
½ teaspoon pepper
1 (15-ounce) can no-salt-added lentils, rinsed
⅔ cup walnuts, toasted and chopped coarse, divided
½ cup fresh cilantro, mint, parsley, and/or tarragon leaves, divided

1 Bring 4 quarts water to boil in large pot. Stir in rice and 2½ teaspoons salt and cook until rice is tender, 22 to 25 minutes. Drain rice and spread onto rimmed baking sheet. Drizzle with 1 tablespoon vinegar and gently fluff with fork to combine; set aside.

2 Heat 1 tablespoon oil in 12-inch skillet over medium-high heat until shimmering. Add mushrooms and ½ teaspoon salt and cook, stirring occasionally, until skillet is dry and mushrooms are browned, 6 to 8 minutes; transfer to plate and let cool.

3 Heat 1 tablespoon oil in now-empty skillet over medium-high heat until shimmering. Add fennel and ¼ teaspoon salt and cook, stirring occasionally, until just browned and crisp-tender, about 4 minutes; transfer to plate with mushrooms and let cool.

4 Whisk shallot, remaining 2 tablespoons oil, pepper, remaining ½ teaspoon salt, and remaining 2 tablespoons vinegar together in large bowl. Add rice, mushroom-fennel mixture, and lentils and toss gently to combine. Let sit for 10 minutes.

5 Add ⅓ cup walnuts and ¼ cup cilantro and toss to combine. Season with salt and pepper to taste. Transfer salad to serving platter, sprinkle with remaining ⅓ cup walnuts and remaining ¼ cup cilantro, and serve.

Chilled Soba Noodle Salad with Spring Vegetables

serves 4 · total time: 30 minutes `FAST`

why this recipe works · Earthy, fiber-rich Japanese soba noodles are made with buckwheat flour. The deeper the color, the more buckwheat the noodles contain (and the richer they taste). Soba noodles are as delicious chilled as they are warm—here we went the chilled route by tossing them in a miso dressing to make a refreshing noodle salad. We cooked the soba noodles in unsalted boiling water until they were tender but still resilient and then rinsed them under cold running water to remove excess starch. We tossed the cooled noodles with the dressing, which clung to and flavored the noodles without overpowering their nutty taste. A mix of raw vegetables—cucumber, snow peas, and radishes—cut into varying sizes provided crunch, color, and an array of nutrients. Strips of toasted nori added more texture and a subtle oceanic flavor. For a spicier dish, use the larger amount of arbol chiles given. If dried arbol chiles are unavailable, you can substitute ¼ to ½ teaspoon red pepper flakes. You can use yellow, red, or brown miso instead of the white.

   3 tablespoons white miso
   3 tablespoons mirin
   2 tablespoons toasted sesame oil
   1 tablespoon sesame seeds
   1 teaspoon grated fresh ginger

1–2 dried arbol chiles (each about 2 inches long), stemmed, seeded, and chopped fine
   8 ounces dried soba noodles
  ⅓ English cucumber, quartered lengthwise, seeded, and sliced thin on bias
   4 ounces snow peas, strings removed, cut lengthwise into matchsticks
   4 radishes, trimmed, halved, and sliced thin
   3 scallions, sliced thin on bias
   1 (8-inch square) sheet nori, toasted and cut into 2-inch-long matchsticks (optional)

1 Whisk miso, mirin, oil, 1 tablespoon water, sesame seeds, ginger, and arbols in large bowl until combined.

2 Meanwhile, bring 4 quarts water to boil in large pot. Add noodles and cook, stirring occasionally, until noodles are cooked through but still retain some chew. Drain noodles and rinse under cold running water until chilled. Drain well and transfer to bowl with dressing. Add cucumber; snow peas; radishes; scallions; and nori, if using, and toss to combine. Season with salt to taste. Serve.

MAKE IT GLUTEN-FREE · For the soba noodles, look for a brand that uses 100% buckwheat flour.

NOTES FROM THE TEST KITCHEN

All About Mirin

The dressing for our soba noodles gets its depth from mirin, a Japanese rice wine that can take different forms. The traditional form is hon-mirin ("real mirin"), a delicately savory-sweet wine that's made exclusively from fermented rice and is available online and in some liquor stores. Supermarkets sell a product labeled "sweet cooking wine," "sweetened sake," or "aji-mirin" ("tastes like mirin") that's made with sweeteners, alcohol, rice, and salt. We have determined that in applications where mirin is a main ingredient, it's worth seeking out the traditional, high-quality mirin. However, in recipes such as this one that call for just a few tablespoons, it's fine to use the supermarket stuff, which is much cheaper: In a taste test, we couldn't tell which batch of noodles contained which type of mirin.

California Chicken Salad Bowls

serves 4 · total time: 25 minutes **FAST**

why this recipe works · You can put avocado on just about anything and call it "Californian," but we wanted to earn our West Coast cred with a healthy, hearty salad that paid respect to the Golden State in every bite. Instead of just throwing on diced avocado, we prepared a luscious, dairy-free dressing with avocado, pureeing the heart-healthy fruit with lemon, garlic, and olive oil. Of course, a California salad should burst with fresh flavors, so we went heavy on green vegetables such as spinach and sugar snap peas. Thinly sliced radishes offered a pop of color, grapes studded the dish with bits of sweetness, and a sprinkling of chopped almonds added welcome crunch and a dose of healthy fats. Then we realized we were missing something quintessentially West Coast (not to mention nutrient-dense): a light, fluffy mound of alfalfa sprouts. We like using our Perfect Poached Chicken (page 92) here, but any cooked chicken will work.

Avocado Ranch Dressing
- 1 avocado, halved, pitted, and cut into ½-inch pieces
- 2 tablespoons extra-virgin olive oil
- 1 teaspoon grated lemon zest plus 3 tablespoons juice
- 1 garlic clove, minced
- ¾ teaspoon table salt
- ¼ teaspoon pepper

Bowls
- 8 ounces (8 cups) baby spinach
- 2 scallions, sliced thin
- 4 cups chopped cooked chicken
- 9 ounces seedless grapes, halved (1½ cups)
- 4 ounces sugar snap peas or snow peas, strings removed, halved
- 8 radishes, trimmed, halved, and sliced thin
- 2 ounces (1 cup) alfalfa sprouts or microgreens
- ¼ cup chopped almonds

1 For the dressing Process all ingredients in food processor until smooth, about 30 seconds, scraping down sides of bowl as needed. Season with salt and pepper to taste.

2 For the bowls Toss spinach, scallions, and half of dressing together in bowl to coat. Season with salt and pepper to taste. Divide spinach mixture among individual serving bowls and top with chicken, grapes, snap peas, and radishes. Drizzle with remaining dressing, top with alfalfa sprouts, and sprinkle with chopped almonds. Serve.

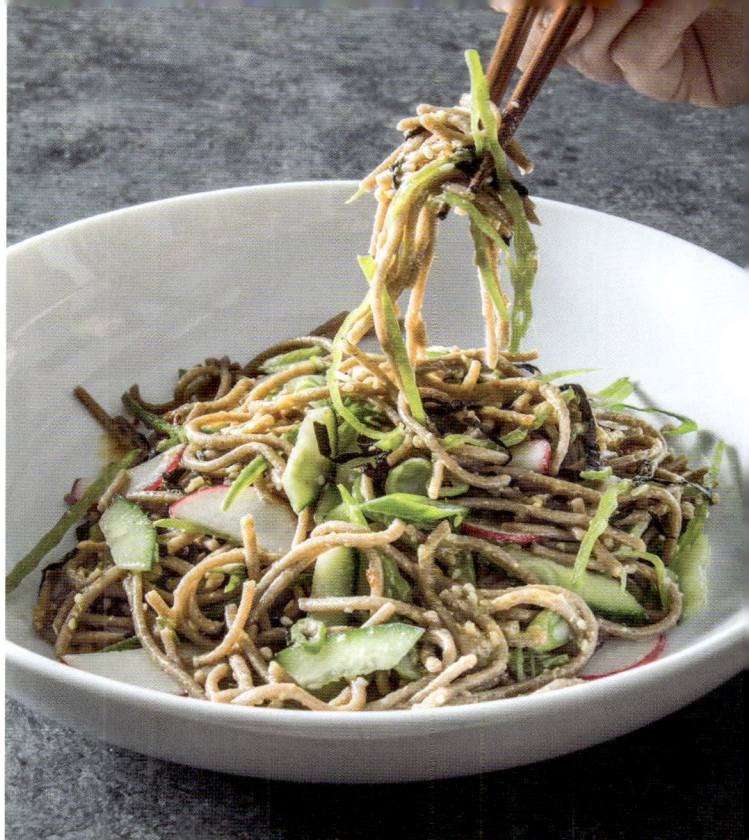

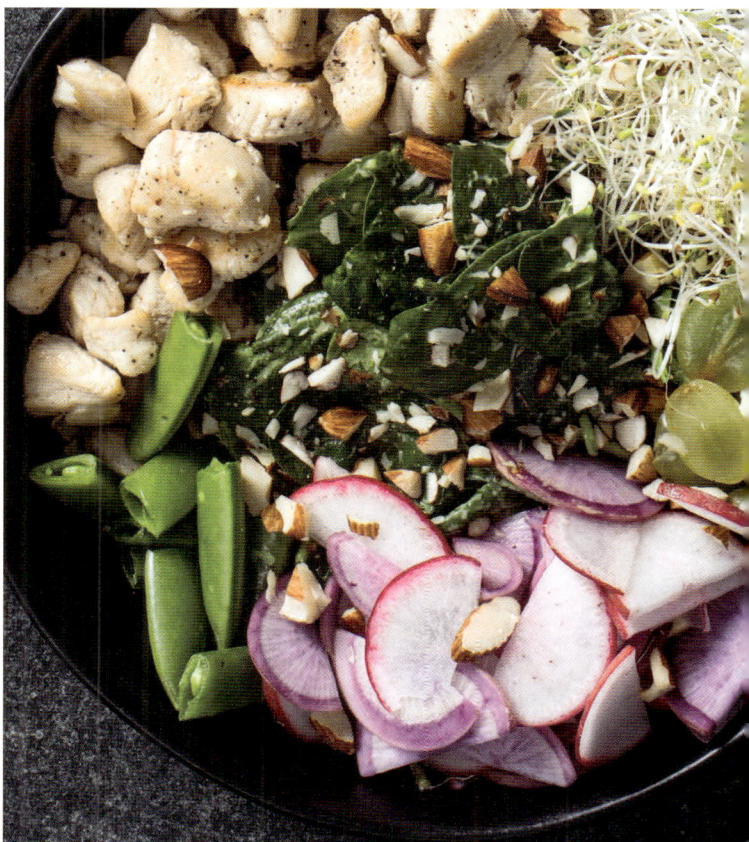

top	*Chilled Soba Noodle Salad with Spring Vegetables*
bottom	*California Chicken Salad Bowl*

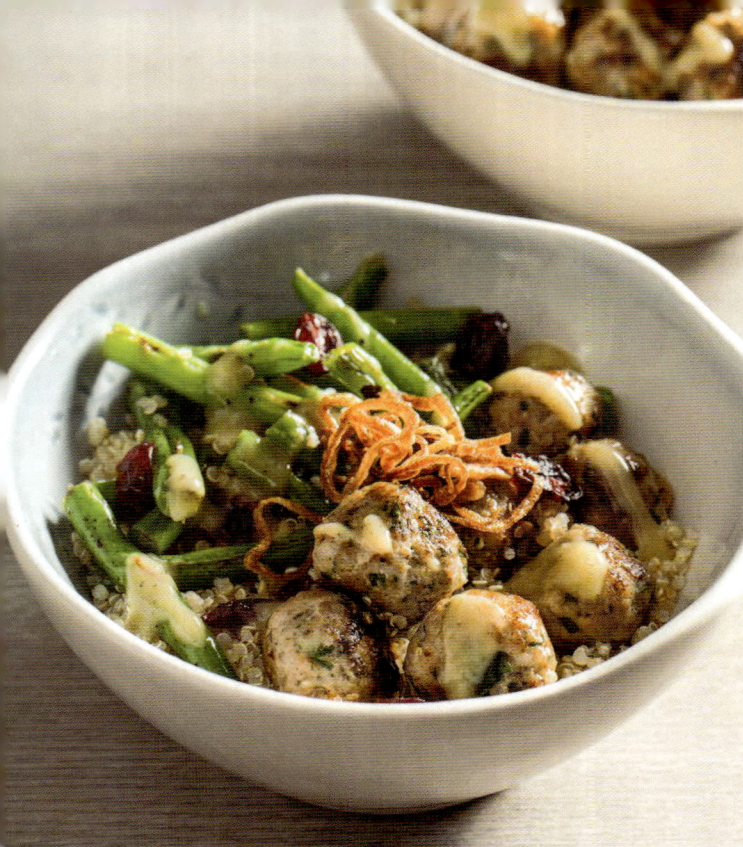

Quinoa Bowls with Turkey Meatballs, Green Beans, and Roasted Garlic Dressing

serves 4 • **total time 1¾ hours**

why this recipe works • With make-ahead options for its major components (mini turkey meatballs, a nutty grain base, and a creamy sauce that ties it all together), this bowl puts Thanksgiving flavors within reach on a regular weeknight. We riffed on traditional stuffing and cranberry sauce with quinoa and dried cranberries for a more anti-inflammatory, yet still delicious, take on those dishes. The green bean "side" couldn't be easier and cooked right in the juices left behind after cooking the meatballs. Be sure to use ground turkey in this recipe, not ground turkey breast (also labeled 99 percent fat-free). If you buy unwashed quinoa (or if you are unsure whether it's been washed), be sure to rinse it before cooking to remove its bitter protective coating (called saponin). You can make microwave-fried shallots for a garnish, if desired: Combine thinly sliced shallots with extra-virgin olive oil and microwave, stirring frequently, until shallots are golden brown.

Roasted Garlic Dressing

- 3 tablespoons Roasted Garlic (recipe follows)
- 2 tablespoons white wine vinegar
- 1½ tablespoons water
- ½ teaspoon Dijon mustard
- ½ teaspoon minced fresh thyme
- ⅛ teaspoon table salt
- ⅛ teaspoon pepper
- ¼ cup extra-virgin olive oil

Bowls

- 1½ cups prewashed white quinoa
- 2½ cups water
- 1⅛ teaspoons table salt, divided
- 1 slice hearty white sandwich bread, crust removed, torn into ¼-inch pieces
- 2 tablespoons milk
- 1 pound ground turkey
- ¼ cup chopped fresh parsley
- 1½ teaspoons ground fennel
- 1½ teaspoons ground sage
- ½ teaspoon pepper
- 4 teaspoons extra-virgin olive oil, divided
- 8 ounces green beans, trimmed and halved crosswise
- ¼ cup dried cranberries

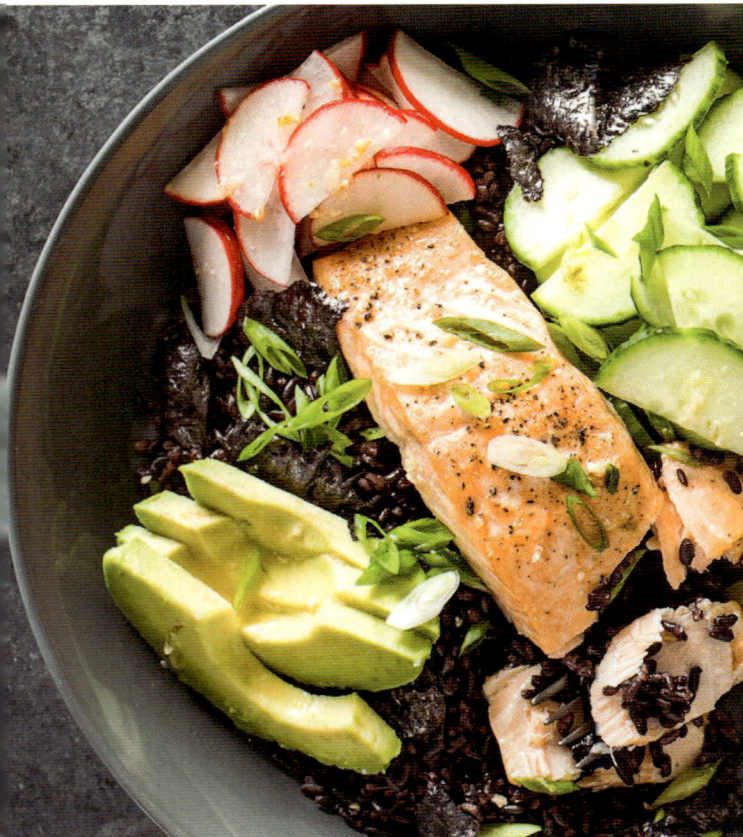

1 For the dressing Using fork, mash garlic into paste in medium bowl. Whisk in vinegar, water, mustard, thyme, salt, and pepper. Whisking constantly, slowly drizzle in oil until emulsified. Season with salt and pepper to taste; set aside.

2 For the bowls Toast quinoa in large saucepan over medium-high heat, stirring often, until very fragrant and quinoa makes continuous popping sound, 5 to 7 minutes. Stir in water and ½ teaspoon salt and bring to simmer. Cover, reduce heat to low, and simmer gently until most of water has been absorbed and quinoa is nearly tender, about 15 minutes. Let sit off heat, covered, for 10 minutes. Spread quinoa onto rimmed baking sheet and let cool for 15 minutes.

3 Using fork, mash bread and milk into paste in large bowl. Break turkey into small pieces over bread mixture and add parsley, fennel, sage, pepper, and ½ teaspoon salt. Lightly knead with your hands until well combined. Pinch off and roll mixture into 18 meatballs (about ½ tablespoon each).

4 Heat 1 teaspoon oil in 12-inch nonstick skillet over medium heat until shimmering. Add half of meatballs and cook until well browned and tender, 5 to 7 minutes. Transfer meatballs to plate; cover with aluminum foil to keep warm. Repeat with 1 teaspoon oil and remaining meatballs. Heat remaining 2 teaspoons oil in now-empty skillet over medium-high heat until shimmering. Add green beans and remaining ⅛ teaspoon salt and cook until green beans are spotty brown, 2 to 4 minutes.

5 Divide quinoa among individual serving bowls, then top with meatballs and green beans. Drizzle with dressing and sprinkle with cranberries. Serve.

MAKE AHEAD • Dressing and cooked quinoa can be refrigerated separately for up to 3 days; whisk dressing to recombine and let dressing and quinoa come to room temperature before assembling bowls. Meatballs can be prepared through step 4 and refrigerated for up to 24 hours.

MAKE IT DAIRY-FREE • Substitute plant-based milk or water for the dairy milk.

Roasted Garlic

makes ⅓ cup • total time: 1¼ hours, plus 20 minutes cooling

   2 large garlic heads
   2 teaspoons extra-virgin olive oil
   ⅛ teaspoon table salt

1 Adjust oven rack to middle position and heat oven to 425 degrees. Cut ½ inch off top of each garlic head to expose most of tops of garlic cloves. Place garlic heads, cut side up, in center of large piece of aluminum foil. Drizzle each with oil, sprinkle with salt, and gather foil tightly around garlic to form packet.

2 Place packet directly on oven rack and roast garlic for 45 minutes. Carefully open just top of foil to expose garlic and continue to roast until garlic is soft and golden brown, about 20 minutes.

3 Remove garlic from oven and let cool for 20 minutes. When cool, squeeze garlic from skins into bowl. (Roasted garlic can be refrigerated in airtight container for up to 1 week.)

Black Rice Bowls with Roasted Salmon and Miso Dressing

serves 4 • total time: 1 hour `SUPERCHARGED`

why this recipe works • Black rice is an ancient grain with a deliciously roasted, nutty flavor, not to mention a great deal of digestion-supporting fiber and satisfying chew. We decided to pair it with meaty salmon, rich avocado, and crisp vegetables for a nutritious, well-rounded meal. Because black rice can be easy to overcook, we boiled it to ensure that all the grains cooked evenly. For the omega-3-packed salmon, we wanted to crisp the exterior while keeping its interior moist. We preheated a baking sheet in a 500-degree oven before reducing the heat to 275 and placing the fish in the oven. The initial blast of heat firmed up the outside, while the interior cooked through gently as the oven temperature slowly dropped. If using wild salmon, cook the fillets until they reach 120 degrees (for medium-rare) and start checking for doneness after 4 minutes. You can substitute brown rice for the black rice but will need to adjust the cooking time.

1½ cups black rice

¼ teaspoon table salt, plus salt for cooking rice

4 (6- to 8-ounce) skin-on salmon fillets, 1 to 1½ inches thick

1 teaspoon avocado oil

⅛ teaspoon pepper

¼ cup unseasoned rice vinegar

¼ cup mirin

1 tablespoon white miso

1 teaspoon grated fresh ginger

½ teaspoon lime zest plus 2 tablespoons juice

1 (8-inch square) sheet toasted nori, crumbled (optional)

4 radishes, trimmed, halved, and sliced thin

1 avocado, sliced thin

1 English cucumber, halved lengthwise and sliced thin

2 scallions, sliced thin

1   Bring 4 quarts water to boil in Dutch oven. Add rice and 1 teaspoon salt and cook until rice is tender, 20 to 25 minutes. Drain rice and transfer to large bowl; cover to keep warm.

2   Meanwhile, adjust oven rack to lowest position, place aluminum foil–lined rimmed baking sheet on rack, and heat oven to 500 degrees. Make 4 or 5 shallow slashes, about 1 inch apart, on skin side of each fillet, being careful not to cut into flesh. Pat salmon dry with paper towels, rub with oil, and sprinkle with salt and pepper.

3   Reduce oven temperature to 275 degrees and remove sheet from oven. Carefully place salmon skin side down on prepared sheet. Roast until center is still translucent when checked with tip of paring knife and registers 125 degrees (for medium-rare), 8 to 12 minutes. Transfer salmon to plate and let cool slightly, about 15 minutes.

4   Whisk vinegar, mirin, miso, ginger, and lime zest and juice in small bowl until miso is fully incorporated. Season with salt and pepper to taste. Measure out ¼ cup dressing, drizzle over rice, and toss to combine.

5   Using 2 forks, flake salmon into rough 2-inch pieces, discarding skin. Divide rice among individual serving bowls and sprinkle with nori, if using. Top with salmon, radishes, avocado, and cucumber. Sprinkle with scallions and drizzle with remaining dressing. Serve.

MAKE AHEAD • Roasted salmon can be refrigerated for up to 3 days.

Nutrition Knowledge   I'm a big fan of black rice—not only for its satisfying chew, but also because it's rich in anthocyanins, powerful antioxidants that help reduce oxidative stress. I like that we pair it here with salmon, one of my favorite sources of heart-healthy omega-3 fatty acids. Miso and ginger round out this anti-inflammatory meal with their gut-healing, inflammation-fighting benefits, courtesy of their probiotics and gingerols.   *—Alicia*

Beet Poke Bowls

serves 4 • total time: 45 minutes, plus 30 minutes chilling

SUPERCHARGED

why this recipe works • When we set out to create a poke-inspired bowl using only plants, we tested a variety of vegetables to find out which one was up to the task. We were thrilled to discover that antioxidant-rich beets—with their sturdy density, absorbent texture, and bright-pink hue (courtesy of anythocyanins)—turned out to be our winner. To start, we chopped the beets into pieces, cooked them in the microwave, and tossed them in a potent savory-sweet marinade featuring classic poke seasonings such as rice vinegar, toasted sesame oil, and fresh ginger. Marinating the beets for at least 30 minutes allowed the flavors to thoroughly infuse them. Rather than the typical rice, we served the beets over micronutrient-rich soba noodles, which we tossed in toasted sesame oil to boost flavor and slurpability. To complete the bowl, we embellished it with nourishing toppings such as carrots, cucumber, avocado, and macadamia nuts. A sprinkle of the Japanese seasoning blend furikake echoed the oceanic notes of traditional poke. There are many different kinds of furikake; we recommend looking for one that has dried seaweed (nori and/or kombu), bonito flakes, and sesame seeds. Look for it at Japanese or Asian grocery stores; you might also find it at some well-stocked supermarkets.

3 scallions, white and green parts separated and sliced thin on bias

2 tablespoons low-sodium soy sauce

2 tablespoons avocado oil

1 tablespoon unseasoned rice vinegar

4 teaspoons toasted sesame oil, divided

2 teaspoons grated fresh ginger

1 garlic clove, minced

¾ teaspoon red pepper flakes

2 pounds beets, trimmed, peeled, and cut into ¾-inch pieces

½ teaspoon table salt

12 ounces dried soba noodles

2 carrots, peeled and cut into 2-inch-long matchsticks

½ seedless English cucumber, halved lengthwise and sliced thin crosswise

1 ripe but firm avocado, halved, pitted, and sliced ¼ inch thick

⅓ cup finely chopped salted dry-roasted macadamia nuts or peanuts

Furikake (optional)

1 Combine scallion whites, soy sauce, avocado oil, vinegar, 2 teaspoons sesame oil, ginger, garlic, and pepper flakes in large bowl; set aside. In separate bowl, toss beets with ⅓ cup water and salt. Cover bowl and microwave until beets can be easily pierced with paring knife, 25 to 30 minutes, stirring halfway through microwaving. Drain beets in colander, transfer to bowl with reserved marinade, and toss to coat. Transfer to refrigerator and let marinate for 30 minutes.

2 Meanwhile, bring 4 quarts water to boil in large pot. Stir in noodles and cook, stirring occasionally, until noodles are cooked through but still retain some chew. Drain noodles and rinse under cold water until chilled. Drain well.

3 Toss noodles with remaining 2 teaspoons sesame oil and divide among individual serving bowls. Top with marinated beets; carrots; cucumber; avocado; macadamia nuts; scallion greens; and furikake, if using. Serve.

MAKE AHEAD · Beets can marinate for up to 24 hours.

MAKE IT GLUTEN-FREE · Substitute low-sodium tamari for the low-sodium soy sauce.

Shrimp Saganaki Zoodle Bowls

serves 4 · total time: 35 minutes · **FAST**

why this recipe works · Shrimp saganaki is a classic Greek dish of shrimp in a rich, zesty tomato sauce sprinkled with herbs and feta cheese. We knew this quick-cooking dish would work well as a bowl, paired with (even quicker-cooking) zucchini noodles. To lighten up the sauce so that it wouldn't weigh down our delicate zoodles, we sautéed cherry tomatoes until they burst with sweet juice and then we added artichoke hearts, fresh dill, and lemon zest to create a chunky topping. Seasoned simply with salt and pepper, the zucchini noodles made a nourishing partner to the sauce and shrimp. Crumbled feta and chopped olives brought bites of brininess. You will need 2 pounds of zucchini to get 1½ pounds of noodles; we prefer to make our own using a spiralizer, but in a pinch you can use store-bought. Cook the zucchini to your desired level of doneness but be careful not to overcook it.

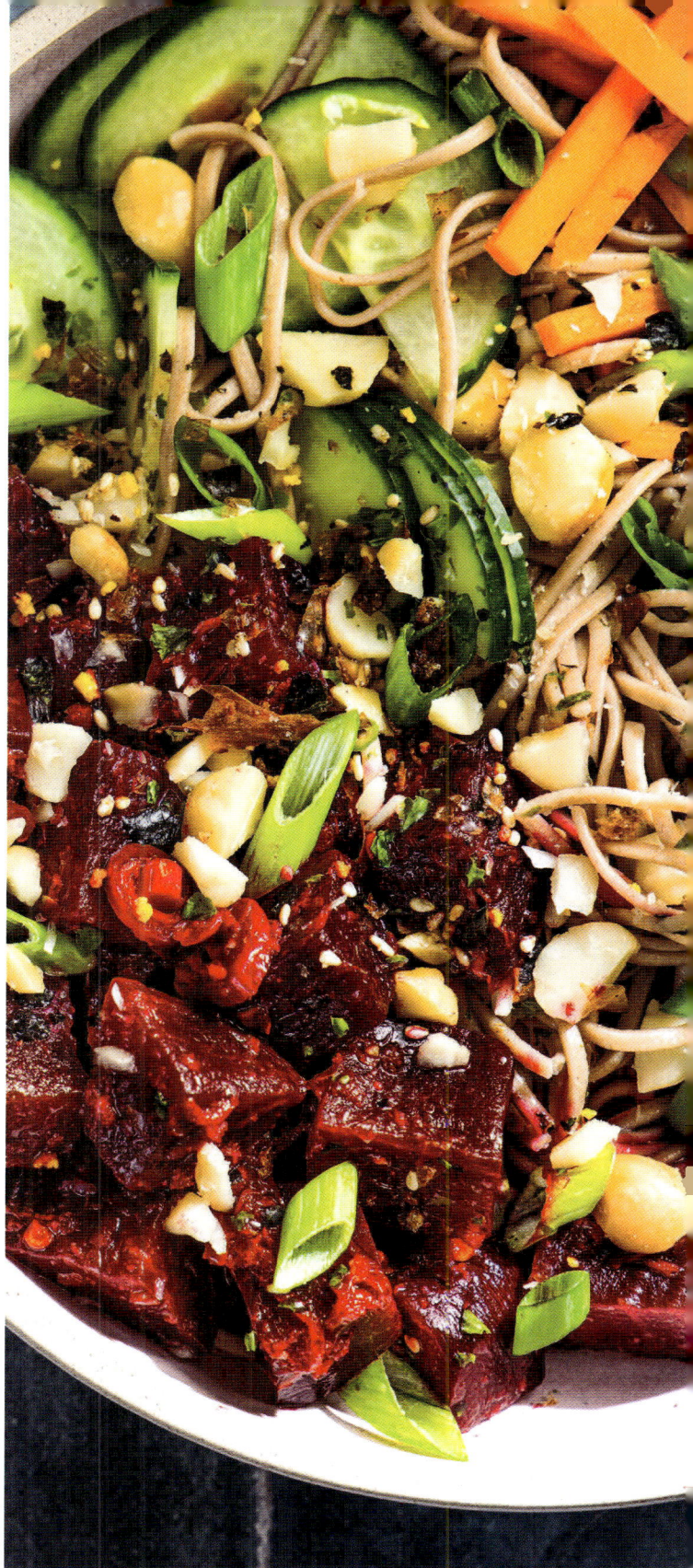

12 ounces extra-large shrimp (21 to 25 per pound), peeled, deveined, and tails removed
¾ teaspoon table salt, divided
¾ teaspoon pepper, divided
1 tablespoon avocado oil
¼ cup extra-virgin olive oil, divided
2 shallots, minced
2 garlic cloves, minced
12 ounces cherry tomatoes, halved
2 cups jarred whole artichoke hearts packed in water, rinsed, patted dry, and halved
1 teaspoon grated lemon zest, plus lemon wedges for serving
2 tablespoons chopped fresh dill
24 ounces zucchini noodles, cut into 6-inch lengths, divided
2 ounces feta cheese, crumbled (½ cup)
¼ cup pitted kalamata olives, chopped

1 Pat shrimp dry with paper towels and sprinkle with ¼ teaspoon salt and ¼ teaspoon pepper. Heat avocado oil in 12-inch nonstick skillet over medium-high heat until just smoking. Add shrimp in single layer and cook, without stirring, until spotty brown and edges turn pink on bottom, about 1 minute. Flip shrimp and continue to cook until all but very center is opaque, about 30 seconds; transfer shrimp to plate and let cool slightly.

2 Heat 2 teaspoons olive oil in now-empty skillet over medium heat until shimmering. Add shallots and garlic and cook until fragrant, about 30 seconds. Stir in tomatoes, artichoke hearts, lemon zest, ¼ teaspoon salt, and ¼ teaspoon pepper and cook, stirring frequently, until tomatoes have softened, 3 to 5 minutes. Transfer to bowl and stir in 2 tablespoons olive oil and dill. Cover with aluminum foil to keep warm and set aside until ready to serve.

3 Wipe skillet clean with paper towels. Heat 2 teaspoons olive oil in now-empty skillet over medium-high heat until shimmering. Add half of zucchini noodles, ⅛ teaspoon salt, and ⅛ teaspoon pepper and cook, tossing frequently, until crisp-tender, about 1 minute. Transfer to individual serving bowls and repeat with remaining 2 teaspoons olive oil, remaining zucchini noodles, remaining ⅛ teaspoon salt, and remaining ⅛ teaspoon pepper. Top zucchini noodles with tomato-artichoke mixture, shrimp, feta, and olives. Serve with lemon wedges.

> **MAKE IT DAIRY-FREE** • Omit the feta cheese or substitute plant-based feta-style cheese.

Fattoush Salad Bowls

serves 4 • total time: 45 minutes   **FAST**

why this recipe works • This Levantine-inspired salad bowl combines fresh cucumbers and tomatoes, crisp pita chips, and bright herbs with nutty, protein-dense chickpeas. We made the pita moisture-repellent by brushing its craggy sides with plenty of heart-healthy olive oil before baking. The oil prevented the pita chips from absorbing so much liquid from the salad that they became soggy but still allowed the chips to pick up flavor from the lemony dressing. However, do serve this salad as soon as you make it so that the pita doesn't sit for too long, as it will get soggy over time. Use ripe, in-season tomatoes if you can find them.

2 (8-inch) pitas
½ cup extra-virgin olive oil, divided
1 garlic clove, minced
½ teaspoon grated lemon zest plus ¼ cup juice (2 lemons)
½ teaspoon ground sumac, plus extra for serving
¾ teaspoon table salt
1 (15-ounce) can no-salt-added chickpeas, rinsed
1 small head escarole (12 ounces), trimmed and cut into 1-inch pieces
½ cup chopped fresh mint
4 scallions, sliced thin
1 pound cherry or grape tomatoes, halved
1 English cucumber, peeled and sliced ⅛ inch thick

1 Adjust oven rack to middle position and heat oven to 375 degrees. Using kitchen shears, cut around perimeter of each pita and separate into 2 thin rounds. Cut each round in half. Place pitas, smooth side down, on wire rack set in rimmed baking sheet. Brush ¼ cup oil over surface of pitas. (Pitas do not need to be uniformly coated. Oil will spread during baking.) Bake until pitas are crisp and pale golden brown, 10 to 14 minutes. Set aside to cool.

2 Meanwhile, whisk remaining ¼ cup oil, garlic, lemon zest and juice, sumac, and salt together in medium bowl. Transfer half of dressing to large bowl; set aside. Add chickpeas to remaining dressing and toss to coat. Let chickpeas sit until flavors meld, about 10 minutes.

3 Toss escarole, mint, and scallions with reserved dressing. Season with salt and pepper to taste. Divide greens among individual serving bowls, then top with tomatoes, cucumber, and chickpeas. Break pitas into ½-inch pieces and sprinkle over top along with extra sumac. Serve.

> **MAKE AHEAD** • Cooled pitas can be stored in zipper-lock bag for up to 24 hours.

All About Escarole

Fiber-rich, inflammation-fighting escarole, a kind of chicory, is a leafy green with a slightly bitter flavor that makes it a great choice for peppery salads, a nice accent for romaine, or an ideal pairing with a simple vinaigrette. Escarole is less assertive than its cousins, Belgian endive and frisée, and is a good choice when you want something slightly, rather than full-on, bitter. Unlike lettuce, escarole stands up well to cooking. Its resilient leaves turn supple but don't fall apart, and the base and spine of each leaf add a little texture. Look for heads bristling with sturdy, unblemished leaves. Use a salad spinner to wash escarole, as the fine, feathery leaves tend to hold a lot of soil.

Tofu Sushi Bowls

serves 4 · total time: 40 minutes **FAST**

why this recipe works · Sushi rolls can be both time-consuming and tedious to make, so we set out to develop a deconstructed version in a bowl that would be easy to assemble at home. For a vegetarian spin, we used tofu, which we browned to crispy perfection. Brown rice isn't typical for sushi rolls, but we liked the added nutritional value and nutty chew in our bowl base. Sushi rice is often seasoned, so we tossed our rice with a sesame-scallion vinaigrette to stand in for the classic sushi rice seasoning. For toppings, we got fresh, satisfying crunch from some thinly sliced radishes and cucumber. We also added creamy, cooling avocado, which offered heart-healthy fats and welcome richness. Some crumbled nori, scattered across the top of our bowl, echoed the sushi vibes. We like this bowl with either warm or room-temperature rice; see page 334 for more information on cooking brown rice. Serve with pickled ginger, if desired.

Vinaigrette

- ¼ cup low-sodium soy sauce
- 2 tablespoons unseasoned rice vinegar
- 2 tablespoons mirin
- 2 tablespoons water
- 1 teaspoon chili oil (optional)
- ½ teaspoon toasted sesame oil
- 1 scallion, minced

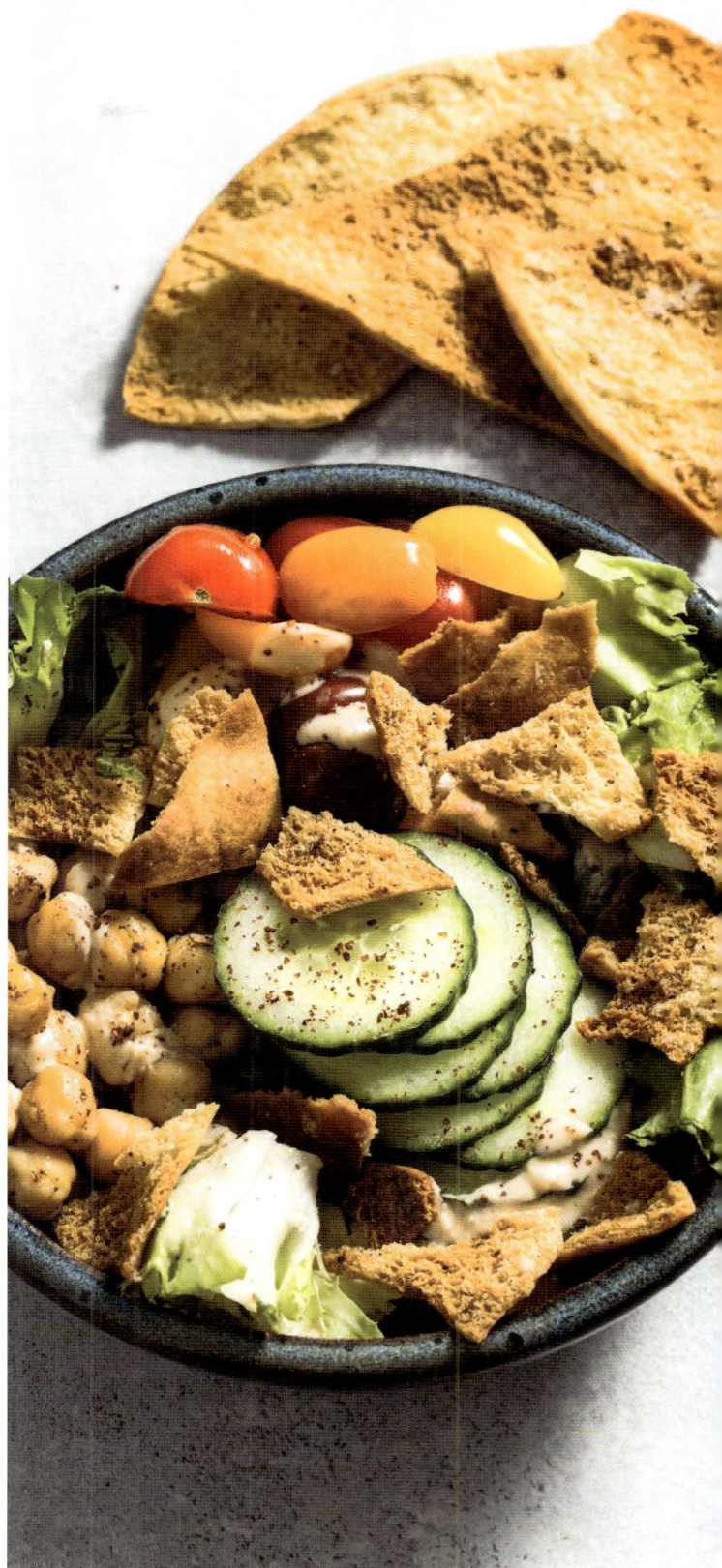

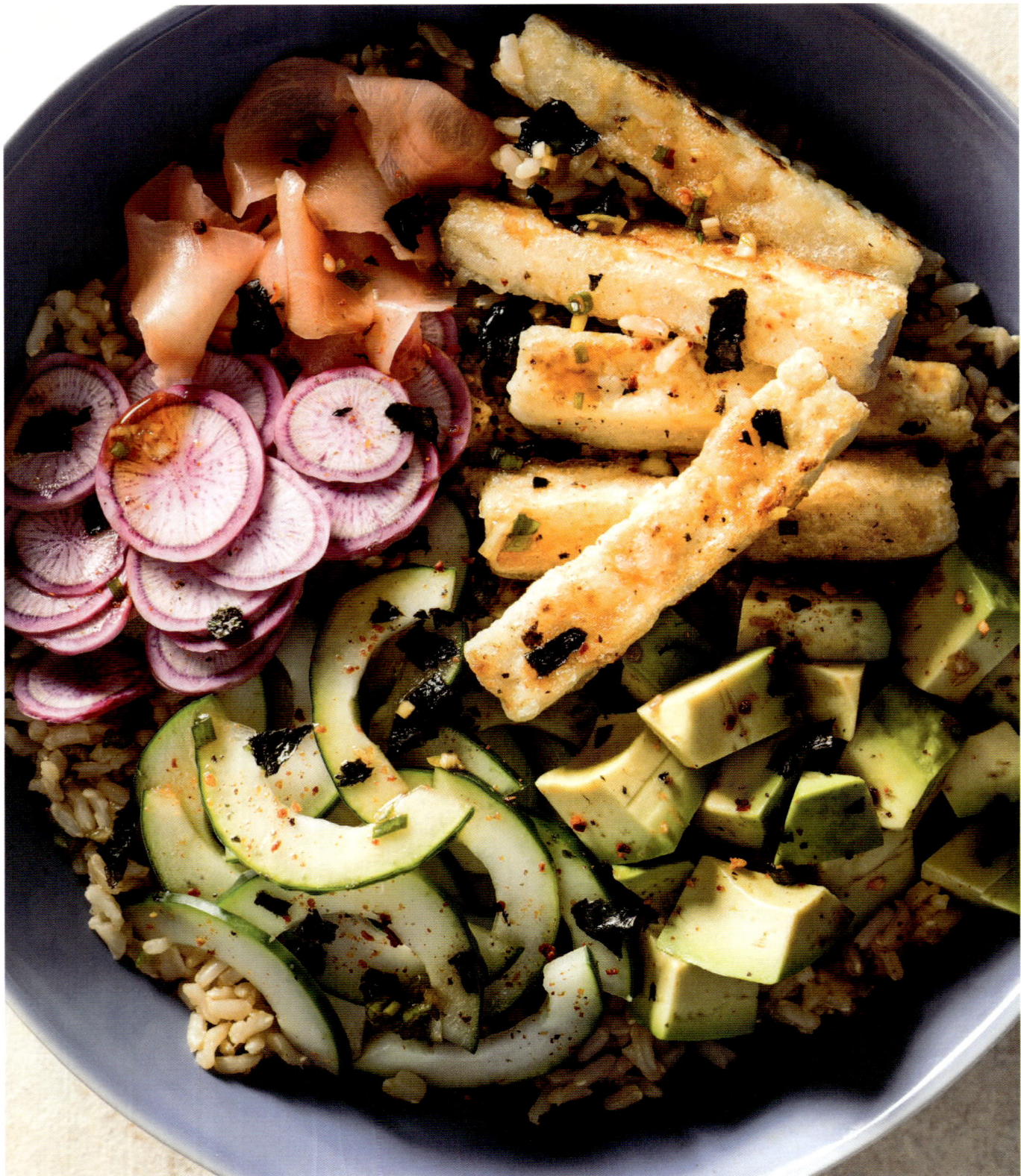

Tofu Sushi Bowls

Bowls

- 14 ounces firm tofu, cut into 3-inch-long by ½-inch-thick fingers
- ¼ teaspoon table salt
- ¼ teaspoon pepper
- 2 tablespoons avocado oil
- 4 cups cooked brown rice
- 6 radishes, sliced thin
- 1 cucumber, halved lengthwise, seeded, and sliced thin
- 1 avocado, halved, seeded, and cut into ¾-inch pieces
- 2 (8-inch square) sheets toasted nori, crumbled

1 For the vinaigrette Whisk all ingredients together in bowl; set aside.

2 For the bowls Spread tofu over paper towel–lined plate and gently pat dry with paper towels. Sprinkle with salt and pepper. Heat oil in 12-inch nonstick skillet over medium-high heat until just smoking. Lightly brown tofu on all sides, 12 to 15 minutes; transfer to clean paper towel–lined plate to drain.

3 Toss rice with half of vinaigrette to coat, then season with salt and pepper to taste. Divide among individual serving bowls, then top with tofu, radishes, cucumber, and avocado. Drizzle with remaining vinaigrette and sprinkle with nori. Serve.

> **MAKE AHEAD** • Vinaigrette can be refrigerated for up to 3 days; whisk to recombine before using.

> **MAKE IT GLUTEN-FREE** • Substitute low-sodium tamari for the low-sodium soy sauce.

Spicy Peanut Noodle Bowls

serves 4 • total time: 40 minutes `FAST`

why this recipe works • This piquant noodle bowl is a stunner, boasting a colorful medley of texturally diverse toppings. We combined tender rice noodles with edamame, pickled carrots, and cabbage and draped it all with a rich peanut sauce. To make some quick pickles, we added rice vinegar to beta-carotene-rich carrots and let them sit while the noodles softened in hot water. We then sautéed the edamame until it was speckled brown but remained crisp-tender. After removing the beans, we finished cooking the noodles in the same pan with half the sauce until the noodles were tender. Once we topped our noodles with the veggies and remaining sauce, we garnished with Thai basil and chopped peanuts. To make this sauce spicier, add the seeds from the chiles. You can use serrano or jalapeño chiles in place of Thai chiles. If you can't find Thai basil, you can substitute regular basil.

- 1 cup shredded carrots
- 5 tablespoons unseasoned rice vinegar, divided
- ½ teaspoon table salt
- 12 ounces (¼-inch wide) rice noodles
- ¼ cup avocado oil, divided
- 2 Thai chiles, stemmed, seeded, and minced
- 3 garlic cloves, minced
- 1 tablespoon grated fresh ginger
- 1½ teaspoons curry powder
- ⅓ cup creamy peanut butter
- 2 tablespoons low-sodium soy sauce
- 1 cup frozen edamame
- 1 cup shredded red cabbage
- ⅓ cup dry-roasted peanuts, chopped
- 2 tablespoons torn fresh Thai basil
  Lime wedges

1 Combine carrots, 2 tablespoons vinegar, and salt in small bowl; set aside. Bring 4 quarts water to boil in large pot. Remove from heat, add noodles, and let sit, stirring occasionally, until soft and pliable but not fully tender. Drain noodles.

2 Meanwhile, heat 1 tablespoon oil in medium saucepan over medium heat until shimmering. Stir in Thai chiles, garlic, ginger, and curry powder and cook until fragrant, about 30 seconds. Stir in ½ cup water, peanut butter, soy sauce, and remaining 3 tablespoons vinegar and bring to simmer. Cook, stirring occasionally, until slightly thickened and flavors meld, about 2 minutes. Adjust consistency as needed with additional water. Transfer sauce to bowl.

3 Heat 1 tablespoon oil in 12-inch nonstick skillet over medium-high heat until just smoking. Add edamame and cook until spotty brown but still bright green, about 2 minutes; transfer to bowl. In now-empty skillet, heat remaining 2 tablespoons oil over medium heat until shimmering. Add drained noodles, 1¼ cups water, and ½ cup peanut sauce and cook until sauce has thickened slightly and noodles are well coated and tender, about 1 minute.

4 Divide noodles among individual serving bowls, then top with carrots, edamame, and cabbage. Drizzle with remaining peanut sauce, sprinkle with peanuts and basil, and serve with lime wedges.

> **MAKE IT GLUTEN-FREE** • Substitute low-sodium tamari for the low-sodium soy sauce.

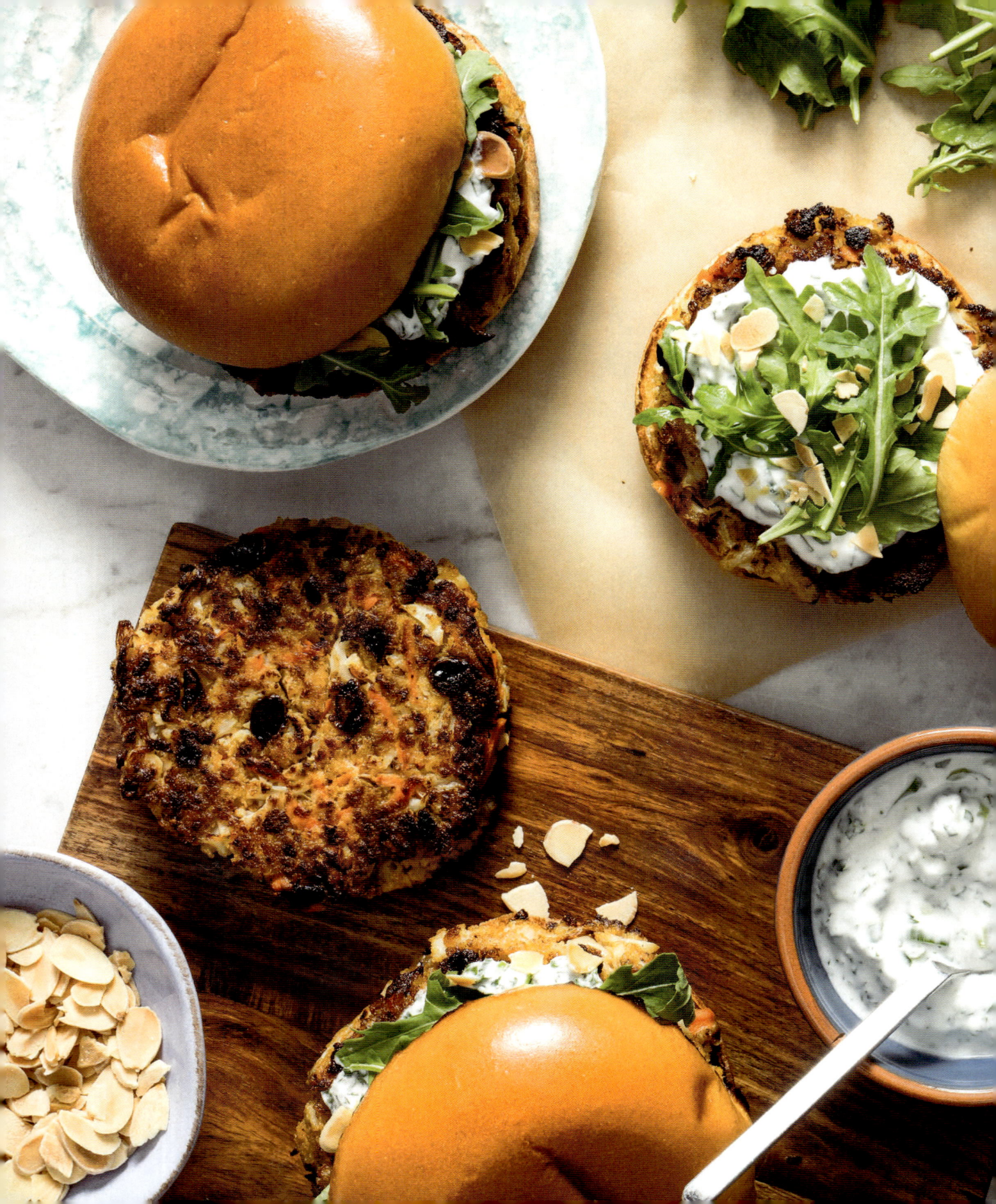

VEGETARIAN MAINS

■ FAST   ■ SUPERCHARGED

Jackfruit Tinga Tacos

serves 6 • total time: 45 minutes **FAST**

why this recipe works • In its ripe form, jackfruit tastes like a combination of papaya, pineapple, and mango. However, immature, green jackfruit is altogether different: vegetal, dense, and very fibrous. When canned in water or brine, green jackfruit tastes more like an artichoke heart than a fruit, and it is widely used in many Asian cuisines as a meat substitute. Once cooked, it shreds beautifully into tender morsels reminiscent of pulled pork or chicken—and uncannily mimics meat in these Mexican-style tinga tacos. After crisping the jackfruit in a skillet, we set it aside and built a savory sauce using tomato sauce enriched with aromatic onion, garlic, and oregano, plus a bit of chipotle chiles in adobo sauce for smoky depth. After a few minutes simmering in the sauce, the jackfruit was tender enough to mash into a hearty taco filling, which we spooned into corn tortillas. To finish, we topped them with a bright, aromatic cabbage-carrot slaw for fiber and crunch, plus avocado pieces for healthy fats and creamy richness. You can find canned jackfruit in most well-stocked supermarkets. Purchase young green (rather than ripe or mature) jackfruit in large pieces (rather than shredded) packed in water, not syrup. Garnish the tacos with fresh cilantro leaves, if desired. You will need a 12-inch nonstick skillet with a tight-fitting lid for this recipe.

3 tablespoons plus 1 teaspoon extra-virgin olive oil, divided
1 tablespoon cider vinegar
2 cups shredded green or red cabbage
1 carrot, peeled and shredded
2 tablespoons minced fresh cilantro
2 scallions, sliced thin
2 (14.5-ounce) cans young green jackfruit packed in water, rinsed and patted dry
1 small onion, chopped fine
3 garlic cloves, minced
1 teaspoon minced canned chipotle chile in adobo sauce
1 teaspoon dried oregano
1 (8-ounce) can no-salt-added tomato sauce
¼ cup water
¾ teaspoon table salt
12 (6-inch) corn tortillas, warmed
1 avocado, halved, pitted, and cut into ½-inch pieces

1 Whisk 2 tablespoons oil and vinegar together in bowl. Add cabbage, carrot, cilantro, and scallions and toss to combine. Season with salt and pepper to taste. Cover slaw and refrigerate until ready to serve.

2 Heat 1 tablespoon oil in 12-inch nonstick skillet over medium-high heat until shimmering. Add jackfruit in single layer and cook until well browned on all sides, flipping occasionally, about 8 minutes. Transfer jackfruit to plate and set aside.

3 Add onion and remaining 1 teaspoon oil to now-empty skillet and cook over medium heat until softened and lightly browned, 5 to 7 minutes. Stir in garlic, chipotle, and oregano and cook until fragrant, about 30 seconds. Stir in tomato sauce, water, and salt and bring to simmer. Add jackfruit to sauce, cover, and cook until jackfruit is very tender, about 8 minutes, flipping jackfruit once halfway through cooking.

4 Remove skillet from heat and, using potato masher, mash jackfruit until thoroughly shredded and well coated in sauce. Divide jackfruit evenly among warm tortillas and top with slaw and avocado. Serve.

Spiced Cauliflower Burgers

serves 4 • total time: 1 hour, plus 30 minutes chilling

why this recipe works • When we set out to develop a veggie burger using a less-expected vegetable, the humble cauliflower made immediate sense. It's creamy and nutty and turns into satisfying patties with tender interiors and crunchy, golden-brown exteriors. The trick to achieving this contrast was to first roast the cauliflower, which took less than 30 minutes; this intensified its flavor and made it easy to crush the florets. Before roasting, we tossed the florets with olive oil and ras el hanout—a lively North African spice blend made with cumin, coriander, cinnamon, and other warm spices. After roasting and processing the cauliflower, we added some panko as a binder, along with shredded carrots and golden raisins for their sweetness and some textural diversity, and formed the mixture into patties. Cooking the patties in olive oil gave them a crisp, well-browned crust. Burger garnishes of peppery baby arugula and herbed yogurt sauce offered fresh bursts of flavor, while a sprinkling of toasted sliced almonds contributed welcome crunch. Use the large holes of a box grater or a food processor fitted with a shredding disk to shred the carrot. We prefer our homemade Ras el Hanout (page 128), but you can use a store-bought blend.

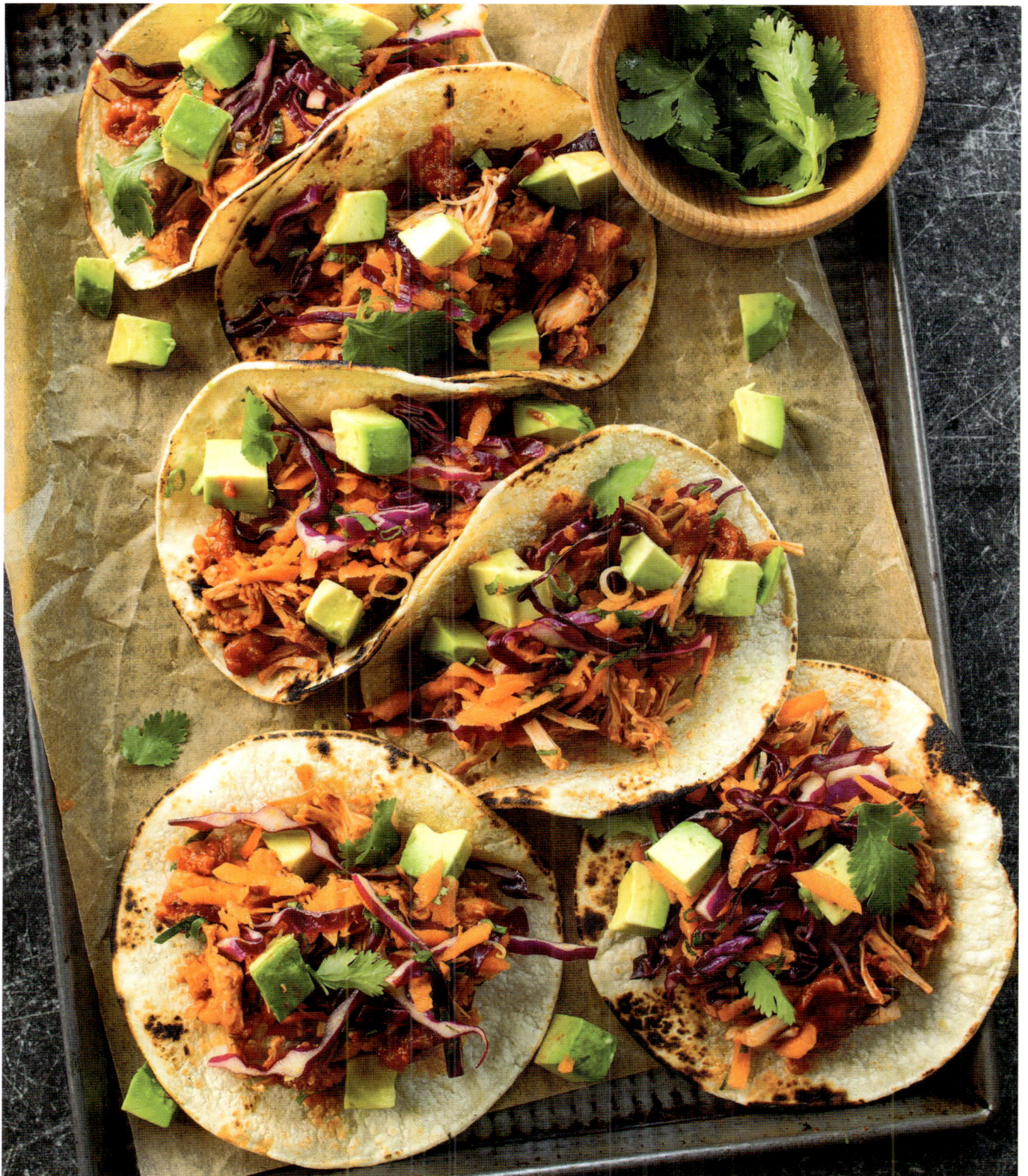

Jackfruit Tinga Tacos

1½ pounds cauliflower florets, cut into 1-inch pieces

3 tablespoons extra-virgin olive oil, divided

1 teaspoon ras el hanout

½ teaspoon table salt

⅛ teaspoon pepper

½ cup panko bread crumbs

1 small carrot, peeled and shredded

¼ cup golden raisins

2 large eggs, lightly beaten

4 hamburger buns, toasted if desired

¼ cup Herb-Yogurt Sauce (page 166)

3 tablespoons sliced almonds, toasted

1 cup baby arugula

1 Adjust oven rack to middle position and heat oven to 450 degrees. Line rimmed baking sheet with aluminum foil. Toss cauliflower with 1 tablespoon oil, ras el hanout, salt, and pepper and spread cauliflower in even layer on prepared sheet. Roast until well browned and tender, about 20 minutes. Let cool slightly and transfer to bowl of food processor.

2 Line clean rimmed baking sheet with parchment paper. Add panko, carrot, raisins, and eggs to cauliflower and pulse until coarsely ground and mixture comes together, about 6 pulses. Divide cauliflower mixture into 4 equal portions. Using your lightly moistened hands, firmly pack each portion into ¾-inch-thick patty and place on prepared sheet. Cover with plastic wrap and refrigerate until patties are firm, at least 30 minutes.

3 Heat remaining 2 tablespoons oil in 12-inch nonstick skillet over medium heat until shimmering. Place patties in skillet and cook until deep golden brown and crisp on first side, 2 to 3 minutes. Using 2 spatulas, gently flip patties and cook until browned and crisp on second side, 2 to 3 minutes. Serve burgers on buns, topped with yogurt sauce, almonds, and arugula.

MAKE AHEAD • Patties can be prepared through step 2 and refrigerated for up to 24 hours.

MAKE IT GLUTEN-FREE • Substitute gluten-free hamburger buns for the hamburger buns and gluten-free panko bread crumbs for the panko bread crumbs.

Ras el Hanout
makes about ½ cup • total time: 10 minutes

16 cardamom pods

4 teaspoons coriander seeds

4 teaspoons cumin seeds

2 teaspoons anise seeds

2 teaspoons ground dried Aleppo pepper

½ teaspoon allspice berries

¼ teaspoon black peppercorns

4 teaspoons ground ginger

2 teaspoons ground nutmeg

2 teaspoons ground cinnamon

Process cardamom pods, coriander, cumin, anise, Aleppo pepper, allspice, and peppercorns in spice grinder until finely ground, about 30 seconds. Stir in ginger, nutmeg, and cinnamon. (Spice blend can be stored at room temperature for up to 1 year.)

Pinto Bean–Beet Burgers
serves 8 • total time: 1 hour 5 minutes SUPERCHARGED

why this recipe works • Did you know that beet juice is sometimes used in plant-based beef for its color? We liked the idea of that but wanted to use beets to their fullest potential. In this modern bean-based burger, we used shredded beets to lighten up the texture and bring sweet-earthy flavor. Bulgur gave the patties heft and pleasing chew, ground nuts offered richness, and garlic and mustard deepened and united all the savory flavors. To bind the burgers, we turned to a surprising ingredient: carrot baby food. The pureed carrots contributed the necessary tackiness to make the patties cohesive, and their subtle sweetness heightened that of the shredded beets. Panko bread crumbs further bound the mixture and helped the patties sear up with a nicely crisp crust. When shopping, don't confuse bulgur with cracked wheat, which has a much longer cooking time and will not work here. Use the large holes of a box grater or a food processor fitted with a shredding disk to shred the beet. This recipe makes a lot of burgers, but they freeze very well. We like to top them with our Crispy Onions (page 159) and/or Quick Pickled Red Onions (page 25), but feel free to use your favorite burger toppings.

1½ teaspoons table salt, plus salt for cooking bulgur

⅔ cup medium-grind bulgur, rinsed

1 large beet (9 ounces), peeled and shredded

¾ cup walnuts

½ cup fresh basil leaves

2 garlic cloves, minced

1 (15-ounce) can no-salt-added pinto beans, rinsed

1 (4-ounce) jar carrot baby food

1 tablespoon whole-grain mustard

½ teaspoon pepper

1½ cups panko bread crumbs

6 tablespoons extra-virgin olive oil, divided

8 hamburger buns, toasted if desired

1   Bring 1½ cups water and ½ teaspoon salt to boil in small saucepan. Off heat, stir in bulgur, cover, and let sit until tender, 15 to 20 minutes. Drain bulgur, spread onto rimmed baking sheet, and let cool slightly.

2   Meanwhile, pulse beet, walnuts, basil, and garlic in food processor until finely chopped, about 12 pulses, scraping down sides of bowl as needed. Add beans, carrot baby food, 2 tablespoons water, mustard, pepper, and salt and pulse until well combined, about 8 pulses. Transfer mixture to large bowl and stir in panko and cooled bulgur.

3   Divide beet-bulgur mixture into 8 equal portions and firmly pack into 3½-inch-wide patties.

4   Adjust oven rack to middle position and heat oven to 200 degrees. Set wire rack in rimmed baking sheet. Heat 3 tablespoons oil in 12-inch nonstick skillet over medium-high heat until shimmering. Place 4 patties in skillet and cook until well browned and crisp on first side, about 4 minutes. Using 2 spatulas, gently flip patties and continue to cook until well browned and crisp on second side, about 4 minutes. Transfer burgers to prepared rack and keep warm in oven. Wipe skillet clean with paper towels and repeat with remaining 3 tablespoons oil and remaining 4 patties. Serve burgers on buns.

MAKE AHEAD • Patties can be prepared through step 3 and refrigerated for up to 3 days or frozen for up to 1 month. To freeze, transfer patties to 2 parchment paper–lined rimmed baking sheets and freeze until firm, about 1 hour. Stack patties, separated by parchment paper; wrap in plastic wrap; and place in zipper-lock freezer bag. Do not thaw patties before cooking.

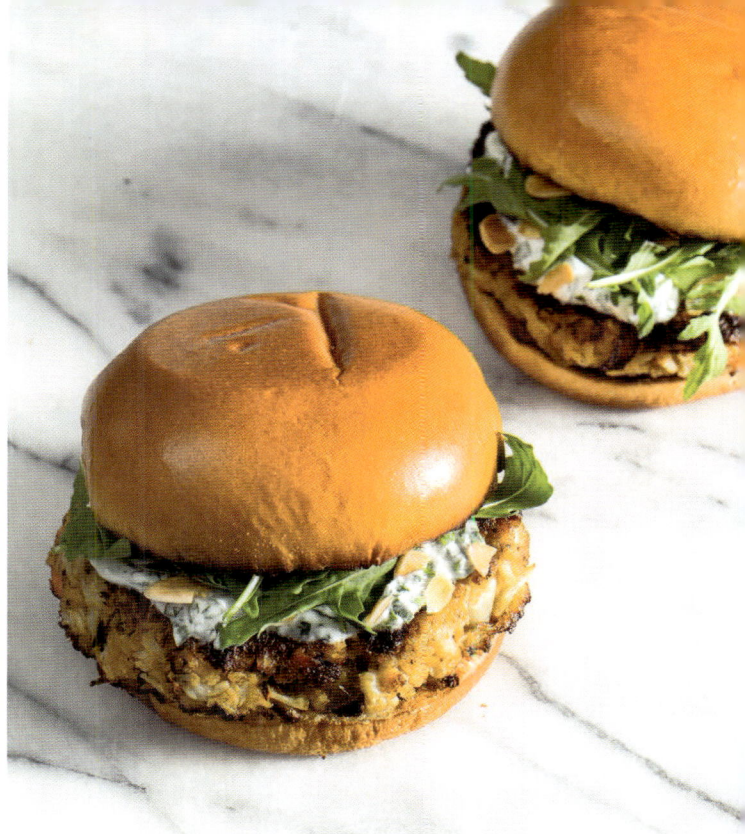

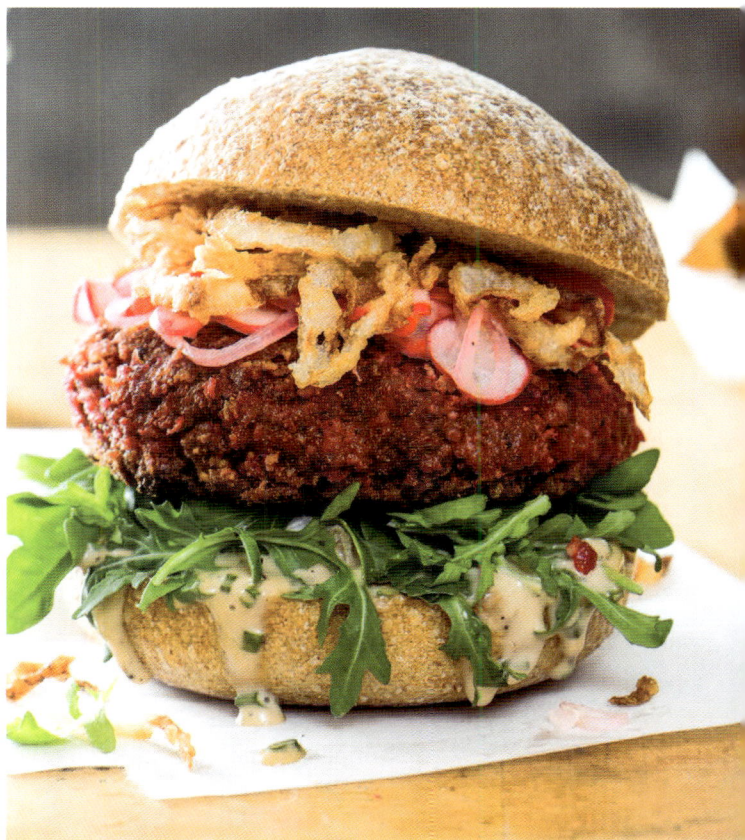

top | *Spiced Cauliflower Burgers*
bottom | *Pinto Bean–Beet Burgers*

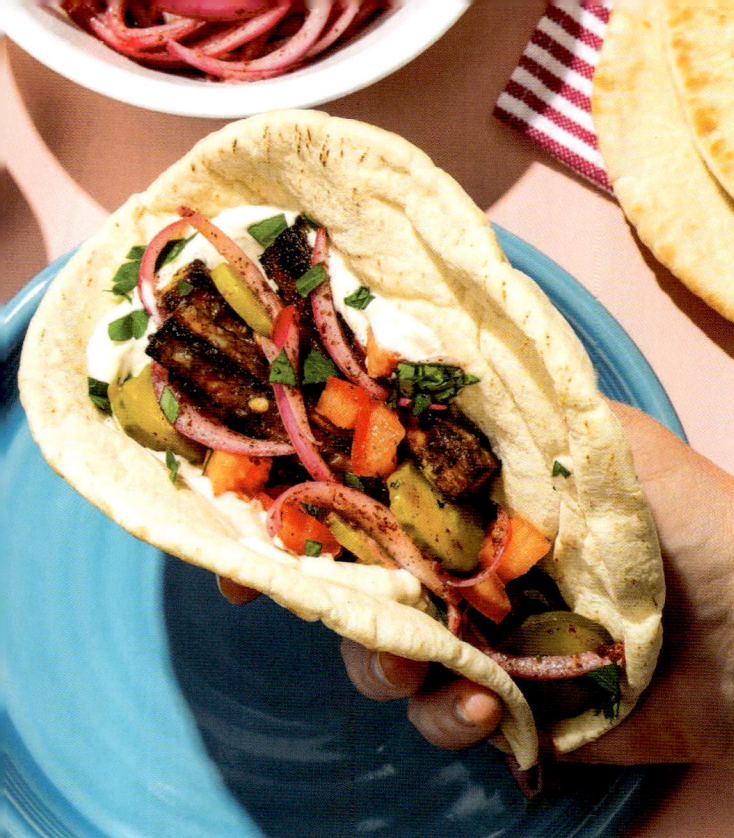

Shawarma-Spiced Tofu Wraps

serves 6 · **total time: 1 hour, plus 1 hour marinating**

SUPERCHARGED

why this recipe works · Crispy charred tofu strips are a delicious plant-powered protein source—and their flavor-absorbing texture is an ideal vehicle for a bevy of antioxidant-rich spices in this satisfying and nutritiously rich vegetarian wrap. We drew inspiration from the flavors of shawarma—popular in street carts throughout the Levant—to make the tofu marinade, combining sumac, fenugreek, paprika, cumin, and garlic. Lemon juice and honey added more complexity; the latter also helped caramelize the tofu. Broiling the tofu bloomed the flavors, infusing the crispy exterior. Tossing the finished tofu in reserved marinade amplified the smoky flavor. We wrapped the tofu in warm pitas (we like whole-wheat for its blood sugar–regulating fiber) and piled on an assortment of toppings typical of shawarma: Tomatoes, sumac onions, pickles, fresh herbs, and a finishing drizzle of cooling, creamy tahini-yogurt sauce made for a nutritionally well-rounded meal. The tofu fingers are delicate and may break while turning; this will not affect the final wraps. We liked to use our Sumac Onions in this recipe, but you can substitute an equal amount of thinly sliced red onion.

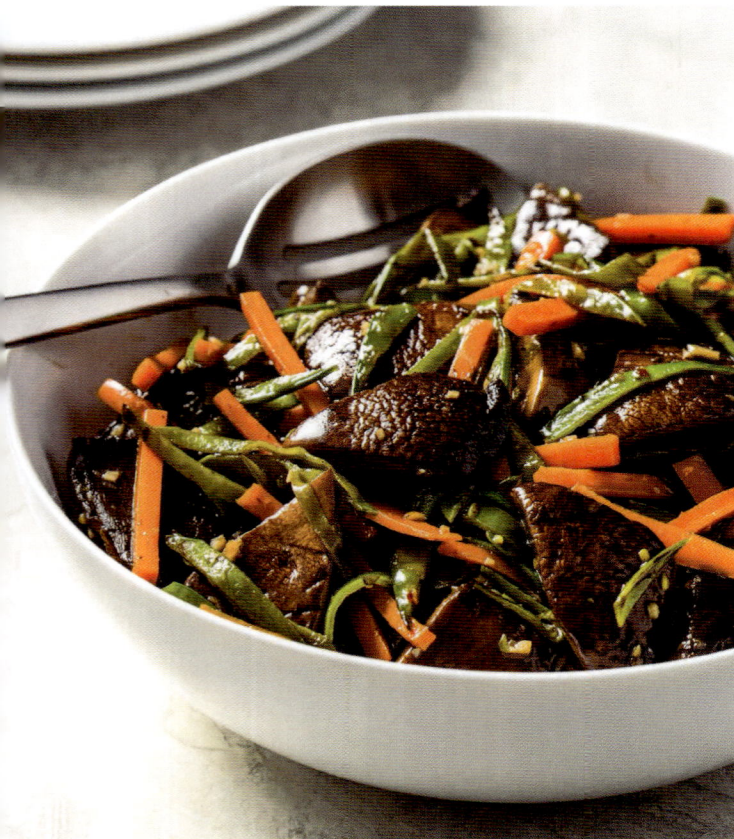

28	ounces firm or extra-firm tofu
½	cup extra-virgin olive oil
6	garlic cloves, minced
1½	tablespoons ground sumac
1	tablespoon ground fenugreek
2	teaspoons smoked paprika
1½	teaspoons ground cumin
1	teaspoon table salt
¼	cup lemon juice (2 lemons)
3	tablespoons honey
6	(8-inch) pitas, warmed
½	cup Tahini-Yogurt Sauce (page 168)
1	tomato, cored and chopped
½	cup chopped fresh parsley and/or mint
½	cup dill pickle slices
½	cup Sumac Onions (recipe follows)

1 Cut tofu crosswise into ½-inch-thick slabs, then slice slabs lengthwise into ½-inch-thick fingers. Spread tofu on paper towel–lined baking sheet and let drain for 20 minutes, then gently press dry with paper towels.

2 Microwave oil, garlic, sumac, fenugreek, paprika, cumin, and salt in medium bowl, stirring occasionally, until fragrant, 30 to 60 seconds. Whisk in lemon juice and honey until honey has dissolved. Measure out and reserve ¼ cup marinade.

3 Arrange tofu in single layer on second rimmed baking sheet and spoon remaining marinade evenly over top. Using your hands, gently turn tofu to coat with marinade. Cover and refrigerate for at least 1 hour.

4 Adjust oven rack 6 inches from broiler element and heat broiler. Line rimmed baking sheet with aluminum foil. Transfer tofu to prepared sheet and arrange in single layer, spaced evenly apart. Broil tofu until well browned on first side, 10 to 15 minutes, rotating sheet halfway through broiling. Gently flip tofu and continue to broil until well browned on second side, 10 to 15 minutes, rotating sheet halfway through broiling. Transfer tofu and reserved ¼ cup marinade to large bowl and toss gently to coat. Spread pitas with tahini sauce, divide tofu evenly among pitas, and top with tomato, parsley, pickles, and sumac onions. Serve.

MAKE AHEAD • Reserved marinade can be refrigerated for up to 24 hours; bring to room temperature and whisk to recombine before using. Marinated tofu can be refrigerated for up to 24 hours.

MAKE IT GLUTEN-FREE • Substitute gluten-free pita for the pita.

Sumac Onions

makes about 2 cups • **total time: 1 hour**

- 1 red onion, halved and sliced ¼ inch thick through root end
- 2 tablespoons lemon juice
- 2 tablespoons red wine vinegar
- 1 tablespoon extra-virgin olive oil
- 1 tablespoon ground sumac
- ½ teaspoon sugar
- ¼ teaspoon table salt

Combine all ingredients in bowl. Let sit, stirring occasionally for 1 hour. (Onions can be refrigerated for up to 1 week.)

Stir-Fried Portobellos with Soy-Maple Glaze

serves 4 to 6 • **total time: 50 minutes**

why this recipe works • Hefty, meaty portobello mushrooms paired with snow peas and carrots make for a supersatisfying vegetable stir-fry that's chewy and crunchy in equal measure. Cooking the mushrooms in two batches not only kept them from steaming in their own juices but also guaranteed even cooking and good browning. Adding a boldly flavored glaze of mirin, soy sauce, and maple syrup gave the mushrooms a sweet-salty flavor boost. We stir-fried the snow peas and carrots until crisp-tender to preserve some crunch, added garlic and ginger and cooked until just fragrant and then finished by stirring in the glazed mushrooms and a simple stir-fry sauce to coat everything in glossy, umami-rich goodness. Serve with rice.

Glaze

- 3 tablespoons maple syrup
- 2 tablespoons mirin
- 1 tablespoon low-sodium soy sauce

Sauce

- ½ cup unsalted vegetable broth
- 2 tablespoons low-sodium soy sauce
- 1½ tablespoons mirin
- 2 teaspoons unseasoned rice vinegar
- 2 teaspoons cornstarch
- 2 teaspoons toasted sesame oil

Vegetables

- 3 tablespoons avocado oil, divided
- 2 garlic cloves, minced
- 2 teaspoons grated fresh ginger
- ¼ teaspoon red pepper flakes
- 2 pounds portobello mushroom caps, gills removed, cut into 2-inch wedges, divided
- 8 ounces snow peas, strings removed and sliced ¼ inch thick on bias
- 2 carrots, peeled and cut into 2-inch-long matchsticks

1 For the glaze Whisk all ingredients together in bowl.

2 For the sauce Whisk all ingredients together in bowl.

3 **For the vegetables** Combine 1 teaspoon oil, garlic, ginger, and pepper flakes in bowl and set aside. Heat 1 tablespoon oil in 12-inch nonstick skillet over high heat until shimmering. Add half of mushrooms and cook, without stirring, until browned on one side, 2 to 3 minutes. Flip mushrooms, reduce heat to medium, and cook until second side is browned and mushrooms are tender, about 5 minutes. Transfer to second bowl. Repeat with 1 tablespoon oil and remaining mushrooms.

4 Return all mushrooms to skillet, add glaze, and cook over medium-high heat, stirring frequently, until glaze is thickened and mushrooms are coated, 1 to 2 minutes. Transfer mushrooms to bowl.

5 Wipe skillet clean with paper towels. Heat remaining 2 teaspoons oil in now-empty skillet over high heat until shimmering. Add snow peas and carrots and cook, stirring occasionally, until vegetables are crisp-tender, about 5 minutes. Clear center of skillet, add garlic mixture, and cook, mashing mixture into skillet, until fragrant, about 30 seconds. Stir garlic mixture into vegetables.

6 Return mushrooms to skillet. Whisk sauce to recombine, then add to skillet. Cook, stirring constantly, until sauce is thickened, 1 to 2 minutes. Serve.

> **MAKE AHEAD** • Vegetables can be prepped up to 24 hours ahead.

> **MAKE IT GLUTEN-FREE** • Substitute low-sodium tamari for the low-sodium soy sauce.

Stir-Fried Tempeh with Orange Sauce

serves 4 • total time: 30 minutes **FAST**

why this recipe works • Tempeh is a firm, dense cake, so it holds its shape when cooked—making it a great plant-based protein choice for stir-fries. For this recipe, we had visions of golden-brown tempeh and crisp vegetables coated in a sweet-sour orange sauce. First we perfected the tempeh, searing cubes of it in a hot skillet with soy sauce to give it an umami flavor boost and crisp brown crust. We added red bell pepper for sweetness and crunch, plus a punch of fiber. Broccoli florets were another great addition; like the bell pepper, they stood up well to the quick, high heat, becoming crisp-tender as they cooked. As for the sauce, we knew we needed a sweeter sauce to stand up to the slightly bitter tempeh but were wary of adding sugar. A tangy,

full-bodied sauce made with orange juice tamed the tempeh and gave us just the right amount of sweetness. A scattering of sliced scallions offered a fresh zing. Serve with rice.

Sauce
- ¼ cup Shaoxing wine or dry sherry
- ¼ cup water
- 2 tablespoons low-sodium soy sauce
- 1 tablespoon cornstarch
- 1 tablespoon grated fresh ginger
- 3 garlic cloves, minced
- 1½ teaspoons toasted sesame oil
- ¼ teaspoon grated orange zest plus ¾ cup juice (2 oranges)

Stir-Fry
- 2 tablespoons avocado oil, divided
- 12 ounces tempeh, cut into ½-inch pieces
- 2 tablespoons low-sodium soy sauce
- 1 pound broccoli, florets cut into ½-inch pieces, stalks peeled, halved, and sliced thin
- 1 red bell pepper, stemmed, seeded, and cut into ¼-inch-wide strips
- 6 scallions, sliced thin on bias
- 1 tablespoon toasted sesame seeds (optional)

1 **For the sauce** Whisk all ingredients together in bowl.

2 **For the stir-fry** Heat 1 tablespoon oil in 12-inch nonstick skillet over high heat until just smoking. Add tempeh and soy sauce and cook, stirring occasionally, until well browned, 4 to 6 minutes; transfer to plate.

3 Heat remaining 1 tablespoon oil in now-empty skillet over high heat until just smoking. Add broccoli and bell pepper and cook, stirring occasionally, until vegetables are spotty brown and crisp-tender, about 4 minutes.

4 Stir in browned tempeh. Whisk sauce to recombine, then add to skillet and cook, stirring constantly, until sauce is thickened, about 30 seconds. Off heat, sprinkle with scallions and sesame seeds, if using. Serve.

> **MAKE AHEAD** • Vegetables can be prepped up to 24 hours ahead.

> **MAKE IT GLUTEN-FREE** • Substitute gluten-free tempeh for the tempeh. Substitute low-sodium tamari for the low-sodium soy sauce.

All About Tempeh

Tempeh is made by fermenting cooked soybeans and then forming the mixture into a firm, dense cake. Some versions also contain beans, grains, and flavorings. It serves as a good meat substitute and is a mainstay of many vegetarian diets—it's particularly popular in Southeast Asia. It has a strong nutty flavor, but it also absorbs other flavors easily. And because it's better than tofu at holding its shape when cooked, it's a versatile choice for many dishes, from sandwiches and tacos to curries. It's also a healthy choice, since it's high in protein, cholesterol-free, and contains many essential vitamins and minerals. Tempeh is sold refrigerated in most supermarkets; we use five-grain tempeh in our recipes, but any plain variety will work. If you are gluten-free, be sure to look for a gluten-free brand.

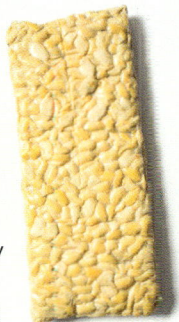

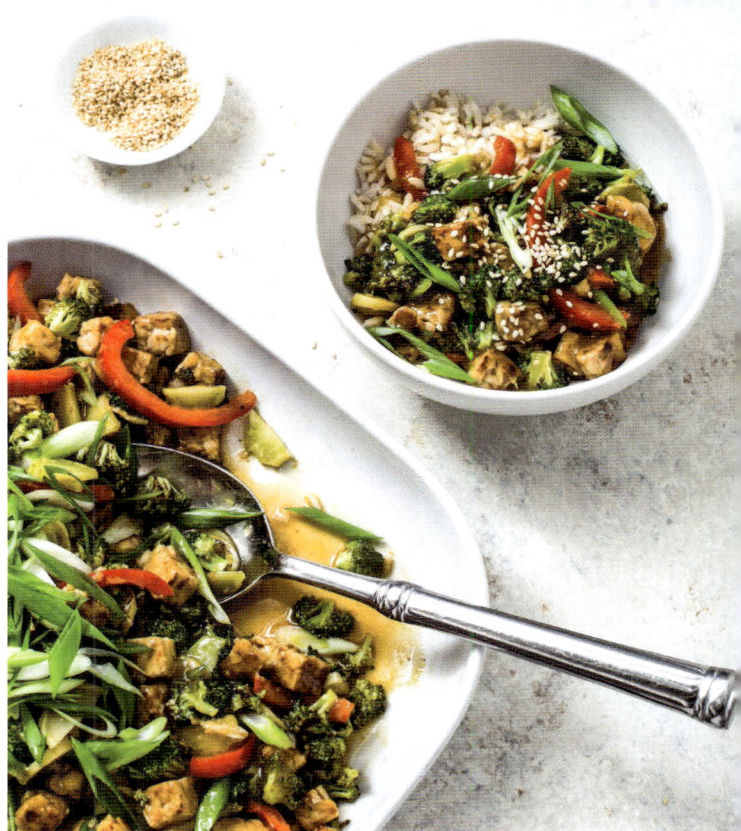

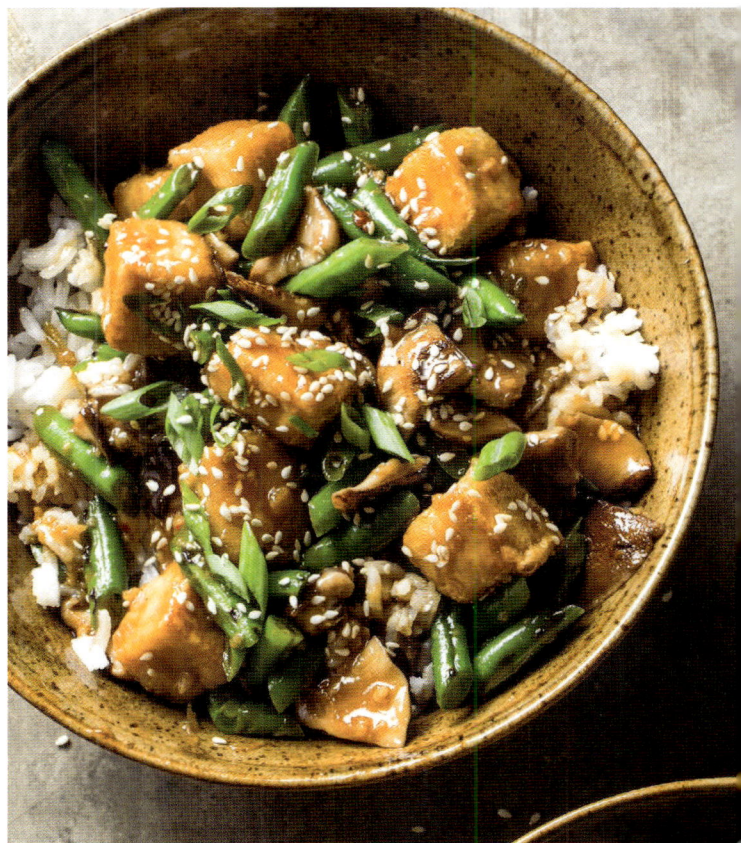

Stir-Fried Tofu, Shiitakes, and Green Beans

serves 4 · total time: 50 minutes, plus 20 minutes draining

why this recipe works · This stir-fry, with its ease of preparation and crowd-pleasing flavors, is a delicious and easy way to prepare tofu. We sliced and drained hearty, protein-packed extra-firm tofu before coating it simply with cornstarch, so the pieces developed a slightly crunchy outer sheath as they browned in the skillet. After transferring the tofu to a plate, we added sturdy green beans and meaty shiitake mushrooms to the skillet, covering them until they softened and then uncovering to brown them. (Make sure not manipulate the tofu or vegetables too much while they're browning, otherwise you won't get that desired sear.) Although we often stir-fry vegetables in batches, here we were able to stir-fry them at the same time; the moisture released from the mushrooms nicely steamed the green beans. For a classic brown sauce, we combined soy sauce, sesame oil, rice vinegar, and a touch of sugar and pepper flakes and then thickened it with cornstarch. Serve with rice.

| top | Stir-Fried Tempeh with Orange Sauce |
| bottom | Stir-Fried Tofu, Shiitakes, and Green Beans |

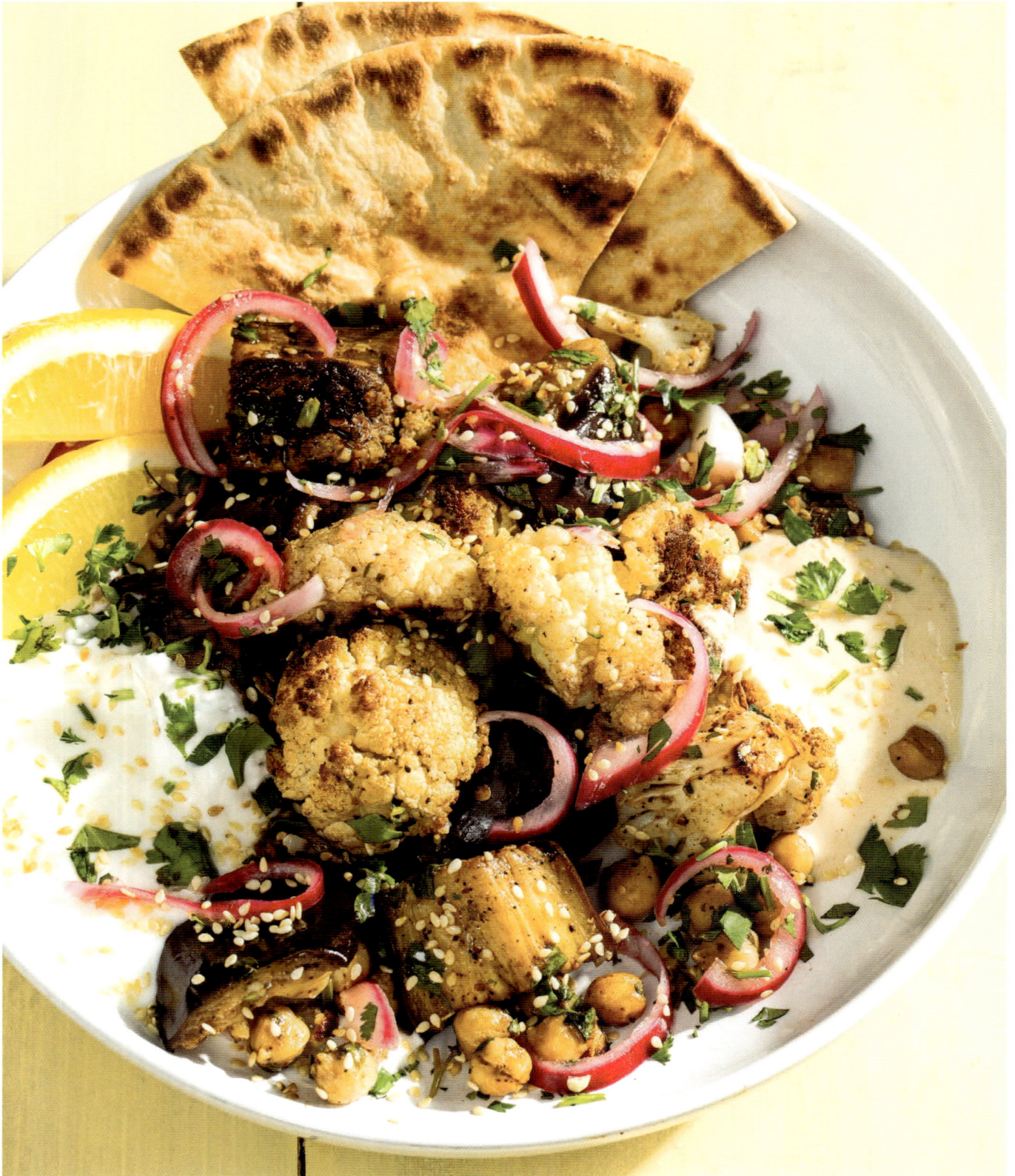

Baharat Cauliflower and Eggplant with Chickpeas

Sauce

- ¾ cup unsalted vegetable broth
- 3 tablespoons low-sodium soy sauce
- 2 tablespoons unseasoned rice vinegar
- 1 tablespoon packed brown sugar
- 2 teaspoons cornstarch
- 1 teaspoon toasted sesame oil
- ⅛ teaspoon red pepper flakes

Stir-Fry

- 14 ounces extra-firm tofu, cut into ¾-inch pieces
- ⅓ cup cornstarch
- 3 tablespoons avocado oil, divided
- 12 ounces green beans, trimmed and cut on bias into 1-inch lengths
- 12 ounces shiitake mushrooms, stemmed and quartered
- 2 scallions, white and green parts separated and sliced thin on bias
- 3 garlic cloves, minced
- 1 tablespoon grated fresh ginger
- 1 tablespoon toasted sesame seeds (optional)

1   For the sauce Whisk all ingredients together in bowl.

2   For the stir-fry Spread tofu over paper towel–lined baking sheet and let drain for 20 minutes. Gently press dry with paper towels. Toss drained tofu with cornstarch in bowl, then transfer to fine-mesh strainer and shake gently to remove excess cornstarch.

3   Heat 2 tablespoons oil in 12-inch nonstick skillet over high heat until shimmering. Add tofu and cook, turning as needed, until crisp and well browned on all sides, 12 to 15 minutes; transfer to paper towel–lined plate to drain.

4   Heat 2 teaspoons oil in now-empty skillet over medium-high heat until shimmering. Add green beans and mushrooms, cover, and cook until mushrooms release their liquid and green beans are bright green and beginning to soften, 4 to 5 minutes. Uncover and continue to cook until vegetables are spotty brown, about 3 minutes.

5   Combine remaining 1 teaspoon oil, scallion whites, garlic, and ginger in bowl. Push vegetables to sides of skillet. Add garlic mixture to center and cook, mashing mixture into pan, until fragrant, about 30 seconds. Stir garlic mixture into vegetables. Add browned tofu and stir to combine. Whisk sauce to recombine, then add to skillet and cook, stirring constantly, until sauce is thickened, about 30 seconds. Transfer to platter and sprinkle with scallion greens and sesame seeds, if using. Serve.

MAKE AHEAD • Vegetables can be prepped up to 24 hours ahead.

MAKE IT GLUTEN-FREE • Substitute low-sodium tamari for the low-sodium soy sauce.

Baharat Cauliflower and Eggplant with Chickpeas

serves 4 • total time: 1¼ hours   SUPERCHARGED

why this recipe works • Cauliflower is a flavor sponge, soaking up any seasoning you throw at it. It also happens to be an inflammation-fighting superstar, loaded with glucosinolates, vitamin C, and quercetin, not to mention fiber. In this sheet-pan recipe, the spice blend baharat brings out the nuttiness and mellow sweetness of cauliflower, which we roasted with eggplant to make the most of their contrasting textures. Stirring in chickpeas amped up the protein (which slows digestion and stabilizes blood sugar) and highlighted the nuttiness of the dish. Serving the mix with a lemony tahini sauce—a little sweet and a little spicy—as well as pickled red onions rounded out the experience of this warm, nourishing dish. We like to use our homemade Baharat (page 136), but you can use a store-bought blend if you prefer. Garnish with toasted sesame seeds, if desired.

- 1½ pounds eggplant, cut into 1½-inch pieces
- 1 teaspoon table salt, divided
- ⅓ cup tahini
- 3 tablespoons water, plus extra as needed
- 5 tablespoons lemon juice, divided, plus lemon wedges for serving
- 1 small garlic clove, grated
- ½ teaspoon honey
- ⅛ teaspoon cayenne pepper (optional)
- 1 small head cauliflower (1½ pounds), cored and cut into 1½-inch florets
- 1 (15-ounce) can no-salt-added chickpeas, rinsed and patted dry
- ¼ cup extra-virgin olive oil
- 1 tablespoon baharat
- ¾ cup chopped fresh cilantro, divided
  Quick Pickled Red Onions (page 25)
  Plain yogurt
- 4 pitas, warmed

1 Adjust oven rack to lower-middle position and heat oven to 450 degrees. Line rimmed baking sheet with aluminum foil and spray with olive oil spray. Toss eggplant with ½ teaspoon salt in colander and let drain for 30 minutes, tossing occasionally. Whisk together tahini, water, 3 tablespoons lemon juice, garlic, honey, and cayenne, if using, until smooth. Season with salt and pepper to taste and set aside until ready to serve. (If needed, add more water 1 teaspoon at a time until sauce is thick but pourable.)

2 Pat eggplant dry with paper towels. Toss eggplant, cauliflower, chickpeas, oil, baharat, and remaining ½ teaspoon salt together in large bowl, then spread in even layer on prepared sheet. Roast until vegetables are very tender and beginning to brown in spots, 30 to 40 minutes, stirring occasionally.

3 Gently toss vegetables with ½ cup cilantro and remaining 2 tablespoons lemon juice and season with salt and pepper to taste. Sprinkle with remaining ¼ cup cilantro and serve with reserved tahini sauce, pickled red onions, yogurt, pitas, and lemon wedges.

MAKE IT GLUTEN-FREE • Substitute gluten-free pita for the pita.

MAKE IT DAIRY-FREE • Substitute plant-based yogurt for the dairy yogurt.

Baharat

makes about ½ cup · total time: 5 minutes

   3 (3-inch) cinnamon sticks, broken into pieces
4¾ teaspoons cumin seeds
1½ tablespoons coriander seeds
   1 tablespoon black peppercorns
   2 teaspoons whole cloves
   1 tablespoon ground cardamom
   2 teaspoons ground nutmeg

Process cinnamon sticks in spice grinder until finely ground, about 30 seconds. Add cumin seeds, coriander seeds, peppercorns, and cloves and process until finely ground, about 30 seconds. Transfer to bowl and stir in cardamom and nutmeg. (Baharat can be stored in airtight container at room temperature for up to 1 year.)

Overstuffed Sweet Potatoes with Tofu and Thai Curry

serves 4 · total time: 55 minutes, plus 20 minutes draining

why this recipe works • This fresh, modern take on stuffed potatoes takes its cue from the tangy and sweet flavors of Thai-style curries. All of the elements—rich, earthy sweet potato halves along with morsels of tofu, broccoli, mushrooms, and bell peppers—are roasted to perfection on a single baking sheet. To create extra-crispy tofu, we dusted pieces with cornstarch and arranged them on one side of an oiled baking sheet, then placed the sweet potato halves on the other side. (Halving the sweet potatoes reduced the roasting time from an hour, for whole potatoes, to a mere 20 minutes.) Once the potatoes were done, we added the other vegetables to the space left on the baking sheet and roasted them until tender in the time it took to finish the crispy tofu. After stuffing the potatoes with the tofu and vegetables, we drizzled them with a curry vinaigrette packed with the bold flavors of lime and curry paste. All this hearty meal needs is a simple green salad. If you can't find Thai basil, you can substitute Italian basil.

14 ounces firm tofu, cut into ¾-inch pieces
   1 teaspoon table salt, divided
   ½ teaspoon pepper, divided
   6 tablespoons cornstarch
   ½ cup plus 1 teaspoon avocado oil, divided
   2 sweet potatoes (12 ounces each), unpeeled, halved lengthwise
   8 ounces broccoli florets, cut into ½-inch pieces
   8 ounces white or cremini mushrooms, trimmed and quartered
   1 red bell pepper, stemmed, seeded, and cut into ¼-inch-wide strips
   1 teaspoon grated lime zest plus 2 tablespoons juice
   2 teaspoons Thai green or red curry paste
   ¼ cup shredded fresh Thai basil

1 Spread tofu on paper towel–lined baking sheet and let drain for 20 minutes. Gently press dry with paper towels. Sprinkle tofu with ½ teaspoon salt and ¼ teaspoon pepper and toss with cornstarch in bowl. Transfer to fine-mesh strainer and shake gently to remove excess cornstarch.

2 Adjust oven rack to lower-middle position and heat oven to 450 degrees. Brush rimmed baking sheet with 3 tablespoons oil. Arrange tofu in even layer on 1 half of sheet. Arrange potato halves cut side down on empty side of sheet and brush skins with 1 teaspoon oil. Roast until potato halves yield to gentle pressure and centers register 200 degrees, 20 to 25 minutes, flipping tofu with spatula halfway through roasting.

3   Toss broccoli, mushrooms, and bell pepper with 1 tablespoon oil, ¼ teaspoon salt, and ⅛ teaspoon pepper in bowl. Remove sheet from oven, transfer potato halves to plate, and tent with aluminum foil to keep warm. Arrange broccoli mixture in even layer on now-empty side of sheet. Roast until vegetables are tender and beginning to brown and tofu is crisp and lightly browned, 10 to 15 minutes, tossing vegetables and flipping tofu halfway through roasting.

4   Whisk lime zest and juice, curry paste, remaining ¼ cup oil, remaining ¼ teaspoon salt, and remaining ⅛ teaspoon pepper together in bowl. Arrange potato halves cut side up on individual serving plates. Using 2 forks, press potato flesh to sides to make room in center for tofu and vegetable mixture. Top potato halves with tofu and vegetable mixture, drizzle with vinaigrette, and sprinkle with basil. Serve.

Loaded Sweet Potato Wedges with Tempeh

serves 4 · total time: 45 minutes   **FAST**

why this recipe works · Sturdy, caramelized wedges of sweet potatoes are excellent as a side dish, but they can also be an incredible base for a hearty plant-based meal. We found that a well-seasoned topping of ground tempeh complemented the sweet tubers with contrasting texture. Sweet cherry tomatoes, crisp radishes, spicy jalapeño, and plenty of fresh cilantro added more fiber, flavor, and color. Serving with yogurt added gut-balancing probiotics. Serve with Quick Pickled Red Onions (page 25) and Avocado-Yogurt Sauce (page 138), if desired.

- 2   pounds sweet potatoes, unpeeled, cut lengthwise into 2-inch-wide wedges
- 5   tablespoons extra-virgin olive oil, divided
- 1   teaspoon table salt, divided
- 8   ounces tempeh, crumbled into pea-size pieces
- 1   teaspoon ground cumin
- 1   teaspoon ground coriander
- 1   teaspoon smoked paprika
- ⅛   teaspoon ground cinnamon
- 4   ounces cherry tomatoes, halved
- 4   radishes, trimmed and sliced thin
- 1   jalapeño, sliced into thin rings
- ¾   cup chopped fresh cilantro
- 3   scallions, sliced thin
-    Plain yogurt
-    Lime wedges

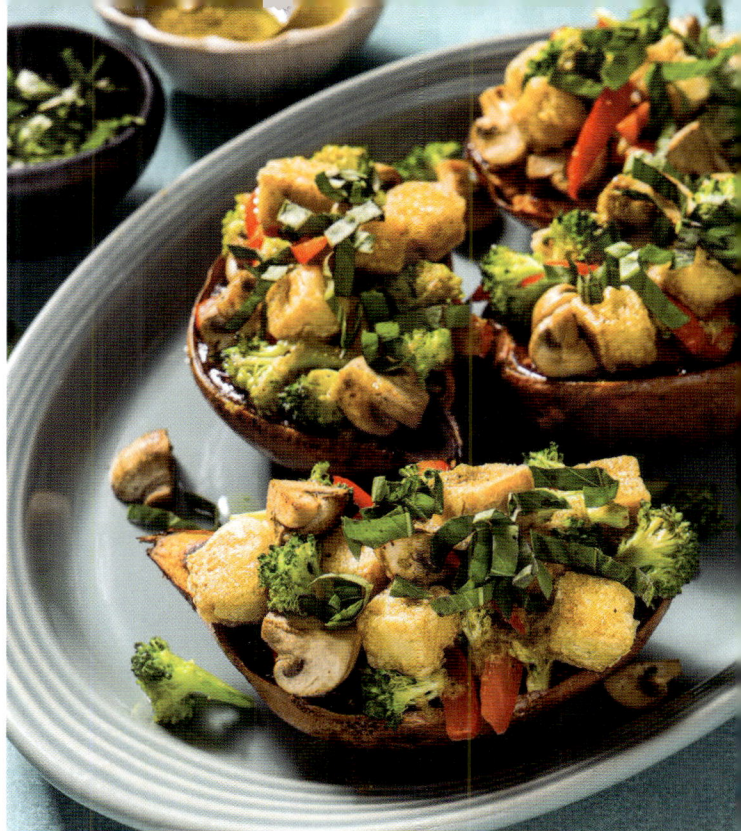

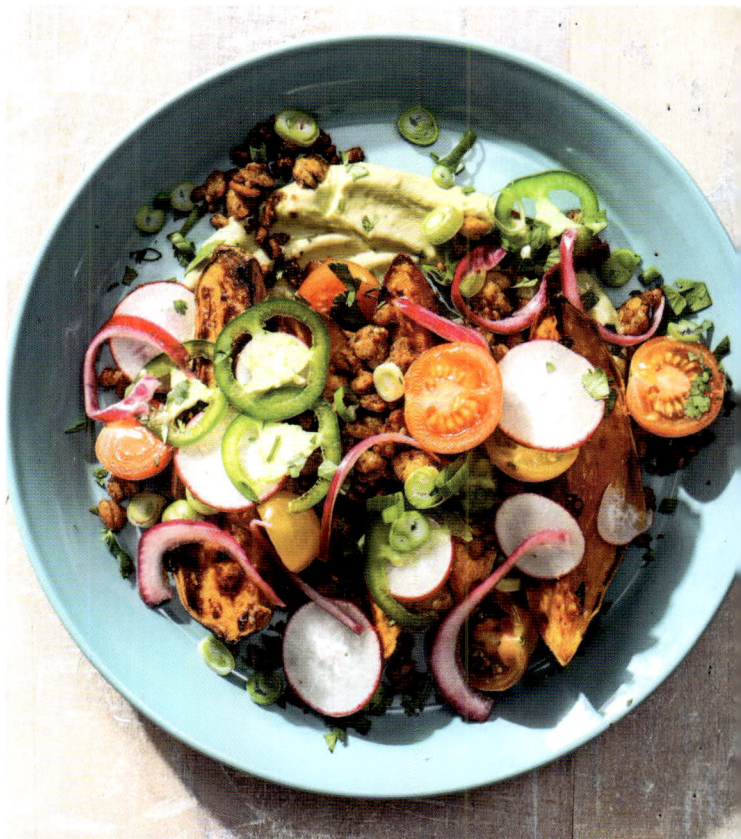

top | *Overstuffed Sweet Potatoes with Tofu and Thai Curry*
bottom | *Loaded Sweet Potato Wedges with Tempeh*

1 Adjust oven rack to middle position and heat oven to 450 degrees. Line rimmed baking sheet with aluminum foil and spray with olive oil spray. Toss potatoes, 1 tablespoon oil, and ½ teaspoon salt together in bowl, then arrange potato wedges, cut sides down, in single layer on prepared sheet. Roast until tender and sides in contact with sheet are well browned, about 30 minutes.

2 Meanwhile, heat remaining ¼ cup oil in 12-inch skillet over medium heat until shimmering. Add tempeh, cumin, coriander, paprika, cinnamon, and remaining ½ teaspoon salt and cook until well browned, 8 to 12 minutes, stirring often; set aside until ready to serve.

3 Transfer sweet potatoes to platter or individual serving plates and top with crispy tempeh, cherry tomatoes, radishes, jalapeño, cilantro, and scallions. Serve with yogurt and lime wedges.

MAKE IT GLUTEN-FREE • Substitute gluten-free tempeh for the tempeh.

MAKE IT DAIRY-FREE • Substitute plant-based yogurt for the dairy yogurt.

Avocado-Yogurt Sauce

makes about 1¼ cups • total time: 10 minutes

- 1 ripe avocado, halved, pitted, and cut into ½-inch pieces
- ¼ cup plain dairy yogurt or plant-based yogurt
- 1 teaspoon lime juice
- ½ teaspoon ground cumin
- ⅛ teaspoon table salt
- ⅛ teaspoon pepper

Using sturdy whisk, mash and stir all ingredients together in bowl until as smooth as possible. Season with salt and pepper to taste. (Sauce can be refrigerated with plastic wrap pressed flush to surface for up to 24 hours.)

NOTES FROM THE TEST KITCHEN

Sweet Potato Varieties

Sweet potatoes, fiber-dense sources of complex carbohydrates, can vary greatly in color, texture, and flavor. The good news is that all these varieties are fairly interchangeable in recipes. If we think a specific variety works best in a recipe, we'll make a note of that.

Beauregard Most often sold as the conventional sweet potato, the Beauregard has dusky red skin and is sweet, moist, and buttery. Its versatility makes it our favorite variety.

Jewel Another favorite of ours that is frequently found in supermarkets, the Jewel sweet potato has copper skin and moist orange flesh.

Red Garnet Named for its red-purple skin, Red Garnets have orange flesh that is more savory and less dense than Beauregards or Jewels.

White Japanese White and White Sweets tend to be less moist and are starchier than the orange-fleshed varieties.

Purple Sweet potatoes such as the Stokes Purple have a dry, dense texture and the highest level of antioxidants of all the sweet potato varieties.

Mushroom Bourguignon

serves 6 to 8 • total time: 1½ hours

why this recipe works • Chunks of portobello mushrooms drenched in a silky, luscious sauce made with shallots, carrots, garlic, and red wine will have you forgetting that traditional French bourguignon has boeuf (beef). We started by cooking portobello mushrooms until they released their savory moisture. We then browned carrots and shallots in oil and added a full cup of red wine, followed by a concoction of miso, soy sauce, and tomato paste, which gave us the umami notes we were after. Use a good-quality light- or medium-bodied red wine, such as a Pinot Noir or Grenache. You can substitute dried shiitake mushrooms for the dried porcini, and yellow or red miso for white miso. Leave the mushroom gills intact; they enhance the stew's color and flavor. Serve over polenta, noodles, or mashed potatoes.

4¾ cups water, divided

¼ cup extra-virgin olive oil, divided

2½ pounds portobello mushroom caps, cut into 1-inch pieces

½ teaspoon table salt

¼ teaspoon pepper

2 carrots, peeled and sliced ¼ inch thick

1 large shallot, chopped

4 garlic cloves, smashed and peeled

3 tablespoons all-purpose flour

1 cup plus 2 tablespoons dry red wine, divided

2 tablespoons white miso

2 tablespoons low-sodium soy sauce

1 tablespoon no-salt-added tomato paste

6 sprigs fresh thyme

2 bay leaves

1 ounce dried porcini mushrooms, rinsed

1 cup frozen pearl onions, thawed

¼ cup minced fresh parsley

1   Add ¼ cup water and 2 tablespoons oil to Dutch oven and bring to simmer over medium-high heat. Add portobello mushrooms, salt, and pepper. Cover and cook, stirring occasionally, until mushrooms have released their moisture, about 10 minutes.

2   Uncover and continue to cook, stirring occasionally, until pot is dry and dark fond forms, 10 to 12 minutes longer. Transfer mushrooms to bowl. Add carrots, shallot, and remaining 2 tablespoons oil to pot and cook, stirring frequently, until vegetables start to brown, 3 to 4 minutes. Add garlic and cook for 1 minute. Stir in flour and cook for 30 seconds. Whisk in 1 cup wine.

3   Add miso, soy sauce, tomato paste, and remaining 4½ cups water and whisk to combine. Add thyme sprigs, bay leaves, and porcini mushrooms and bring to boil over high heat. Reduce heat to maintain vigorous simmer and cook, stirring occasionally and scraping bottom of pot to loosen any browned bits, until sauce is reduced and has consistency of heavy cream, about 25 minutes.

4   Strain sauce through fine-mesh strainer set over large bowl, pressing on solids to extract as much liquid as possible; discard solids. You should have 2 cups sauce. (If you have more, return sauce to pot and continue to cook over medium heat until reduced. If you have less, add enough water to yield 2 cups.) Return sauce to pot. Stir in portobello mushrooms, onions, and remaining 2 tablespoons wine. Cover and cook over low heat, stirring occasionally, until onions are tender, about 20 minutes. Stir in parsley. Season with salt and pepper to taste, and serve.

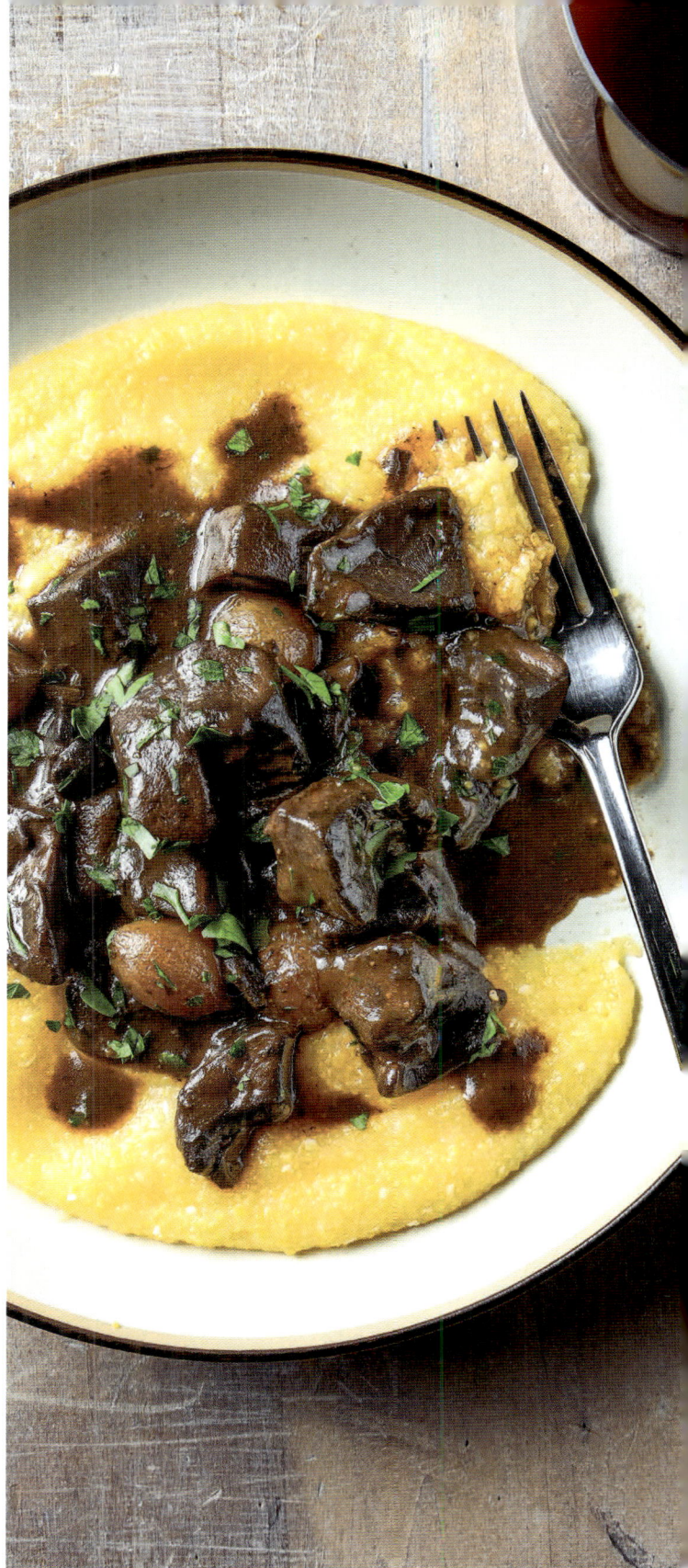

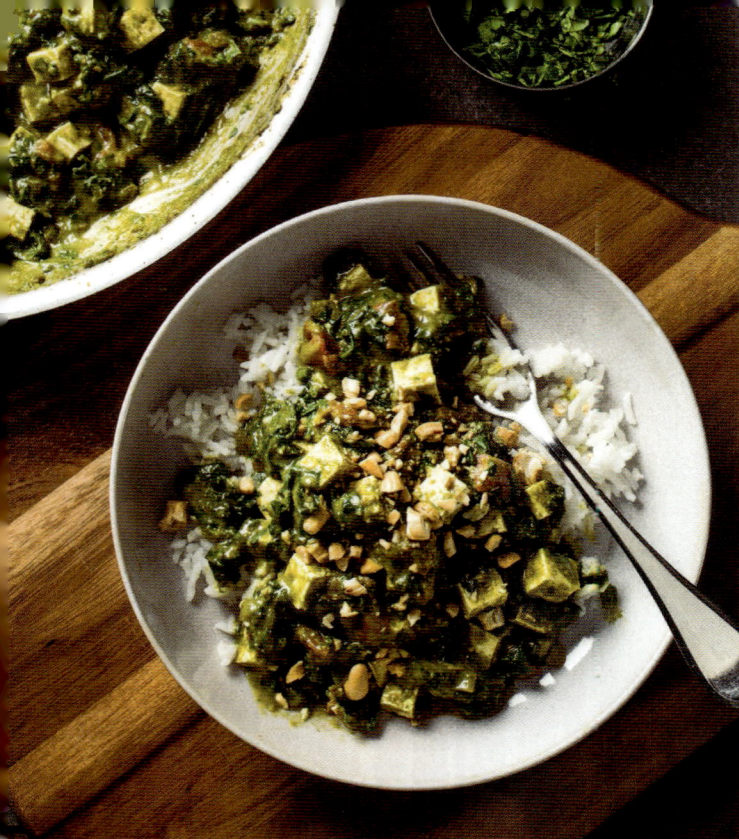

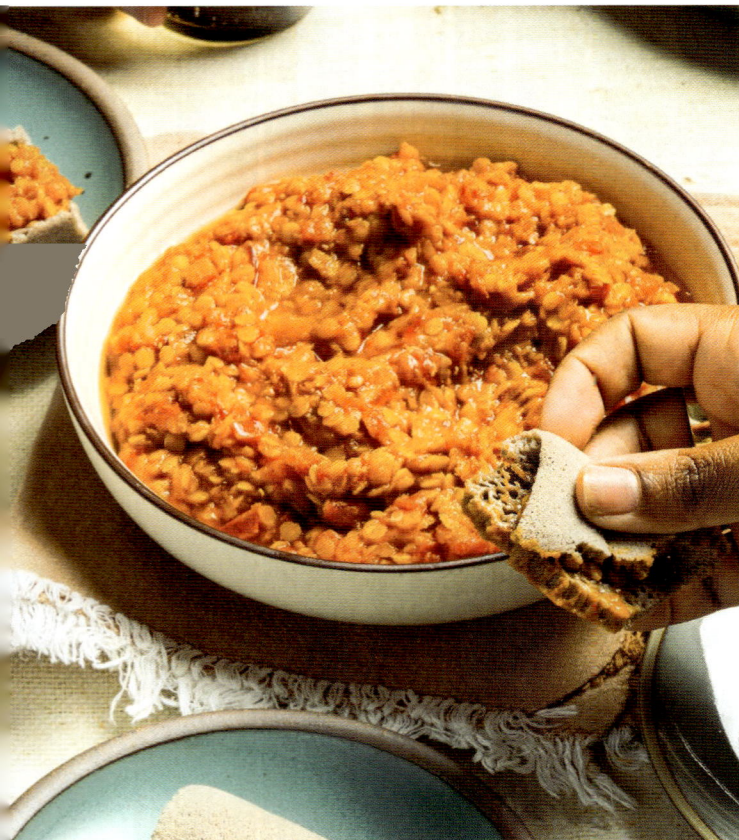

Saag Tofu

serves 4 • total time: 1 hour   **SUPERCHARGED**

why this recipe works • Saag paneer features stewed, pureed spinach cooked with pieces of fresh cheese. The mild cheese reminded us of firm tofu, so we thought a rendition made with tofu would make for a great spin on the classic Indian dish. We built layers of flavor—and packed in antioxidants—with a bevy of aromatics: onion, jalapeño, garlic, ginger, and tomatoes. Mustard greens, often featured in saag paneer in northern India, added pungency, hearty chew, and inflammation-fighting vitamin K. Cashews, pureed into the sauce with milk and also sprinkled on top for serving, added butteriness and body, plus a dose of mono-unsaturated fats. All we needed to do with the tofu was heat it in the sauce until it took on a creamy consistency. We prefer firm tofu here, but you can substitute extra-firm tofu. For a spicier dish, include the ribs and seeds from the jalapeño. Serve over rice.

14 ounces firm tofu, cut into ½-inch pieces
1⅛ teaspoons table salt, divided
  Pinch pepper
12 ounces curly-leaf spinach, stemmed
12 ounces mustard greens, stemmed
 3 tablespoons avocado oil
 1 teaspoon cumin seeds
 1 teaspoon ground coriander
 1 teaspoon paprika
 ½ teaspoon ground cardamom
 ¼ teaspoon ground cinnamon
 1 onion, chopped fine
 1 jalapeño chile, stemmed, seeded, and minced
 3 garlic cloves, minced
 1 tablespoon grated fresh ginger
 1 (14.5-ounce) can no-salt-added diced tomatoes, drained and chopped
1½ cups milk, divided
 ½ cup roasted cashews, chopped, divided
 1 teaspoon sugar
1½ tablespoons lemon juice
 3 tablespoons minced fresh cilantro

1 Spread tofu over paper towel–lined baking sheet and let drain for 20 minutes. Gently press dry with paper towels. Sprinkle tofu with ⅛ teaspoon salt and pepper and set aside.

2 Meanwhile, microwave spinach in bowl, covered, until wilted, about 3 minutes; transfer ½ cup spinach to blender. Chop remaining spinach and set aside. Microwave mustard greens in now-empty bowl, covered, until wilted, about 4 minutes; transfer ½ cup to blender with spinach. Chop remaining mustard greens and set aside.

3 Heat oil in 12-inch skillet over medium-high heat until shimmering. Add cumin seeds, coriander, paprika, cardamom, and cinnamon and cook until fragrant, about 30 seconds. Add onion and remaining 1 teaspoon salt and cook, stirring frequently, until softened, about 3 minutes. Stir in jalapeño, garlic, and ginger and cook until lightly browned and just beginning to stick to pan, about 3 minutes. Stir in tomatoes, scraping up any browned bits, and cook until pan is dry and tomatoes are beginning to brown, about 4 minutes.

4 Transfer half of onion-tomato mixture, ¾ cup milk, ¼ cup cashews, and sugar to blender with greens and process until smooth, about 1 minute. Transfer pureed mixture to skillet with remaining onion-tomato mixture and add chopped greens, lemon juice, and remaining ¾ cup milk. Bring to simmer over medium-high heat. Reduce heat to low and season with salt and pepper to taste. Stir in tofu and cook until warmed through, about 2 minutes. Transfer to serving platter, sprinkle with cilantro and remaining ¼ cup cashews, and serve.

MAKE IT DAIRY-FREE • Substitute plant-based milk for the dairy milk.

Misir Wot

serves 4 • total time: 45 minutes `FAST` `SUPERCHARGED`

why this recipe works • One of Ethiopia's most famous vegetarian dishes, misir wot is a deeply flavored, nutrient-packed lentil dish. It's traditionally seasoned with the antioxidant-rich spice blend berbere, which delivers intense warmth alongside sweet and citrusy notes. Since berbere is not always easy to find, we made it ourselves. Premade berbere often contains powdered ginger, which has a strong peppery aroma; we wanted to work in the floral sweetness of fresh ginger. To start, we cooked some red onion and then added umami-rich tomato paste, fresh ginger, garlic, and our berbere blend—paprika, coriander, cardamom, cumin, and cayenne. Cooking the mixture until fragrant allowed the flavors to bloom. Next came quick-cooking red lentils, as well as some plum tomatoes, which brought a welcome freshness and

an almost cooling effect to this complex dish. We finished with a drizzle of red wine vinegar, the acidity of which helped cut through the layers of delicious heat. Do not substitute other types of lentils for the red lentils here; they have a very different texture. Adjust the amount of cayenne according to your preference. Be sure to bloom the spices for the full minute; otherwise, you'll be left with a raw, dusty texture in the finished dish. Serve with injera.

3 tablespoons extra-virgin olive oil
1 red onion, chopped fine
2 tablespoons no-salt-added tomato paste
4 teaspoons grated fresh ginger
3 garlic cloves, minced
2½ teaspoons paprika
1¼ teaspoons ground coriander
¾ teaspoon ground cardamom
¾ teaspoon ground cumin
½–1 teaspoon cayenne pepper
2 cups water
1 cup dried red lentils, picked over and rinsed
4 plum tomatoes, cored and chopped fine
1 teaspoon table salt
Red wine vinegar

1 Heat oil in large saucepan over medium-high heat until shimmering. Add onion and cook, stirring occasionally, until softened and lightly browned, 5 to 7 minutes. Add tomato paste, ginger, garlic, paprika, coriander, cardamom, cumin, and cayenne and cook until fragrant, about 1 minute.

2 Stir in water, lentils, tomatoes, and salt and bring to simmer. Reduce heat to low and simmer, stirring occasionally, until lentils are tender and beginning to break down, 15 to 25 minutes. Season with salt, pepper, and vinegar to taste. Serve.

Nutrition Knowledge Lentils are an excellent source of beta-glucan, which supports heart health and blood sugar balance. Misir wot makes a great showcase for the protein-rich ingredient, thanks to a bevy of delicious (and inflammation-fighting) supporting ingredients: Tomatoes deliver lycopene, a powerful antioxidant that helps combat oxidative stress; garlic and ginger provide potent compounds such as allicin and gingerols to reduce inflammation; and onions pack quercetin, a flavonoid that blocks the release of pro-inflammatory cytokines. —*Alicia*

Chana Masala

serves 4 • total time: 50 minutes **SUPERCHARGED**

why this recipe works • Chana masala (spiced chickpeas) is arguably one of North India's best-known vegetarian dishes. It also makes a star out of chickpeas, an anti-inflammatory power-house loaded with plant-powered polyphenols. We used canned chickpeas because their flavor and texture are nearly indistinguish-able from those cooked from dried. Plus, the canning liquid adds body and savory depth. A paste made from onion, garlic, ginger, and chile, along with pureed canned tomatoes, formed the base sauce. We simmered the chickpeas in the sauce until they turned soft. Adding cumin, turmeric, and fennel seeds at the start of cook-ing helped them permeate the dish; delicate garam masala went in toward the end to preserve its aroma. Serve with rice or naan.

 1 small red onion, quartered, divided
10 sprigs fresh cilantro, stems and leaves separated
 1 (1½-inch) piece ginger, peeled and chopped coarse
 2 garlic cloves, chopped coarse
 2 serrano chiles, stemmed, halved, seeded, and
      chopped, divided
 3 tablespoons avocado oil
 1 (14.5-ounce) can no-salt-added whole peeled tomatoes
 1 teaspoon paprika
 1 teaspoon ground cumin
 ½ teaspoon ground turmeric
 ½ teaspoon fennel seeds
 2 (15-ounce) cans no-salt-added chickpeas, undrained
1½ teaspoons garam masala
 1 teaspoon table salt
      Lime wedges

1 Coarsely chop three-quarters of onion; reserve remaining quarter for garnish. Cut cilantro stems into 1-inch lengths and reserve leaves for garnish. Process chopped onion, cilantro stems, ginger, garlic, and half of serranos in food processor until finely chopped, about 20 seconds, scraping down sides of bowl as necessary. Cook onion mixture and oil in large saucepan over medium-high heat, stirring frequently, until onion is fully softened and beginning to stick to saucepan, 5 to 7 minutes.

2 While onion mixture cooks, process tomatoes and their juice in now-empty food processor until smooth, about 30 seconds. Add paprika, cumin, turmeric, and fennel seeds to onion mixture and cook, stirring constantly, until fragrant, about 1 minute. Stir in processed tomatoes and chickpeas and their liquid and bring to boil. Adjust heat to maintain simmer, then cover and simmer for 15 minutes. While mixture cooks, finely chop reserved onion.

3 Stir garam masala and salt into chickpea mixture and continue to cook, uncovered and stirring occasionally, until chickpeas are softened and sauce is thickened, 8 to 12 minutes. Season with salt to taste. Transfer to wide, shallow serving bowl. Sprinkle with chopped onion, remaining serranos, and cilantro leaves and serve, passing lime wedges separately.

Vindaloo-Style Potatoes

serves 4 • total time: 1 hour 5 minutes

why this recipe works • Vindaloo is a complex dish that draws on Portuguese and Indian cuisines in a potent braise featuring warm spices, chiles, wine vinegar, tomatoes, onions, garlic, and mustard seeds. It's often made with pork, lamb, or chicken as the main ingredient, but here we wanted to translate its comfort-food appeal into a satisfying vegan stew. Centering our dish on a com-bination of sweet potatoes and red potatoes gave us just the right hearty base. To give the stew exceptionally deep flavor, we sim-mered an antioxidant-rich mix of Indian spices, along with bay leaves and mustard seeds, with tomatoes, vinegar, and the pota-toes. However, after 45 minutes of simmering, the potatoes still weren't fully cooked. A second look at our ingredients suggested why: Perhaps the acidic environment created by the tomatoes and vinegar was preventing the potatoes from becoming tender. To test our theory, we whipped up another batch, this time leaving out the tomatoes and vinegar until near the end and cooking them just enough to mellow their flavors. Sure enough, after just 15 minutes, the potatoes were perfectly tender.

 2 tablespoons avocado oil
 2 onions, chopped fine
 1 pound sweet potatoes, peeled and cut into ½-inch pieces
 1 pound red potatoes, unpeeled, cut into ½-inch pieces
1½ teaspoons table salt, divided
10 garlic cloves, minced
 4 teaspoons paprika
 1 teaspoon ground cumin
 ¾ teaspoon ground cardamom
 ½ teaspoon cayenne pepper
 ¼ teaspoon ground cloves
2½ cups water
 2 bay leaves
 1 tablespoon mustard seeds
 1 (28-ounce) can no-salt-added diced tomatoes
2½ tablespoons red wine vinegar
 ¼ cup minced fresh cilantro

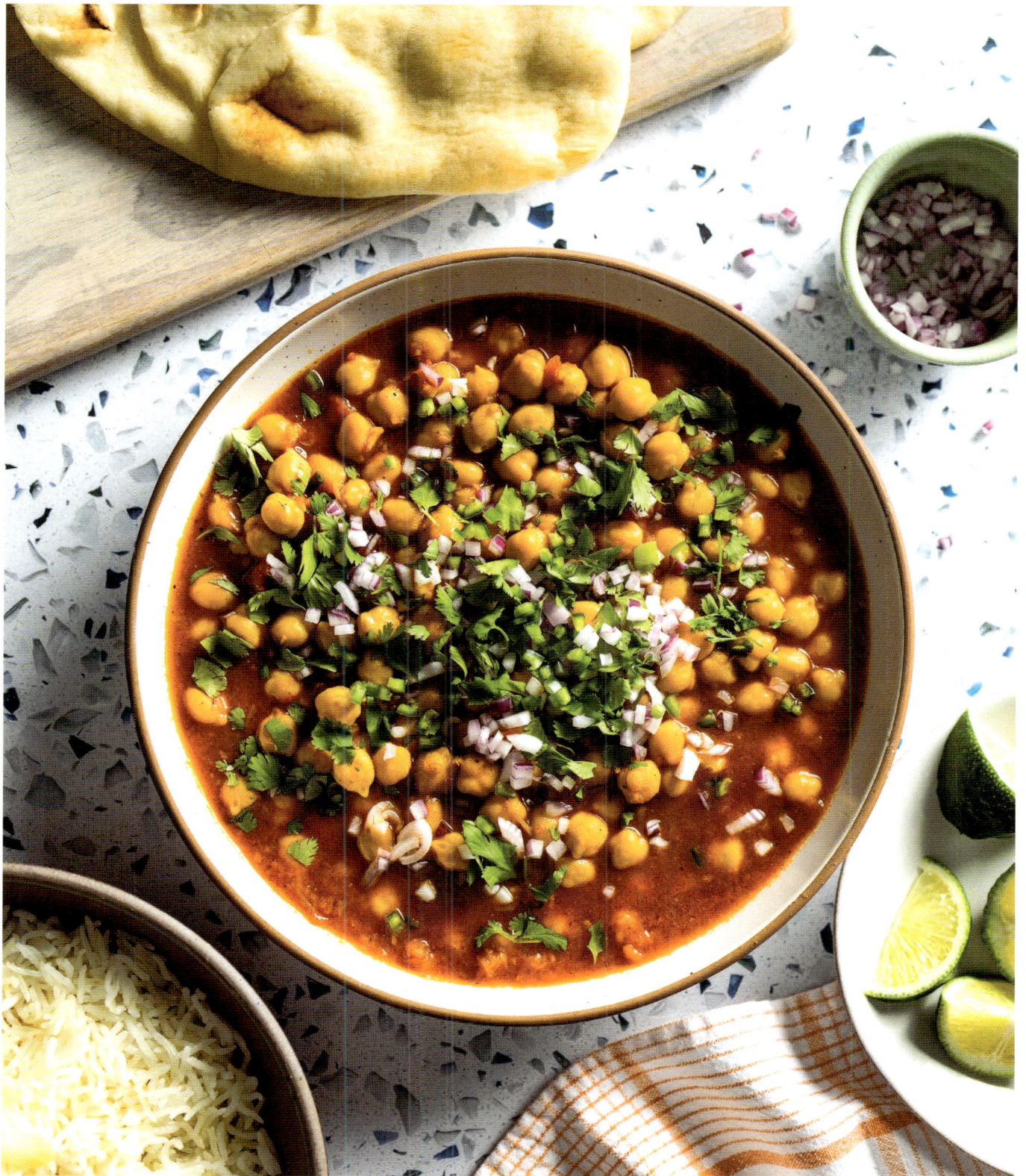

1 Heat oil in Dutch oven over medium heat until shimmering. Add onions, sweet potatoes, red potatoes, and ½ teaspoon salt and cook, stirring occasionally, until onions are softened and potatoes begin to soften at edges, 10 to 12 minutes.

2 Stir in garlic, paprika, cumin, cardamom, cayenne, and cloves and cook until fragrant and vegetables are well coated, about 2 minutes. Gradually stir in water, scraping up any browned bits. Stir in bay leaves, mustard seeds, and remaining 1 teaspoon salt and bring to simmer. Cover, reduce heat to medium-low, and cook until potatoes are tender, 15 to 20 minutes.

3 Stir in tomatoes and their juice and vinegar and continue to simmer, uncovered, until flavors meld and sauce has thickened slightly, about 15 minutes. Discard bay leaves. Stir in cilantro, season with salt and pepper to taste, and serve.

Mexican-Style Spaghetti Squash Casserole

serves 4 • total time: 1½ hours

why this recipe works • Since it's frequently used as a substitute for pasta, spaghetti squash is often paired with Italian ingredients. But we wanted to show off the squash's versatility in two different ways: using it as the base for a casserole and jazzing it up with bright Mexican flavors. First we roasted the oblong yellow squash until the delicately sweet strands could be easily shredded from the skins. Minced garlic, smoked paprika, and cumin built an aromatic base for our casserole, and incorporating black beans, corn, tomatoes, and scallions contributed to the Mexican-inspired flavor profile, with minced jalapeño providing just the right amount of gentle heat. We mixed everything together and baked it to meld the flavors. To finish it off, we served our squash with creamy avocado and a squeeze of lime. The queso fresco, if you use it, adds more creamy richness.

1 (2½- to 3-pound) spaghetti squash, halved lengthwise and seeded
3 tablespoons extra-virgin olive oil, divided
1¼ teaspoons table salt, divided
¼ teaspoon pepper
2 garlic cloves, minced
½ teaspoon smoked paprika
½ teaspoon ground cumin
1 (15-ounce) can no-salt-added black beans, rinsed
1 cup frozen corn
6 ounces cherry tomatoes, halved
6 scallions (4 minced, 2 sliced thin)
1 jalapeño chile, stemmed, seeded, and minced
1 avocado, halved, pitted, and cut into ½-inch pieces
2 ounces queso fresco, crumbled (½ cup) (optional)
Lime wedges

1 Adjust oven rack to middle position and heat oven to 375 degrees. Spray 8-inch square baking dish with olive oil spray. Brush cut sides of squash with 1 tablespoon oil and sprinkle with ½ teaspoon salt and pepper. Place squash cut side down in prepared dish (squash will not sit flat in dish) and roast until just tender, 40 to 45 minutes. Remove from oven, flip squash cut side up, and let sit until cool enough to handle, about 20 minutes.

2 While squash roasts, combine garlic, paprika, cumin, remaining ¾ teaspoon salt, and remaining 2 tablespoons oil in large bowl and microwave until fragrant, about 30 seconds. Stir in beans, corn, tomatoes, minced scallions, and jalapeño until well combined.

3 Using fork, scrape squash into strands over bowl with bean mixture. Stir to combine, then spread mixture evenly in now-empty dish and cover tightly with aluminum foil. Bake until warmed through, 20 to 25 minutes.

4 Remove dish from oven. Sprinkle with avocado; queso fresco, if using; and sliced scallions. Serve with lime wedges.

> **MAKE AHEAD** • Squash can be prepared through step 1 and refrigerated for up to 2 days.

SHREDDING SPAGHETTI SQUASH

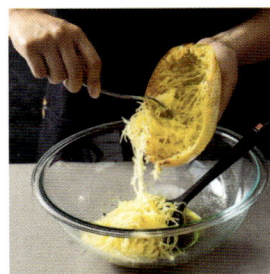

Holding roasted squash half with clean dish towel over large bowl, use fork to scrape squash flesh from skin, shredding flesh into fine strands.

Big-Batch Meatless Meat Sauce with Chickpeas and Mushrooms

makes 6 cups; enough for 2 pounds pasta • total time: 1 hour

why this recipe works • A big batch of red sauce can be a life-saver on busy nights—it's a tasty and versatile canvas for all sorts of add-ins. Instead of a meat-based sauce, though, we decided to take a vegan approach. For our primary protein, we chose chopped chickpeas. To punch up the umami flavor, we turned to cremini mushrooms and tomato paste—both rich sources of savory glutamates. Extra-virgin olive oil pulled double duty, both enriching the sauce and helping to toast the aromatics: garlic, dried oregano, and red pepper flakes. To thin the sauce without diluting its flavor, we added vegetable broth. Make sure to rinse the chickpeas after pulsing them in the food processor or the sauce will be too thick.

- 10 ounces cremini mushrooms, trimmed
- 1 onion, chopped
- 1 (15-ounce) can no-salt-added chickpeas, rinsed
- 6 tablespoons extra-virgin olive oil, divided
- 1½ teaspoons table salt
- ¼ cup no-salt-added tomato paste
- 5 garlic cloves, minced
- 1¼ teaspoons dried oregano
- ¼ teaspoon red pepper flakes
- 1 (28-ounce) can no-salt-added crushed tomatoes
- 2 cups unsalted vegetable broth
- 2 tablespoons chopped fresh basil

1 Working in batches, pulse mushrooms in food processor until pieces are no larger than ⅛ to ¼ inch, 7 to 10 pulses, scraping down sides of bowl as necessary; transfer to bowl. Pulse onion in now-empty food processor until finely chopped, 7 to 10 pulses, scraping down sides of bowl as necessary; set aside separately. Pulse chickpeas in again-empty food processor until chopped into ¼-inch pieces, 7 to 10 pulses. Transfer chickpeas to fine-mesh strainer and rinse under cold running water until water runs clear; drain well.

2 Heat 5 tablespoons oil in Dutch oven over medium-high heat until shimmering. Add mushrooms and salt and cook, stirring occasionally, until mushrooms are browned and fond has formed on bottom of pot, about 8 minutes.

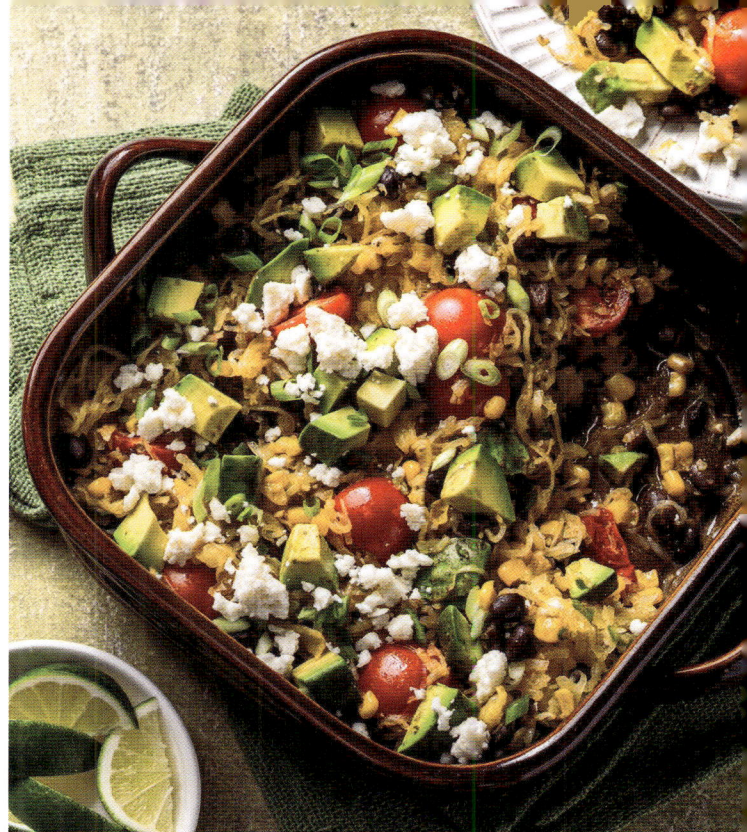

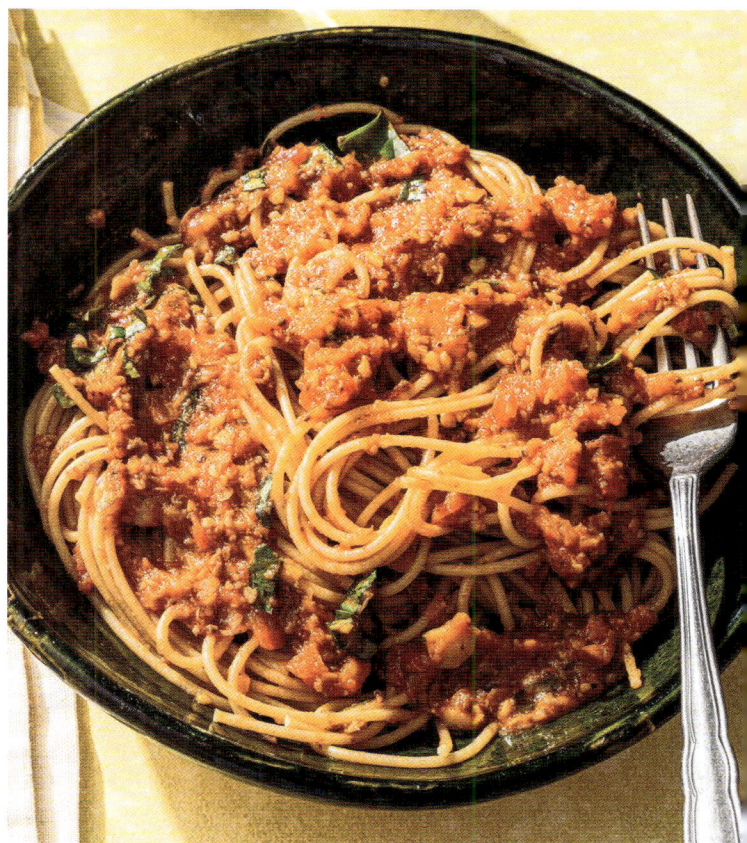

top	Mexican-Style Spaghetti Squash Casserole
bottom	*Big-Batch Meatless Meat Sauce with Chickpeas and Mushrooms*

3   Stir in onion and cook until softened, about 5 minutes. Add tomato paste and cook, stirring constantly, until mixture is rust-colored, 1 to 2 minutes. Reduce heat to medium and push vegetables to sides of pot. Add remaining 1 tablespoon oil, garlic, oregano, and pepper flakes to center and cook, stirring constantly, until fragrant, about 30 seconds. Stir in tomatoes and broth and bring to simmer over high heat. Reduce heat to low and simmer sauce for 5 minutes, stirring occasionally.

4   Stir drained chickpeas into sauce in pot and simmer until sauce is slightly thickened, about 15 minutes. Stir in basil, season with salt and pepper to taste, and serve.

> **MAKE AHEAD** • Sauce can be refrigerated for up to 2 days or frozen for up to 1 month.

Fava Bean Pesto Pasta

serves 4 to 6 • total time: 40 minutes **FAST**

why this recipe works • Don't be fooled by fava beans' delicate appearance—they're rich in protein and packed with soluble fiber. We took advantage of their buttery consistency and transformed the legumes into a creamy pesto-like sauce in just minutes. We seasoned the favas with Pecorino Romano and fresh dill and blended them with toasted walnuts, a great source of omega-3 fatty acids. The nuts gave the mixture body as they melded with the beans. To mellow the flavor of raw garlic, we toasted it, skin on, before adding the flesh to the food processor with the other ingredients, where it infused the pesto with a roasty aroma. Reserving some whole beans to toss in at the end brought welcome pops of color and bite to the pasta. Using frozen favas, which are already blanched, eliminated the task of shelling fresh beans. If your favas still have the sheath (outer leathery skin), remove it by making a small cut on the side and then gently squeezing to release the bean.

½   cup walnuts
1   garlic clove, unpeeled
1½   cups frozen shelled fava beans, thawed, sheaths removed, divided
¾   cup plus 2 tablespoons fresh dill, divided
1   ounce Pecorino Romano cheese, grated (½ cup)
6   tablespoons extra-virgin olive oil
1   teaspoon table salt, plus salt for cooking pasta
1   pound spaghetti
1   tablespoon grated lemon zest

1   Toast walnuts in 8-inch skillet over medium heat, stirring frequently, until just golden and fragrant, about 5 minutes; transfer to food processor. Add garlic to now-empty skillet and toast over medium heat, shaking skillet occasionally, until fragrant and garlic skin is browned in spots, about 7 minutes. Let garlic cool slightly, then peel and add to processor.

2   Transfer one-third fava beans to small bowl. Add remaining beans to food processor along with ¾ cup dill, Pecorino, oil, and salt. Process until thick and mostly smooth, about 1 minute, scraping down sides of bowl halfway through processing. Transfer pesto to large bowl.

3   Meanwhile, bring 4 quarts water to boil in large pot. Add pasta and 1 tablespoon salt and cook, stirring often, until al dente. Reserve 2 cups cooking water, then drain pasta.

4   Add lemon zest and 1½ cups cooking water to pesto and whisk until combined. Add pasta and remaining fava beans and toss until pasta is coated in creamy, lightly thickened sauce, 1 to 2 minutes, adjusting consistency with remaining cooking water as needed. Sprinkle with remaining 2 tablespoons dill and season with salt to taste. Serve immediately.

> **MAKE AHEAD** • Pesto can be refrigerated, with plastic wrap pressed flush to surface, for up to 2 days or frozen for up to 1 month.

> **MAKE IT GLUTEN-FREE** • Substitute gluten-free spaghetti for the spaghetti.

Whole-Wheat Spaghetti with Greens, Beans, and Tomatoes

serves 4 to 6 • total time: 50 minutes

why this recipe works • This rustic trio of pasta, greens, and beans is another fine example of the knack Italian cooks have for transforming humble ingredients into elevated meals. Here we used spinach, along with canned diced tomatoes and cannellini beans, for a meal that is feasible enough for a busy weeknight but elegant enough for guests. To create a strong savory presence that wasn't dependent on cheese, we employed a one-two punch of white miso and cheesy-tasting nutritional yeast. This duo not only contributed intense umami but also added a complexity that belied the simplicity of the ingredients. To ensure that everything would fit in one pan, we wilted half the spinach before adding the rest with the tomatoes and broth. We braised the spinach for a few minutes and then added the beans, plus some olives for a briny pop that contributed a pleasantly sharp counterpoint and brightened the overall profile. This mixture simmered with al dente pasta for just a couple minutes to create a harmonious dish. The skillet will be very full when you add all the spinach in step 2, but the greens will become manageable as they wilt.

- ¼ cup extra-virgin olive oil, divided, plus extra for serving
- 8 garlic cloves, peeled (5 sliced thin, 3 minced)
  Pinch plus ¾ teaspoon table salt, divided, plus salt for cooking pasta
- 1 onion, chopped fine
- ½ teaspoon red pepper flakes
- 1¼ pounds curly-leaf spinach, stemmed and cut into 1-inch pieces, divided
- ¾ cup unsalted vegetable broth
- 2 tablespoons white miso
- 2 tablespoons nutritional yeast
- 1 (14.5-ounce) can no-salt-added diced tomatoes, drained
- 1 (15-ounce) can no-salt-added cannellini beans, rinsed
- ¾ cup pitted kalamata olives, chopped coarse
- 1 pound whole-wheat spaghetti
  Parmesan cheese, grated (optional)

1 Cook 3 tablespoons oil and sliced garlic in 12-inch skillet over medium heat, stirring often, until garlic turns golden but not brown, about 3 minutes. Using slotted spoon, transfer garlic to paper towel–lined plate; sprinkle with pinch salt.

2 Add onion to oil left in skillet and cook over medium heat until softened and just beginning to brown, 5 to 7 minutes. Stir in minced garlic and pepper flakes and cook until fragrant, about 30 seconds. Add half of spinach and cook, tossing occasionally, until beginning to wilt, about 2 minutes. Whisk broth, miso, and nutritional yeast together in bowl, then add to skillet along with tomatoes, remaining spinach, and remaining ¾ teaspoon salt. Bring to simmer, then cover and cook, tossing occasionally, until spinach is completely wilted, about 10 minutes (mixture will be somewhat loose and watery at this point). Stir in beans and olives, then remove skillet from heat and cover to keep warm.

3 Meanwhile, bring 4 quarts water to boil in large pot. Add pasta and 1 tablespoon salt and cook, stirring often, until nearly al dente. Reserve ½ cup cooking water, then drain pasta and return it to pot. Stir in spinach mixture and cook over medium heat, tossing to combine, until pasta is al dente and most of liquid is absorbed, about 2 minutes.

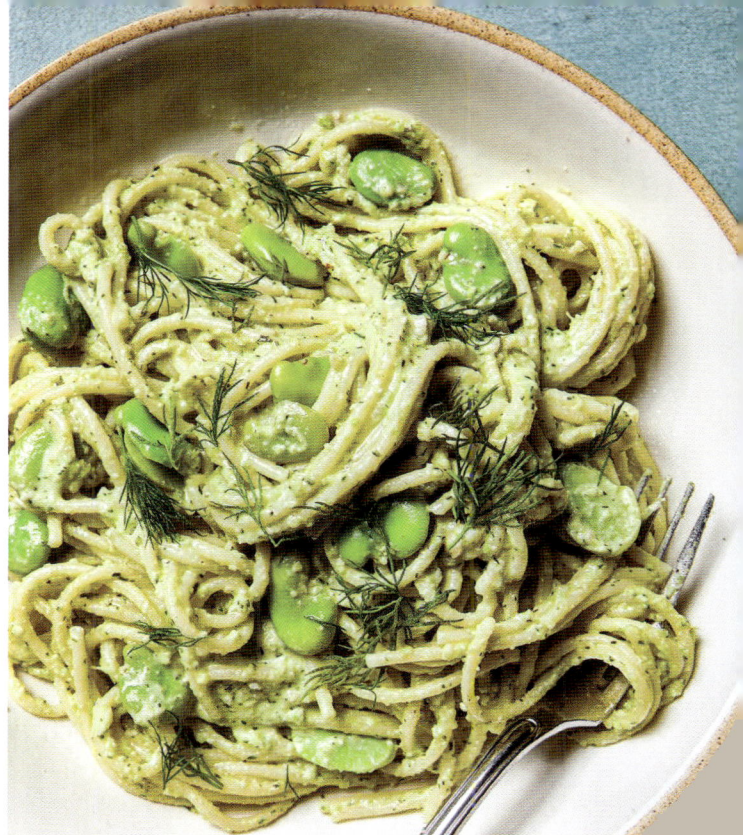

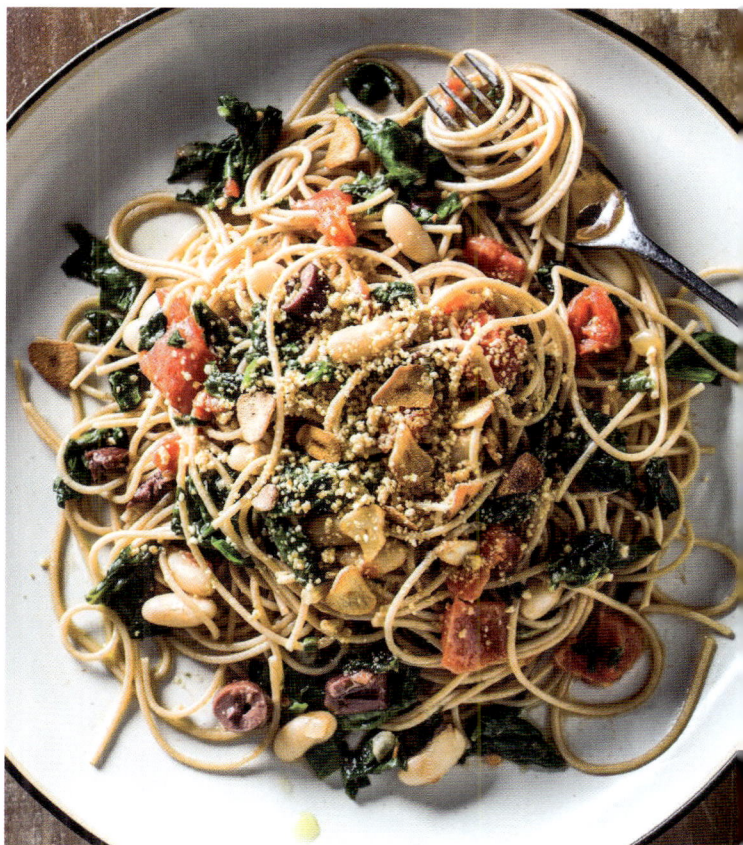

top	*Fava Bean Pesto Pasta*
bottom	*Whole-Wheat Spaghetti with Greens, Beans, and Tomatoes*

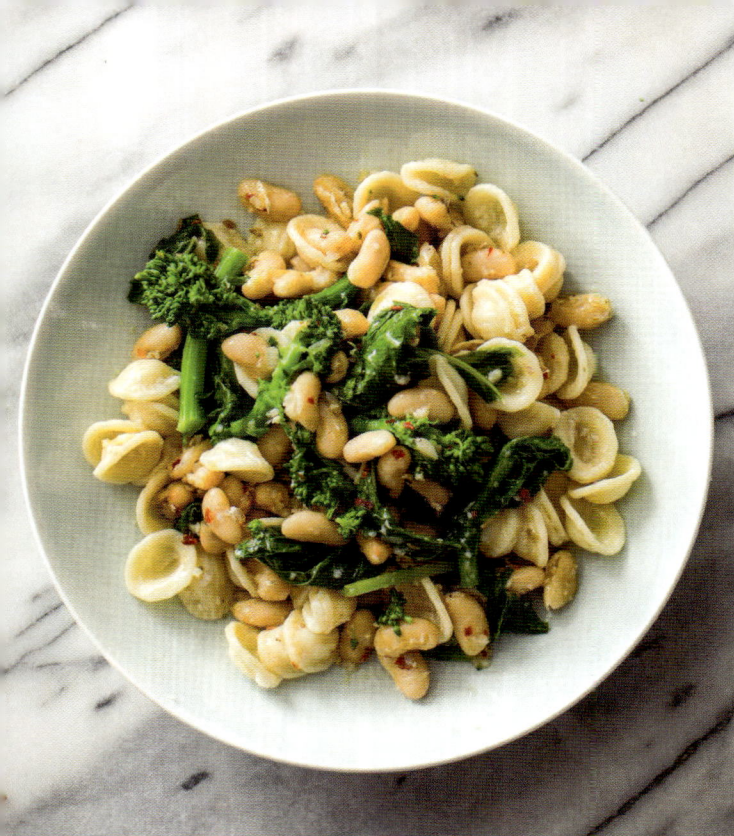

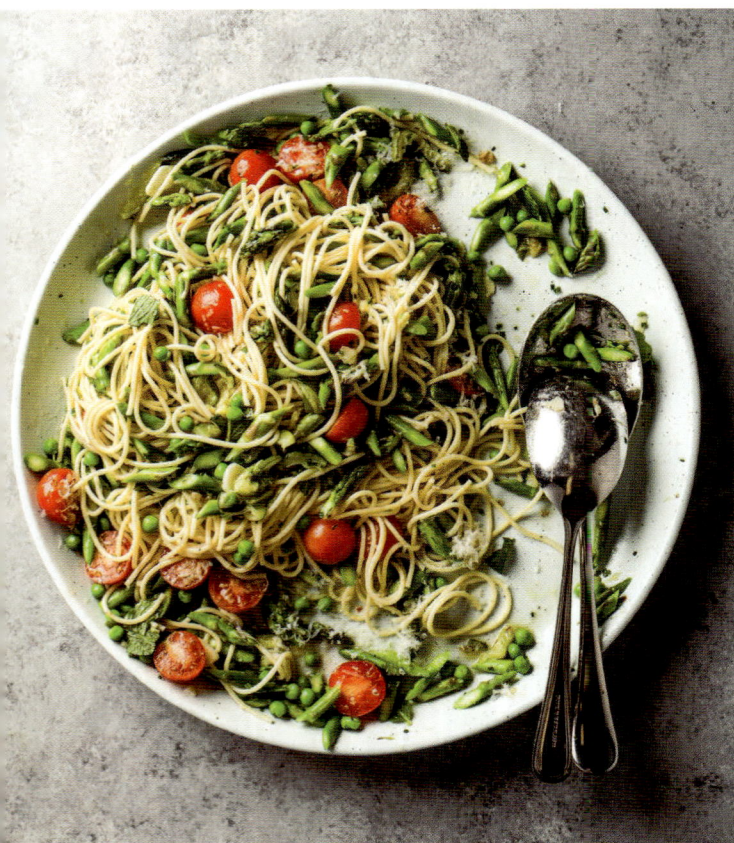

4 Off heat, stir in remaining 1 tablespoon oil. Adjust consistency with reserved cooking water as needed and season with salt and pepper to taste. Serve, sprinkling individual portions with garlic chips and Parmesan, if using, and drizzling with extra oil.

> **MAKE IT GLUTEN-FREE** • Substitute gluten-free spaghetti for the whole-wheat spaghetti.

Farfalle and Summer Squash with Tomatoes, Basil, and Pine Nuts

serves 4 to 6 • **total time: 35 minutes, plus 30 minutes salting**

why this recipe works • This summery pasta dish is light and flavorful. We kept the skin on the squash to keep the pieces intact (and for a color and nutrition boost), then salted the squash to release excess liquid and concentrate the vegetable's flavor. This step was essential to prevent a watery finished sauce. It also encouraged good browning; it took just 5 minutes in a hot skillet to lightly char each batch. To accompany the squash, we chose halved grape tomatoes, fresh basil, and crunchy pine nuts. We finished the sauce with balsamic vinegar to give it a tangy kick. For our pasta shape, we chose farfalle, which trapped all the flavor-packed ingredients. A combination of zucchini and summer squash make for a nice mix of colors, but you can stick to just one, if you prefer. We prefer kosher salt in this recipe because residual grains are easily wiped away from the squash. If using table salt, be sure to reduce all of the salt amounts in the recipe by half.

2 pounds summer squash and/or zucchini, halved lengthwise and sliced ½ inch thick
  Kosher salt for salting squash and cooking pasta
5 tablespoons extra-virgin olive oil, divided
3 garlic cloves, minced
½ teaspoon red pepper flakes
1 pound farfalle
12 ounces grape tomatoes, halved
½ cup chopped fresh basil
¼ cup pine nuts, toasted
2 tablespoons balsamic vinegar

1 Toss squash with 1 tablespoon salt in colander and let drain for 30 minutes. Pat squash dry with paper towels and carefully wipe away any residual salt.

2 Heat 1 tablespoon oil in 12-inch nonstick skillet over high heat until just smoking. Add half of squash and cook, stirring occasionally, until golden brown and slightly charred, 5 to 7 minutes, reducing heat if skillet begins to scorch; transfer to large plate. Repeat with 1 tablespoon oil and remaining squash.

3 Heat 1 tablespoon oil in now-empty skillet over medium heat until shimmering. Add garlic and pepper flakes and cook until fragrant, about 30 seconds. Stir in browned squash and cook until warmed through, about 30 seconds.

4 Meanwhile, bring 4 quarts water to boil in large pot. Add pasta and 2 tablespoons salt and cook, stirring often, until al dente. Reserve ½ cup cooking water, then drain pasta and return it to pot. Add squash mixture, tomatoes, basil, pine nuts, vinegar, and remaining 2 tablespoons oil and toss to combine. Before serving, adjust consistency with reserved cooking water as needed and season with salt and pepper to taste.

MAKE IT GLUTEN-FREE • Substitute gluten-free farfalle for the farfalle.

Orecchiette with Broccoli Rabe and White Beans

serves 4 to 6 • total time: 30 minutes **FAST**

why this recipe works • Orecchiette is a quintessential pasta shape of Puglia, the heel of the Italian boot. It is often served with leafy greens, traditionally turnip tops, though broccoli rabe is also frequently used. Sometimes the dish includes sausage to add richness and offset the slight bitterness of the greens For this meat-free rendition, we swapped in buttery, creamy white beans, which achieved the same effect in conjunction with some Parmesan. To boost the beans' flavor, we cooked a shallot with garlic, oregano, and fennel seeds before adding the beans. To ensure that the thick stalks, tender leaves, and small florets of the broccoli rabe all cooked evenly, we boiled them briefly, pulling them from the pot just as they turned crisp-tender. You can substitute 2 pounds of broccoli, cut into 1-inch florets, for the broccoli rabe.

¼ cup extra-virgin olive oil
1 shallot, minced
6 garlic cloves, minced
1 teaspoon minced fresh oregano or ¼ teaspoon dried

½ teaspoon table salt, plus salt for cooking vegetables and pasta
½ teaspoon fennel seeds, crushed
¼ teaspoon red pepper flakes
1 (15-ounce) can no-salt-added cannellini beans, rinsed
1 pound broccoli rabe, trimmed and cut into 1½-inch pieces
1 pound orecchiette
2 ounces Parmesan cheese, grated (1 cup)

1 Heat oil in 12-inch nonstick skillet over medium heat until shimmering. Add shallot and cook until softened, about 2 minutes. Stir in garlic, oregano, salt, fennel seeds, and pepper flakes and cook until fragrant, about 30 seconds. Stir in beans and cook until warmed through, about 2 minutes; set aside.

2 Meanwhile, bring 4 quarts water to boil in large pot. Add broccoli rabe and 1 tablespoon salt and cook, stirring often, until crisp-tender, about 2 minutes. Using slotted spoon, transfer broccoli rabe to skillet with bean mixture.

3 Return water to boil, add pasta, and cook, stirring often, until al dente. Reserve 1 cup cooking water, then drain pasta and return to pot. Add bean–broccoli rabe mixture, Parmesan, and ⅓ cup reserved cooking water and toss to combine. Before serving, adjust consistency with remaining reserved ⅔ cup cooking water as needed and season with salt and pepper to taste.

MAKE IT GLUTEN-FREE • Substitute gluten-free orecchiette for the orecchiette.

MAKE IT DAIRY-FREE • Substitute plant-based Parmesan cheese for the dairy Parmesan.

Spaghetti with Spring Vegetables

serves 4 to 6 • total time: 35 minutes **FAST**

why this recipe works • For this spin on Italian American pasta primavera, we made inventive use of zucchini by overcooking it with olive oil and aromatics to break it down into a silky, creamy—yet cream-free—sauce. The sauce nicely coated asparagus and peas (two of our favorite spring veggies) and the noodles. We marinated cherry tomatoes with oil and garlic and spooned them over the pasta and then added a sprinkling of fresh mint to finish off our dish with a pop of color and freshness. The zucchini slices will break down as they cook to create a base for the sauce; do not be alarmed when the slices turn soft and creamy and lose their shape.

6 ounces cherry tomatoes, halved

6 tablespoons extra-virgin olive oil, divided

5 garlic cloves (1 small, minced; 4 sliced thin)

¾ teaspoon table salt, divided, plus salt for cooking pasta

¼ teaspoon pepper

1 pound spaghetti

1 zucchini, halved lengthwise and sliced ¼ inch thick

⅛ teaspoon red pepper flakes

1 pound asparagus, trimmed and cut on bias into 1-inch lengths

1 cup frozen peas, thawed

¼ cup minced fresh chives

1 tablespoon lemon juice

¼ cup grated Pecorino Romano cheese

2 tablespoons torn fresh mint leaves

1 Toss tomatoes, 1 tablespoon oil, minced garlic, ¼ teaspoon salt, and pepper together in bowl; set aside. Bring 4 quarts water to boil in large Dutch oven. Add pasta and 1 tablespoon salt and cook, stirring often, until al dente. Drain pasta and return to pot.

2 Meanwhile, heat 3 tablespoons oil in 12-inch nonstick skillet over medium-low heat until shimmering. Add zucchini, pepper flakes, sliced garlic, and remaining ½ teaspoon salt and cook, covered, until zucchini softens and breaks down, 10 to 15 minutes, stirring occasionally. Add asparagus, peas, and ¾ cup water and bring to simmer over medium-high heat. Cover and cook until asparagus is crisp-tender, about 2 minutes.

3 Add vegetable mixture, chives, lemon juice, and remaining 2 tablespoons oil to pasta and toss to combine; season with salt and pepper to taste. Transfer to serving bowl and sprinkle with Pecorino Romano cheese. Spoon tomatoes and their juices over top, sprinkle with mint, and serve.

MAKE IT GLUTEN-FREE • Substitute gluten-free spaghetti for the spaghetti.

MAKE IT DAIRY-FREE • Substitute plant-based Pecorino Romano cheese for the dairy Pecorino Romano cheese.

Baked Ziti with Creamy Leeks, Kale, and Sun-Dried Tomatoes

serves 4 to 6 • **total time: 1¼ hours**

why this recipe works • This take on baked ziti, which is gratifyingly vegetable-forward, gives star billing to aromatic leeks. We sautéed 2 pounds until they began to caramelize, deglazed with a splash of white wine and then simmered them in broth until the leeks were meltingly soft and ready to be blended into a velvety sauce. After parcooking our pasta, we used the same pot to sauté kale and sun-dried tomatoes, mixed in our sauce and pasta, and baked it all so that the ziti could finish cooking while absorbing the sauce. For a crispy topping, we sprinkled on panko, Parmesan, and lemon zest and then broiled it to perfection. If you can't find baby kale, substitute 8 ounces kale, stemmed and chopped.

½ cup panko bread crumbs

¼ cup grated Parmesan cheese

¼ cup extra-virgin olive oil, divided

½ teaspoon grated lemon zest, plus lemon wedges for serving

2 pounds leeks, white and light green parts only, halved lengthwise, sliced thin, and washed thoroughly

1 teaspoon table salt, divided, plus salt for cooking pasta

⅛ teaspoon pepper

2 teaspoons minced fresh thyme or ¾ teaspoon dried

½ cup dry white wine

2 cups unsalted vegetable broth

1 pound ziti

6 garlic cloves, minced

¼ teaspoon red pepper flakes

6 ounces (6 cups) baby kale

¼ cup oil-packed sun-dried tomatoes, chopped coarse

2 tablespoons chopped fresh parsley

1 Adjust oven rack to upper-middle position and heat oven to 450 degrees. Combine panko, Parmesan, 1 tablespoon oil, and lemon zest in bowl; set aside.

2 Heat 2 tablespoons oil in Dutch oven over medium heat until shimmering. Stir in leeks, ½ teaspoon salt, and pepper and cook until softened and lightly browned, 8 to 12 minutes. Stir in thyme and cook until fragrant, about 30 seconds. Stir in wine, scraping up any browned bits, and cook until evaporated, about 2 minutes. Stir in broth and bring to boil. Reduce heat to low, cover, and simmer until leeks are very tender, about 8 minutes. Process leek mixture in blender on high speed until very smooth, about 2 minutes. Season with salt and pepper to taste.

3 Meanwhile, bring 4 quarts water to boil in Dutch oven. Add pasta and 1 tablespoon salt and cook, stirring often, until nearly al dente. Reserve 1½ cups cooking water, then drain pasta. Cook remaining 1 tablespoon oil, garlic, and pepper flakes in now-empty pot over medium heat until fragrant, about 1 minute. Stir in kale, sun-dried tomatoes, and remaining ½ teaspoon salt and cook, stirring occasionally, until kale is wilted and tomatoes are softened, about 3 minutes. Off heat, stir in cooked pasta, leek mixture, and 1 cup reserved cooking water; season with salt and pepper to taste. Adjust consistency with remaining ½ cup cooking water as needed (sauce should be thick but still creamy).

4 Transfer pasta mixture to broiler-safe 13 by 9-inch baking dish, smoothing top with silicone spatula. Cover tightly with aluminum foil and bake until sauce is bubbling, 10 to 12 minutes. Remove baking dish from oven and heat broiler. Remove aluminum foil and sprinkle panko mixture evenly over pasta. Broil until panko mixture is golden brown, about 2 minutes. Sprinkle with parsley and serve with lemon wedges.

> **MAKE IT GLUTEN-FREE** • Substitute gluten-free panko bread crumbs and gluten-free ziti for the panko bread crumbs and ziti.

> **MAKE IT DAIRY-FREE** • Substitute plant-based Parmesan cheese for the dairy Parmesan cheese.

Thai Curry Rice Noodles with Crispy Tofu and Broccoli

serves 4 • total time: 1 hour

why this recipe works • Crispy tofu, tender vegetables, and hearty rice noodles mingle with a coconut-curry sauce in this dish that's a cinch to prepare. While the noodles hydrated in hot water, we crisped our tofu after dusting the pieces with cornstarch. After wiping the skillet, we sautéed our vegetables, stirred in curry paste, and built the sauce with coconut milk, water, and a bit of brown sugar. We added the softened noodles to the skillet with the vegetables and sauce and simmered everything until the noodles were cooked through and the sauce was thickened. To finish, we topped the noodles with the crispy tofu, followed by a generous helping of fresh Thai basil. If you can't find Thai basil, you can substitute Italian basil.

- 8 ounces (¼-inch-wide) rice noodles
- 14 ounces firm tofu, cut into ¾-inch pieces
- ½ teaspoon table salt, divided
- ⅛ teaspoon pepper
- 3 tablespoons cornstarch
- 3 tablespoons avocado oil, divided
- 6 ounces broccoli, florets cut into 1-inch pieces, stalks peeled and cut into ½-inch pieces
- 1 red bell pepper, stemmed, seeded, and cut into ½-inch pieces
- 4 scallions, white parts cut into 1-inch lengths, green parts sliced thin, separated
- ¼ cup Thai red curry paste
- ½ cup canned coconut milk
- ½ cup water
- 1 teaspoon packed brown sugar
- ¼ cup chopped fresh Thai basil
  Lime wedges

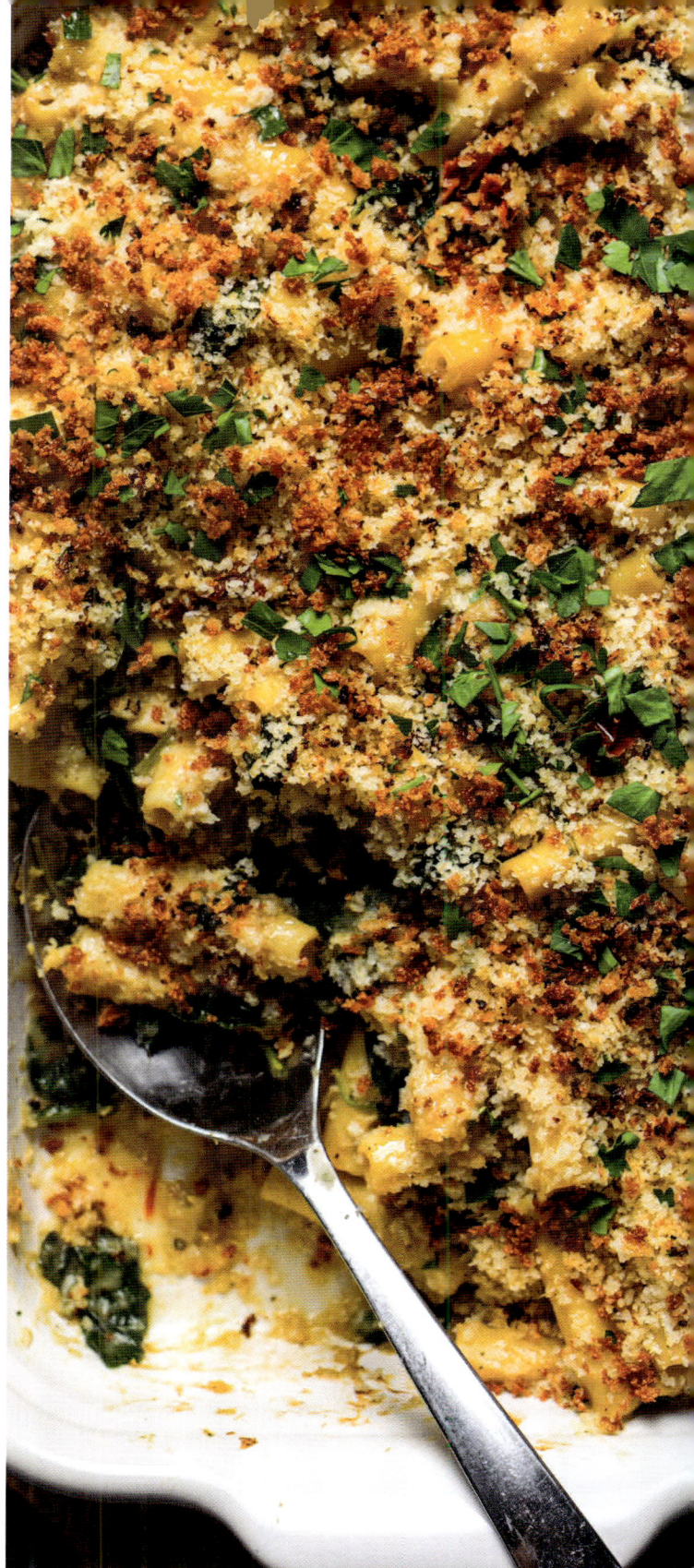

Baked Ziti with Creamy Leeks, Kale, and Sun-Dried Tomatoes

1   Bring 2 quarts water to boil in large pot. Remove from heat, add noodles, and let sit, stirring occasionally, until soft and pliable but not fully tender, 8 to 10 minutes. Drain noodles and rinse with cold water until water runs clear. Drain noodles again and set aside. While noodles soak, spread tofu over paper towel–lined baking sheet and let drain for 20 minutes. Gently pat tofu dry with paper towels.

2   Sprinkle tofu with ¼ teaspoon salt and pepper, then toss with cornstarch in bowl. Heat 2 tablespoons oil in 12-inch nonstick skillet over medium-high heat until just smoking. Add tofu and cook, turning as needed, until crisp and browned on all sides, 8 to 10 minutes; transfer to paper towel–lined plate to drain.

3   Wipe out now-empty skillet with paper towels, add remaining 1 tablespoon oil, and heat over medium heat until shimmering. Add broccoli florets and stalks, bell pepper, scallion whites, and remaining ¼ teaspoon salt and cook until softened and lightly browned, 3 to 5 minutes. Push vegetables to sides of skillet. Add curry paste to center and cook, mashing paste into skillet, until fragrant, about 30 seconds. Stir curry paste into vegetables, then stir in coconut milk, water, and sugar, scraping up any browned bits, and bring to simmer.

4   Add drained rice noodles and toss to combine. Cook, tossing gently, until sauce has thickened slightly and noodles are well coated and tender, about 3 minutes. Season with salt and pepper to taste and top with crispy tofu, scallion greens, and basil. Serve with lime wedges.

Sweet Potato Noodles with Shiitakes and Spinach

serves 4 · **total time: 35 minutes**   FAST

why this recipe works · One of Korea's most beloved celebratory dishes, japchae, combines sweet potato starch noodles and vegetables for a result that is both stunning and delicious. The flavorful, balanced sauce—made with sesame oil, soy sauce, sugar, sesame seeds, and garlic—makes it clear why, throughout much of history, Korean royalty kept this dish to themselves. Opting for a variety of vegetables, we found that we needed to stagger their cooking times to ensure that they were properly cooked. After cooking the noodles, we stir-fried earthy shiitake mushrooms, carrots, and onion. We then added scallions, which needed less time to cook, and spinach, which helped bulk up the vegetable ratio in this simple but luxurious noodle dish. If you can't find sweet potato noodles (sometimes sold as sweet potato starch noodles or sweet potato glass noodles), substitute cellophane noodles.

8   ounces (⅛-inch-wide) dried sweet potato noodles, broken into 12-inch lengths
2   teaspoons plus 2 tablespoons toasted sesame oil, divided
3   garlic cloves, minced, divided
2   teaspoons plus 1 tablespoon avocado oil, divided
¼   cup low-sodium soy sauce
3   tablespoons sugar
1   tablespoon sesame seeds, toasted
8   ounces shiitake mushrooms, stemmed and sliced thin
2   carrots, peeled and cut into 2-inch-long matchsticks
1   small onion, halved and sliced ½ inch thick
2   scallions, sliced thin
8   ounces (8 cups) baby spinach

1   Bring 2 quarts water to boil in large pot. Remove from heat, add noodles, and let sit, stirring occasionally, until noodles are soft and pliable but not fully tender, 5 to 10 minutes. Drain noodles and rinse under cold running water until chilled. Drain noodles again and toss with 2 teaspoons sesame oil; set aside.

2   Combine two-thirds of garlic and 2 teaspoons avocado oil in small bowl; set aside. Whisk soy sauce, sugar, sesame seeds, remaining 2 tablespoons sesame oil, and remaining garlic in second small bowl until sugar has dissolved; set sauce aside.

3   Heat remaining 1 tablespoon avocado oil in 12-inch skillet over high heat until just smoking. Add mushrooms, carrots, and onion and cook, stirring constantly, until onion and carrots are crisp-tender, 4 to 6 minutes. Add scallions and spinach and cook until wilted, about 2 minutes.

4   Push vegetables to 1 side of skillet. Add garlic mixture to clearing and cook, mashing mixture into skillet, until fragrant, about 30 seconds. Stir garlic mixture into vegetables. Add noodles and sauce and cook, stirring constantly, until mixture is thoroughly combined and noodles are well coated and tender, 2 to 4 minutes. Serve.

MAKE IT GLUTEN-FREE · Substitute low-sodium tamari for the low-sodium soy sauce.

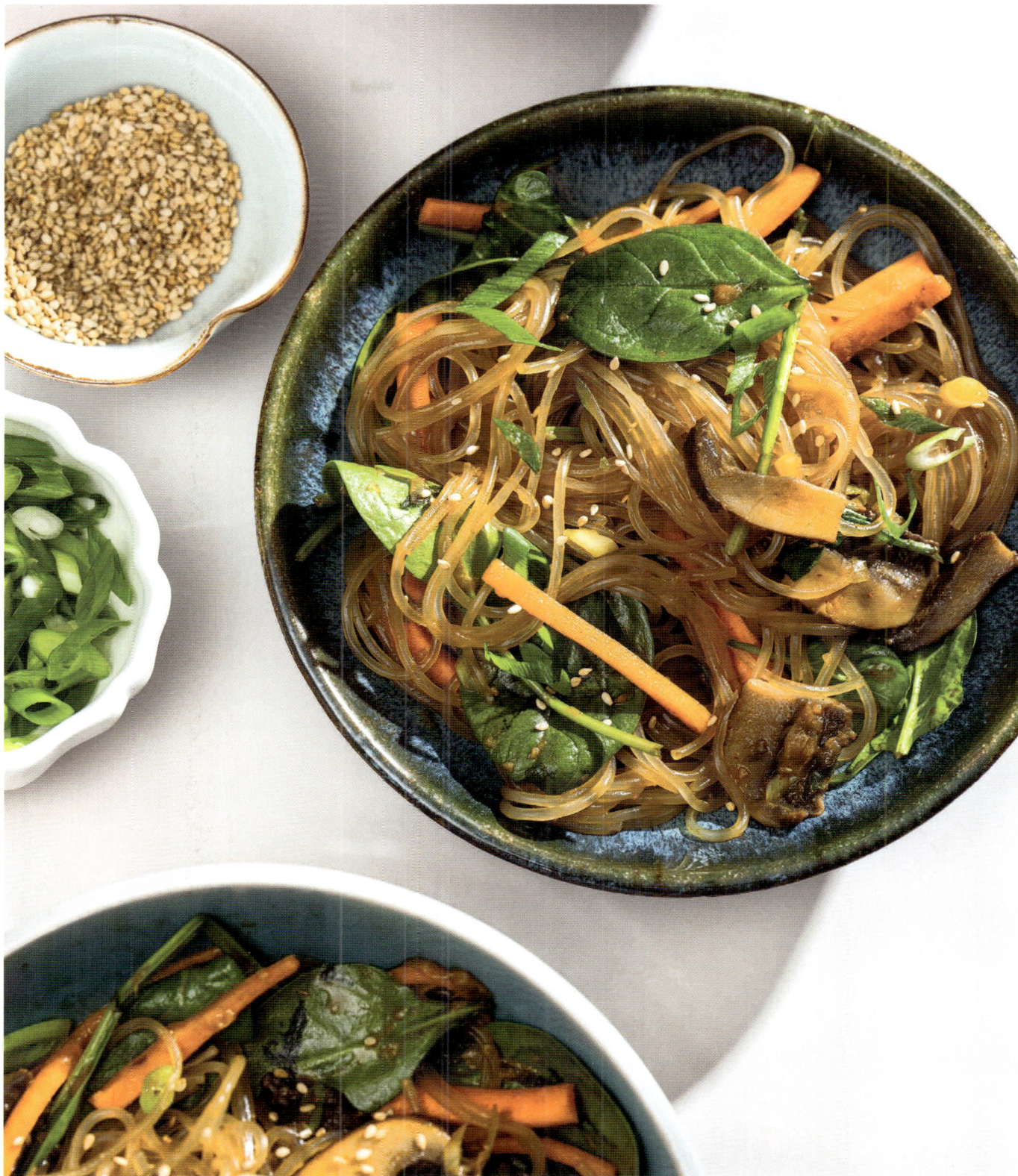

Sweet Potato Noodles with Shiitakes and Spinach

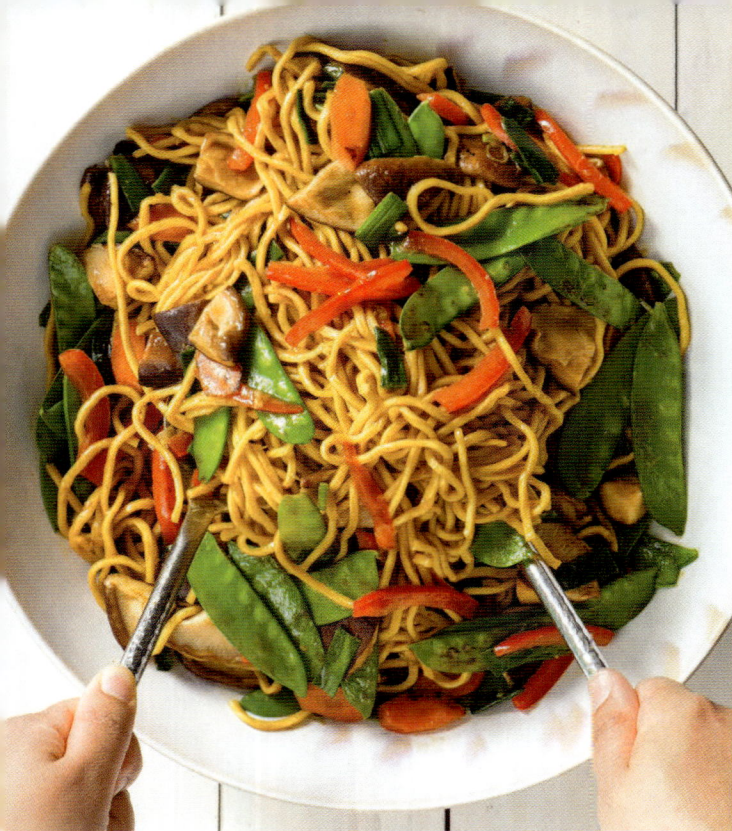

Vegetable Lo Mein

serves 4 • total time: 45 minutes **FAST**

why this recipe works • Tender and bouncy tangles of fresh Chinese noodles are traditionally the star of lo mein, which may get its name from the Cantonese "lou minh," meaning "stirred noodles." Variations of this comforting dish spread around the world in the 20th century, but it actually dates back thousands of years in China. The idea is simple: Cooked egg (or wheat) noodles are tossed with a savory sauce and stir-fried meat and/or vegetables. Part of the fun of lo mein is that it's endlessly customizable with mix-ins. For this vegetable rendition, we chose ingredients with plenty of bite—shiitake mushrooms, snow peas, bell pepper, and carrot. We coated the vegetables and noodles in a mix of soy, oyster, and hoisin sauces for a salty, sweet, spicy dish dripping with umami. This dish progresses quickly, so it's important that all of your ingredients are ready to go when you start cooking. You will need a 14-inch flat-bottomed wok or 12-inch nonstick skillet for this recipe.

Sauce

- ½ cup unsalted vegetable broth
- 3 tablespoons low-sodium soy sauce
- 2 tablespoons vegetarian oyster sauce
- 2 tablespoons hoisin sauce
- 1 tablespoon toasted sesame oil
- 1 teaspoon cornstarch
- ¼ teaspoon five-spice powder

Noodles and Vegetables

- 3 tablespoons avocado oil, divided
- 4 teaspoons grated fresh ginger
- 3 garlic cloves, minced
- 1 pound shiitake mushrooms, stemmed and halved if small or quartered if large
- 10 scallions, white parts sliced thin and green parts cut into 1-inch pieces
- 2 red bell peppers, stemmed, seeded, and sliced into ¼-inch-wide strips
- ½ small head napa cabbage, halved, cored, and cut into ½-inch pieces (4 cups)
- ¼ cup Shaoxing wine or dry sherry
- 1 pound fresh Chinese noodles
- 1 tablespoon chili-garlic sauce

1 For the sauce Whisk all ingredients together in bowl.

2 For the noodles and vegetables Combine 1 tablespoon oil, ginger, and garlic in bowl and set aside. Heat 1 tablespoon oil in 14-inch flat-bottomed wok or 12-inch nonstick skillet over medium heat

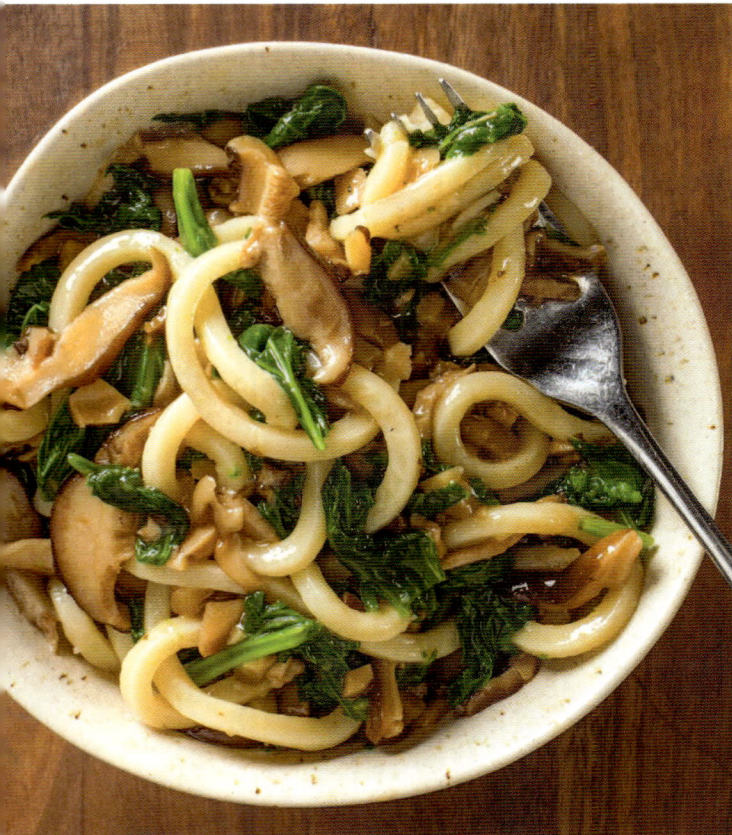

top | *Vegetable Lo Mein*

bottom | *Udon Noodles and Mustard Greens with Shiitake-Ginger Sauce*

until just smoking. Add mushrooms and cook, tossing slowly but constantly, until lightly browned, 6 to 8 minutes. Stir in scallions and cook until wilted, 2 to 3 minutes; transfer to separate bowl.

3 Add remaining 1 tablespoon oil, bell peppers, and cabbage to now-empty wok and cook, stirring constantly, until spotty brown, about 8 minutes. Push vegetables to 1 side of wok. Add garlic mixture to clearing and cook, mashing mixture into wok, until fragrant, about 30 seconds. Stir garlic mixture into vegetables.

4 Stir in Shaoxing wine and cook until liquid is nearly evaporated, 30 to 60 seconds. Stir in mushroom mixture and sauce and simmer until thickened, 1 to 2 minutes; cover and set aside.

5 Bring 4 quarts water to boil in large pot. Add noodles and cook, stirring often, until tender. Drain noodles and return them to pot. Add cabbage mixture and chili-garlic sauce and toss to combine. Serve.

> **MAKE AHEAD** • Vegetables can be prepped up to 24 hours ahead.

> **MAKE IT GLUTEN-FREE** • Substitute low-sodium tamari and gluten-free vegetarian oyster sauce, hoisin sauce, and noodles for the soy sauce, vegetarian oyster sauce, hoisin sauce, and Chinese noodles.

Udon Noodles and Mustard Greens with Shiitake-Ginger Sauce

serves 4 • total time: 35 minutes **FAST**

why this recipe works • Noodles and greens are a common pairing throughout Asia. Here, the spicy bite of mustard greens and the resilient chew of udon noodles make a great partnership that's delicate yet filling. Since udon noodles are starchy and a bit sweet, they stand up well to savory sauces; so we made a highly aromatic and flavorful base from Asian pantry staples, first browning meaty fresh shiitake mushrooms for flavor and then adding water and mirin along with rice vinegar, soy sauce, smashed garlic cloves, and a chunk of smashed fresh ginger. Dried shiitake mushrooms, sesame oil, and chili-garlic sauce rounded out the flavors. After this mixture simmered and reduced, we had a sauce that was light and brothy but super-savory—perfect for pairing with our cooked noodles and greens. Because fresh noodles cook so quickly, make sure to add the greens to the pot before the noodles. Do not substitute other types of noodles for the udon noodles here.

1 tablespoon avocado oil
8 ounces shiitake mushrooms, stemmed and sliced thin
¼ cup mirin
3 tablespoons unseasoned rice vinegar
3 tablespoons low-sodium soy sauce
2 garlic cloves, smashed and peeled
1 (1-inch) piece ginger, peeled, halved, and smashed
½ ounce dried shiitake mushrooms, rinsed and minced
1 teaspoon toasted sesame oil
1 teaspoon chili-garlic sauce
1 pound mustard greens, stemmed and cut into 2-inch pieces
Table salt for cooking noodles and greens
1 pound fresh udon noodles

1 Heat avocado oil in Dutch oven over medium-high heat until shimmering. Add fresh mushrooms and cook, stirring occasionally, until softened and lightly browned, about 5 minutes. Stir in 2 cups water, mirin, vinegar, soy sauce, garlic, ginger, dried mushrooms, sesame oil, and chili-garlic sauce and bring to simmer. Reduce heat to medium-low and simmer until sauce has reduced by half, 8 to 10 minutes. Off heat, discard garlic and ginger and cover pot to keep sauce warm.

2 Meanwhile, bring 4 quarts water to boil in large pot. Add mustard greens and 1 tablespoon salt and cook until greens are nearly tender, about 5 minutes. Add noodles and cook until greens and noodles are tender, about 2 minutes. Reserve ⅓ cup cooking water, drain noodles and greens, and return them to pot. Add sauce and reserved cooking water and toss to combine. Cook over medium-low heat, tossing constantly, until sauce clings to noodles, about 1 minute. Season with salt and pepper to taste, and serve.

> **NOTES FROM THE TEST KITCHEN**
>
> ### Fresh Shiitake Substitute
>
> You can substitute cremini mushrooms for shiitakes, but keep in mind that they will have a softer texture and less intense flavor. Be sure to sauté or stir-fry cremini for a few extra minutes, since they release more liquid than shiitakes.

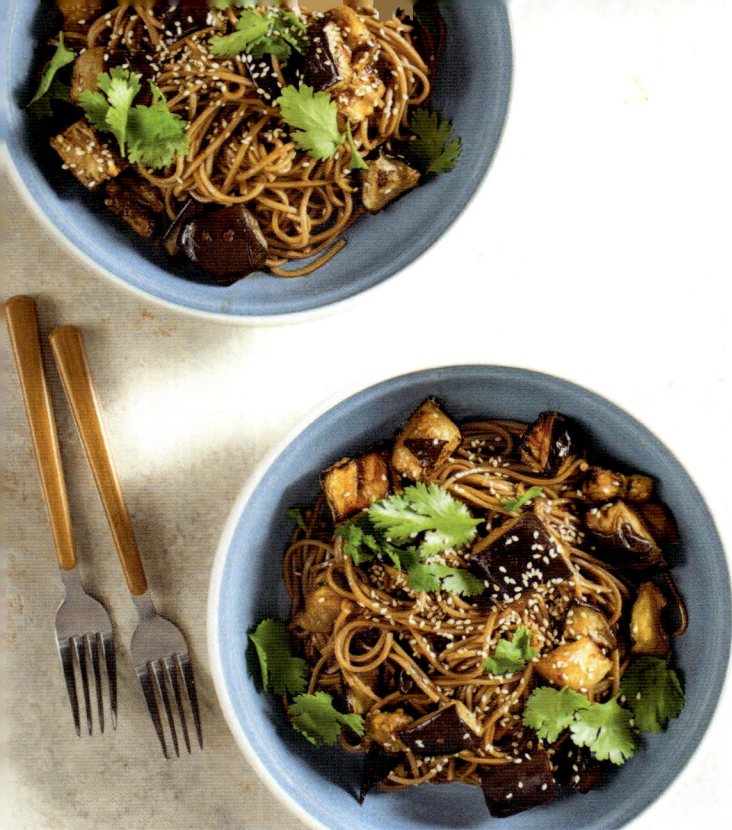

Soba Noodles with Roasted Eggplant and Sesame

serves 4 • total time: 40 minutes **FAST**

why this recipe works • When you power up your plate with heaps of whole grains and vegetables, all you need for a well-rounded meal is a little flavor-enhancing kick. Case in point: this simple combination of soba noodles and roasted eggplant, dressed with a savory mixture of vegetarian oyster sauce, soy sauce, sake, and sesame oil. We took a hands-off approach to cooking the eggplant and simply tossed it with some oil before sending it into a hot oven. The roasted vegetable pieces were soft, silky, and lightly caramelized. Don't forget to reserve some noodle cooking water for adjusting the consistency of the dish. For a gluten-free dish, make sure the soba noodles you purchase do not contain gluten.

- 3 pounds eggplant, cut into 1-inch pieces
- ¼ cup avocado oil
- 3 tablespoons vegetarian oyster sauce
- 3 tablespoons toasted sesame oil
- 5 teaspoons sake
- 1 tablespoon low-sodium soy sauce
  Pinch red pepper flakes (optional)
- 12 ounces dried soba noodles
- ¾ cup fresh cilantro leaves
- 2 teaspoons sesame seeds, toasted

1 Adjust oven racks to upper-middle and lower-middle positions and heat oven to 450 degrees. Line 2 rimmed baking sheets with aluminum foil and spray with avocado oil spray. Toss eggplant with avocado oil and spread on prepared sheets. Roast until well browned and tender, 25 to 30 minutes, stirring and switching sheets halfway through.

2 Combine oyster sauce, sesame oil, 2 tablespoons water, sake, soy sauce, and pepper flakes, if using, in small saucepan. Cook over medium heat, stirring often, about 1 minute; cover and set aside.

3 Meanwhile, bring 4 quarts water to boil in large pot. Add noodles and cook, stirring often, until tender. Reserve ½ cup cooking water, then drain noodles and return to pot. Add reserved sauce and roasted eggplant and toss to combine, adding reserved cooking water as needed to adjust consistency. Serve, sprinkling individual portions with cilantro and sesame seeds.

MAKE IT GLUTEN-FREE • Substitute low-sodium tamari and gluten-free vegetarian oyster sauce for the low-sodium soy sauce and vegetarian oyster sauce.

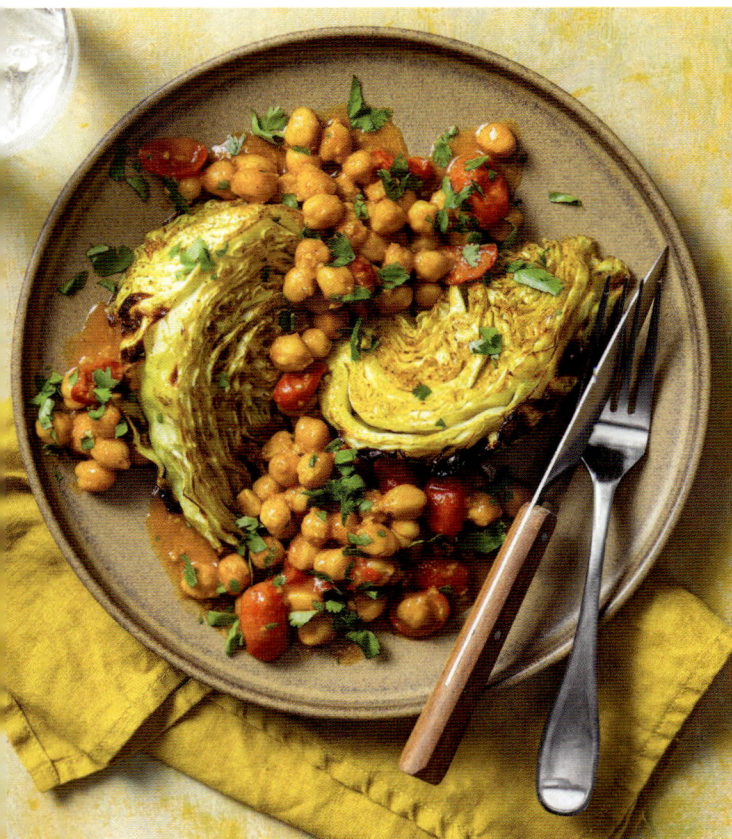

Curry Roasted Cabbage Wedges with Tomatoes and Chickpeas

serves 4 • total time: 50 minutes

why this recipe works • Roasting cabbage wedges transforms the vegetable into something fabulous, with crispy edges and tender inner layers. First we brushed them with a curry powder–infused oil, plus a little sugar to enhance browning. We then covered them with foil before roasting, which steamed the wedges. We found that we didn't need to flip the wedges, but simply uncovered them to crisp the upper sides while they continued to brown underneath. As the cabbage cooked, we simmered an aromatic chickpea-tomato curry on the stovetop to spoon over the crispy wedges. When slicing the cabbage, be sure to slice through the core, leaving it intact so that the wedges don't fall apart. Smaller cabbages work best here; if you have a larger cabbage, you can remove the outer leaves until it weighs about 2 pounds, though it may not brown as well. We like to serve the cabbage with our Herb Yogurt Sauce (page 166).

- 7 tablespoons avocado oil, divided
- 1 tablespoon curry powder, divided
- 1½ teaspoons sugar
- 1 teaspoon table salt
- ¼ teaspoon pepper
- 1 head green cabbage (2 pounds)
- 2 garlic cloves, minced
- 2 teaspoons grated fresh ginger
- 2 (15-ounce) cans no-salt-added chickpeas, undrained
- 10 ounces grape tomatoes, halved
- ¼ cup chopped fresh cilantro

1 Adjust oven rack to lowest position and heat oven to 500 degrees. Combine ¼ cup oil, 2 teaspoons curry powder, sugar, salt, and pepper in small bowl. Halve cabbage through core and cut each half into 4 approximately 2-inch-wide wedges, leaving core intact (you will have 8 wedges).

2 Arrange cabbage wedges in even layer on rimmed baking sheet, then brush cabbage all over with oil mixture. Cover tightly with aluminum foil and roast for 10 minutes. Remove foil and drizzle 2 tablespoons oil evenly over wedges. Return cabbage to oven and roast, uncovered, until cabbage is tender and sides touching sheet are well browned, 12 to 15 minutes.

3 Meanwhile, heat remaining 1 tablespoon oil in 12-inch skillet over medium-high heat until shimmering. Add garlic, ginger, and remaining 1 teaspoon curry powder and cook, mashing mixture into skillet, until fragrant, about 30 seconds. Add chickpeas and

their liquid and tomatoes and bring to simmer. Cook, stirring frequently, until tomatoes begin to break down and mixture has thickened slightly, 7 to 9 minutes.

4 Divide cabbage among individual plates and spoon chickpea mixture over top. Sprinkle with cilantro and serve.

Lentils and Roasted Broccoli with Lemony Bread Crumbs

serves 4 to 6 • total time: 1 hour 20 minutes

why this recipe works • This supersavory dish elevates earthy French green lentils and humble broccoli to a whole new level. We opted for classic aromatics to create our flavorful base: onion, garlic, and herbaceous thyme. By preheating the baking sheet in a 500-degree oven and arranging the broccoli in a single layer on the hot sheet, we were able to impart deep, flavorful browning to the stalks and florets in a short amount of time. While the lentils cooked, we quickly made a bright, crispy, lemony bread crumb topping in a skillet. Using the same skillet, we reduced some balsamic vinegar, transforming its flavor from sharp and assertive to luxurious and sweet. We then assembled our bowls: lentils topped with broccoli and bread crumbs, all drizzled with balsamic reduction. Lentilles du Puy (or French green lentils) hold their shape quite well during cooking; we do not recommend substituting other types of lentils in this dish.

- 6 tablespoons avocado oil, divided
- 1 onion, chopped fine
- 1 teaspoon table salt, divided
- 2 garlic cloves, minced
- 1 teaspoon minced fresh thyme or ½ teaspoon dried
- 12 ounces (1¾ cups) dried lentilles du Puy (French green lentils), picked over and rinsed
- 3¾ cups water
- ½ cup panko bread crumbs
- 2 teaspoons grated lemon zest
- ½ cup balsamic vinegar
- 2 pounds broccoli, florets cut into 1-inch pieces, stalks peeled and sliced lengthwise into ½-inch-thick planks

1 Adjust oven rack to lowest position, place aluminum foil–lined rimmed baking sheet on rack, and heat oven to 500 degrees. Heat 1 tablespoon oil in large saucepan over medium heat until shimmering. Add onion and ½ teaspoon salt and cook until softened, about 5 minutes. Stir in garlic and thyme and cook until fragrant, about 30 seconds.

2 Stir in lentils and water and bring to simmer over high heat. Reduce heat to low, cover, and simmer, stirring occasionally, until lentils are just tender, about 25 minutes. Uncover, increase heat to medium, and continue to cook until lentils are completely tender and most of liquid has evaporated, 10 to 15 minutes. Season with salt and pepper to taste, cover to keep warm, and set aside.

3 While lentils cook, combine panko and 2 tablespoons oil in 8-inch skillet, stirring to coat. Cook over medium-low heat, stirring frequently, until light golden brown, 5 to 7 minutes; transfer to bowl and stir in lemon zest. Wipe skillet clean with paper towels. Simmer vinegar in now-empty skillet, scraping bottom of skillet with silicone spatula, until thickened and reduced to 2 tablespoons, about 5 minutes.

4 Toss broccoli with remaining 3 tablespoons oil and remaining ½ teaspoon salt in bowl. Working quickly, lay broccoli in single layer, flat sides down, on preheated sheet. Roast until florets are browned, 9 to 11 minutes. Divide lentils among individual serving bowls and top with broccoli mixture. Sprinkle with panko mixture, drizzle with balsamic reduction, and serve.

> **MAKE AHEAD** • Cooked lentils can be refrigerated for up to 3 days.

> **MAKE IT GLUTEN-FREE** • Substitute gluten-free panko bread crumbs for the panko bread crumbs.

Koshari

serves 4 to 6 • total time: 2 hours

why this recipe works • Considered the national dish of Egypt, koshari evolved from a way to use up leftovers to became a popular street food. The hearty dish usually features lentils, rice, pasta, and chickpeas smothered in a spiced tomato sauce and topped with fried onions. Although the dish takes some time to put together, each element is fairly simple. We cooked the lentils and the pasta separately in boiling water, drained them and then set them aside while we prepared the rice and sauce. Soaking the rice in hot water before blooming spices in oil (then toasting the rice in the fragrant oil) eliminated excess starch, so the grains didn't clump. Using the same spices (coriander, cumin, cinnamon, nutmeg, and cayenne) from the rice to make a vinegar-spiked tomato sauce built a layered flavor profile. Adding the chickpeas directly to the sauce to simmer infused them with flavor. The finishing touch: a generous amount of ultrasavory, crunchy fried onions.

Large green or brown lentils both work well in this recipe; do not use French green lentils, or lentilles du Puy. Long-grain white, jasmine, or Texmati rice can be substituted for the basmati. You can use store-bought crispy onions and ¼ cup avocado oil in place of the crispy onions and their oil, if you prefer.

- 4 ounces (1 cup) elbow macaroni
- 1 teaspoon table salt, divided, plus salt for cooking pasta and lentils
- 1 cup dried green or brown lentils, picked over and rinsed
- 1 recipe Crispy Onions (recipe follows), plus ¼ cup reserved oil, divided
- 4 garlic cloves, minced, divided
- 1½ teaspoons ground coriander, divided
- 1½ teaspoons ground cumin, divided
- ¾ teaspoon ground cinnamon, divided
- ¼ teaspoon ground nutmeg, divided
- ¼ teaspoon cayenne pepper, divided
- 1 (28-ounce) can no-salt-added tomato sauce
- 1 (15-ounce) can no-salt-added chickpeas, rinsed
- 1 cup basmati rice
- 1 tablespoon red wine vinegar
- 3 tablespoons minced fresh parsley

1 Bring 2 quarts water to boil in Dutch oven. Add macaroni and 1½ teaspoons salt and cook, stirring often, until al dente. Drain macaroni, rinse with water, then drain again. Transfer to bowl and set aside.

2 Meanwhile, bring lentils, 4 cups water, and 1 teaspoon salt to boil in medium saucepan over high heat. Reduce heat to low and cook until lentils are just tender, 15 to 17 minutes. Drain and set aside.

3 Cook 1 tablespoon reserved onion oil, 1 teaspoon garlic, ½ teaspoon coriander, ½ teaspoon cumin, ¼ teaspoon cinnamon, ⅛ teaspoon nutmeg, ⅛ teaspoon cayenne, and ½ teaspoon salt in now-empty saucepan over medium heat until fragrant, about 1 minute. Stir in tomato sauce and chickpeas, bring to simmer, and cook until slightly thickened, about 10 minutes. Remove from heat and cover sauce to keep warm.

4 While sauce cooks, place rice in medium bowl, cover with hot tap water by 2 inches, and let sit for 15 minutes. Using your hands, gently swish grains to release excess starch. Carefully pour off water, leaving rice in bowl. Repeat adding and pouring off cold water 4 or 5 times, until water runs almost clear. Drain rice in fine-mesh strainer.

5   Cook remaining 3 tablespoons reserved onion oil, remaining garlic, remaining 1 teaspoon coriander, remaining 1 teaspoon cumin, remaining ½ teaspoon cinnamon, remaining ⅛ teaspoon nutmeg, and remaining ⅛ teaspoon cayenne in now-empty pot over medium heat until fragrant, about 2 minutes. Add rice and cook, stirring occasionally, until grain edges begin to turn translucent, about 3 minutes. Stir in 2 cups water and remaining ½ teaspoon salt and bring to boil. Stir in lentils, reduce heat to low, cover, and simmer gently until all liquid is absorbed, about 12 minutes.

6   Off heat, sprinkle macaroni over rice mixture. Cover, laying clean dish towel underneath lid, and let sit for 10 minutes.

7   Return sauce to simmer over medium heat. Stir in vinegar and season with salt and pepper to taste. Fluff rice and lentils with fork and stir in parsley and half of onions. Transfer to serving platter and top with half of sauce and remaining onions. Serve, passing remaining sauce separately.

MAKE IT GLUTEN-FREE • Substitute gluten-free elbow macaroni for the elbow macaroni.

Crispy Onions

makes 1½ cups • **total time: 35 minutes**

It is crucial to thoroughly dry the microwaved onions after rinsing. Be sure to reserve enough oil to use in Koshari or Mujaddara (page 160). Any remaining oil tastes great in salad dressings, sautéed vegetables, eggs, and pasta sauces.

    2 pounds onions, halved and sliced crosswise into
       ¼-inch-thick pieces
    2 teaspoons table salt
  1½ cups avocado oil

1   Toss onions and salt together in large bowl. Microwave for 5 minutes. Rinse thoroughly, transfer to paper towel–lined baking sheet, and dry well.

2   Heat onions and oil in Dutch oven over high heat, stirring frequently, until onions are golden brown, 25 to 30 minutes. Drain onions in colander set in large bowl; reserve oil. Transfer onions to paper towel–lined baking sheet to drain. (Oil may be stored in airtight container and refrigerated for up to 4 weeks.)

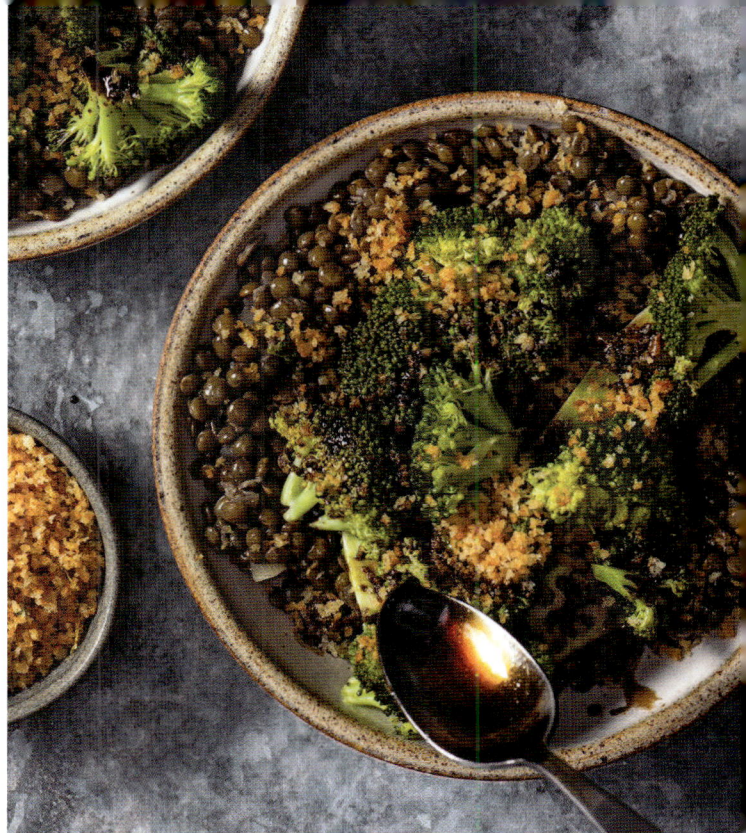

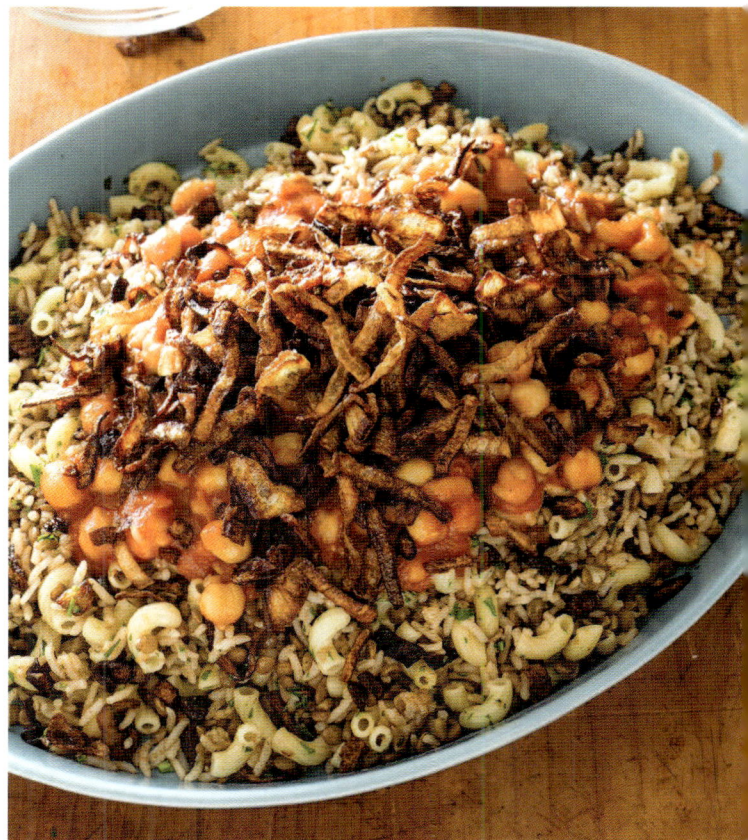

top | *Lentils and Roasted Broccoli with Lemony Bread Crumbs*
bottom | *Koshari*

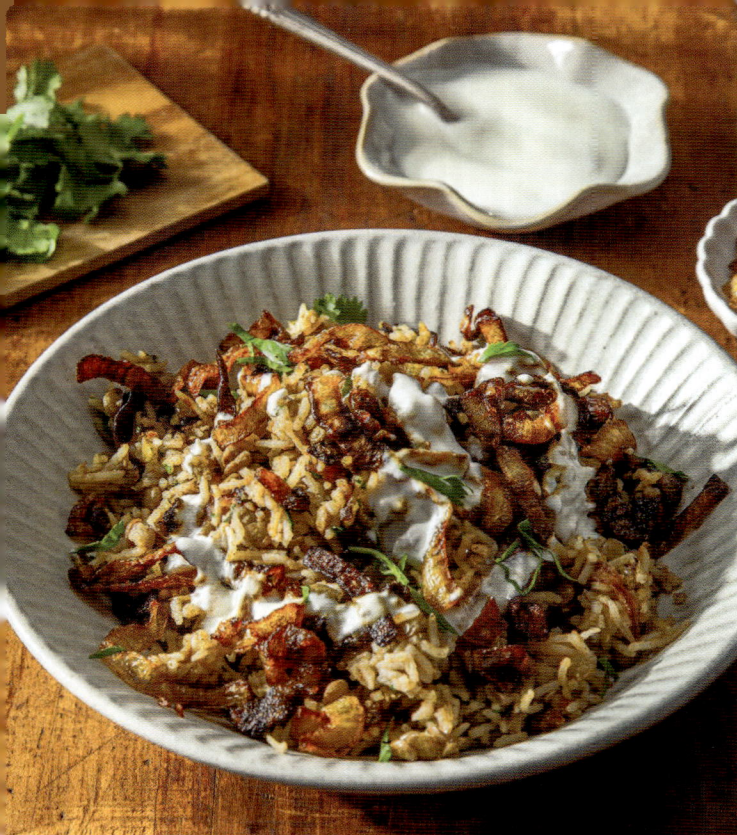

Mujaddara

serves 4 to 6 • **total time: 1 hour 25 minutes**

why this recipe works • This classic Levantine dish is a spectacular example of how a few humble ingredients can add up to something both nourishing and satisfying. Mujaddara typically consists of tender basmati rice and lentils seasoned with warm spices and minced garlic and topped with fried onions. To ensure that the rice and lentils finished cooking at the same time, we par-cooked the lentils and then set them aside while we prepared the rice. We soaked the rice in hot water to ensure that the grains turned out fluffy, not sticky, then toasted the grains along with the spices in some of the flavorful frying oil from the onions. Finished with a bracing garlicky yogurt sauce, this pilaf is as comforting as it is nutritious. Large green or brown lentils both work well in this recipe; do not use French green lentils, or lentilles du Puy. Long-grain white, jasmine, or Texmati rice can be substituted for the basmati. You can use store-bought crispy onions and 3 tablespoons avocado oil in place of the crispy onions and their oil, if you prefer.

Yogurt Sauce

- 1   cup plain yogurt
- 2   tablespoons lemon juice
- ½   teaspoon minced garlic
- ½   teaspoon table salt

Rice and Lentils

- 8¾   ounces (1¼ cups) dried green or brown lentils, picked over and rinsed
- 1   teaspoon table salt, plus salt for cooking lentils
- 1¼   cups basmati rice
- 1   recipe Crispy Onions (page 159), plus 3 tablespoons reserved oil
- 3   garlic cloves, minced
- 1   teaspoon ground coriander
- 1   teaspoon ground cumin
- ½   teaspoon ground cinnamon
- ½   teaspoon ground allspice
- ¼   teaspoon pepper
- ⅛   teaspoon cayenne pepper
- 1   teaspoon sugar
- 3   tablespoons minced fresh cilantro

1   For the yogurt sauce Whisk all ingredients together in bowl and refrigerate until ready to serve.

2   For the rice and lentils Bring lentils, 4 cups water, and 1 teaspoon salt to boil in medium saucepan over high heat. Reduce heat to low and cook until lentils are just tender, 15 to 17 minutes. Drain and set aside.

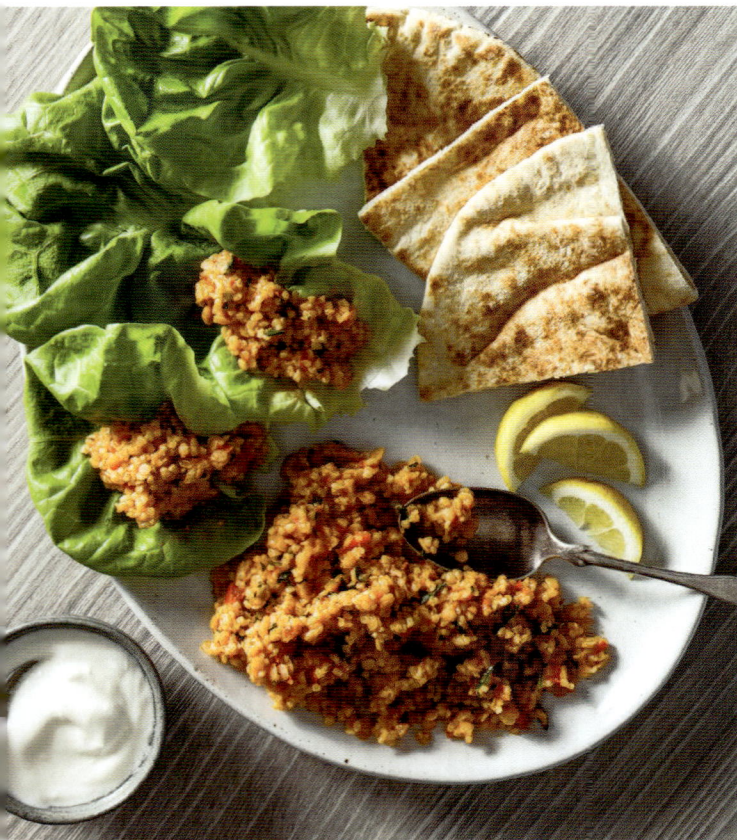

3 Meanwhile, place rice in medium bowl, cover with hot tap water by 2 inches, and let sit for 15 minutes. Using your hands, gently swish grains to release excess starch. Carefully pour off water, leaving rice in bowl. Repeat adding and pouring off cold water 4 or 5 times, until water runs almost clear. Drain rice in fine-mesh strainer.

4 Cook reserved onion oil, garlic, coriander, cumin, cinnamon, allspice, pepper, and cayenne in Dutch oven over medium heat until fragrant, about 2 minutes. Add rice and cook, stirring occasionally, until grain edges begin to turn translucent, about 3 minutes. Stir in 2¼ cups water, sugar, and 1 teaspoon salt and bring to boil. Stir in lentils, reduce heat to low, cover, and simmer gently until all liquid is absorbed, about 12 minutes.

5 Off heat, cover, laying clean dish towel underneath lid, and let sit for 10 minutes. Fluff rice and lentils with fork and stir in cilantro and half of onions. Transfer to serving platter and top with remaining onions. Serve with yogurt sauce.

MAKE AHEAD • Yogurt sauce can be refrigerated for up to 3 days.

MAKE IT DAIRY-FREE • Substitute plant-based yogurt for the dairy yogurt.

Red Lentil Kibbeh

serves 4 to 6 • total time: 1 hour   `SUPERCHARGED`

why this recipe works • Kibbeh is a popular Middle Eastern dish made from bulgur, minced onions, various spices, and often ground meat. During Lent, though, the meal is often prepared with lentils as the main protein. We wanted to turn this nutrient-packed, plant-powered version of the dish into something that could be served on its own with Bibb lettuce and yogurt, or as a showstopping addition to a larger spread. We chose red lentils—which are quick cooking, iron-rich, and dense with prebiotics—and enhanced both their color and flavor with two red pastes: Tomato paste brought sweetness and umami, while harissa added complexity. We gave the bulgur a head start before adding the lentils to the same saucepan, so both finished cooking at the same time. To balance the deeply flavorful aromatics and pastes, we stirred in lemon juice and fresh parsley at the end. We like to use our homemade Harissa (page 106); you can use store-bought, though spiciness can vary greatly by brand. If your harissa is spicy, omit the cayenne. Serve with warmed pita.

3 tablespoons extra-virgin olive oil, divided
1 onion, chopped fine
1 red bell pepper, stemmed, seeded, and chopped fine
1⅛ teaspoons table salt
2 tablespoons harissa
2 tablespoons no-salt-added tomato paste
½ teaspoon cayenne pepper (optional)
1 cup medium-grind bulgur
4 cups water
¾ cup dried red lentils, picked over and rinsed
½ cup chopped fresh parsley
2 tablespoons lemon juice, plus lemon wedges for serving
1 head Bibb lettuce (8 ounces), leaves separated
½ cup plain yogurt

1 Heat 1 tablespoon oil in large saucepan over medium heat until shimmering. Add onion, bell pepper, and salt and cook until softened, about 5 minutes. Stir in harissa, tomato paste, and cayenne, if using, and cook, stirring frequently, until fragrant, about 1 minute.

2 Stir in bulgur and water and bring to simmer. Reduce heat to low, cover, and simmer gently until bulgur is barely tender, about 8 minutes. Stir in lentils, cover, and continue to cook, stirring occasionally, until lentils and bulgur are tender, 8 to 10 minutes.

3 Off heat, lay clean dish towel underneath lid and let mixture sit for 10 minutes. Stir in 1 tablespoon oil, parsley, and lemon juice and stir vigorously until mixture is cohesive. Season with salt and pepper to taste. Transfer to platter and drizzle with remaining 1 tablespoon oil. Spoon kibbeh into lettuce leaves and drizzle with yogurt. Serve with lemon wedges.

MAKE AHEAD • Kibbeh can be refrigerated for up to 2 days; adjust consistency with hot water as needed before serving.

MAKE IT DAIRY-FREE • Substitute plant-based yogurt for the dairy yogurt.

Nutrition Knowledge   The red lentils and bulgur in this kibbeh dish make a powerful duo. Slow-digesting lentils regulate blood sugar, while bulgur is a whole grain rich in magnesium and iron, key inflammation-fighting minerals. Top it off with another potent combo, harissa and cayenne, and you've got a double dose of capsaicin—and a delicious, inflammation-fighting powerhouse of a dish. —*Alicia*

Burst Cherry Tomato Puttanesca with Roman Beans

serves 4 · total time: 40 minutes   **FAST**

why this recipe works · Creamy Roman beans (also called cranberry beans) turn punchy puttanesca sauce into a one-pan meal. For a fresh tomato sauce, we used sweet cherry tomatoes: We blistered them in a skillet and then added the beans and classic puttanesca ingredients—capers, olives, and pepper flakes, plus a vegetarian anchovy substitute—and cooked it all until the tomatoes turned juicy. Panko with lemon and basil made for a crunchy, flavorful topping. Make sure the cherry tomatoes are no larger than 1 inch in diameter or they won't burst in the given time range.

- 3 tablespoons extra-virgin olive oil, divided, plus extra for drizzling
- ½ cup panko bread crumbs
- ¼ cup chopped fresh basil
- 1 teaspoon grated lemon zest
- ⅛ teaspoon pepper
- 1 pound cherry tomatoes
- 2 (15-ounce) cans no-salt-added Roman beans, rinsed
- ½ cup pitted kalamata olives, chopped coarse
- 3 tablespoons capers, rinsed and minced
- 3 teaspoons anchovy substitute (recipe follows)
- 3 garlic cloves, minced
- ½ teaspoon table salt
- ¼ teaspoon red pepper flakes
- ¼ teaspoon sugar

1 Heat 1 tablespoon oil and panko in 12-inch skillet over medium heat, stirring occasionally, until panko is golden brown, 4 to 5 minutes. Transfer to medium bowl and let cool to room temperature, about 10 minutes. Stir in basil, lemon zest, and pepper. Wipe skillet clean.

2 Heat remaining 2 tablespoons oil in now-empty skillet over medium heat until shimmering. Add tomatoes and stir to coat evenly in oil. Cook, partially covered, without stirring, until tomatoes have blistered on bottom, about 3 minutes.

3 Stir in beans, olives, capers, anchovy substitute, garlic, salt, pepper flakes, and sugar and continue to cook until beans are warmed through and tomato juices have formed a light sauce, about 3 minutes. Serve, topping individual portions with panko mixture and drizzling with extra oil.

MAKE IT GLUTEN-FREE · Substitute gluten-free panko bread crumbs for the panko bread crumbs.

Anchovy Substitute

makes ¼ cup · total time: 5 minutes

Anchovies play a subtle but unmistakably helpful supporting role in many recipes, lending savory funk. For a vegetarian expression of that flavor, we developed this substitute. Use 1 teaspoon anchovy substitute to replace either 1 anchovy fillet or ½ teaspoon anchovy paste. If you can't find nori powder, you can grind 1 sheet of toasted nori in a spice grinder to a fine powder (do not use snack-size sheets).

- ¼ cup white miso
- 1 teaspoon nori powder

Combine miso and nori powder in small bowl. (Anchovy substitute can be refrigerated for up to 2 months.)

Spicy Braised Chickpeas and Turnips with Couscous

serves 4 to 6 · total time: 55 minutes

why this recipe works · For this plant-powered braise, we took inspiration from Tunisian cuisine, which is known for being quite spicy and deeply flavorful. While the combo of chickpeas and braised turnips may be new to some, the two work great together. Turnips have a peppery bite akin to radishes when raw, but when cooked their spiciness mellows, and they develop a dense, creamy texture reminiscent of potatoes, but with less starch. Including the aquafaba—the starchy, seasoned liquid from canned chickpeas—instead of draining it away gave the braising liquid enough body and flavor to turn it into a velvety sauce. A base of fluffy couscous made the perfect bed for our savory braise.

- 3 tablespoons extra-virgin olive oil, divided
- 2 onions, chopped
- 2 red bell peppers, stemmed, seeded, and chopped
- 1 teaspoon table salt, divided
- ¼ teaspoon pepper
- ¼ cup no-salt-added tomato paste
- 1 jalapeño chile, stemmed, seeded, and chopped
- 5 garlic cloves, minced
- ¾ teaspoon ground cumin
- ¼ teaspoon cayenne pepper
- 2 (15-ounce) cans no-salt-added chickpeas, undrained

12   ounces turnips, peeled and cut into ½-inch pieces

2¼   cups water, divided, plus extra hot water as needed

1½   cups couscous

¼   cup chopped fresh parsley

2   tablespoons lemon juice, plus lemon wedges for serving

1   Heat 2 tablespoons oil in Dutch oven over medium heat until shimmering. Add onions, bell peppers, ¾ teaspoon salt, and pepper and cook until softened and lightly browned, 5 to 7 minutes. Stir in tomato paste, jalapeño, garlic, cumin, and cayenne and cook until fragrant, about 30 seconds.

2   Stir in chickpeas and their liquid, turnips, and ¾ cup water. Bring to simmer and cook until turnips are tender and sauce has thickened, 25 to 35 minutes.

3   Meanwhile, heat remaining 1 tablespoon oil in medium saucepan over medium-high heat until shimmering. Add couscous and cook, stirring frequently, until grains are just beginning to brown, 3 to 5 minutes. Stir in remaining 1½ cups water and remaining ¼ teaspoon salt. Cover, remove saucepan from heat, and let sit until couscous is tender, about 7 minutes. Fluff couscous with fork.

4   Stir parsley and lemon juice into braised turnips. Season with salt and pepper to taste. Adjust consistency with hot water as needed. Serve chickpea-turnip mixture over couscous with lemon wedges.

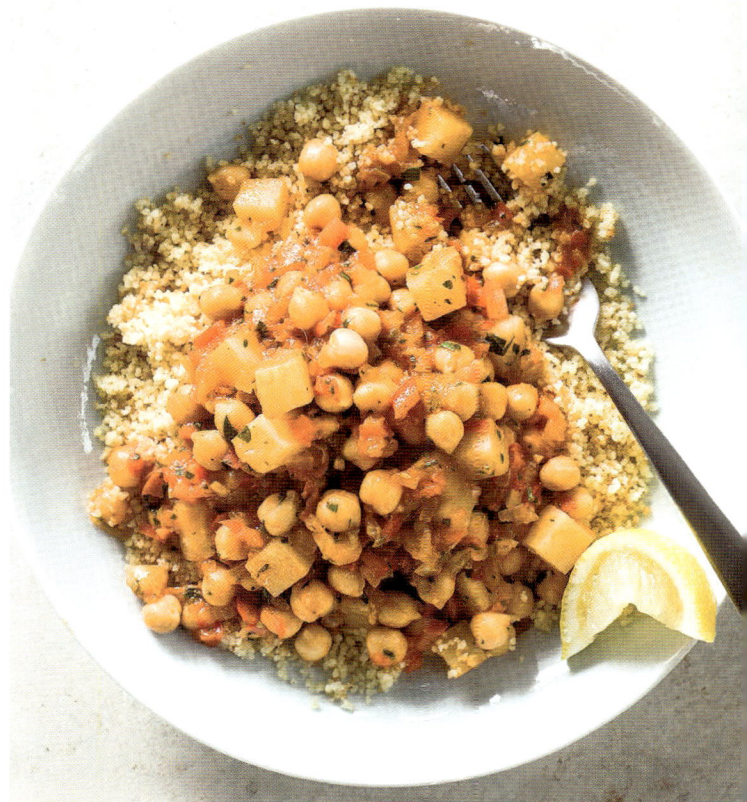

Stuffed Delicata Squash

serves 4 · total time: 45 minutes   FAST

why this recipe works · Delicata squash offers earthy, autumnal sweetness similar to acorn or butternut squash, but with none of the elbow grease required to prepare those varieties. Delicata's tender skin is thin and perfectly edible. Here, we halved the squash to create boats—ideal for holding a hearty stuffing. To start, we simply seasoned the squash halves and microwaved them until the flesh was tender and the skin was softened—no shell removal required. We then stuffed the squash halves with a savory, nutty filling: We cooked mushrooms, onion, and spinach in olive oil to imbue the vegetables with richness and stirred in bulgur, toasted pecans, and shredded cheddar for a mixture with plenty of bite and savory flavor. Before broiling the squash, we brushed the surfaces of the filling with additional oil to encourage flavorful browning (and contribute more healthy fats).

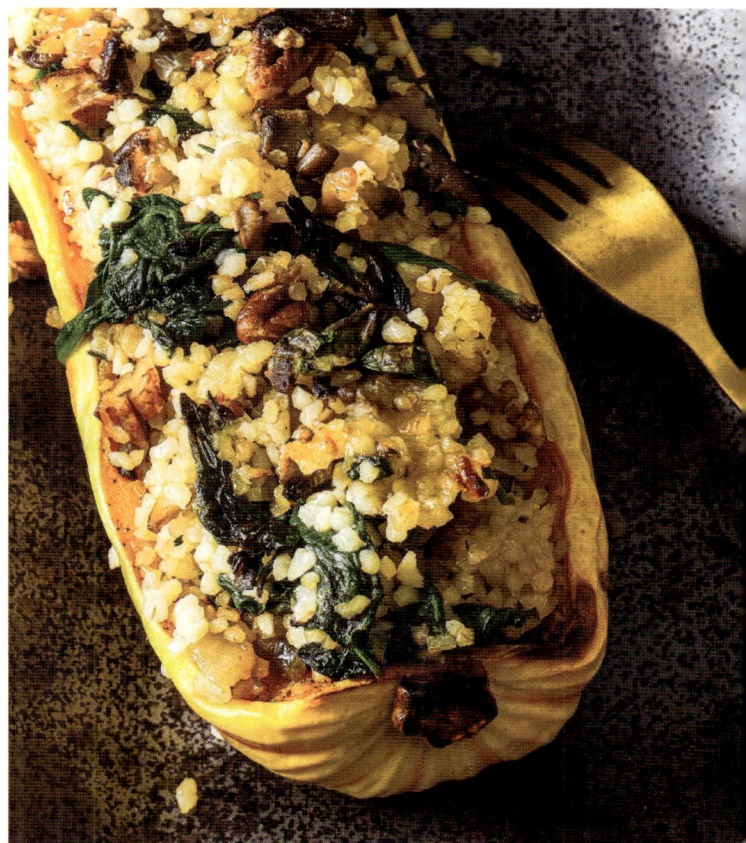

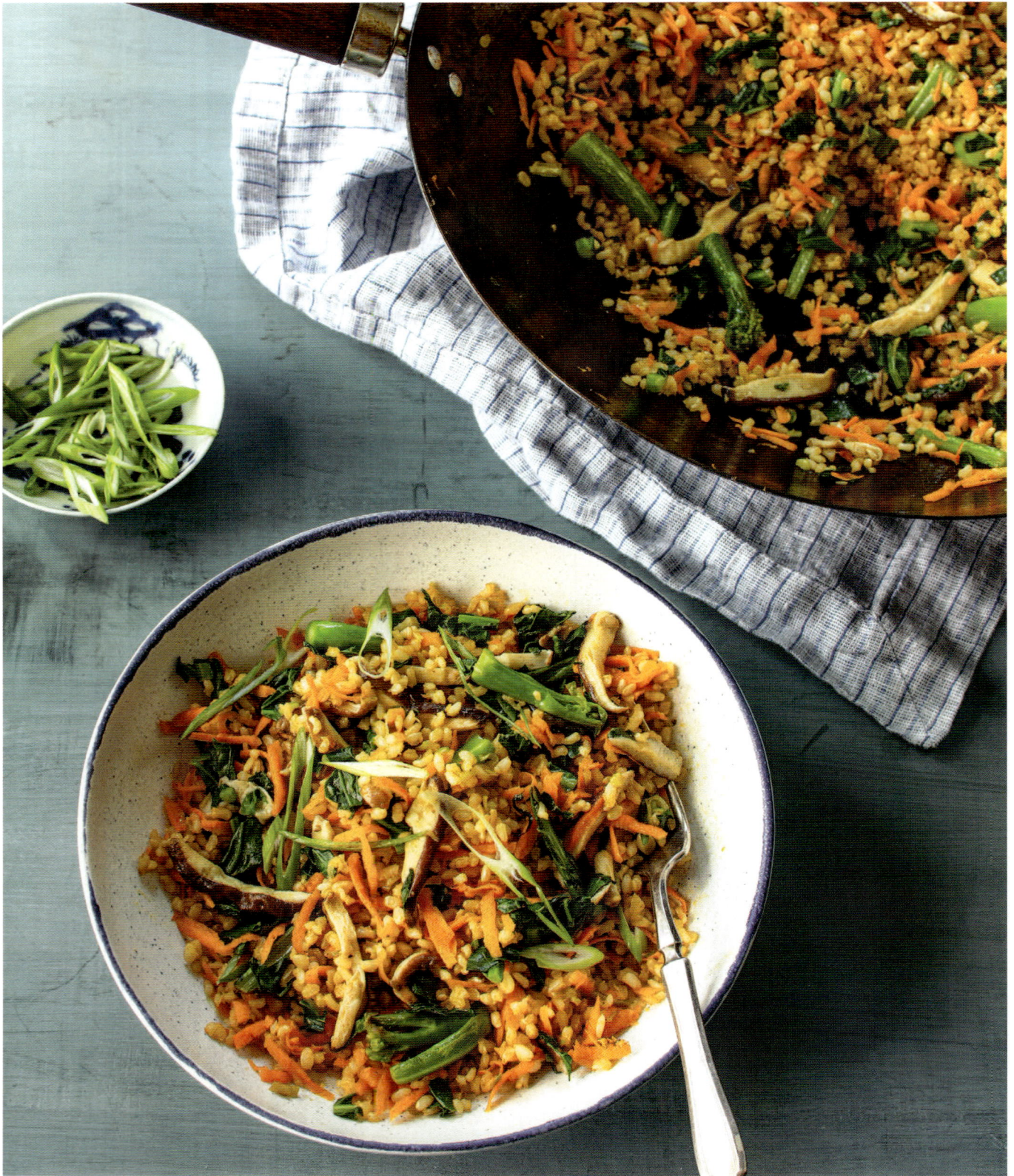

Vegetable Fried Rice with Gai Lan and Shiitake Mushrooms

2 delicata squashes (about 1 pound each), halved lengthwise and seeded
1½ teaspoons table salt, divided, plus salt for cooking bulgur
½ teaspoon pepper
1 cup medium-grind bulgur
6 tablespoons extra-virgin olive oil, divided
10 ounces cremini mushrooms, trimmed and chopped
1 onion, chopped
5 ounces (5 cups) baby spinach, chopped coarse
1 teaspoon minced fresh thyme
½ cup chopped toasted pecans
1 ounce sharp cheddar cheese, shredded (¼ cup)

1 Sprinkle cut sides of squash with 1 teaspoon salt and pepper. Microwave in large covered bowl until tender, 12 to 15 minutes. Bring 2 quarts water to boil in large saucepan. Add bulgur and 1 teaspoon salt. Reduce heat to medium-low and simmer until tender, 5 to 8 minutes. Drain.

2 Meanwhile, heat ¼ cup oil in 12-inch nonstick skillet over medium-high heat until shimmering. Add mushrooms, onion, and remaining ½ teaspoon salt and cook, stirring occasionally, until vegetables are browned, about 10 minutes. Stir in spinach and thyme and cook until wilted, about 3 minutes. Off heat, stir in bulgur, pecans, and cheddar.

3 Adjust oven rack 8 inches from broiler element and heat broiler. Transfer squash, cut side up, to rimmed baking sheet. Tightly pack bulgur mixture into squash halves, mounding bulgur mixture up over squash rims. Brush filling with remaining 2 tablespoons oil. Broil until lightly browned, 4 to 5 minutes. Serve.

MAKE IT DAIRY-FREE • Substitute plant-based cheddar cheese for the dairy cheddar cheese or omit.

Vegetable Fried Rice with Gai Lan and Shiitake Mushrooms

serves 4 • total time: 1 hour

why this recipe works • We wanted to develop a quick plant-based spin on fried rice, for which it's always important to use leftover rice (which doesn't clump like fresh). For a faux leftover rice, minus the wait, we boiled it like pasta. For a hearty vegetable, we quickly sautéed gai lan, followed by the cooked rice, then stirred in a sauce. A 14-inch wok ensures that the vegetables don't retain too much moisture and allows more space to toss the rice, but you can also use a 12-inch nonstick skillet.

1½ cups short-grain brown rice
½ teaspoon table, salt plus salt for cooking rice
1 tablespoon Chinese black vinegar or sherry vinegar
2 tablespoons low-sodium soy sauce
1 tablespoon Shaoxing wine or dry sherry
¼ teaspoon white pepper
¼ cup avocado oil, divided
6 scallions, white and green parts sliced thin, separated
2 garlic cloves, minced
2 teaspoons grated fresh ginger
12 ounces Chinese broccoli, trimmed, leaves roughly chopped, stalks cut into 2-inch pieces, leaves and stalks separated
8 ounces shiitake mushrooms, stemmed and sliced ¼ inch thick
2 carrots, peeled and shredded
1 tablespoon toasted sesame oil

1 Bring 2 quarts water to boil in large pot. Add rice and 2 teaspoons salt and cook, stirring occasionally, until rice is tender, 30 to 40 minutes. Drain well and set aside.

2 Meanwhile, whisk vinegar, soy sauce, Shaoxing wine, salt, and white pepper together in small bowl; set aside. Combine 2 tablespoons avocado oil, scallion whites, garlic, and ginger in second small bowl; set aside.

3 Heat 1 tablespoon avocado oil in 14-inch flat-bottomed wok or 12-inch nonstick skillet over medium heat until just smoking. Add broccoli stalks and 2 tablespoons water (water will sputter), cover, and cook until broccoli is bright green, 1 to 2 minutes. Uncover, increase heat to high, and continue to cook, tossing slowly but constantly, until water has evaporated and stalks are crisp-tender, 1 to 3 minutes; transfer to medium bowl.

4 Heat remaining 1 tablespoon avocado oil in now-empty wok over high heat until just smoking. Add broccoli leaves and mushrooms and cook, tossing vegetables slowly but constantly, until mushrooms are softened and broccoli leaves are completely wilted, 3 to 5 minutes; transfer to bowl with broccoli stalks.

5 Add reserved scallion mixture to again-empty wok and cook over medium heat, mashing mixture into wok, until fragrant, about 30 seconds. Add reserved rice, reserved vinegar mixture, carrots, sesame oil, and reserved vegetable mixture and increase heat to high. Cook, tossing rice constantly, until mixture is thoroughly combined and warmed through, about 3 minutes. Sprinkle scallion greens over top and serve.

MAKE AHEAD • Cooked rice can be refrigerated for up to 3 days.

Saffron Cauliflower Rice

serves 4 · **total time: 50 minutes**

why this recipe works · Biryani places fragrant long-grain basmati center stage, enriching it with saffron and a variety of fresh herbs and pungent spices. However, traditional recipes take a long time to develop deep flavor by steeping whole spices and cooking each component on its own before marrying them. We wanted to deconstruct this dish to make it easier and faster while staying true to its warmth and home-style appeal. Drawing inspiration from biryani, we decided to pair our basmati rice with sweet, earthy cauliflower, so we cut the cauliflower into small florets and tossed them with warm spices in a skillet to give them deep flavor. We added cooked rice and currants to this flavorful mixture so that all the flavors could meld. The residual heat also helped plump the currants and bloom the saffron. Finally, we stirred in lots of bright mint and cilantro along with our roasted cauliflower. Biryani is traditionally served with a cooling yogurt sauce; ideally, you should make it before starting the biryani to allow the flavors in the sauce to meld. We like to serve this with our Herb-Yogurt Sauce (recipe follows), but you can omit if you prefer. You will need a 12-inch nonstick skillet with a tight-fitting lid for this recipe.

- 1½ cups brown basmati rice
- 1 teaspoon table salt, plus salt for cooking rice
- ¼ cup extra-virgin olive oil, divided
- 1 head cauliflower (2 pounds), cored and cut into 1-inch florets
- 4 garlic cloves, minced
- 1 serrano chile, stemmed, seeded, and minced
- ½ teaspoon ground cardamom
- ½ teaspoon ground cumin
- ¼ teaspoon ground cinnamon
- ¼ teaspoon ground ginger
- ¼ teaspoon pepper
- ⅛ teaspoon saffron threads, lightly crumbled
- ¼ cup dried currants or raisins
- ¼ cup chopped fresh cilantro
- ¼ cup chopped fresh mint
- ¼ cup chopped cashews, toasted

1 Bring 2 quarts water to boil in large pot. Add rice and 2 teaspoons salt and cook, stirring occasionally, until rice is tender, 25 to 35 minutes. Drain well and set aside.

2 Meanwhile, heat 2 tablespoons oil in 12-inch nonstick skillet over medium-high heat until shimmering. Add cauliflower florets, cover, and cook until florets start to brown and edges just start to become translucent, about 5 minutes.

3 Remove lid and add remaining 2 tablespoons oil, garlic, serrano, cardamom, cumin, cinnamon, ginger, salt, pepper, and saffron. Continue to cook, stirring frequently, until florets are tender and golden brown in many spots, 4 to 8 minutes.

4 Add reserved rice and currants to skillet with cauliflower, stirring to combine, and cook until warmed through, about 1 minute. Sprinkle with cilantro, mint, and cashews and season with salt and pepper to taste. Serve.

> **MAKE AHEAD** · Cooked rice can be refrigerated for up to 3 days.

Herb-Yogurt Sauce

makes 1 cup · **total time: 5 minutes, plus 30 minutes resting**

- 1 cup plain dairy yogurt or plant-based yogurt
- 2 tablespoons minced fresh cilantro
- 2 tablespoons minced fresh mint
- 1 garlic clove, minced

Whisk all ingredients together in bowl and season with salt and pepper to taste. Let sit until flavors meld, at least 30 minutes. (Sauce can be refrigerated for up to 3 days.)

Beet Barley Risotto

serves 6 · **total time: 1¼ hours**

why this recipe works · Hearty pearl barley holds its own against the sweet earthiness of beets and sturdy beet greens in this robust, comforting risotto. Pearl barley, which has its outer husk removed to expose the starchy interior, helped the cooking liquid thicken into an irresistibly velvety sauce as it simmered. Cooking the grains with white wine and vegetable broth imbued the barley with complex flavor and savoriness. And simmering the barley until the grains were just cooked but still somewhat firm in the center helped them retain some of their satisfying bite. We stirred raw grated beets into the barley in two parts—half at the beginning for a base of flavor, and half at the end for freshness, color, and pleasant chew—which gave each bite textural interest. A bit of Parmesan, folded in at the end, gave the risotto a rich, buttery aroma without pushing the saturated fat over the edge. A scattering of parsley made the perfect fresh garnish. Do not substitute hulled, hull-less, quick-cooking, or presteamed barley (read the package label to determine this) in this recipe. If you can't find beets with their greens attached or the greens aren't in good shape, use 10 ounces beets and 2 cups stemmed and chopped Swiss chard. Use a box grater or the shredding disk on a food processor to shred the beets. You might not need to use all of the broth when cooking the risotto.

- 3 cups unsalted vegetable broth
- 3 cups water
- 2 tablespoons extra-virgin olive oil
- 1 pound beets with greens attached, beets peeled and grated, divided; greens stemmed and cut into 1-inch pieces (2 cups)
- 1 onion, chopped
- ¾ teaspoon table salt
- 1½ cups pearl barley, rinsed
- 4 garlic cloves, minced
- 1 teaspoon minced fresh thyme or ¼ teaspoon dried
- 1 cup dry white wine
- 1 ounce Parmesan cheese, grated (½ cup)
- 2 tablespoons chopped fresh parsley

1 Bring broth and water to simmer in medium saucepan. Reduce heat to lowest setting and cover to keep warm.

2 Heat oil in large saucepan over medium heat until shimmering. Add half of grated beets, onion, and salt and cook until vegetables are softened, 5 to 7 minutes. Stir in barley and cook, stirring often, until aromatic, about 4 minutes. Stir in garlic and thyme and cook until fragrant, about 30 seconds. Stir in wine and cook until fully absorbed, about 2 minutes.

3 Stir in 3 cups warm broth. Simmer, stirring occasionally, until liquid is absorbed and bottom of pan is dry, 22 to 25 minutes. Stir in 2 cups warm broth and simmer, stirring occasionally, until liquid is absorbed and bottom of pan is dry, 15 to 18 minutes.

4 Add beet greens and continue to cook, stirring often and adding remaining broth as needed to prevent pan bottom from becoming dry, until greens are softened and barley is cooked through but still somewhat firm in center, 5 to 10 minutes. Off heat, stir in remaining grated beets and Parmesan. Season with salt and pepper to taste and sprinkle with parsley. Serve.

MAKE IT DAIRY-FREE • Substitute plant-based Parmesan cheese for the dairy Parmesan cheese.

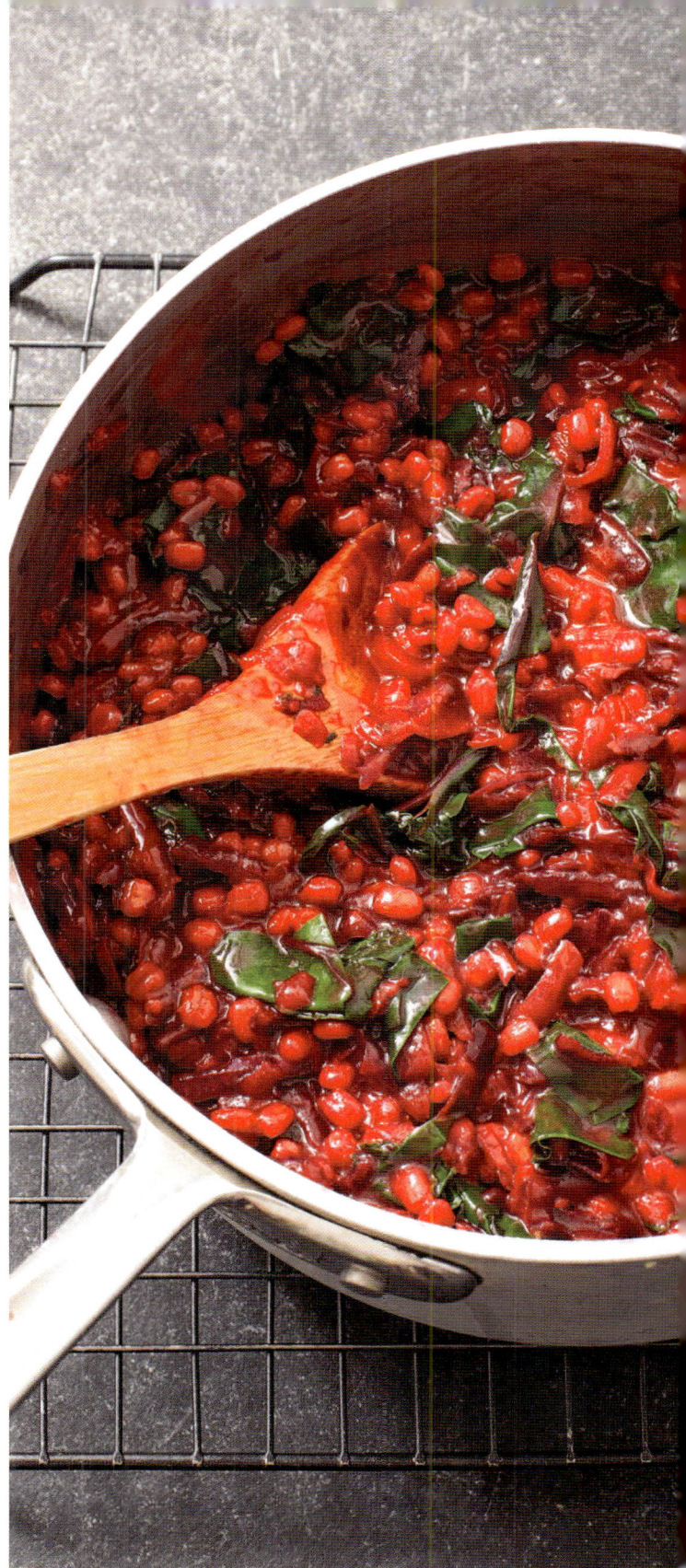

Beet Barley Risotto

Barley with Lentils, Mushrooms, and Tahini-Yogurt Sauce

serves 4 · total time: 50 minutes

why this recipe works · We love black lentils for their nutty, robust flavor and ability to hold their shape once cooked. They shone when we paired them with equally sturdy barley; we cooked both together in the same Dutch oven. For our mushroom go-withs, we opted to use a large nonstick skillet to cook meaty portobellos with umami-rich dried porcini; its broad surface area allowed for more browning and faster cooking. Our tangy tahini-yogurt sauce balanced all the hearty flavors, while fresh dill and strips of lemon zest brightened the earthy notes. Do not substitute hulled, hull-less, quick-cooking, or presteamed barley (read the package label to determine this) in this recipe. Green or brown lentils can be substituted for the black lentils.

- ½ ounce dried porcini mushrooms, rinsed
- 1 cup pearl barley, rinsed
- ½ cup black lentils, picked over and rinsed
- ½ teaspoon table salt, plus salt for cooking barley and lentils
- 2 tablespoons extra-virgin olive oil
- 1 onion, chopped fine
- 2 large portobello mushroom caps, cut into 1-inch pieces
- 3 (2-inch) strips lemon zest, sliced thin lengthwise
- ¾ teaspoon ground coriander
- ¼ teaspoon pepper
- 2 tablespoons chopped fresh dill
- ½ cup Tahini-Yogurt Sauce (recipe follows)

1 Microwave 1½ cups water and porcini mushrooms in covered bowl until steaming, about 1 minute. Let sit until softened, about 5 minutes. Drain mushrooms in fine-mesh strainer lined with coffee filter set over bowl. Reserve soaking liquid, chop mushrooms, and set aside.

2 Bring 4 quarts water to boil in Dutch oven and add barley, lentils, and 1 tablespoon salt. Return to boil and cook until tender, 20 to 40 minutes. Drain barley and lentils, return to now-empty pot, and cover to keep warm.

3 Meanwhile, heat oil in 12-inch nonstick skillet over medium heat until shimmering. Add onion and cook until softened, about 5 minutes. Stir in portobello mushrooms, cover, and cook until portobellos have released their liquid and begin to brown, about 4 minutes.

4 Uncover, stir in lemon zest, coriander, salt, and pepper, and cook until fragrant, about 30 seconds. Stir in porcini and porcini

soaking liquid, bring to boil, and cook, stirring occasionally, until liquid is thickened slightly and reduced to ½ cup, about 5 minutes. Stir mushroom mixture and dill into barley-lentil mixture and season with salt and pepper to taste. Serve, drizzling individual portions with tahini-yogurt sauce.

MAKE AHEAD · Cooked barley and lentils can be refrigerated for up to 3 days.

Tahini-Yogurt Sauce

makes 1 cup · total time: 5 minutes, plus 30 minutes resting

- ⅓ cup tahini
- ⅓ cup plain dairy yogurt or plant-based yogurt
- ¼ cup water
- 3 tablespoons lemon juice
- 1 garlic clove, minced
- ¾ teaspoon table salt

Whisk all ingredients together in bowl and season with salt and pepper to taste. Let sit until flavors meld, about 30 minutes. (Sauce can be refrigerated for up to 3 days.)

Farro and Broccoli Rabe Gratin

serves 4 to 6 · total time: 50 minutes

why this recipe works · Setting out to create a fresh, modern gratin, we chose Italian flavors, accenting nutty farro with creamy white beans and slightly bitter broccoli rabe. Toasting the farro first gave it extra nuttiness and jump-started the cooking process, resulting in more evenly cooked grains. Small white beans blended nicely with the farro while adding creaminess and protein. Blanching the broccoli rabe in salted water tamed its bitterness. We then tossed it with olive oil infused with garlic and red pepper flakes for extra flavor. The addition of sun-dried tomatoes gave us the extra pop of umami we were after, with their sweetness providing a counterpoint to the assertive broccoli rabe. Cheese is typically used to bind a gratin filling into a cohesive whole, but we found that miso paste created a supercreamy sauce when mixed with cooked grains, adding a subtle backbone of flavor. Finally, a combo of panko bread crumbs and Parmesan was transformed into a burnished, crunchy topping after a quick spell under the broiler. We prefer the flavor and texture of whole farro in this recipe. Do not substitute pearled, quick-cooking, or presteamed farro (read the package label to determine this) for the whole farro in this recipe.

   3   tablespoons extra-virgin olive oil, divided
   1   onion, chopped fine
   ¼   teaspoon table salt, plus salt for cooking vegetables
1½   cups whole farro, rinsed
   2   cups unsalted vegetable broth
   2   tablespoons white miso
   ½   cup panko bread crumbs
   ¼   cup grated Parmesan cheese
   1   pound broccoli rabe, trimmed and cut into 2-inch pieces
   6   garlic cloves, minced
   ⅛   teaspoon red pepper flakes
   1   (15-ounce) can no-salt-added small white beans or navy beans, rinsed
   ¾   cup oil-packed sun-dried tomatoes, chopped

1   Heat 1 tablespoon oil in large saucepan over medium heat until shimmering. Add onion and salt and cook until softened and lightly browned, 5 to 7 minutes. Stir in farro and cook until lightly toasted, about 2 minutes. Stir in 2½ cups water, broth, and miso. Bring to simmer and cook, stirring often, until farro is just tender and remaining liquid is thickened and creamy, 25 to 35 minutes.

2   Meanwhile, toss panko with 1 tablespoon oil in bowl and microwave, stirring occasionally, until golden brown, 1 to 2 minutes. Stir in Parmesan and set aside.

3   Bring 4 quarts water to boil in Dutch oven. Add broccoli rabe and 1 tablespoon salt and cook until just tender, about 2 minutes. Drain broccoli rabe and set aside. Combine remaining 1 tablespoon oil, garlic, and pepper flakes in now-empty pot and cook over medium heat until fragrant and sizzling, 1 to 2 minutes. Stir in broccoli rabe and cook until well coated, about 2 minutes. Off heat, stir in beans, sun-dried tomatoes, and farro. Season with salt and pepper to taste.

4   Adjust oven rack 10 inches from broiler element and heat broiler. Transfer bean-farro mixture to broiler-safe 3-quart gratin dish (or broiler-safe 13 by 9-inch baking dish) and sprinkle with panko mixture. Broil until lightly browned and hot, 1 to 2 minutes. Serve.

MAKE IT DAIRY-FREE • Substitute plant-based Parmesan cheese for the Parmesan cheese or omit.

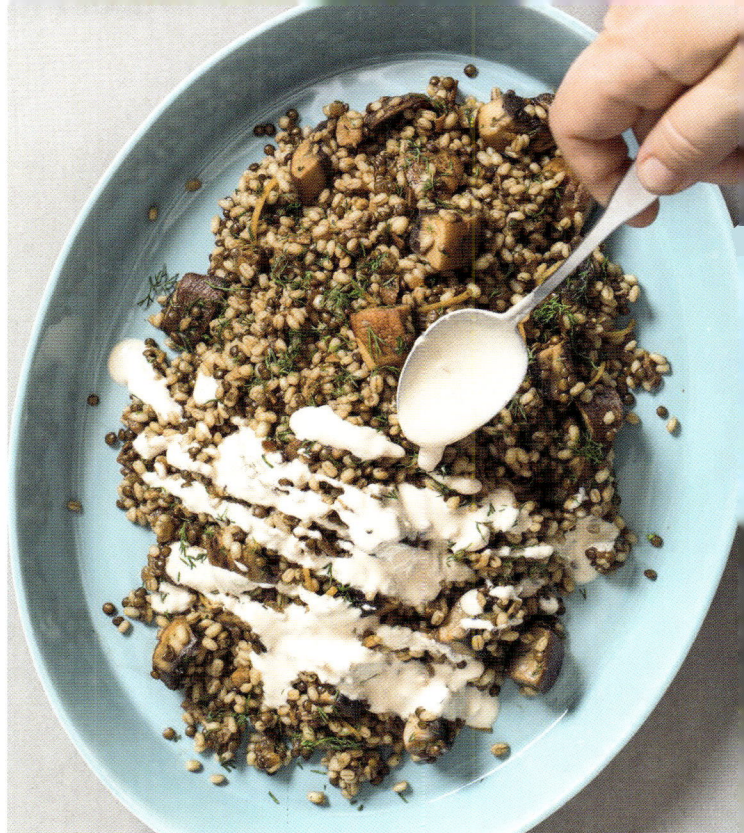

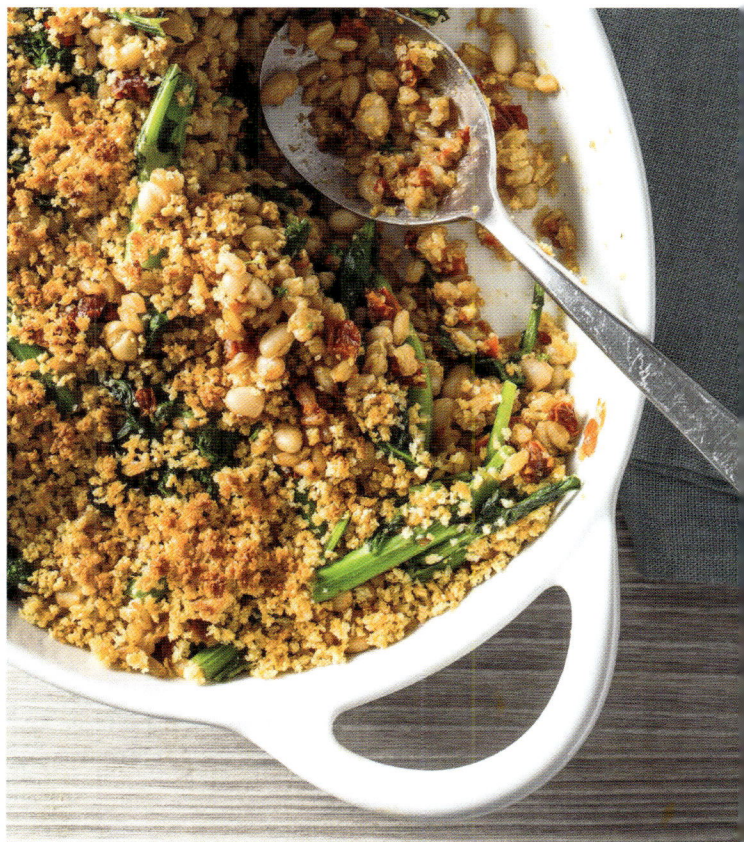

top | *Barley with Lentils, Mushrooms, and Tahini-Yogurt Sauce*
bottom | *Farro and Broccoli Rabe Gratin*

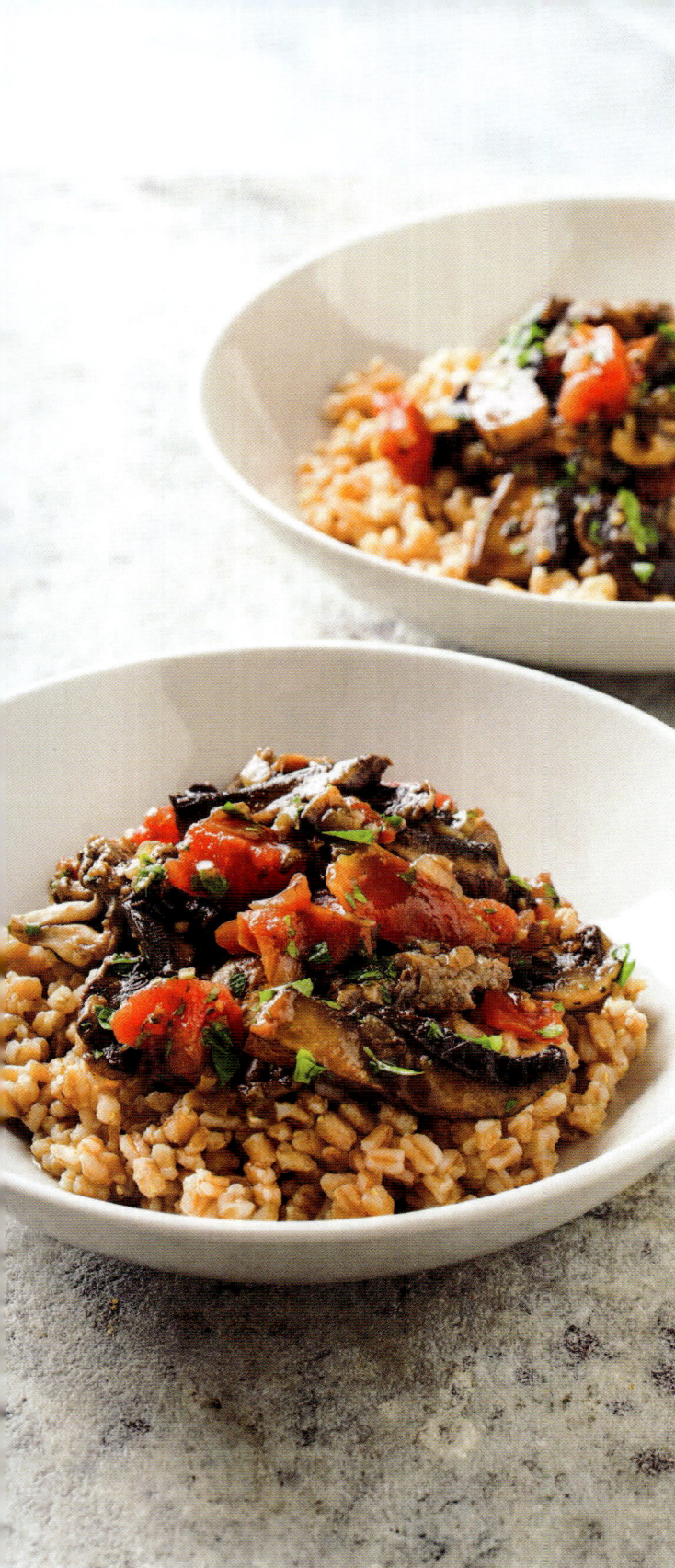

Wild Mushroom Ragout with Farro

serves 4 • total time: 45 minutes **FAST**

why this recipe works • We love whole-grain farro for its slightly sweet, nutty flavor and chewy texture. Since the ingredient is popular in Italy, we decided to pair it with a mushroom ragout. Chunks of portobellos and other assorted mushrooms added texture, while dried porcini contributed flavor and depth. For the best flavor, we prefer to use a combination of white, shiitake, and oyster mushrooms; however, you can choose just one or two varieties if you like. The woody stems of shiitakes are unpleasant to eat, so be sure to remove them. Drizzle individual portions with good balsamic vinegar before serving, if desired. We prefer the flavor and texture of whole farro in this recipe: Do not use pearl, quick-cooking, or presteamed farro (read the package label to determine this) for the whole farro in this recipe.

3½ cups unsalted vegetable broth

1½ cups whole farro, rinsed

1 pound portobello mushroom caps, halved and sliced ½-inch-thick crosswise

18 ounces assorted mushrooms, trimmed and halved if small or quartered if large

2 tablespoons extra-virgin olive oil

1 onion, chopped fine

½ ounce dried porcini mushrooms, rinsed and minced

¾ teaspoon table salt

3 garlic cloves, minced

1 teaspoon minced fresh thyme or ¼ teaspoon dried

¼ cup dry Madeira

1 (14.5-ounce) can no-salt-added diced tomatoes, drained and chopped

2 tablespoons minced fresh parsley

1 Combine broth and farro in large saucepan and bring to simmer over medium heat. Cook until farro is tender and creamy, 20 to 25 minutes. Season with salt and pepper to taste; cover and keep warm.

2 Meanwhile, microwave portobello and assorted mushrooms in covered bowl until tender, 6 to 8 minutes. Drain, reserving mushroom liquid.

3 Heat oil in Dutch oven over medium-high heat until shimmering. Add onion, porcini, and salt and cook until softened and lightly browned, 5 to 7 minutes. Stir in drained mushrooms and cook, stirring often, until mushrooms are dry and lightly browned, about 5 minutes.

4 Stir in garlic and thyme and cook until fragrant, about 30 seconds. Stir in Madeira and reserved mushroom liquid, scraping up any browned bits. Stir in tomatoes and simmer gently until sauce is slightly thickened, about 8 minutes. Off heat, stir in parsley and season with salt and pepper to taste. Portion farro into individual serving bowls and top with mushroom mixture. Serve.

> **MAKE AHEAD** • Farro can be prepared through step 1 and refrigerated for up to 3 days. Rewarm and thin with warm water before serving.

Teff-Stuffed Acorn Squash with Lime Crema and Roasted Pepitas

serves 4 • total time: 1 hour

why this recipe works • Teff is a gluten-free whole grain indigenous to Ethiopia and Eritrea that has a mildly nutty, earthy flavor. It is packed with nutrients and ranges in color from dark brown to red to white. Although the tiny grains of teff are typically ground into flour to make the flatbread known as injera in Ethiopia, we wanted to embrace teff as a whole grain by cooking it pilaf-style to make a base for a savory stuffing to spoon into roasted acorn squash. We chose brown teff, which tends to be the most readily available in U.S. supermarkets. To showcase the grain's versatility, we put a Southwestern spin on our stuffing by incorporating the warm and bright flavors of chopped green chiles, chipotle chile powder, cumin, coriander, and oregano. After spooning the stuffing into the squash, we topped it off with lime crema and toasted pepitas.

Lime Crema
- ½ cup sour cream
- 2 teaspoons grated lime zest plus 3 tablespoons juice (2 limes)
- ¼ teaspoon table salt

Teff-Stuffed Acorn Squash
- 1 tablespoon extra-virgin olive oil
- 1 tablespoon chipotle chile powder
- 1 teaspoon table salt, divided
- ½ teaspoon ground cumin
- ½ teaspoon ground coriander
- ½ teaspoon pepper
- ¼ teaspoon dried oregano
- 2 acorn squashes (1½ pounds each), quartered lengthwise and seeded

- 2 cups unsalted vegetable broth
- 1 cup teff
- 2 (4-ounce) cans chopped green chiles, drained
- ½ cup minced fresh cilantro
- ¼ cup roasted pepitas

1 **For the lime crema** Whisk all ingredients together in bowl; set aside until ready to serve.

2 **For the teff-stuffed acorn squash** Adjust oven rack to middle position and heat oven to 400 degrees. Line rimmed baking sheet with aluminum foil. Combine oil, chipotle chile powder, ¾ teaspoon salt, cumin, coriander, pepper, and oregano in bowl. Brush flesh side of squash evenly with spice mixture. Place wedges cut side down on prepared sheet and roast until browned on first side, about 20 minutes.

3 Flip wedges so second cut sides are in contact with sheet and roast until second sides are browned and tip of paring knife slips easily into flesh, about 15 minutes.

4 Meanwhile, bring broth to boil in medium saucepan. Stir in teff and remaining ¼ teaspoon salt, reduce heat to medium-low, cover, and simmer until broth is absorbed, 15 to 20 minutes. Remove from heat and let sit, covered, for 10 minutes. Fluff grains with fork and set aside.

5 Using spoon, scoop flesh from each squash wedge, leaving about ¼-inch thickness of flesh in each shell. Chop squash flesh into rough ½-inch pieces and transfer to large bowl. Gently fold reserved teff, green chiles, and cilantro into squash in bowl, then gently mound teff-squash mixture evenly in squash shells. Drizzle reserved lime crema over top and sprinkle with pepitas. Serve.

> **MAKE AHEAD** • Lime crema can be refrigerated for up to 3 days.

> **MAKE IT DAIRY-FREE** • Substitute plant-based sour cream for the dairy sour cream.

Joloff-Inspired Fonio

serves **4 to 6** · total time: **40 minutes** **FAST**

why this recipe works · The foundational ingredients of joloff rice, a beloved West African specialty, are rice, tomatoes, onions, and spices, though many variations are prevalent throughout the region. We wanted to apply joloff's signature bright, savory flavors to fonio, an ancient variety of millet that also hails from West Africa. We began by blitzing canned tomatoes and an assortment of aromatics in a blender to create a smooth, flavorful cooking liquid for the fonio. As the grains simmered, the fonio took on a rouge color, characteristic of joloff rice, and drank up the tomatoes' savory brightness. We enriched this concoction with a bit of olive oil and topped it with sweet, soft caramelized onions and fresh parsley. Hearty, comforting, and deeply flavorful, this dish works equally well as a substantial side or a meal on its own.

- 3 cups unsalted vegetable broth, divided
- 1 (14.5-ounce) can no-salt-added whole peeled tomatoes
- 1 red onion (½ onion quartered, ½ onion sliced thin)
- 4 garlic cloves, peeled
- 1 teaspoon packed brown sugar
- 1 teaspoon table salt
- ½ teaspoon red pepper flakes
- 6 tablespoons extra-virgin olive oil, divided
- 1 cup fonio
- 2 bay leaves
- 2 tablespoons chopped fresh parsley

1 Process 1 cup broth, tomatoes and their juice, quartered onion, garlic, sugar, salt, and pepper flakes in blender on high speed until smooth, 1 to 2 minutes. Heat 2 tablespoons oil in 12-inch nonstick skillet over medium heat until shimmering. Add tomato mixture and cook, stirring occasionally, until slightly thickened, 5 to 7 minutes.

2 Add fonio, bay leaves, and remaining 2 cups broth and stir well. Cook, stirring occasionally, until most of liquid has been absorbed, 3 to 4 minutes. Stir in 2 tablespoons oil, remove from heat, and cover. Let stand until all liquid has been absorbed, 10 to 15 minutes.

3 While fonio stands, heat remaining 2 tablespoons oil in 10-inch nonstick skillet over medium heat until shimmering. Add sliced onion and cook, stirring occasionally, until it begins to brown at edges, 2 to 3 minutes. Reduce heat to low and continue to cook, stirring occasionally, until onion is soft and deeply brown, 15 to 20 minutes.

4 Transfer fonio to serving dish, discard bay leaves, and top with caramelized onions and parsley. Serve.

Curried Fonio with Roasted Vegetables and Hibiscus Vinaigrette

serves **4** · total time: **1 hour** **SUPERCHARGED**

why this recipe works · Tiny but mighty, fonio is a perfect grain for pilaf: The gluten-free and nutrient-rich West African relative of millet not only cooks up quickly, but it is also light and fluffy and absorbs flavors well. To create a punchy and flavorful foundation for a fonio pilaf meal, we used curry powder along with fresh garlic and ginger. Sweet butternut squash, red onion, and grassy okra roasted at the same time in the oven, but on separate baking sheets so that we could first cover the okra to steam before uncovering it to turn crispy and brown in the oven's heat. We added extra crunch and richness by stirring in chopped roasted cashews to finish and then drizzled everything with a sweet-tart vinaigrette made with dried hibiscus flowers. The bright fuchsia flowers—from a plant related to okra and native to Africa—added a unique cranberry-like flavor and color that pulled this striking plate together. It's best to use whole dried hibiscus flowers, not ones that have been cut and sifted. If you can find only cut and sifted hibiscus, use the weight listed (¼ ounce), not the volume. For an accurate measurement of boiling water, bring a kettle of water to a boil and then measure out the desired amount. If you're looking for another way to use hibiscus flowers, try our recipe for Hibiscus Iced Tea on page 387.

Hibiscus Vinaigrette
- ¼ ounce (¼ cup) whole dried hibiscus flowers
- ¼ cup boiling water
- ¼ cup extra-virgin olive oil
- 1 tablespoon red wine vinegar
- 1 tablespoon sugar
- ½ teaspoon Dijon mustard
- ½ teaspoon table salt
- ¼ teaspoon pepper
- 1½ teaspoons minced shallot

Fonio and Vegetables
- 1 pound butternut squash, peeled, seeded, and cut into ¾-inch pieces
- 1 red onion, cut through root end into 1-inch wedges
- 2 tablespoons plus 2 teaspoons extra-virgin olive oil, divided
- 1 teaspoon table salt, divided
- ¼ teaspoon pepper, divided
- 12 ounces okra, trimmed and halved lengthwise
- 2 garlic cloves, minced
- 1½ teaspoons curry powder

1 teaspoon grated fresh ginger
2 cups water
1 cup fonio
⅓ cup roasted cashews, chopped
¼ cup chopped fresh parsley

1 For the hibiscus vinaigrette Combine hibiscus flowers and boiling water in blender jar and let sit for 10 minutes. Add oil, vinegar, sugar, mustard, salt, and pepper and process until only small pieces of flowers remain, about 1 minute. Transfer to small bowl and stir in shallot.

2 For the fonio and vegetables Adjust oven racks to upper-middle and lower-middle positions and heat oven to 425 degrees. Line 2 rimmed baking sheets with aluminum foil. Toss squash and onion with 1 tablespoon oil, ½ teaspoon salt, and ⅛ teaspoon pepper in bowl, then arrange in even layer on one prepared sheet. Toss okra with 2 teaspoons oil, ¼ teaspoon salt, and remaining ⅛ teaspoon pepper in now-empty bowl, then arrange cut side down on second prepared sheet. Cover sheet with okra tightly with foil.

3 Place sheet with squash and onions on lower rack and sheet with okra on upper rack. Roast for 15 minutes, then remove foil from sheet with okra. Continue to roast vegetables until squash and onions are tender and browned and cut sides of okra are well browned, 7 to 12 minutes.

4 Meanwhile, heat remaining 1 tablespoon oil in medium saucepan over medium heat until shimmering. Add garlic, curry powder, and ginger and cook until fragrant, about 30 seconds. Stir in water, fonio, and remaining ¼ teaspoon salt and bring to simmer. Cover, reduce heat to low, and simmer until liquid is absorbed, about 3 minutes. Off heat, let fonio sit, covered, for 10 minutes, then gently fluff with fork, breaking up any large clumps. Stir in cashews.

5 Divide fonio among individual serving bowls. Top with roasted vegetables and drizzle with vinaigrette. Sprinkle with parsley and serve.

MAKE AHEAD · Hibiscus vinaigrette can be refrigerated for up to 5 days.

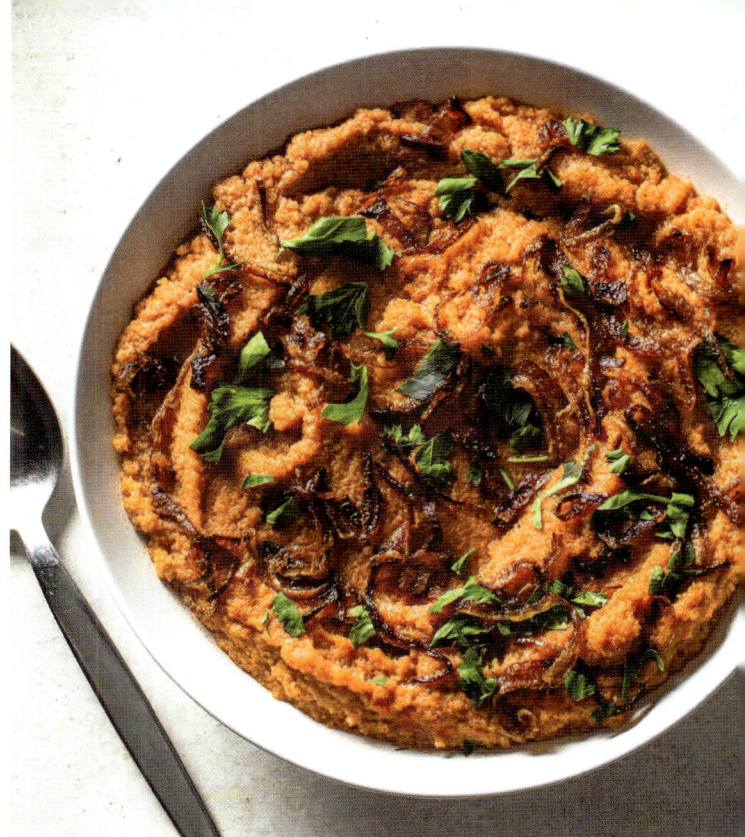

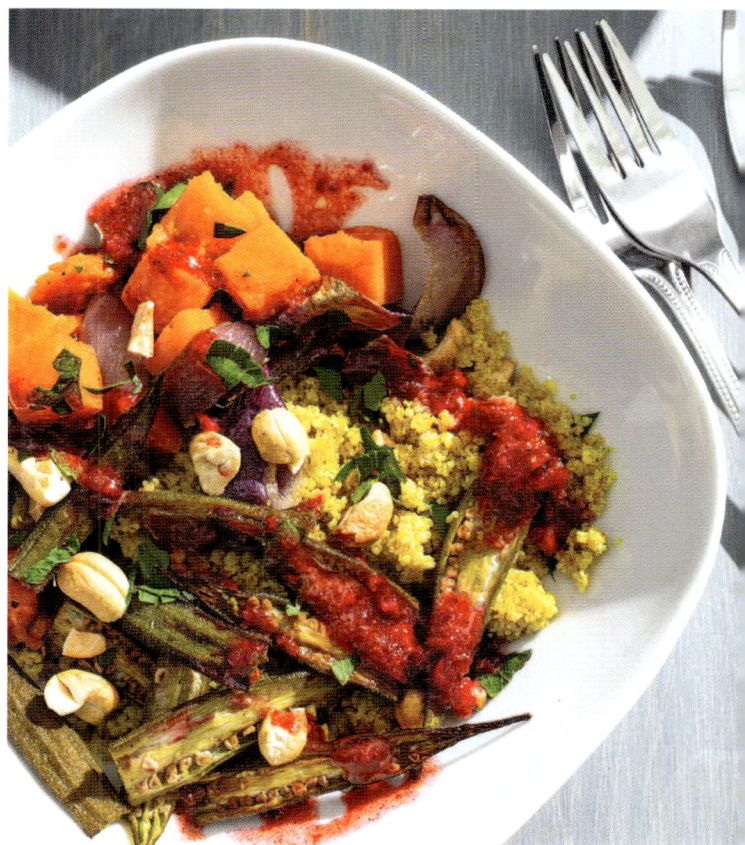

top | Joloff-Inspired Fonio
bottom | Curried Fonio with Roasted Vegetables and Hibiscus Vinaigrette

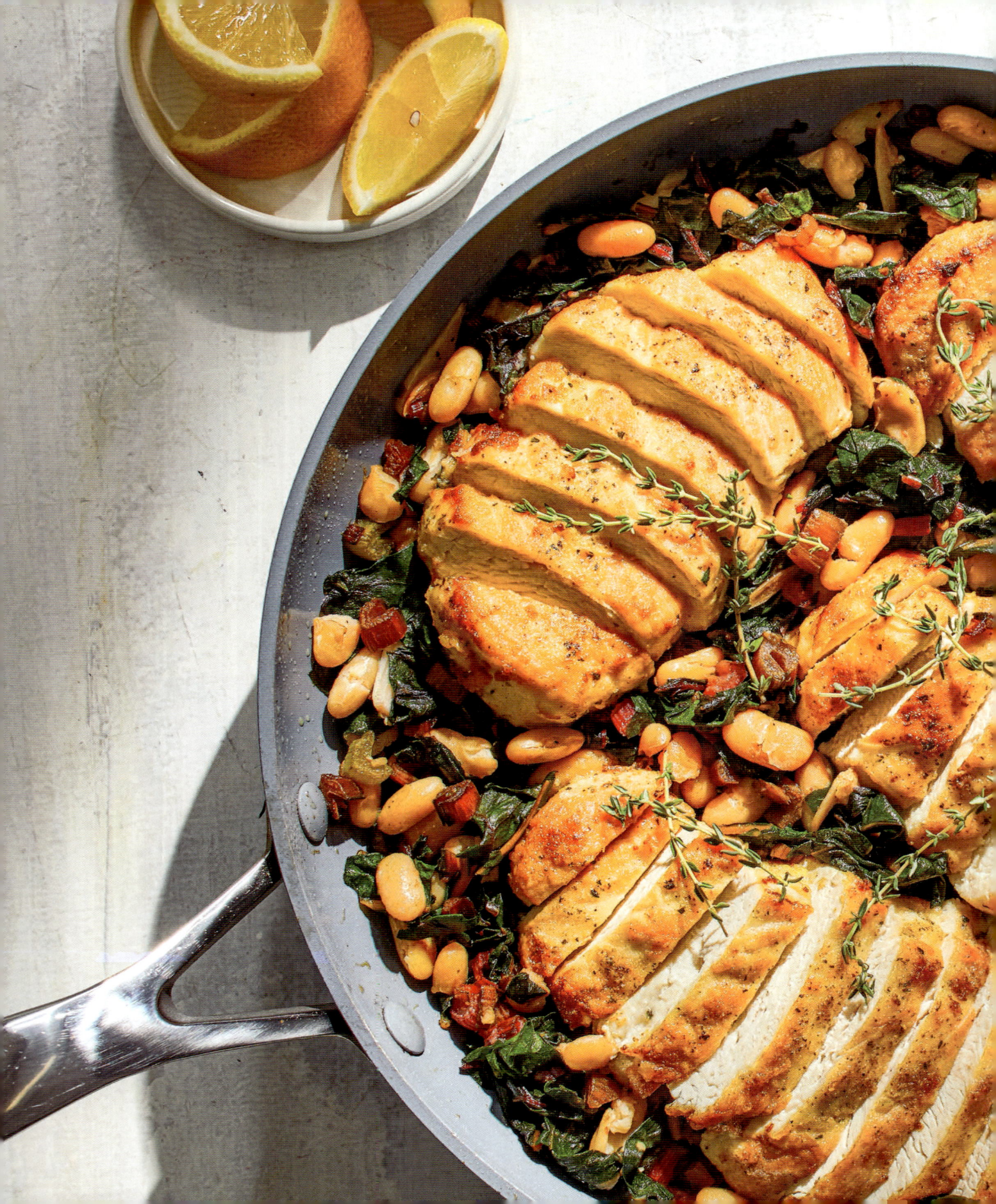

POULTRY

■ FAST　　■ SUPERCHARGED

Perfect Poached Chicken with Warm Tomato-Ginger Vinaigrette

serves 4 • total time: 55 minutes

why this recipe works • As a source of lean protein, boneless chicken breasts can't be beat for their endless versatility and quick prep. But they easily overcook. Poaching might be the most foolproof way to ensure juicy, tender meat, and this approach guarantees succulent chicken while boosting flavor. We arranged the breasts in a steamer basket and submerged the basket in our poaching liquid—a flavorful mix of soy sauce, garlic, and water. We heated the liquid to 175 degrees and then shut off the heat, covered the pot, and let the chicken cook gently in the residual heat to a perfect 160 degrees. A warm vinaigrette of ginger, shallot, and cherry tomatoes brought bold flavor and antioxidants. This is poached chicken reimagined—bright, aromatic, and anything but dry or stringy. Don't balk at the amount of soy sauce used: Most of it is drained away after poaching the chicken, so the amount of sodium you'll actually consume is minimal.

Chicken

- 4 (6- to 8-ounce) boneless, skinless chicken breasts, trimmed
- ½ cup low-sodium soy sauce
- 6 garlic cloves, smashed and peeled

Vinaigrette

- 2 tablespoons extra-virgin olive oil, divided
- 1 small shallot, minced
- 1 teaspoon grated fresh ginger
  Pinch ground cumin
  Pinch ground fennel
- 6 ounces cherry tomatoes, halved
- ⅛ teaspoon table salt
- 1 tablespoon chopped fresh cilantro
- 1½ teaspoons red wine vinegar

1 For the chicken Gently pound thicker end of each breast until ½ inch thick. Whisk 4 quarts water, soy sauce, and garlic together in Dutch oven. Arrange breasts, skinned side up, in steamer basket, making sure not to overlap them, then submerge steamer basket in water.

2 Heat pot over medium heat, stirring liquid occasionally to even out hot spots, until water registers 175 degrees, 15 to 20 minutes. Turn off heat, cover pot, and remove from burner; let sit until chicken registers 160 degrees, 17 to 22 minutes. Transfer breasts to plate, tent with aluminum foil, and discard poaching liquid. Let chicken rest while preparing vinaigrette.

3 For the vinaigrette Heat 1 tablespoon oil in 10-inch nonstick skillet over medium heat until shimmering. Add shallot, ginger, cumin, and fennel and cook until fragrant, about 15 seconds. Stir in tomatoes and salt and cook, stirring frequently, until tomatoes have softened, 3 to 5 minutes. Off heat, stir in remaining 1 tablespoon oil, cilantro, and vinegar. Season with pepper to taste. Spoon vinaigrette evenly over each breast before serving.

> **MAKE AHEAD** • Cooked chicken can be refrigerated for up to 3 days.

> **MAKE IT GLUTEN-FREE** • Substitute low-sodium tamari for the low-sodium soy sauce.

Cold-Start Pan-Seared Chicken Breasts with Sun-Dried Tomato Relish

serves 4 • total time: 35 minutes **FAST**

why this recipe works • Our tried-and-true cold-start cooking method ensures that boneless, skinless chicken breasts cook up golden-brown on the outside and juicy on the inside. (You'll find this method used in a number of recipes in this chapter.) Gently flattening the thick part of the breast with a meat pounder encourages even cooking, while lightly brushing oil on both sides of the breast allows for even browning without splattering. We put the oiled chicken in an unheated dry skillet, set it over high heat, and flip the breasts regularly (dropping the heat partway through to ensure more even cooking). Flipping frequently means that the meat cooks gently: The exterior slowly develops a deep, brown crust while the interior remains juicy. Removing the chicken from the pan when it reaches 155 degrees and letting it rest for 10 minutes to climb to a 165-degree serving temperature allows time for whipping up a tasty relish in the pan. For the best results, buy similar-size chicken breasts weighing up to 8 ounces each. The relish is meant to be started after you have seared chicken in a skillet. Do not wash the skillet after searing—any remaining browned bits add important flavor to the sauce.

Chicken

- 4 (6- to 8-ounce) boneless, skinless chicken breasts, trimmed
- 2 tablespoons extra-virgin olive oil
- ½ teaspoon table salt

Sun-Dried Tomato Relish

- ½ cup unsalted chicken broth
  Pinch red pepper flakes
- ¼ cup oil-packed sun-dried tomatoes, rinsed, patted dry, and minced
- 2 tablespoons extra-virgin olive oil
- 1 tablespoon capers, rinsed and minced
- 1 teaspoon lemon juice
- 2 tablespoons minced fresh parsley
- 1 tablespoon minced fresh mint

1 For the chicken Gently pound thicker end of each breast until ½ inch thick. Pat breasts dry with paper towels. Brush both sides of breasts with oil and sprinkle with salt. Place breasts, skinned side down, in cold 12-inch nonstick skillet, arranging narrow parts of breasts opposite wider parts. Place skillet over high heat and cook for 2 minutes. Flip breasts and cook for 2 minutes (there should be light browning).

2 Flip breasts, reduce heat to medium, and continue to cook, flipping breasts every 2 minutes, until exterior is well browned and thickest part of breast registers 155 degrees, 6 to 8 minutes longer. Transfer breasts, skinned side up, to platter. Tent with aluminum foil and let rest while making relish.

3 For the relish Pour off any fat from skillet and add broth and pepper flakes, scraping up any browned bits. Cook over medium heat until liquid is reduced to 2 tablespoons, about 5 minutes. Stir in tomatoes, oil, capers, and lemon juice and bring to simmer. Off heat, stir in parsley, mint, and any accumulated chicken juices from platter. Season with pepper to taste. Spoon relish evenly over each breast before serving.

> **MAKE AHEAD** • Relish can be refrigerated for up to 2 days and cooked chicken can be refrigerated for up to 3 days.

VARIATION

Cold-Start Pan-Seared Chicken Breasts with Chimichurri

Omit sun-dried tomato relish. Combine 2 tablespoons hot water, 1 teaspoon dried oregano, and ¼ teaspoon table salt in small bowl; let sit for 5 minutes to soften oregano. Pulse ½ cup fresh parsley leaves, ¼ cup fresh cilantro leaves, 3 minced garlic cloves, and ¼ teaspoon red pepper flakes in food processor until coarsely chopped, about 10 pulses. Add oregano mixture and 2 tablespoons red wine vinegar and pulse briefly to combine. Transfer mixture to medium bowl and slowly whisk in ¼ cup extra-virgin olive oil until incorporated. Cover and let sit at room temperature for at least 1 hour to allow flavors to meld. Season with pepper to taste.

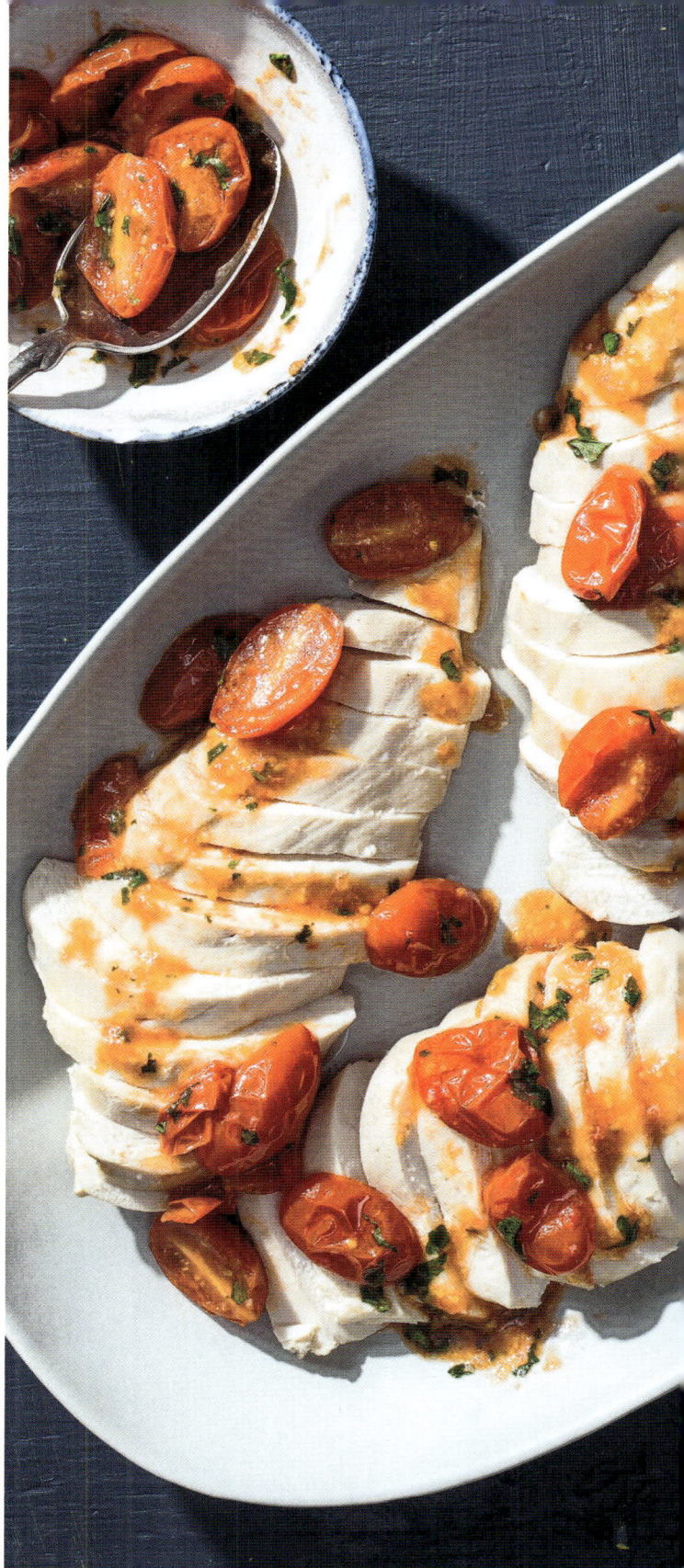

Perfect Poached Chicken with Warm Tomato-Ginger Vinaigrette

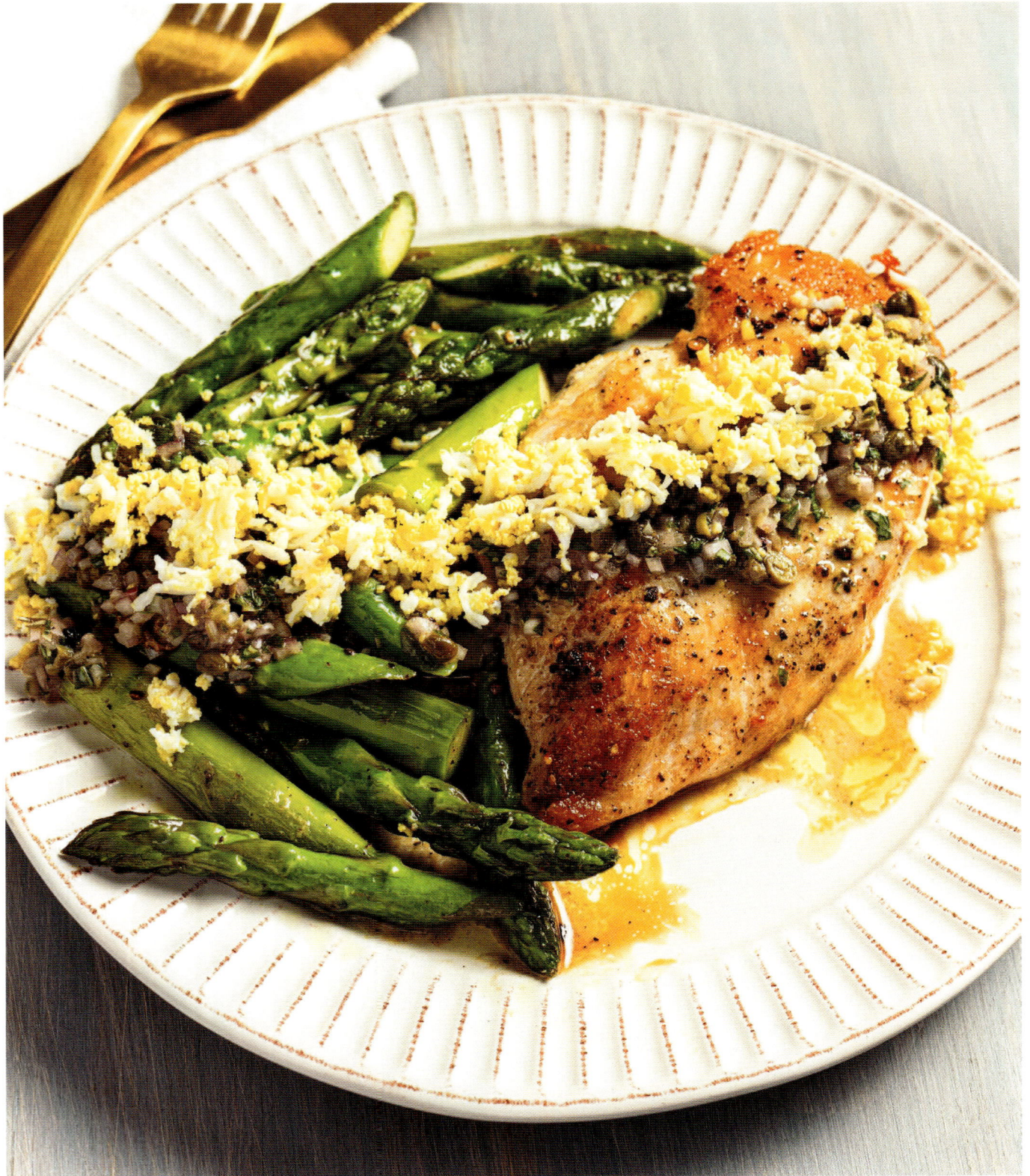

Chicken Breasts and Asparagus Mimosa

Chicken Breasts and Asparagus Mimosa

serves 4 · total time: 40 minutes   **FAST**

why this recipe works · Classic French asparagus mimosa is a dish that celebrates contrast and balance—tender asparagus, a source of gut-nourishing prebiotics, paired with a sharp, mustardy vinaigrette and finished with finely grated hard-boiled eggs for richness and texture. It's traditionally served as a light starter; we turned this elegant dish into a satisfying meal by incorporating lean protein in the form of seared chicken breasts. We cooked everything in one skillet for an easy, nutrient-dense weeknight dinner. The vinaigrette—punched up with red wine vinegar, briny capers, and fresh tarragon—added contrast and elevated the simplicity of the ingredients. Finely grated hard-boiled eggs are the traditional garnish for this take on a classic French dish, but they can be omitted, if desired.

- 2 tablespoons red wine vinegar
- 1 tablespoon capers, rinsed and chopped
- 1 tablespoon minced shallot
- 1 tablespoon minced fresh tarragon
- 2 teaspoons Dijon mustard
- 1¼ teaspoons table salt, divided
- ¾ teaspoon pepper, divided
- 5 tablespoons extra-virgin olive oil, divided
- 4 (6- to 8-ounce) boneless, skinless chicken breasts, trimmed
- 1½ pounds asparagus, trimmed and cut on bias into 2-inch lengths
- 2 large Easy Peel Hard-Cooked Eggs (page 31), peeled (optional)

1 Whisk vinegar, capers, shallot, tarragon, mustard, ½ teaspoon salt, and ½ teaspoon pepper together in bowl. Slowly whisk in 2 tablespoons oil until incorporated.

2 Gently pound thicker end of each breast until ½ inch thick. Pat breasts dry with paper towels. Brush both sides of breasts with 2 tablespoons oil and sprinkle with ½ teaspoon salt. Place breasts, skinned side down, in cold 12-inch nonstick skillet, arranging narrow parts of breasts opposite wider parts. Place skillet over high heat and cook for 2 minutes. Flip breasts and cook for 2 minutes (there should be light browning).

3 Flip breasts, reduce heat to medium, and continue to cook, flipping breasts every 2 minutes, until exterior is well browned and thickest part of breast registers 155 degrees, 6 to 8 minutes longer. Transfer breasts, skinned side up, to platter. Tent with aluminum foil and let rest while cooking asparagus.

4 Add asparagus, remaining 1 tablespoon oil, remaining ¼ teaspoon salt, and remaining ¼ teaspoon pepper to now-empty skillet and cook until crisp-tender, 5 to 7 minutes. Transfer asparagus to platter with chicken. Drizzle vinaigrette over chicken and asparagus. Grate eggs on small holes of box grater over chicken and asparagus. Serve.

MAKE AHEAD · Cooked chicken can be refrigerated for up to 3 days.

Seared Chicken Breasts with Chickpea Salad

serves 4 · total time: 35 minutes   **FAST**

why this recipe works · This simple yet nourishing meal combines well-browned chicken breasts with a chickpea salad for a well-rounded, inflammation-fighting dinner. Chickpeas bring fiber and plant-based protein to support gut health and keep blood sugar stable. Using a cold-start searing method, we started cooking the breasts in a cold nonstick skillet and flipped them periodically for good browning and a moist interior. For a punchy vinaigrette to toss with the salad and drizzle over the meat, we combined olive oil and a squeeze of lemon for heart-healthy fats and vitamin C, adding zingy paprika and cumin for antioxidants and some honey for subtle sweetness. Either smoked sweet or smoked hot paprika can be used in this recipe.

- 4 (6- to 8-ounce) boneless, skinless chicken breasts, trimmed
- ¼ cup plus 2 tablespoons extra-virgin olive oil, divided
- 1 teaspoon table salt, divided
- ½ teaspoon plus ⅛ teaspoon pepper, divided
- ¼ cup lemon juice (2 lemons)
- 1 teaspoon honey
- 1 teaspoon smoked paprika
- ½ teaspoon ground cumin
- 2 (15-ounce) cans no-salt-added chickpeas, rinsed
- ½ red onion, sliced thin
- ¼ cup chopped fresh mint

1 Gently pound thicker end of each breast until ½ inch thick. Pat breasts dry with paper towels. Brush both sides of breasts with 2 tablespoons oil and sprinkle with ½ teaspoon salt and ⅛ teaspoon pepper. Place breasts, skinned side down, in 12-inch nonstick skillet, arranging narrow parts of breasts opposite wider parts. Place skillet over high heat and cook for 2 minutes. Flip breasts and cook for 2 minutes (there should be light browning).

2 Flip breasts, reduce heat to medium, and continue to cook, flipping breasts every 2 minutes, until exterior is well browned and thickest part of breast registers 155 degrees, 6 to 8 minutes longer. Transfer breasts, skinned side up, to platter and tent with aluminum foil. Let rest for 10 minutes.

3 Meanwhile, whisk lemon juice, honey, paprika, cumin, remaining ¼ cup oil, remaining ½ teaspoon salt, and remaining ½ teaspoon pepper together in large bowl until combined. Reserve 3 tablespoons dressing in small bowl for serving. Add chickpeas, onion, and mint to remaining dressing and toss to combine. Season with salt and pepper to taste. Drizzle reserved dressing over chicken and serve with salad.

> **MAKE AHEAD** • Cooked chicken can be refrigerated for up to 3 days.

Sautéed Chicken with Cherry Tomatoes, Olives, and Feta

serves 4 • total time: 45 minutes `FAST`

why this recipe works • Quick sautéed chicken breasts are an excellent blank canvas for bright flavors. We lightly browned chicken breasts using our cold-start method, then prepared a warm relish that is part sauce/part side in the same pan to take advantage of all the flavorful brown bits. Halving and cooking cherry tomatoes released some of their liquid, while olives provided a salty contrast to the sweet tomatoes. To finish, feta cheese contributed a creaminess and tang, and shredded mint added color and freshness.

- 4 (6- to 8-ounce) boneless, skinless chicken breasts, trimmed
- 3 tablespoons extra-virgin olive oil, divided
- ¾ teaspoon table salt, divided
- ¼ teaspoon pepper
- 2 garlic cloves, minced
- 12 ounces cherry tomatoes, halved
- ⅓ cup pitted kalamata olives, chopped
- 2 tablespoons water
- 1 ounce feta cheese, crumbled (¼ cup)
- ¼ cup shredded fresh mint

1 Gently pound thicker end of each breast until ½ inch thick. Pat breasts dry with paper towels. Brush both sides of breasts with 2 tablespoons oil and sprinkle with ½ teaspoon salt and pepper. Place breasts, skinned side down, in 12-inch nonstick

skillet, arranging narrow parts of breasts opposite wider parts. Place skillet over high heat and cook for 2 minutes. Flip breasts and cook for 2 minutes (there should be light browning).

2 Flip breasts, reduce heat to medium, and continue to cook, flipping breasts every 2 minutes, until exterior is well browned and thickest part of breast registers 155 degrees, 6 to 8 minutes longer. Transfer breasts, skinned side up, to platter. Tent with aluminum foil and let rest while making relish.

3 Cook remaining 1 tablespoon oil and garlic in now-empty skillet over medium heat until fragrant, about 30 seconds. Stir in tomatoes, olives, water, and remaining ¼ teaspoon salt, scraping up any browned bits, and cook until tomatoes are just softened, about 2 minutes. Stir in any accumulated chicken juices from platter and season with salt and pepper to taste. Spoon relish over chicken, sprinkle with feta and mint, and serve.

> **MAKE AHEAD** • Cooked chicken can be refrigerated for up to 3 days.

> **MAKE IT DAIRY-FREE** • Substitute plant-based feta for the dairy feta or omit the cheese.

Chicken Baked in Foil with Fennel and Sun-Dried Tomatoes

serves 4 • total time: 1 hour, plus 1 hour chilling
`SUPERCHARGED`

why this recipe works • Baking food in foil packets (a technique known as en papillote) promises an easy one-dish meal—and bonus points awarded because the foil contains the mess for minimal cleanup. It is especially well-suited for lean proteins like chicken breasts that are prone to drying out. To ensure that our quick-cooking chicken breasts were seasoned throughout, we sprinkled them with salt before assembling the packets and refrigerated the packets for at least an hour. Leaving headroom at the top of the packets allowed maximum steam circulation for even cooking, and checking the temperature of the chicken through the foil let us monitor its progress. We layered sliced potatoes under the chicken to insulate the delicate meat from the hot pan and then arranged the rest of our vegetables around the meat and added a drizzle of seasoned extra-virgin olive oil before closing up the packets. Two convenient pantry products—olives and sun-dried tomatoes—lent the chicken bold flavor, as did a final boost of balsamic vinegar and fresh basil. Make sure to buy chicken breasts that are roughly the same size to ensure even cooking.

5 tablespoons extra-virgin olive oil

6 garlic cloves, sliced thin

1 teaspoon minced fresh thyme

¼ teaspoon red pepper flakes

12 ounces Yukon Gold potatoes, unpeeled, sliced crosswise ¼ inch thick

1 fennel bulb, stalks discarded, bulb halved, cored, and cut into ½-inch-thick wedges, layers separated

½ large red onion, sliced ½ inch thick, layers separated

¼ cup oil-packed sun-dried tomatoes, rinsed, patted dry, and chopped fine

¼ cup pitted kalamata olives, chopped fine

¾ teaspoon table salt, divided

4 (6- to 8-ounce) boneless, skinless chicken breasts, trimmed

¼ teaspoon pepper

2 tablespoons balsamic vinegar

2 tablespoons shredded fresh basil

1 Spray centers of four 20 by 12-inch sheets of aluminum foil with avocado oil spray. Combine oil, garlic, thyme, and pepper flakes in large bowl and microwave until garlic begins to brown, about 1 minute. Add potatoes, fennel, onion, tomatoes, olives, and ½ teaspoon salt to bowl with garlic oil and toss to combine.

2 Gently pound thicker end of each breast until ½ inch thick. Pat chicken dry with paper towels and sprinkle with remaining ¼ teaspoon salt and pepper. Position 1 piece of prepared foil with long side parallel to counter edge. In center of foil, arrange one-quarter of potato slices in 2 rows perpendicular to counter edge. Lay 1 chicken breast on top of potato slices. Place one-quarter of vegetables around chicken. Repeat with remaining prepared foil, remaining potato slices, remaining chicken, and remaining vegetables. Drizzle any remaining oil mixture from bowl over chicken.

3 Bring short sides of foil together and crimp to seal tightly. Crimp remaining open ends of packets, leaving as much head-room as possible inside packets. Refrigerate for at least 1 hour.

4 Adjust oven rack to lowest position and heat oven to 475 degrees. Place packets on rimmed baking sheet and bake until chicken registers 160 degrees, 18 to 23 minutes. (To check temperature, poke thermometer through foil of 1 packet and into chicken.) Let chicken rest in packets for 3 minutes.

5 Transfer chicken packets to individual serving plates, open carefully (steam will escape), and slide contents onto plates. Drizzle vinegar over chicken and vegetables, sprinkle with basil, and serve.

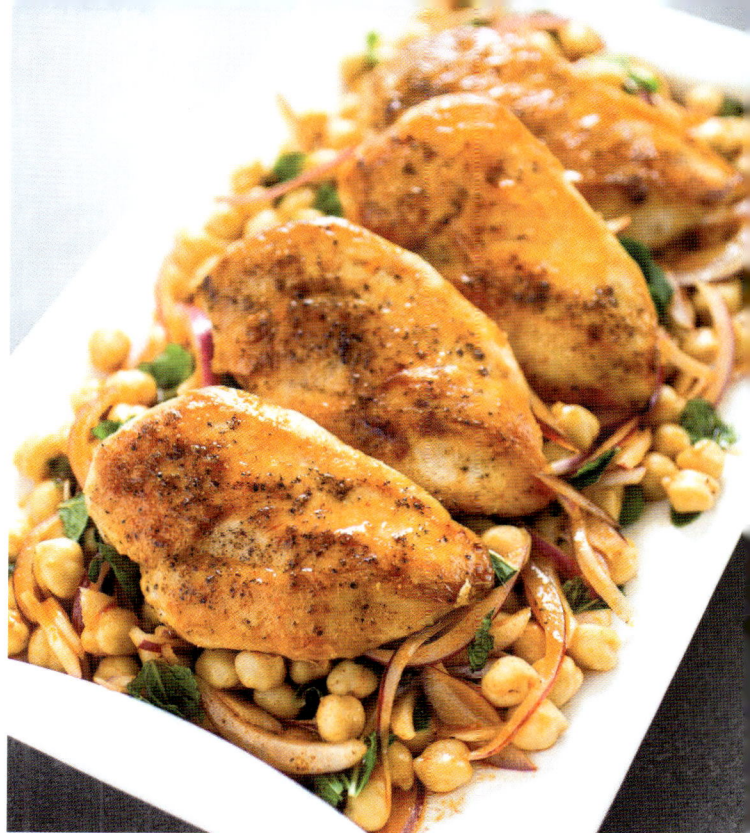

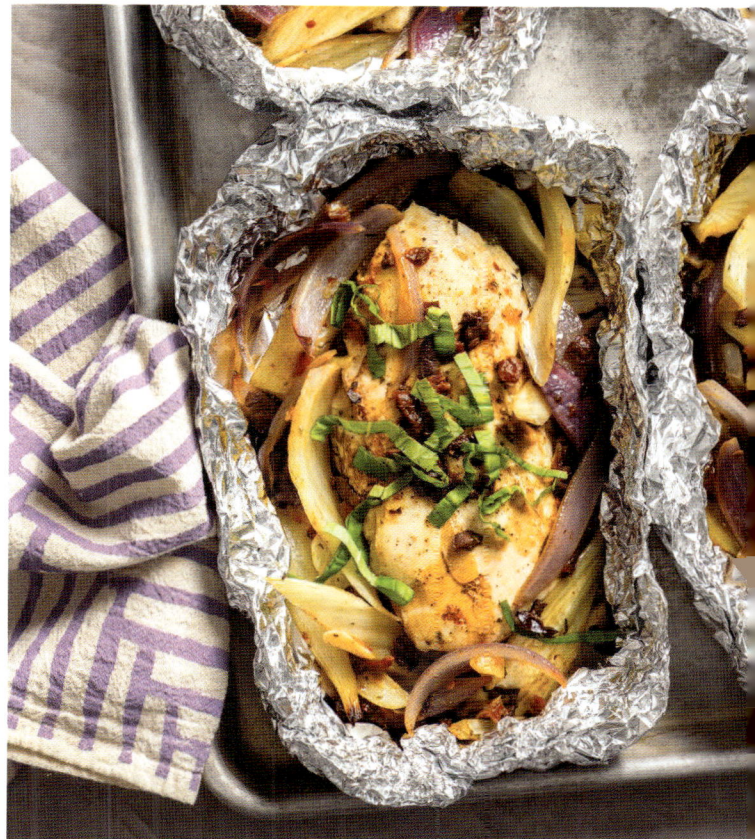

top | *Seared Chicken Breasts with Chickpea Salad*
bottom | *Chicken Baked in Foil with Fennel and Sun-Dried Tomatoes*

Chicken Baked in Foil with Potatoes and Carrots

Omit sun-dried tomatoes and olives. Substitute 2 carrots (peeled, quartered lengthwise and cut into 2-inch lengths) for fennel, lemon juice for balsamic vinegar, and chives for basil.

Chicken Baked in Foil with Sweet Potato and Radish

Omit olives. Substitute 1 tablespoon grated fresh ginger for thyme, 12 ounces sweet potato (peeled and sliced ¼ inch thick) for Yukon Gold potatoes, 4 radishes (trimmed and quartered) for fennel, 2 celery ribs (quartered lengthwise and cut into 2-inch lengths) for tomatoes, unseasoned rice vinegar for balsamic vinegar, and cilantro for basil.

MAKE AHEAD • Assembled packets, prepared through step 3, can be refrigerated for up to 24 hours.

Lemon-Thyme Chicken with Garlicky Greens and White Beans

serves 4 • total time: 45 minutes **FAST**

why this recipe works • Beans and greens are a classic pairing, offering both antioxidants and fiber. To take them up a notch, we served them with lemon-and-thyme-seasoned chicken breasts. Cooking our side dish in the skillet we first used to cook the chicken allowed the greens—Swiss chard—to soak up the fond left behind. Adding some anchovies to the pan brought umami and healthy fats. We gave our chard stems a head start on the leaves to ensure that they become tender and then added the leaves and a can of cannellini beans along with their liquid. The starchy bean liquid created a full-bodied sauce in the time it took the chard to wilt.

 2 teaspoons minced fresh thyme or ¾ teaspoon dried
 1 teaspoon grated lemon zest, plus lemon wedges for serving
 ¾ teaspoon table salt, divided
 ¼ teaspoon pepper, divided
 4 (6- to 8-ounce) boneless, skinless chicken breasts, trimmed
 ¼ cup extra-virgin olive oil, divided
 4 anchovy fillets, rinsed, patted dry, and minced
 1 pound Swiss chard, stems chopped, leaves cut into 1-inch pieces
 4 garlic cloves, sliced thin
 ¼ teaspoon red pepper flakes
 1 (15-ounce) can no-salt-added cannellini or Great Northern beans, undrained

1 Combine thyme, lemon zest, ½ teaspoon salt, and ⅛ teaspoon pepper in bowl. Gently pound thicker end of each breast until ½ inch thick. Pat breasts dry with paper towels. Brush both sides of breasts with 2 tablespoons oil and sprinkle with thyme mixture. Place breasts, skinned side down, in cold 12-inch nonstick skillet, arranging narrow parts of breasts opposite wider parts. Place skillet over high heat and cook for 2 minutes. Flip breasts and cook for 2 minutes (there should be light browning).

2 Flip breasts, reduce heat to medium, and continue to cook, flipping breasts every 2 minutes, until exterior is well browned and thickest part of breast registers 155 degrees, 6 to 8 minutes longer. Transfer breasts, skinned side up, to platter and tent with aluminum foil. Let rest while cooking greens.

3 Cook anchovies and remaining 2 tablespoons oil in now-empty skillet over medium heat until fragrant and beginning to brown, about 30 seconds. Add chard stems and cook until softened, 3 to 5 minutes. Stir in garlic, pepper flakes, remaining ¼ teaspoon salt, and remaining ⅛ teaspoon pepper and cook until fragrant, about 30 seconds. Stir in beans and their liquid and any accumulated chicken juices from platter, scraping up any browned bits, then stir in chard leaves, one handful at a time. Cover and cook, stirring occasionally, until chard is tender, about 4 minutes. Serve chicken with chard mixture, passing lemon wedges separately.

MAKE AHEAD • Cooked chicken can be refrigerated for up to 3 days.

Chicken and Couscous with Fennel, Apricots, and Orange

serves 4 • total time: 1 hour

why this recipe works • For a change of pace from the usual chicken and rice, couscous (a tiny pasta made from semolina wheat) offers the perfect choice for a quick supper. This recipe streamlines the cooking because you can cook both the protein and starch in one skillet. We coated chicken breasts in olive oil before browning to guard against dryness and give them a nice crust. The fond left in the pan provided a flavor base for our vegetables, aromatic fennel and red onion, which we sautéed to soften slightly before adding the couscous. Toasting the couscous briefly not only brought out its nutty aroma but also helped prevent it from clumping. While couscous is often hydrated with water or broth, for even more flavor we supplemented broth with orange juice. The citrusy flavor brightened the entire dish and gave it a gently sweet tang that paired beautifully with the savory ingredients. The orange juice, plus dried apricots, also made marvelous complements to fennel—the fruits' acidic sweetness brought out more of the fennel's flavor. A sprinkle of cilantro contributed a fresh, herbal lift. Drizzling the dish at the very end with a dressing of more orange juice, olive oil, and cayenne made for a fragrant flavor boost.

4 (6- to 8-ounce) boneless, skinless chicken breasts, trimmed
½ cup extra-virgin olive oil, divided
1 teaspoon table salt, divided
¼ teaspoon pepper
1 red onion, sliced thin
1 fennel bulb, stalks discarded, bulb halved, cored, and sliced thin
1 cup couscous
3 garlic cloves, minced
⅛ teaspoon cayenne pepper, divided
1 cup orange juice (2 oranges), divided
¾ cup unsalted chicken broth
½ cup coarsely chopped dried apricots
¼ cup minced fresh cilantro, divided

1 Gently pound thicker end of each breast until ½ inch thick. Pat breasts dry with paper towels. Brush both sides of breasts with 2 tablespoons oil and sprinkle with ½ teaspoon salt and pepper. Place breasts, skinned side down, in cold 12-inch non-stick skillet, arranging narrow parts of breasts opposite wider parts. Place skillet over high heat and cook for 2 minutes. Flip breasts and cook for 2 minutes (there should be light browning).

2 Flip breasts, reduce heat to medium, and continue to cook, flipping breasts every 2 minutes, until exterior is well browned and thickest part of breast registers 155 degrees, 6 to 8 minutes longer. Transfer breasts, skinned side up, to platter. Tent with aluminum foil and let rest while cooking couscous and vegetables.

3 Heat 1 tablespoon oil in now-empty skillet over medium heat until shimmering. Add onion, fennel, and remaining ½ teaspoon salt and cook until vegetables are softened, 5 to 7 minutes. Stir in couscous, garlic, and pinch cayenne and cook until fragrant, about 30 seconds. Stir in ¾ cup orange juice, broth, and apricots and bring to simmer. Off heat, cover and let sit until liquid is absorbed, about 5 minutes.

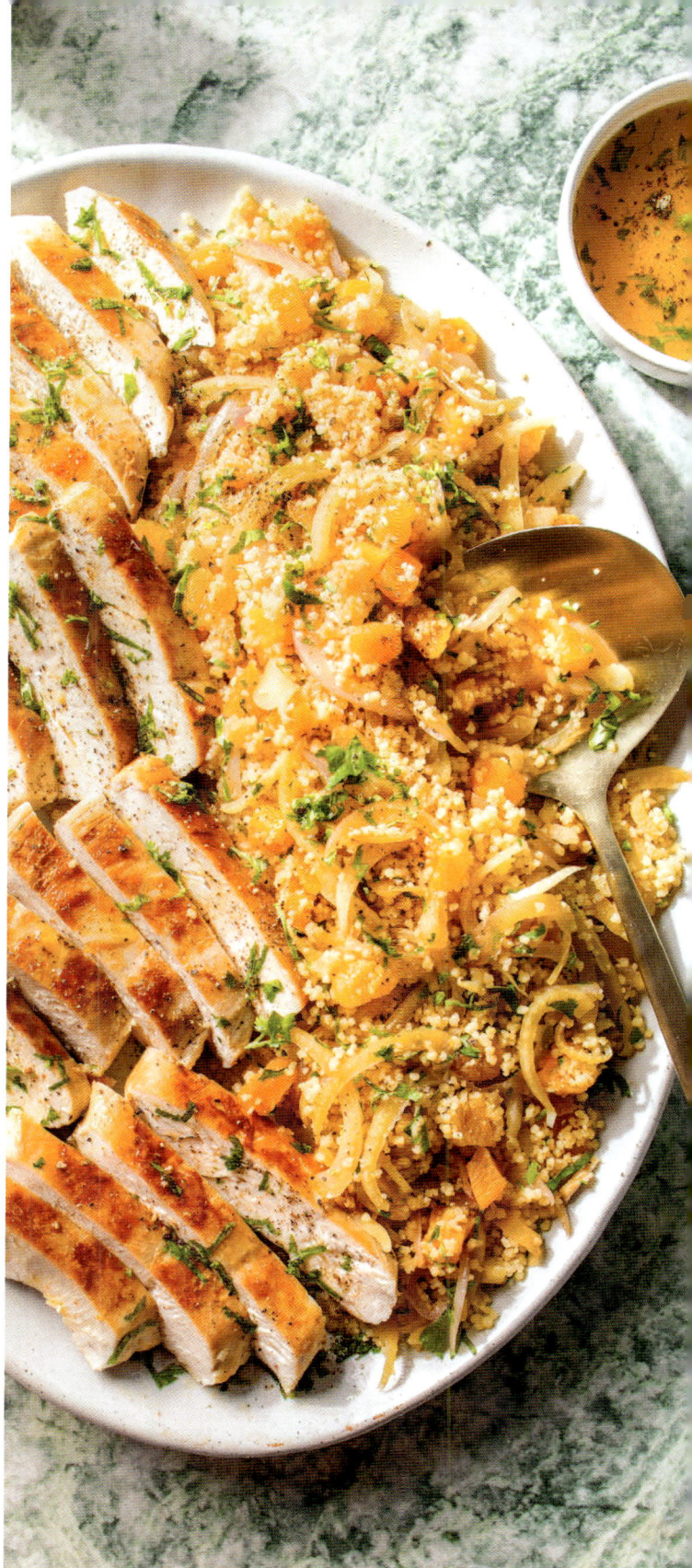

Chicken and Couscous with Fennel, Apricots, and Orange

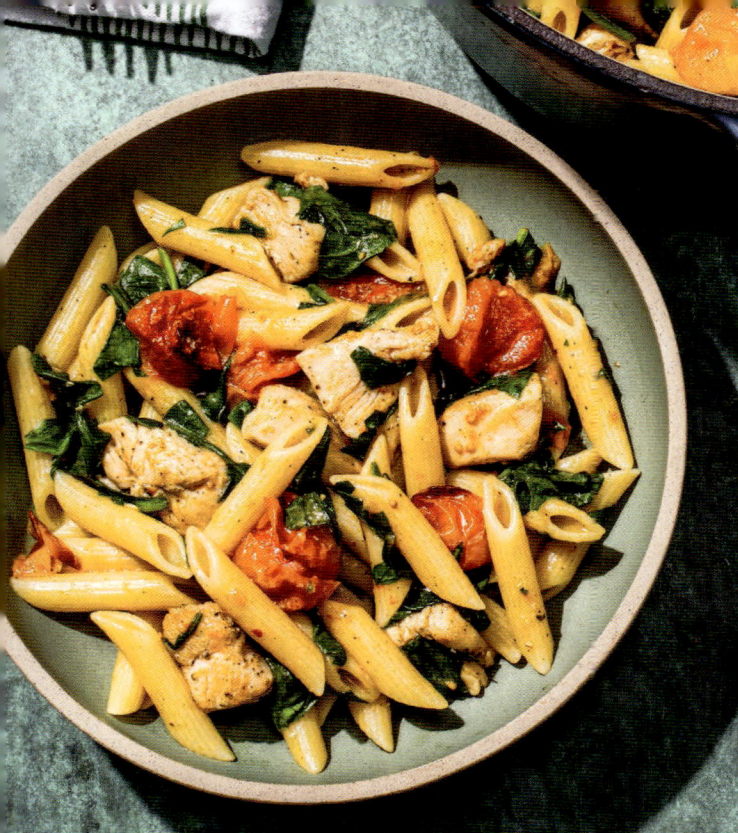

4 Whisk 2 tablespoons cilantro, remaining 5 tablespoons oil, remaining pinch cayenne, and remaining ¼ cup orange juice together in bowl. Add remaining 2 tablespoons cilantro to cous-cous and gently fluff with fork to combine. Season with salt and pepper to taste. Drizzle oil–orange juice mixture over chicken and couscous before serving.

> **MAKE AHEAD** · Cooked chicken and couscous-vegetable mixture can be refrigerated for up to 3 days.

Penne with Chicken, Roasted Cherry Tomatoes, and Spinach

serves 4 · total time: 45 minutes   **FAST**

why this recipe works · Spinach and tomatoes are the light, fresh stars of this summery pasta dish. After searing pieces of chicken breast and setting them aside, we used the fond in the skillet to cook shallots and red pepper flakes, then deglazed with chicken broth. This simple step added layers of savory depth and ensured that no flavor went to waste. Cooking the pasta in this flavorful liquid made a glossy, rich-tasting sauce, which we rounded out with oven-roasted cherry tomatoes. The tomatoes also provided a dose of lycopene, a powerful antioxi-dant known for reducing inflammation and supporting heart health. Stirring in baby spinach at the end wilted the greens, studding the pasta with vibrant pops of green. You can top this pasta with chopped fresh basil or grated Parmesan cheese, if desired.

1½ pounds cherry tomatoes
5 tablespoons extra-virgin olive oil, divided
1¼ teaspoons table salt, divided
1 pound boneless, skinless chicken breasts, trimmed and cut into ¾-inch pieces
½ teaspoon pepper
2 shallots, chopped
¼ teaspoon red pepper flakes
2 cups unsalted chicken broth
2 cups water
12 ounces (3¾ cups) penne
5 ounces (5 cups) baby spinach, chopped coarse

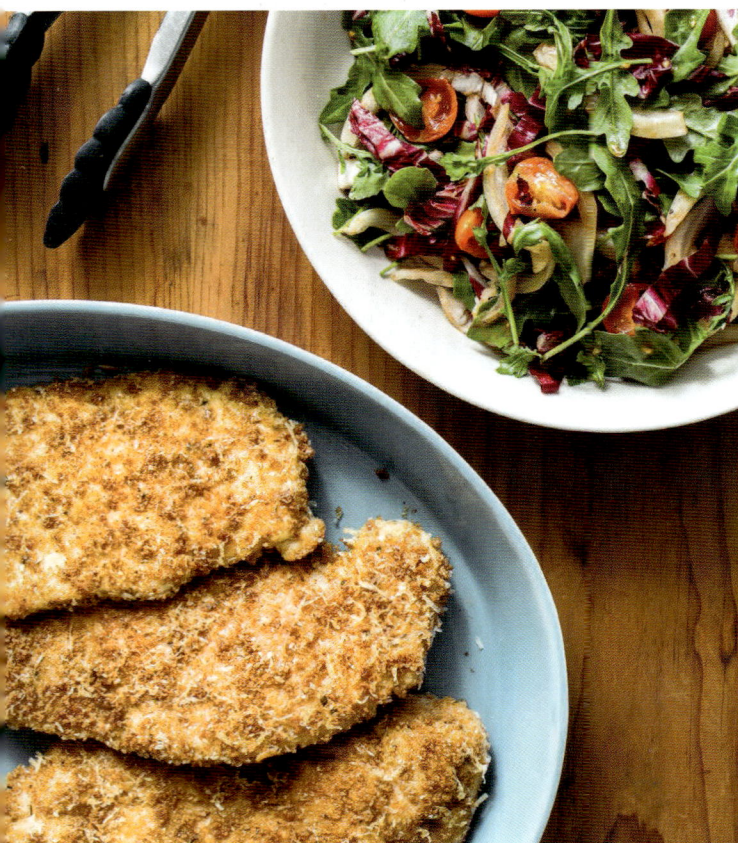

top | Penne with Chicken, Roasted Cherry Tomatoes, and Spinach
bottom | Parmesan Chicken with Warm Arugula, Radicchio, and Fennel Salad

1   Adjust oven rack to middle position and heat oven to 500 degrees. Line rimmed baking sheet with parchment paper. Toss tomatoes, 2 tablespoons oil, and ½ teaspoon salt together on prepared sheet. Roast until tomatoes are blistered and browned, 15 to 20 minutes.

2   Meanwhile, pat chicken dry with paper towels, then sprinkle with ¼ teaspoon salt and pepper. Heat 2 tablespoons oil in Dutch oven over medium-high heat until shimmering. Add chicken and cook, stirring occasionally, until just cooked through, about 5 minutes; transfer to bowl.

3   Add shallots, pepper flakes, and remaining 1 tablespoon oil to pot and cook until softened, 1 to 2 minutes. Stir in broth, water, pasta, and remaining ½ teaspoon salt and bring to boil over high heat. Reduce heat to medium-low, cover, and simmer, stirring occasionally, until pasta is al dente, 10 to 14 minutes (some liquid will remain in bottom of pot). Stir in roasted tomatoes, chicken and any accumulated juices, and spinach and cook, stirring constantly, until spinach is wilted, about 1 minute. Season with salt and pepper to taste, and serve.

MAKE AHEAD • Roasted tomatoes can be refrigerated for up to 24 hours.

MAKE IT GLUTEN-FREE • Substitute gluten-free pasta for the pasta.

Parmesan Chicken with Warm Arugula, Radicchio, and Fennel Salad

serves 4 • total time: 1 hour

why this recipe works • Chicken Parmesan is often sopped with oil, smothered with cheese, and served over a mountain of pasta. While undeniably indulgent, this approach can feel heavy, pushing saturated fat higher than is optimal for an anti-inflammatory eating pattern. For a modern twist that turns an eye toward anti-inflammation, we served our flavorful cutlets with a fresh salad. Instead of a layer of cheese, we added a smaller amount of grated Parmesan to the breading and then boosted the flavor with classic seasonings like garlic powder and oregano. Using a nonstick skillet helped us brown the cutlets perfectly while keeping the meat nice and moist. To bring in more nutrients, we then used the skillet to soften fennel and cherry tomatoes before tossing them with radicchio and baby arugula in a simple vinaigrette

for a warm, gently wilted salad. The cooked vegetables helped mellow the bitterness of the radicchio, while the vinaigrette added just the right amount of acidity. The slight bitterness of the greens also contrasted well with the rich and savory chicken, creating a well-balanced, nutrient-dense, inflammation-fighting spin on an Italian American favorite.

  2 (6- to 8-ounce) boneless, skinless chicken breasts, trimmed, halved horizontally, and pounded ½ inch thick
  ½ teaspoon table salt, divided
  ½ cup all-purpose flour
  2 large eggs
  ½ cup panko bread crumbs
  1 ounce Parmesan cheese, grated (½ cup)
  ½ teaspoon garlic powder
  ½ teaspoon dried oregano
  5 tablespoons extra-virgin olive oil, divided
  1 fennel bulb, stalks discarded, bulb halved, cored, and sliced thin
  1 tablespoon white wine vinegar
  1½ teaspoons minced shallot
  ½ teaspoon Dijon mustard
     Pinch pepper
  12 ounces cherry tomatoes, halved
  ½ head radicchio (5 ounces), cored and sliced thin
  2 ounces (2 cups) baby arugula

1   Adjust oven rack to middle position and heat oven to 200 degrees. Sprinkle cutlets with ¼ teaspoon salt; let stand at room temperature for 20 minutes.

2   Spread flour in shallow dish. Beat eggs in second shallow dish. Combine panko, Parmesan, garlic powder, and oregano in third shallow dish. Pat chicken dry with paper towels. Working with 1 cutlet at a time, dredge in flour, dip in egg, then coat with panko mixture, pressing gently to adhere.

3   Heat 3 tablespoons oil in 12-inch nonstick skillet over medium heat until shimmering. Add 2 cutlets to skillet and cook until chicken is tender, golden brown, and crisp, 3 to 4 minutes per side. Transfer to paper towel–lined plate and place in oven to keep warm. Repeat with remaining 2 cutlets.

4   Wipe out skillet with paper towels. Heat 1 tablespoon oil in now-empty skillet over medium heat until shimmering. Add fennel and cook until softened and just beginning to brown, about 5 minutes.

5 Meanwhile, whisk vinegar, shallot, mustard, remaining ¼ teaspoon salt, and pepper together in large bowl. Whisking constantly, slowly drizzle in remaining 1 tablespoon oil until emulsified. Transfer cooked fennel to bowl with vinaigrette. Add tomatoes to now-empty skillet and cook until softened, about 2 minutes; transfer to bowl with fennel along with radicchio and arugula, tossing gently to combine. Season salad with salt and pepper to taste and serve with chicken.

MAKE IT DAIRY-FREE • Substitute plant-based Parmesan cheese for the dairy Parmesan cheese.

Za'atar Chicken Cutlets with Sweet Potato Wedges and Cabbage Salad

serves 4 • total time: 55 minutes

why this recipe works • Crispy chicken cutlets hold so much appeal that we wanted to find a way to enjoy them in a satisfying anti-inflammatory meal. Rather than top them with cheese or a creamy sauce, we opted for two nutrient-dense sides: Thick roasted sweet potato wedges and a crunchy cabbage salad (perked up with a hefty amount of antioxidant-rich parsley) delivered a double dose of fiber. With such hearty vegetables on the plate, a single crispy cutlet was all we needed to complete the meal. To give each cutlet a punch of bright flavor as well as a boost of anti-oxidants, we seasoned our panko coating with a ¼ cup of za'atar, the Middle Eastern spice blend made with sumac, dried herbs, and toasted sesame seeds. Pan-frying the cutlets in extra-virgin olive oil kept saturated fat in check for a meal that was both nutritious and comforting. We prefer to use our homemade Za'atar (page 186), but you can use store-bought if you prefer.

- 1½ pounds sweet potatoes, unpeeled, cut into 1½-inch-wide wedges
- 2 tablespoons extra-virgin olive oil, divided
- ¾ teaspoon plus ⅛ teaspoon table salt, divided
- 1 small head green cabbage (1¼ pounds), halved, cored, and shredded (4 cups)
- ¾ cup fresh parsley or tarragon leaves
- 3 tablespoons red wine vinegar
- 1 large egg
- 1 cup panko bread crumbs
- ¼ cup za'atar
- 2 (6- to 8-ounce) boneless, skinless chicken breasts, trimmed
- ½ cup extra-virgin olive oil, for frying
  Lemon wedges

1 Adjust oven rack to middle position and heat oven to 450 degrees. Spray aluminum foil–lined rimmed baking sheet with avocado oil spray. Toss potatoes with 1 tablespoon oil and ¼ teaspoon salt. Arrange potatoes cut side down in even layer on prepared sheet. Roast until potato bottoms are well browned, 20 to 25 minutes. Transfer to serving platter and tent with foil to keep warm.

2 Meanwhile, toss cabbage, parsley, vinegar, 1 tablespoon oil, and ⅛ teaspoon salt together and refrigerate until ready to serve.

3 Lightly beat egg in shallow dish. Combine panko and za'atar in second shallow dish. Halve chicken breasts horizontally to form 4 cutlets of even thickness. Place 1 cutlet between 2 sheets of plastic wrap and pound to ¼-inch thickness. Repeat with remaining cutlets. Pat cutlets dry with paper towels and sprinkle with remaining ½ teaspoon salt. Working with 1 cutlet at a time, dip in egg, allowing excess to drip off, then coat with panko mixture, pressing gently to adhere.

4 Line second rimmed baking sheet with double layer of paper towels. Heat ½ cup oil in 12-inch nonstick skillet over medium-high heat until shimmering. Place 2 cutlets in skillet and cook until deep golden brown, 2 to 3 minutes per side. Transfer cutlets to prepared sheet and repeat with remaining 2 cutlets. Season with salt and pepper to taste. Serve chicken with potatoes, cabbage salad, and lemon wedges.

MAKE IT GLUTEN-FREE • Substitute gluten-free panko for the panko.

Za'atar

makes about ⅓ cup • total time: 10 minutes

- 2 tablespoons dried thyme
- 1 tablespoon dried oregano
- 1½ tablespoons sumac
- 1 tablespoon sesame seeds, toasted
- ¼ teaspoon salt

Process thyme and oregano in spice grinder or mortar and pestle until finely ground and powdery. Transfer to bowl and stir in sumac, sesame seeds, and salt. (Za'atar can be stored at room temperature in airtight container for up to 1 year.)

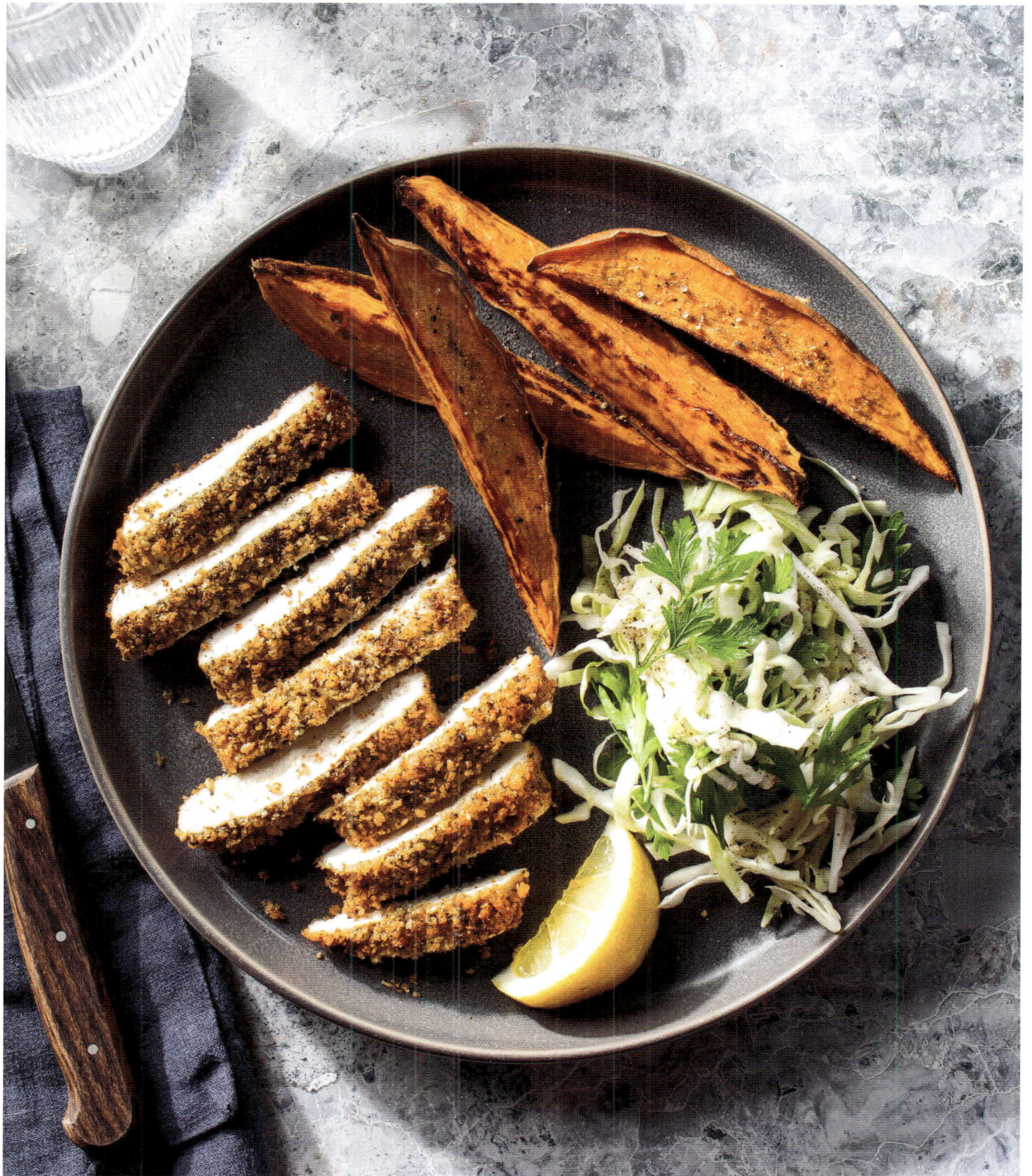

Za'atar Chicken Cutlets with Sweet Potato Wedges and Cabbage Salad

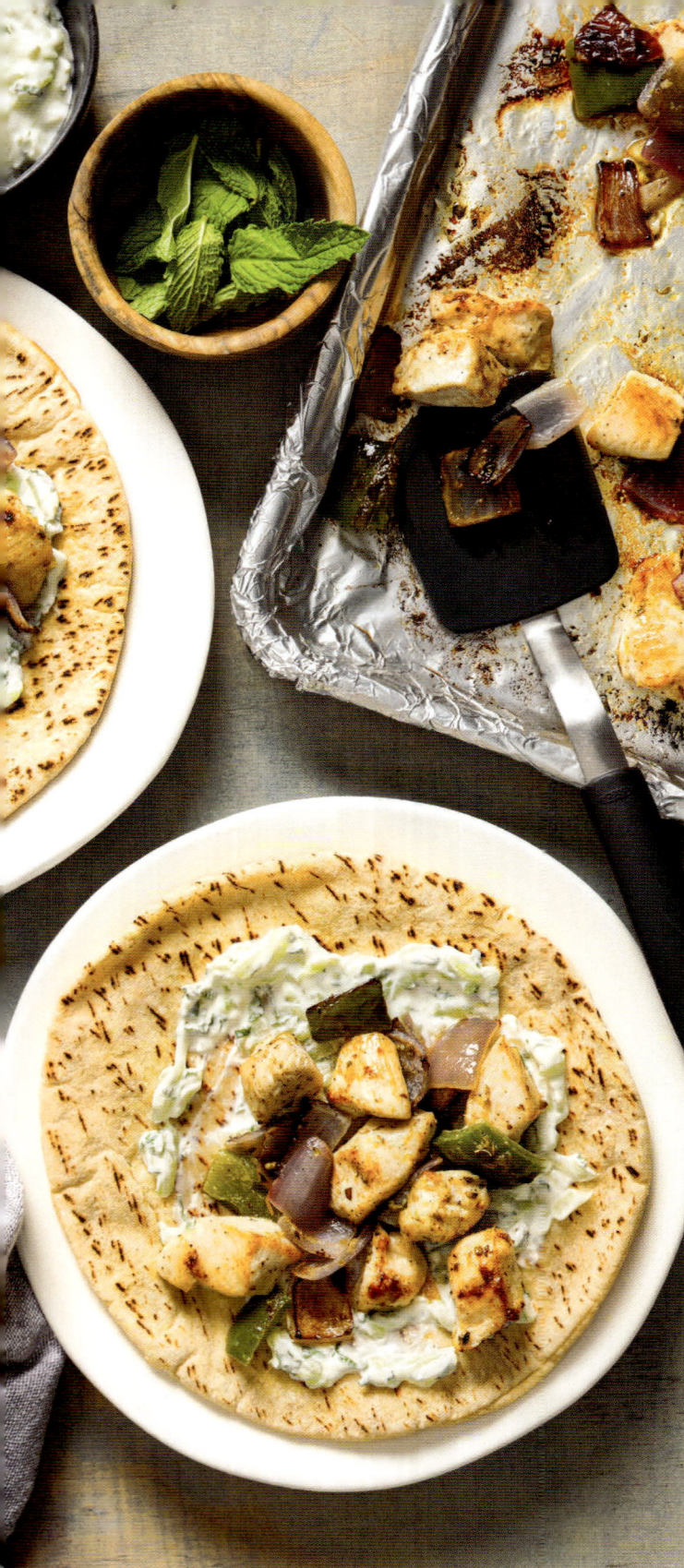

Sheet-Pan Chicken Souvlaki

serves 4 • total time: 30 minutes **FAST**

why this recipe works • If you want to be transported to the tiny eateries lining the back streets of Athens, where souvlaki is king, try this version using a baking sheet—no grill, rotisserie, or fussy skewering required. Bright lemon flavor and moist, evenly cooked meat are the hallmarks of good slouvlaki, which is traditionally made with chunks of pork. Here, we used also-popular boneless, skinless chicken breast pieces for a lean protein and a baking sheet and the broiler to give us more control, ensuring that the chicken turned juicy and spotty brown and that the vegetables were crisp-tender. A quick toss beforehand in a flavorful marinade of lemon, olive oil, and herbs also helped eliminate the chance that the chicken would dry out; we set some aside to create a vinaigrette to toss with the chicken just before wrapping it in pita. You can use Persian cucumber in place of the English cucumber and skip the seeding. We like parsley and mint in the accompanying tzatziki, but you can substitute any leafy herb; if substituting woodsy herbs like thyme, oregano, or marjoram, use one-third the amount.

Tzatziki
- ½ cup English cucumber, halved lengthwise, seeded, and shredded
- ½ cup plain Greek yogurt
- 2 teaspoons lemon juice
- 2 tablespoons chopped fresh mint
- 2 tablespoons chopped fresh parsley
- ⅛ teaspoon table salt
- 1 garlic clove, minced
- ¼ teaspoon pepper

Chicken and Vegetables
- 5 tablespoons extra-virgin olive oil
- 1 teaspoon grated lemon zest plus 2 tablespoons juice
- 1 teaspoon dried oregano
- 1 teaspoon table salt
- ½ teaspoon pepper
- 1 pound boneless, skinless chicken breasts, trimmed and cut into 1-inch pieces
- 1 green bell pepper, cut into 1-inch pieces
- 1 small red onion, cut into 1-inch pieces
- 4 (8-inch) whole-wheat pita bread, warmed

1 For the tzatziki Combine all ingredients in bowl and season with salt and pepper to taste. Refrigerate until ready to serve.

2 For the chicken and vegetables Adjust oven rack 6 inches from broiler element and heat broiler. Spray aluminum foil–lined rimmed baking sheet with avocado oil spray. Whisk oil, lemon zest, oregano, salt, and pepper together in large bowl. Measure out and reserve 3 tablespoons oil mixture, then whisk lemon juice into remaining oil mixture in bowl to make a vinaigrette; set vinaigrette aside. Toss chicken, bell pepper, and onion with reserved oil mixture in bowl, then spread into even layer on prepared sheet.

3 Broil until chicken is spotty brown on top side, 4 to 6 minutes. Stir chicken and vegetables, then redistribute into even layer and continue to broil until chicken is spotty brown on second side and vegetables are tender, 4 to 6 minutes.

4 Whisk reserved vinaigrette to recombine, then drizzle over roasted chicken and vegetables on sheet; toss to combine, gently scraping up any fond from sheet. Lay each pita on 12-inch square of foil. Divide tzatziki evenly among pitas, spreading over half pita, then place one-quarter chicken and vegetables in center of each pita. Roll into wrap, using foil to hold shape, and serve.

> **MAKE AHEAD** • Tzatziki can be refrigerated for up to 2 days.

> **MAKE IT GLUTEN-FREE** • Substitute gluten-free pita for the pita.

> **MAKE IT DAIRY-FREE** • Substitute plant-based Greek yogurt for the dairy Greek yogurt.

Smoked Paprika Chicken and Corn Salad with Lime

serves 4 • total time: 40 minutes **FAST**

why this recipe works • This summery one-skillet meal of smoky chicken with a warm, citrusy salad of corn, tomato, and edamame is low-effort, high-reward. An anti-inflammatory spice blend of smoked paprika, cumin, and cayenne livened up chicken breasts, which we kept tender and juicy by employing our trusty cold-start cooking method. Pounding the thicker end of each breast and frequently flipping the meat in a skillet ensured that the lean protein cooked evenly. After cooking the chicken, we softened red onion in the flavorful fond before adding corn and edamame to warm in the pan for a colorful salad packed with protein. Adding tomatoes gave us a welcome dose of brightness and tang, plus some antioxidants. A rasp-style grater makes quick work of turning the garlic into a paste.

- 2 teaspoons smoked paprika
- 1½ teaspoons table salt, divided
- 1 teaspoon ground cumin
- ½ teaspoon pepper, divided
- ¼ teaspoon cayenne pepper
- 5 tablespoons extra-virgin olive oil, divided
- 1 tablespoon grated lime zest plus 2 tablespoons juice (2 limes), plus lime wedges for serving
- 1 small garlic clove, minced to paste
- 4 (6- to 8-ounce) boneless, skinless chicken breasts, trimmed
- 1 red onion, chopped fine
- 2½ cups frozen corn, thawed
- 1 cup frozen shelled edamame, thawed
- 12 ounces cherry tomatoes, halved
- ½ cup chopped fresh cilantro, divided

1 Combine paprika, 1 teaspoon salt, cumin, ¼ teaspoon pepper, and cayenne together in bowl; set aside. Whisk 2 tablespoons oil, lime zest and juice, garlic, ¼ teaspoon salt, and remaining ¼ teaspoon pepper together in large bowl; set aside.

2 Gently pound thicker end of each breast until ½ inch thick. Pat breasts dry with paper towels. Brush both sides of breasts with 2 tablespoons oil and evenly sprinkle with reserved paprika mixture. Place breasts, skinned side down, in cold 12-inch non-stick skillet, arranging narrow parts of breasts opposite wider parts. Place skillet over high heat and cook for 2 minutes. Flip breasts and cook for 2 minutes (there should be light browning).

3 Flip breasts, reduce heat to medium, and continue to cook, flipping breasts every 2 minutes, until exterior is well browned and thickest part of breast registers 155 degrees, 6 to 8 minutes longer. Transfer breasts, skinned side up, to platter and tent with aluminum foil. Let rest while making corn salad.

4 Heat remaining 1 tablespoon oil in now-empty skillet over medium-high heat until shimmering. Add onion and remaining ¼ teaspoon salt and cook, stirring occasionally, until softened, 3 to 5 minutes. Stir in corn and edamame and cook until warmed through, 3 to 5 minutes. Add corn mixture, tomatoes, and 6 tablespoons cilantro to bowl with reserved dressing and toss to combine. Sprinkle chicken and corn salad with remaining 2 tablespoons cilantro and serve with lime wedges.

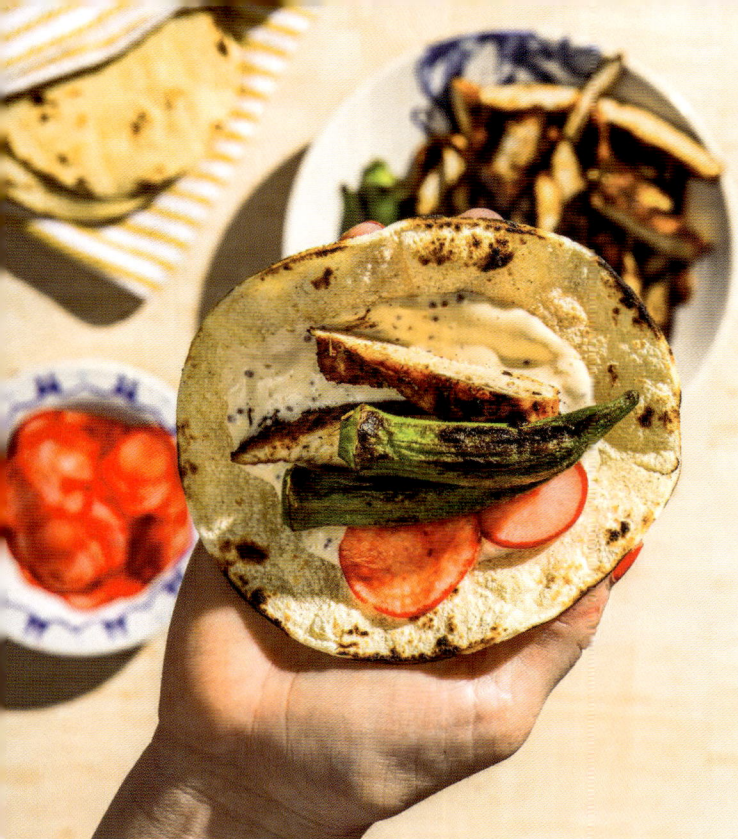

Cajun-Spiced Chicken and Okra Tacos

serves 6 • total time: 45 minutes   **FAST**

why this recipe works • Seared okra is the star of these veggie-forward tacos: The plump, crisp pods offer up a smoky, vegetal flavor that's balanced by a modest amount of chicken. To get the most flavor out of our chicken, we turned to bold flavor Cajun seasonings and opted to make our own blend to have control over the amount of salt in the recipe. We coated our cutlets in the spice rub and then seared them in a preheated cast-iron skillet, which cooked the thin cutlets in a flash while creating a spiced crust. The meat's spicy aroma made a fantastic foil for the fiberful okra. We found that quickly cooking whole pods over medium-high heat minimized the release of their mucilage and maximized their crispness. For brightness, we lightly smeared corn tortillas with a remoulade-inspired sauce, then piled on the chicken and okra and topped off the tacos with slices of lemon-pickled radishes. Okra pods less than 3 inches long will be the most tender; cut any pods longer than 4 inches in half crosswise. For a spicier dish, use the larger amount of cayenne. A rasp-style grater makes quick work of turning the garlic into a paste.

6	radishes, trimmed and sliced thin
¼	teaspoon grated lemon zest plus 2½ tablespoons juice, divided
⅓	cup mayonnaise
2	teaspoons whole-grain mustard
1	teaspoon Worcestershire sauce
¼	teaspoon garlic, minced to paste
1	tablespoon paprika
1½	teaspoons garlic powder
1½	teaspoons dried thyme
1	teaspoon table salt, divided
¾	teaspoon pepper
¼–½	teaspoon cayenne pepper
2	(6- to 8-ounce) boneless, skinless chicken breasts, trimmed
2	tablespoons avocado oil, divided
1	pound okra, stemmed
12	(6-inch) corn tortillas, warmed

1   Combine radishes and 2 tablespoons lemon juice in small bowl; set aside. Whisk mayonnaise, mustard, Worcestershire, garlic, lemon zest, and remaining 1½ teaspoons lemon juice in separate bowl; set sauce aside. Combine paprika, garlic powder, thyme, ¾ teaspoon salt, pepper, and cayenne in wide, shallow bowl.

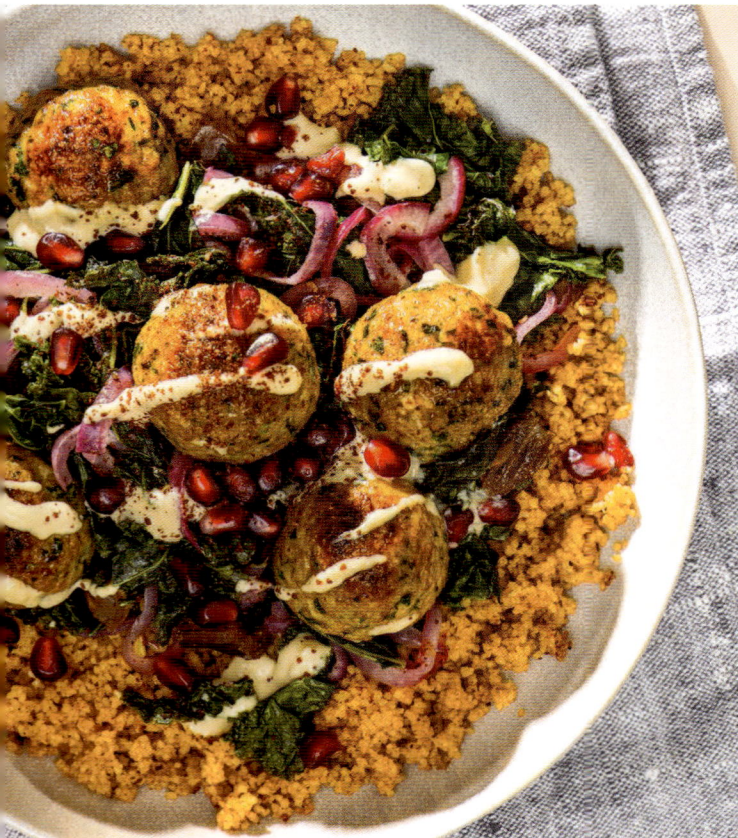

2 Working with 1 chicken breast at a time, halve breast cross-wise, then cut thick half in half horizontally, creating 3 cutlets of similar thickness. Place cutlets between sheets of plastic wrap and gently pound to even ⅓-inch thickness. Pat cutlets dry with paper towels. Working with 1 cutlet at a time, dredge thoroughly in spice mixture, pressing to adhere. Shake off excess spice mixture and place cutlets in single layer on rimmed baking sheet.

3 Heat 12-inch cast-iron skillet over medium heat for 3 minutes. Add 1 tablespoon oil and heat until just smoking. Add cutlets to skillet in single layer, press on each firmly with spatula, and cook undisturbed for 2 minutes. Flip cutlets, then press cutlets against skillet with spatula and cook for 1 minute. Remove skillet from heat and transfer cutlets to cutting board. Tent loosely with aluminum foil and let rest while cooking okra.

4 Wipe out skillet with paper towels to remove any debris. Heat remaining 1 tablespoon oil in now-empty skillet over medium-high heat until just smoking. Add okra and remaining ¼ teaspoon salt and cook, stirring occasionally, until crisp-tender and well charred on most sides, 5 to 7 minutes (okra may not fit in single layer to start; that is OK). Transfer okra to bowl.

5 Thinly slice chicken. Divide reserved sauce evenly among tortillas; top with chicken, okra, and reserved radishes; and serve.

MAKE AHEAD • Cooked chicken can be refrigerated for up to 3 days. Radish–lemon juice mixture and sauce can be refrigerated for up to 24 hours.

HOW TO STEM OKRA

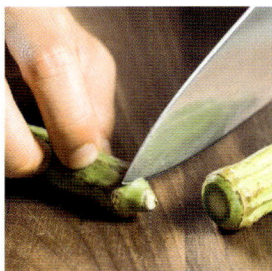

To stem okra, trim the stems from the okra pods, making sure to leave the top "cap" on each pod intact. This minimizes slip and prevents the okra from becoming gooey as it cooks.

Bulgur Bowls with Chicken Meatballs and Sumac Kale

serves 4 to 6 • total time: 1 hour SUPERCHARGED

why this recipe works • This flavor-packed, inflammation-fighting bowl made with chicken, bulgur, and antioxidant-rich spices comes together with the ease of just one baking sheet. Bulgur pulls double duty: After soaking it in a harissa-spiked brew and seasoning it with sumac, we used a portion as a binder to make chicken meatballs and then broiled the rest alongside them on the sheet pan. We used the same pan to roast kale with red onion and dates before dressing the melange with lemon juice and more sumac. A tahini sauce, pomegranate molasses, and pomegranate seeds were perfect finishers. Be sure to use ground chicken, not ground chicken breast (also labeled 99 percent fat-free). We prefer our homemade Harissa (page 106), but you can use store-bought.

2	tablespoons harissa
2	teaspoons table salt, divided
3½	cups boiling water
1¾	cups fine-grind bulgur
4	teaspoons ground sumac, divided, plus extra for sprinkling
1	pound ground chicken
3	tablespoons plain whole-milk yogurt
3	tablespoons minced fresh parsley
2	garlic cloves, minced
1½	teaspoons ground cumin
¾	teaspoon ground coriander
1	pound curly kale, stemmed, leaves torn into 1½- to 2-inch pieces
5	tablespoons extra-virgin olive oil, divided
1	red onion, halved and sliced thin
¼	cup chopped pitted dates
1	tablespoon lemon juice
1	recipe Tahini-Garlic Sauce (page 192)
⅓	cup pomegranate seeds
	Pomegranate molasses

1 Adjust oven rack 6 inches from broiler element and heat oven to 400 degrees. Whisk harissa, ¾ teaspoon salt, and boiling water together in large bowl. Stir in bulgur, cover, and let sit until grains are tender, about 15 minutes.

2 Drain bulgur (you may not have excess liquid), then toss with 2 teaspoons sumac in bowl. Combine ¾ cup bulgur-sumac mixture, ground chicken, yogurt, parsley, garlic, cumin, coriander, and ½ teaspoon salt in separate bowl. Using wet hands, pinch off about 2 tablespoons and roll into sixteen 1½-inch-wide meatballs; transfer to large plate and set aside.

3 Spread kale over rimmed baking sheet, then drizzle with 2 tablespoons oil and sprinkle with ½ teaspoon salt. Vigorously squeeze and massage kale with your hands until leaves are uniformly darkened and slightly wilted, about 1 minute. Toss onion and dates with 1 tablespoon oil and remaining ¼ teaspoon salt in bowl, then scatter over top of kale on sheet. Roast until kale and onion are tender, about 10 minutes. Transfer to bowl, stir in lemon juice and remaining 2 teaspoons sumac, and cover to keep warm. Wipe sheet clean, then spray with avocado oil spray. Heat broiler.

4 Transfer remaining bulgur-sumac mixture to one half of now-empty sheet, spreading into even layer. Transfer reserved meatballs to second half of sheet, then brush top of bulgur with remaining 2 tablespoons oil. Broil until top layer of bulgur is lightly browned and crisp in spots and meatballs are cooked through and lightly browned, 7 to 12 minutes, rotating sheet halfway through broiling.

5 Divide bulgur among individual serving bowls, then top with reserved kale mixture and meatballs. Drizzle with Tahini-Garlic sauce and sprinkle with pomegranate seeds. Serve, topping with pomegranate molasses and extra sumac, if desired.

MAKE AHEAD • Meatballs and bulgur can be prepared through step 2 and refrigerated for up to 24 hours.

MAKE IT DAIRY-FREE • Substitute plant-based yogurt for the dairy yogurt.

Tahini-Garlic Sauce

makes 1 cup • **total time: 10 minutes**

- ⅓ cup tahini
- 3 tablespoons plain dairy yogurt or plant-based yogurt
- 2 tablespoons lemon juice
- 2 tablespoons water
- 2 teaspoons pomegranate molasses
- 1 garlic clove, minced
- ½ teaspoon table salt

Whisk all ingredients together in bowl until well combined. Season with salt and pepper to taste. (Sauce can be refrigerated for up to 3 days. Thin with extra water as needed before serving.)

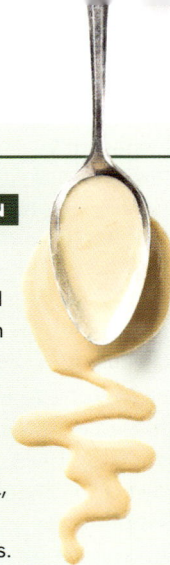

One Big Cast-Iron Chicken and Chard Enchilada

serves 6 • **total time: 1¼ hours**

why this recipe works • For a weeknight-friendly take on a Mexican favorite, we skipped rolling individual tortillas and instead made one big enchilada in a cast-iron skillet. The fun format not only saved time but also left lots of room for a savory, vegetable-packed filling of ground chicken, antioxidant-rich Swiss chard and bell peppers, and fiberful beans. Instead of frying corn tortillas, we dry-toasted them in the piping-hot skillet, amplifying the corn flavor. Preheating the skillet for 5 minutes was the key to perfectly toasty tortillas that didn't dry out. A savory chile sauce came together quickly with pantry ingredients. We folded some of it into the filling and spooned the rest over the tortillas. A judicious amount of Monterey Jack cheese and generous sprinkling of minced fresh jalapeño made for a satisfying, crowd-pleasing dinner. Be sure to use ground chicken, not ground chicken breast (also labeled 99 percent fat-free) in this recipe. Serve with sliced radish, extra chopped onion, and extra chopped cilantro, if desired.

- 6 (6-inch) corn tortillas
- 2 tablespoons extra-virgin olive oil, divided
- 2 onions, chopped fine, divided
- 1¾ teaspoons table salt, divided
- 6 garlic cloves, minced, divided
- 1 tablespoon chili powder
- 1 teaspoon ground cumin
- ½ teaspoon pepper, divided

- 1 (15-ounce) can no-salt-added tomato sauce
- 1 cup unsalted chicken broth
- 1 pound ground chicken
- 1 pound Swiss chard, stemmed and sliced into ½-inch-wide strips
- 2 yellow bell peppers, stemmed, seeded, and cut into 2-inch-long matchsticks
- 1 (15-ounce) can no-salt-added pinto beans, rinsed and coarsely mashed
- ¾ cup chopped fresh cilantro leaves and tender stems, divided
- 4 ounces Monterey Jack cheese, shredded (1 cup)
- 1 jalapeño chile, stemmed, seeded, and minced
  Lime wedges

1 Adjust oven rack to middle position and heat oven to 450 degrees. Heat 12-inch cast-iron skillet over medium-high heat for 5 minutes. Reduce heat to medium and, working in batches, toast tortillas in hot skillet until lightly browned, about 1 minute per side; transfer to plate and cover with dish towel.

2 Heat 1 tablespoon oil in large saucepan over medium heat until shimmering. Add half of onions and ¾ teaspoon salt and cook until softened, about 5 minutes. Stir in half of garlic, chili powder, cumin, and ¼ teaspoon pepper and cook until fragrant, about 30 seconds. Stir in tomato sauce and broth, bring to simmer, and cook until slightly thickened, about 3 minutes. Set sauce aside.

3 Meanwhile, heat remaining 1 tablespoon oil in now-empty skillet over medium-high heat until shimmering. Add chicken and cook, breaking up meat with wooden spoon, until no longer pink and lightly browned, about 5 minutes. Add remaining onion, remaining 1 teaspoon salt, and remaining ¼ teaspoon pepper and cook until softened and just beginning to brown, about 5 minutes. Add remaining garlic and cook until fragrant, about 30 seconds. Add chard, one handful at a time, then bell peppers. Cover and cook until chard is tender, 6 to 8 minutes. Off heat, stir in beans, 1½ cups reserved sauce, and ½ cup cilantro. Season filling with salt and pepper to taste.

4 Arrange toasted tortillas over filling in pinwheel pattern and top with remaining reserved sauce, leaving some exposed edges. Sprinkle evenly with Monterey Jack and jalapeño. Bake until cheese is melted and spotty brown and tortillas are browned around the edges, about 15 minutes. Transfer skillet to wire rack and let cool for 10 minutes. Sprinkle with remaining ¼ cup cilantro and serve with lime wedges.

MAKE IT DAIRY-FREE • Substitute plant-based Monterey Jack or mozzarella cheese for the Monterey Jack cheese.

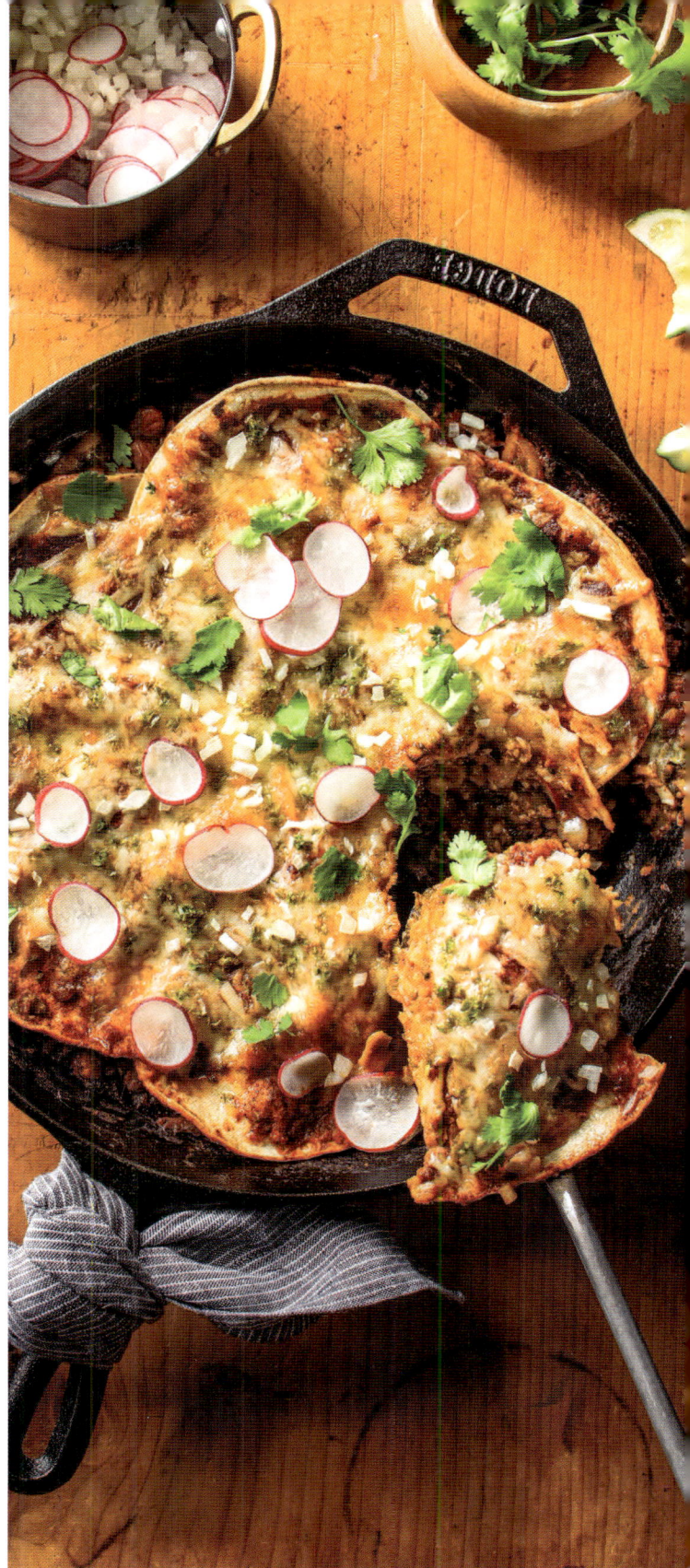

One Big Cast-Iron Chicken and Chard Enchilada

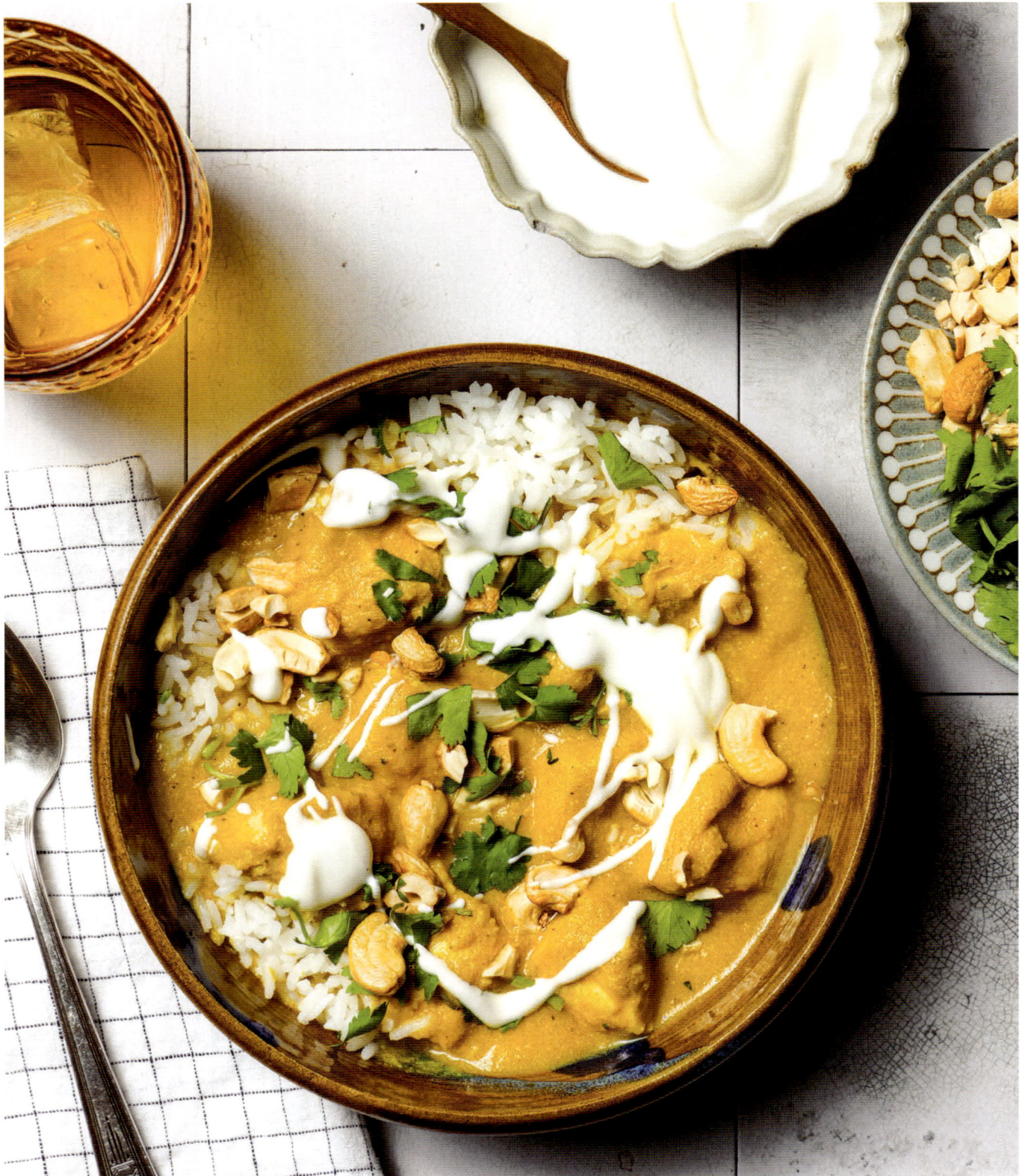

Golden Chicken Korma

Golden Chicken Korma

serves 4 • total time: 1 hour 5 minutes `SUPERCHARGED`

why this recipe works • Korma is a savory, saucy South Asian dish that generally features meat or vegetables simmered in a richly flavored sauce, frequently thickened with nuts, yogurt, coconut, or cream. The name comes from the Urdu word for "braise," describing the gentle process of simmering the dish over low heat and exemplifying the wide variety of styles and types of kormas eaten throughout South Asia. Our korma started with processing soaked cashews, browned onions, and tomato into a savory, velvety sauce full of healthy fats and antioxidants. We then bloomed a bevy of anti-inflammatory spices and aromatics—cloves, cinnamon, cardamom, turmeric, ginger, garlic, and cayenne—for maximum flavor and added the cashew-based sauce. Finally, in went lean chicken breast pieces to simmer gently in the sauce, so the meat stayed succulent. A sprinkle of cilantro and a drizzle of yogurt brought freshness and tang, respectively, to our finished dish. A rasp-style grater makes quick work of turning the garlic into a paste. Serve with rice.

- 3 tablespoons whole roasted cashews, plus 2 tablespoons chopped, divided
- ¾ cup hot water, plus ¾ cup tap water, divided
- 5 tablespoons extra-virgin olive oil, divided
- 2 onions, chopped fine
- 1½ teaspoons table salt, divided
- 1 tomato, cored and chopped coarse
- 4 (6- to 8-ounce) boneless, skinless chicken breasts, trimmed and cut into 1½-inch pieces
- 3 whole cloves
- 2 (3-inch) cinnamon sticks
- 2 bay leaves
- 4 garlic cloves, minced to paste
- 1 teaspoon grated fresh ginger
- 1 teaspoon ground coriander
- 1 teaspoon ground turmeric
- ½ teaspoon pepper
- ¼ teaspoon ground cardamom
- ¼ teaspoon cayenne pepper
- 1 cup coarsely chopped cilantro leaves and tender stems
  Plain yogurt

1 Process whole cashews in blender on low speed to consistency of fine gravel mixed with sand, 10 to 15 seconds. Add hot water and process on low speed until combined, about 5 seconds. Scrape down sides of blender jar and let mixture sit for 15 minutes.

2 Meanwhile, heat 3 tablespoons oil in Dutch oven over medium heat until shimmering. Add onions and ¼ teaspoon salt and cook, stirring occasionally, until dark golden brown, adjusting heat as needed if beginning to scorch, 10 to 15 minutes.

3 Transfer onions to blender jar along with tomato and process on low speed until coarse puree forms, about 1 minute. Scrape down sides of blender jar, then process on high speed until sauce is completely smooth, about 1 minute.

4 Pat chicken dry with paper towels and sprinkle with 1 teaspoon salt. Heat remaining 2 tablespoons oil in now-empty pot over medium heat until shimmering. Add cloves, cinnamon sticks, and bay leaves and cook, stirring occasionally, until fragrant, 30 to 60 seconds. Add garlic, ginger, coriander, turmeric, pepper, cardamom, and cayenne and cook until fragrant, 30 to 60 seconds. Add cashew-onion mixture, tap water, and remaining ¼ teaspoon salt and stir, scraping up any brown bits from bottom of pot. Bring to simmer, then reduce heat to low, cover, and simmer gently for 10 minutes.

5 Stir in chicken, increase heat to medium, and return to simmer. Reduce heat to medium-low, cover, and simmer gently until chicken registers 160 degrees, 10 to 15 minutes. Discard bay leaves and cinnamon. Sprinkle korma with cilantro and chopped cashews and serve with yogurt.

Nutrition Knowledge   I love that this boldly spiced chicken dish is more than just comforting—it's packed with anti-inflammatory power. Golden turmeric brings curcumin, a polyphenol known to ease inflammation at the cellular level, while fresh ginger and garlic deliver gingerol and allicin, compounds that support immunity and fight oxidative stress. Slow-cooked onions offer quercetin, a natural antihistamine, and juicy tomato adds a dose of lycopene, a carotenoid linked to reduced inflammation.

—*Alicia*

Skillet-Roasted Chicken Breasts with Garlic-Ginger Broccoli

serves 4 • total time: 50 minutes

why this recipe works • This simple yet satisfying recipe turns humble broccoli into a delicious vehicle for flavor. After roasting bone-in chicken breasts in the oven, we cooked garlic and fresh ginger in the juices left behind, maximizing all that meaty flavor. (Bonus: Garlic and ginger are excellent inflammation fighters.) From there, we added broccoli and water and let the cruciferous vegetable simmer. As the liquid reduced, the broccoli became coated in a luxuriously flavorful sauce. Be sure to remove excess fatty skin from the thick ends of the breasts when trimming. You will need a 12-inch ovensafe nonstick skillet with a tight-fitting lid for this recipe.

- 4 (10- to 12-ounce) bone-in split chicken breasts, trimmed
- 1¼ teaspoons table salt, divided
- 3 garlic cloves, sliced thin
- 2 teaspoons grated fresh ginger
- 2 teaspoons toasted sesame oil
- 1½ pounds broccoli, florets cut into ¾-inch pieces, stalks trimmed, peeled, and sliced on bias ¼ inch thick
- ½ cup water

1 Adjust oven rack to lower-middle position and heat oven to 325 degrees. Pat chicken dry with paper towels and sprinkle with ½ teaspoon salt. Place chicken skin side down in cold 12-inch ovensafe nonstick skillet. Cook over medium heat until skin is well browned, 5 to 7 minutes. Carefully flip chicken and transfer skillet to oven. Roast until chicken registers 160 degrees, 25 to 40 minutes.

2 Using potholders, remove skillet from oven. Being careful of hot skillet handle, transfer chicken to plate. Add garlic, ginger, oil, and remaining ¾ teaspoon salt to liquid left in skillet and cook over medium-high heat, stirring occasionally and scraping up any browned bits, until moisture has evaporated and mixture begins to sizzle, 2 to 4 minutes.

3 Add broccoli and water and bring to simmer. Cover skillet, reduce heat to medium, and cook until broccoli is crisp-tender, 5 minutes, stirring halfway through cooking. Uncover and continue to cook, stirring frequently, until broccoli is fully tender and sauce coats broccoli, 2 to 4 minutes. Add any accumulated chicken juices to skillet and toss to combine. Season with salt to taste. Serve chicken with broccoli.

MAKE AHEAD • Cooked chicken can be refrigerated for up to 3 days.

Skillet-Roasted Chicken Breasts with Harissa-Mint Carrots

serves 4 • total time: 1 hour

why this recipe works • Pairing spices with herbs is a great way to build flavor while boosting your meal with anti-inflammatory compounds. Here, spicy harissa and cooling mint add complex, balanced flavor to a skillet dinner of roasted bone-in chicken breasts and carrots. We cooked the dish in stages, first roasting bone-in chicken breasts until crispy, then cooking the carrots along with a shallot and harissa in the leftover juices. Be sure to remove excess fatty skin from the thick ends of the breasts when trimming. We prefer to use our homemade Harissa (page 106), but you can use store-bought. You will need a 12-inch ovensafe skillet with a tight-fitting lid in this recipe.

- 4 (10- to 12-ounce) bone-in split chicken breasts, trimmed
- 1 teaspoon table salt, divided
- 1 shallot, sliced thin
- 2 teaspoons harissa
- 1½ pounds carrots, peeled and sliced on bias ¼ inch thick
- ½ cup water
- 2 teaspoons lemon juice
- 1 tablespoon chopped fresh mint, divided

1 Adjust oven rack to lower-middle position and heat oven to 325 degrees. Pat chicken dry with paper towels and sprinkle with ½ teaspoon salt. Place chicken skin side down in cold 12-inch ovensafe nonstick skillet. Cook over medium heat until skin is well browned, 5 to 7 minutes. Carefully flip chicken and transfer skillet to oven. Roast until chicken registers 160 degrees, 25 to 40 minutes.

2 Using potholders, remove skillet from oven. Being careful of hot skillet, transfer chicken to cutting board. Add shallot, harissa, and remaining ½ teaspoon salt to liquid left in skillet and cook over medium-high heat, stirring occasionally and scraping up any browned bits, until moisture has evaporated and mixture begins to sizzle, 2 to 4 minutes.

3 Add carrots and water and bring to simmer. Cover skillet and cook until carrots are tender, 10 to 12 minutes, stirring halfway through cooking. Uncover and continue to cook, stirring frequently, until sauce begins to coat carrots, 2 to 4 minutes. Add lemon juice, 1½ teaspoons mint, and any accumulated chicken juices to skillet and toss to combine. Season with salt to taste and sprinkle with remaining 1½ teaspoons mint. Serve chicken with carrots.

MAKE AHEAD • Cooked chicken can be refrigerated for up to 3 days.

Skillet-Roasted Chicken Breasts with Garlicky Green Beans

serves 4 • total time: 1 hour

why this recipe works • This recipe is another twofer from one skillet. We pan-roasted bone-in chicken breasts, starting them in a cold skillet, which allowed the skin to brown without overcooking the interior, and then moved the chicken to the oven to finish. While the meat rested, we added garlic and red pepper flakes to the pan to cook briefly before adding green beans and some water. We covered the beans at first so that they could cook through and then uncovered the pan to allow the savory liquid to thicken into a sauce. Be sure to remove excess fatty skin from the thick ends of the breasts when trimming. You will need a 12-inch ovensafe skillet with a tight-fitting lid for this recipe.

- 4 (10- to 12-ounce) bone-in split chicken breasts, trimmed
- 1 teaspoon table salt, divided
- 3 garlic cloves, sliced thin
- ¼ teaspoon red pepper flakes
- 1¼ pounds green beans, trimmed
- ⅓ cup water
- 1½ ounces Parmesan cheese, shredded (½ cup) (optional)

1 Adjust oven rack to lower-middle position and heat oven to 325 degrees. Pat chicken dry with paper towels and sprinkle with ½ teaspoon salt. Place chicken skin side down in cold 12-inch ovensafe nonstick skillet. Cook over medium heat until skin is well browned, 5 to 7 minutes. Carefully flip chicken and transfer skillet to oven. Roast until chicken registers 160 degrees, 25 to 40 minutes.

2 Using potholders, remove skillet from oven. Being careful of hot skillet, transfer chicken to plate. Add garlic, pepper flakes, and remaining ½ teaspoon salt to liquid left in skillet and cook over medium-high heat, stirring occasionally and scraping up any browned bits, until moisture has evaporated and mixture begins to sizzle, 2 to 4 minutes.

3 Add green beans and water and bring to simmer. Cover skillet, reduce heat to medium, and cook until green beans are tender, 8 to 10 minutes, stirring halfway through cooking. Uncover and continue to cook, stirring frequently, until sauce begins to coat green beans, 2 to 4 minutes. Add any accumulated chicken juices to skillet and toss to combine. Season with salt to taste. Transfer green beans to serving platter and sprinkle with Parmesan, if using. Top with chicken and serve.

MAKE AHEAD • Cooked chicken can be refrigerated for up to 3 days.

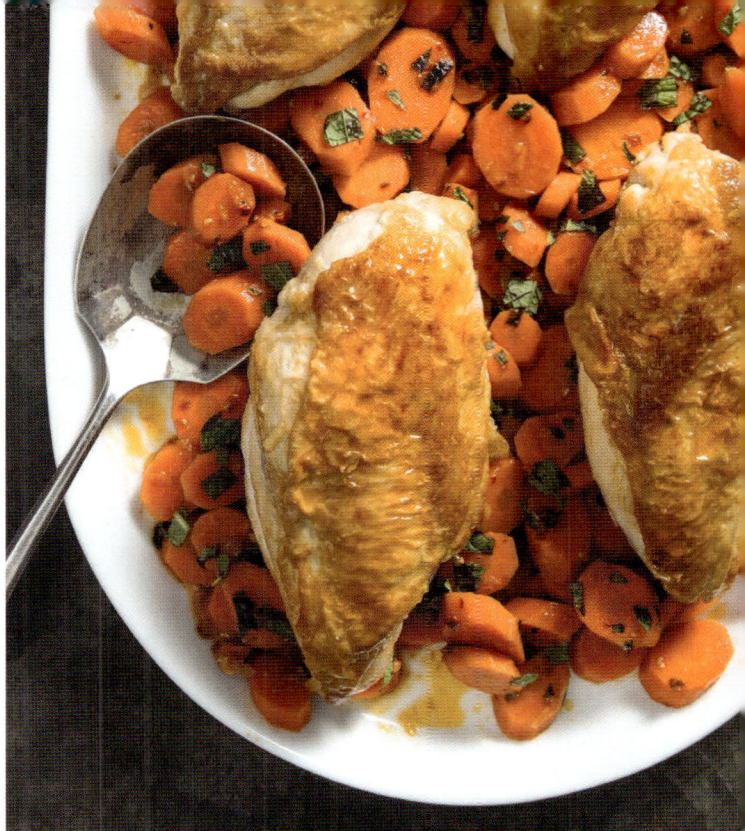
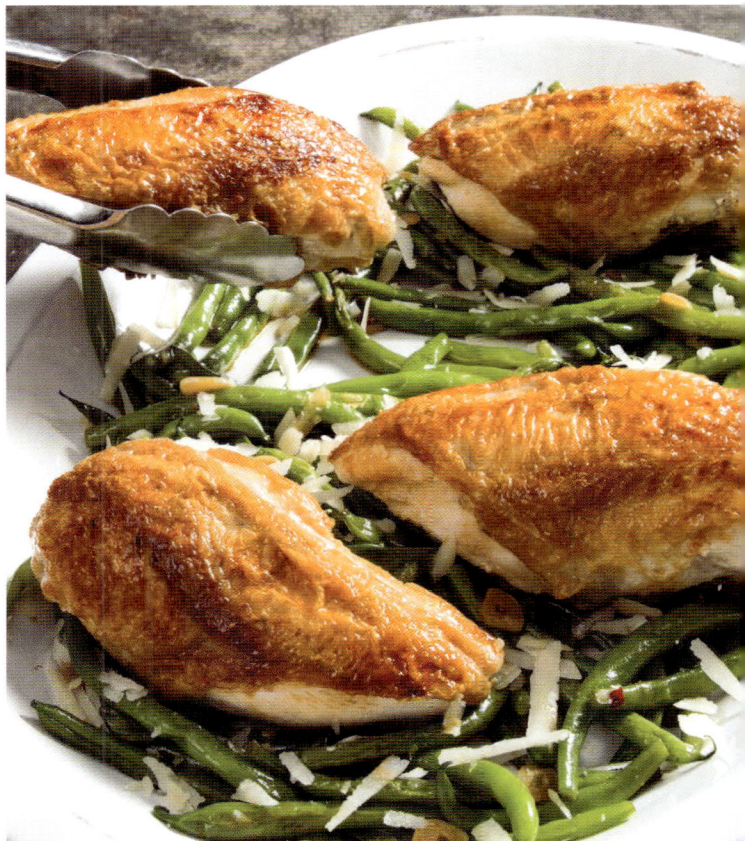

top | *Skillet-Roasted Chicken Breasts with Harissa-Mint Carrots*
bottom | *Skillet-Roasted Chicken Breasts with Garlicky Green Beans*

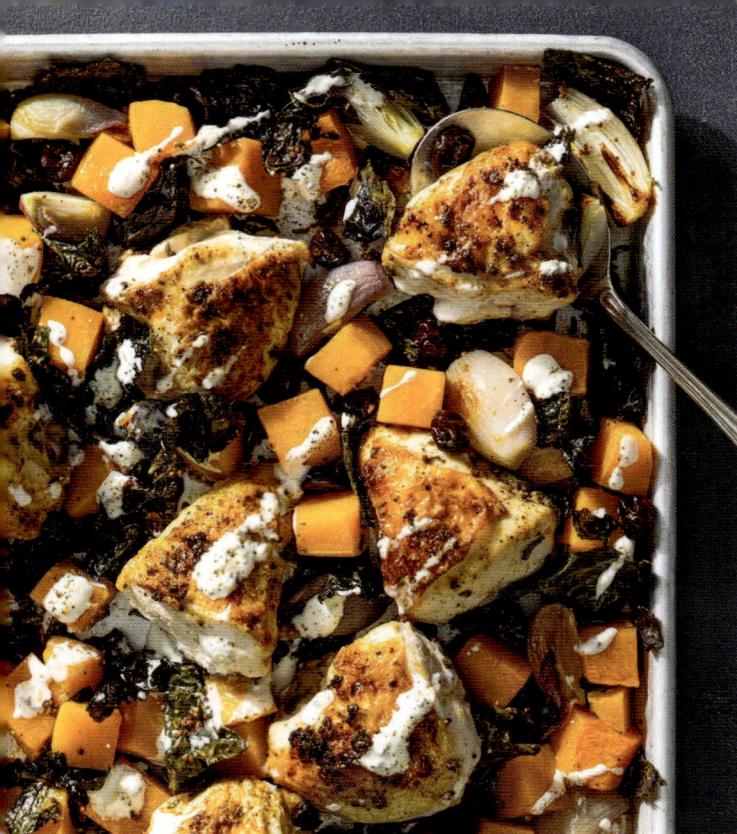

One-Pan Chicken with Butternut Squash and Kale

serves 4 · total time: 1 hour

why this recipe works · A baking sheet full of roast chicken, kale, and butternut squash promised a satisfying, nutrient-dense meal with minimal cleanup. However, in order to combine sturdy squash, dark leafy greens, and chicken in a single pan, we needed to get them to cook at the same rate. We used bone-in split chicken breasts, a relatively lean cut that also wouldn't smother the vegetables underneath and cause them to steam. A simple sage marinade seasoned both the chicken and vegetables. After just half an hour of roasting, we had crisp chicken, tender squash, and lightly crispy kale. A sprinkle of dried tart cherries—a source of flavonoids, which bring anti-inflammatory benefits—added sweet-tangy chew to the mix. We topped our chicken with a drizzle of light, creamy yogurt sauce accented with orange zest to bring the dish into harmony. Both curly and lacinato kale will work here.

- 6 tablespoons extra-virgin olive oil, divided
- 3 tablespoons minced fresh sage, divided
- 1 tablespoon whole-grain mustard
- 1 teaspoon table salt, divided
- ½ teaspoon pepper, divided
- ¾ cup plain yogurt
- 2 teaspoons grated orange zest, divided
- 8 ounces kale, stemmed and cut into 2-inch pieces
- 2 pounds butternut squash, peeled, seeded, and cut into 1-inch pieces (6 cups)
- 8 shallots, peeled and halved
- ½ cup dried tart cherries
- 4 (10- to 12-ounce) bone-in split chicken breasts, trimmed and halved crosswise

1 Adjust oven rack to upper-middle position and heat oven to 475 degrees. Whisk 5 tablespoons oil, 2 tablespoons sage, mustard, ½ teaspoon salt, and ¼ teaspoon pepper together in large bowl until well combined. In separate bowl, whisk together yogurt, 1 teaspoon orange zest, and 1 tablespoon oil mixture, then season with salt and pepper to taste; set sauce aside.

2 Vigorously squeeze and massage kale with hands in large bowl until leaves are uniformly darkened and slightly wilted, about 1 minute. Add squash, shallots, cherries, and remaining oil mixture and toss to combine. Spread into single layer on rimmed baking sheet. Combine remaining 1 tablespoon oil, remaining 1 tablespoon sage, remaining 1 teaspoon orange zest, remaining ½ teaspoon salt, and remaining ¼ teaspoon pepper in now-empty

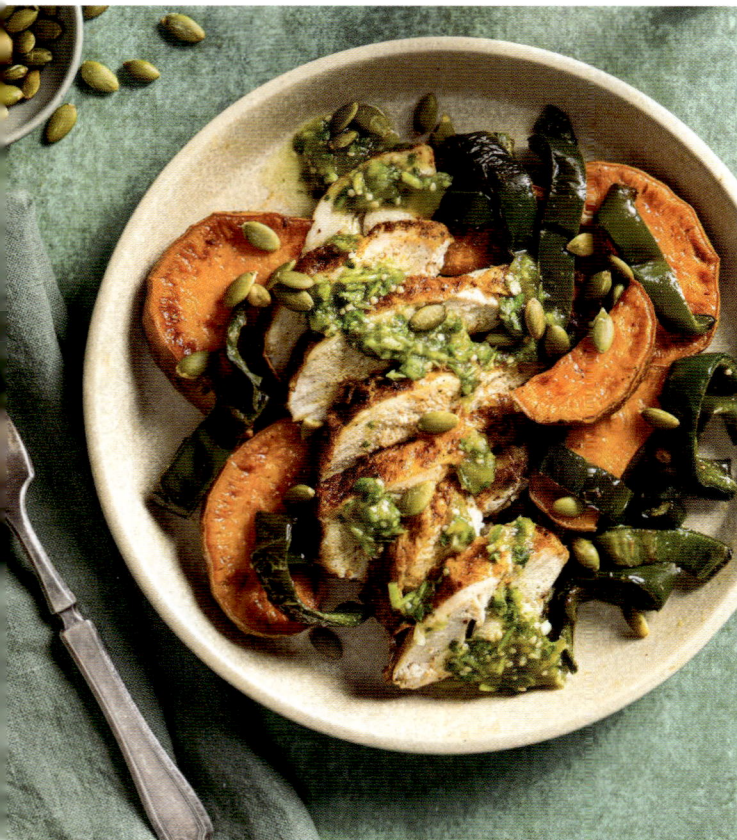

top | *One-Pan Chicken with Butternut Squash and Kale*
bottom | *One-Pan Roasted Chicken Breasts with Sweet Potatoes, Poblanos, and Tomatillo Salsa*

bowl, then add chicken and toss to coat. Place chicken, skin side up, on top of vegetables on sheet. Transfer sheet to oven and roast until chicken registers 160 degrees, 25 to 35 minutes, rotating sheet halfway through baking.

3 Transfer chicken to serving platter, tent with aluminum foil, and let rest for 10 minutes. Toss vegetables with any accumulated chicken juices on sheet, then transfer to platter with chicken. Drizzle ¼ cup yogurt sauce over chicken and vegetables and serve, passing remaining yogurt sauce separately.

MAKE AHEAD • Cooked chicken-vegetable mixture and yogurt sauce can be refrigerated for up to 3 days.

MAKE IT DAIRY-FREE • Substitute plant-based yogurt for the dairy yogurt.

One-Pan Roasted Chicken Breasts with Sweet Potatoes, Poblanos, and Tomatillo Salsa

serves 4 • total time: 1 hour   **SUPERCHARGED**

why this recipe works • For this Southwest-inspired anti-inflammatory sheet-pan dinner, we started with bone-in chicken breasts—a lean yet still flavorful cut. The skin and bone added flavor and moisture that kept the meat tender and juicy even while roasting. Seasoned with a mixture of inflammation-fighting spices like fruity ancho chili powder, warming cumin, and herbaceous oregano, the chicken roasted over strips of poblano chiles, which are full of antioxidants. Bright-orange sweet potatoes made for a creamy, fiberful starch, while tomatillos added tartness and complexity. We removed the tomatillos from the oven when they began to burst and processed them into a quick salsa that contributed bright acidity, not to mention a phytonutrient boost. A final sprinkling of roasted pepitas offered pops of crunch plus a dose of healthy fats. The result was a well-rounded, utterly delicious meal. A rasp-style grater makes quick work of turning the garlic into a paste.

- 1½ pounds sweet potatoes, unpeeled, halved lengthwise, and sliced crosswise ¾ inch thick
- 3 poblano chiles, stemmed, halved, seeded, and cut crosswise into ½-inch-wide strips
- 8 ounces tomatillos, husks and stems removed, rinsed well and dried

- 2 tablespoons extra-virgin olive oil
- 1¼ teaspoons table salt, divided
- 1 teaspoon ancho chili powder
- 1 teaspoon ground cumin
- 1 teaspoon dried oregano
- ¼ teaspoon pepper
- 4 (10- to 12-ounce) bone-in split chicken breasts, trimmed
- 1 cup coarsely chopped fresh cilantro leaves and tender stems
- ½ serrano chile, stemmed and chopped
- 1 small garlic clove, minced to paste
- 2 tablespoons roasted pepitas

1 Adjust oven rack to middle position and heat oven to 475 degrees. Spray rimmed baking sheet with avocado oil spray. Toss sweet potatoes, poblanos, tomatillos, oil, and ½ teaspoon salt together on prepared sheet. Arrange sweet potatoes and tomatillos around perimeter of sheet and poblanos in center of sheet in even layer.

2 Combine chili powder, cumin, oregano, pepper, and ½ teaspoon salt in bowl. Pat chicken dry with paper towels, sprinkle all over with spice mixture, and place skin side up over poblanos on sheet. Roast until tomatillos are lightly browned and split, 15 to 20 minutes.

3 Remove sheet from oven and transfer tomatillos to food processor workbowl. Return sheet with sweet potatoes, chicken, and poblanos to oven and continue to roast until chicken registers 160 degrees, 15 to 20 minutes longer.

4 Meanwhile, let tomatillos cool 10 minutes. Add cilantro, serrano, garlic, and remaining ¼ teaspoon salt to processor bowl with tomatillos. Pulse until slightly chunky, 10 to 12 pulses; set salsa aside until ready to serve.

5 Remove sheet from oven and transfer chicken to large platter. Return vegetables still on sheet to oven and continue to roast until poblanos are completely softened, 5 to 7 minutes.

6 Toss vegetables with juices on sheet, then transfer to platter with chicken. Sprinkle with pepitas and serve with reserved tomatillo salsa.

MAKE AHEAD • Cooked chicken and vegetables and prepared salsa can be refrigerated for up to 2 days.

One-Pan Ratatouille with Chicken

serves 4 • total time: 1¾ hours

why this recipe works • This one-pan ratatouille jazzes up lean bone-in chicken breasts with a colorful array of vegetables, creating a well-rounded meal. The traditional ratatouille mix of eggplant, squash, bell peppers, and tomatoes offered an impressive range of antioxidants and phytonutrients; we opted to roast them on a baking sheet until they turned soft and juicy. We then removed the sheet from the oven, scooted the vegetables over to one side, and added the chicken, minimizing clean-up and taking advantage of the already-hot oven. A sprinkling of lemon zest and thyme enhanced the ratatouille with warm flavor and anti-inflammatory benefits.

- 1 pound eggplant, peeled and cut into 1-inch pieces
- 12 ounces yellow summer squash, cut into 1-inch pieces
- 2 red bell peppers, stemmed, seeded, and cut into 1-inch pieces
- 10 ounces grape tomatoes
- 6 shallots, sliced thin
- 1 tablespoon extra-virgin olive oil
- 3 garlic cloves, sliced thin
- 1¼ teaspoons table salt, divided
- 1¼ teaspoons pepper, divided
- 4 (10- to 12-ounce) bone-in split chicken breasts, trimmed
- ½ cup pitted kalamata olives, halved
- ¼ cup chopped fresh basil
- 2 teaspoons grated lemon zest, plus lemon wedges for serving
- 2 teaspoons minced fresh thyme

1 Adjust oven rack to middle position and heat oven to 450 degrees. Toss eggplant, squash, bell peppers, tomatoes, shallots, oil, garlic, ¾ teaspoon salt, and 1 teaspoon pepper together on rimmed baking sheet and spread into even layer. Roast until vegetables are slightly softened and beginning to char in spots, about 25 minutes, stirring halfway through roasting.

2 Pat chicken dry with paper towels and sprinkle with remaining ½ teaspoon salt and remaining ¼ teaspoon pepper. Remove sheet from oven. Using silicone spatula, push vegetables to 1 side of sheet. Arrange chicken, skin side up, on now-empty side of sheet. Roast until chicken registers 160 degrees and vegetables are completely softened, about 25 minutes, stirring vegetables and rotating sheet halfway through roasting.

3 Remove sheet from oven, tent with aluminum foil, and let rest for 5 minutes. Transfer chicken to cutting board, carve chicken from bones (discard bones), and slice chicken ½ inch thick. Stir vegetables and pan juices until juices are almost completely absorbed and vegetables are well coated, about 1 minute. Stir in olives and basil and top with chicken. Combine lemon zest and thyme in small bowl and sprinkle over chicken. Serve with lemon wedges.

MAKE AHEAD • Cooked chicken and vegetables can be refrigerated for up to 2 days.

Spiced Ginger Chicken with Potatoes, Cauliflower, and Pickled Onions

serves 4 • total time: 1 hour

why this recipe works • This zingy and warmly spiced sheet-pan meal starts by blooming a fragrant, antioxidant-rich mix of garlic, paprika, ginger, coriander, and cayenne in oil using the microwave—an easy way to intensify their flavors. We used half of this spiced oil to coat cauliflower wedges and thick-cut potato slices, which we roasted at 500 degrees; the high temperature enabled the vegetables to develop deep and flavorful caramelization. We then nudged the vegetables to one side of the pan to make room for halved boneless chicken breasts, which we tossed with the remaining spiced oil to infuse the meat with bold, smoky flavor. After everything roasted to golden perfection, pickled red onion introduced a bright, tangy contrast, while a cooling yogurt sauce laced with lime zest and fresh herbs balanced the mild heat.

- ½ cup plain yogurt
- ¼ cup chopped fresh cilantro, dill, mint, and/or parsley
- ½ teaspoon grated lime zest
- 6 tablespoons avocado oil
- 8 garlic cloves, minced
- 4 teaspoons paprika
- 2 teaspoons ground coriander
- 2 teaspoons ground ginger
- 1¼ teaspoons table salt
- ½ teaspoon cayenne pepper
- 4 (6- to 8-ounce) boneless, skinless chicken breasts, trimmed
- 1 head cauliflower (2 pounds)
- 1½ pounds Yukon Gold potatoes, unpeeled, sliced ¾ inch thick
- ½ English cucumber, cut into ¾-inch pieces
- 1 recipe Quick Pickled Red Onions (page 25)

1   Adjust oven rack to upper-middle position and heat oven to 500 degrees. Combine yogurt, cilantro, and lime zest in bowl. Adjust consistency with water and season with salt and pepper to taste; refrigerate until ready to serve.

2   Combine oil, garlic, paprika, coriander, ginger, salt, and cayenne in medium bowl. Microwave until fragrant and bubbling, about 30 seconds. Transfer half of spiced oil to large bowl; set aside. Gently pound thicker ends of breasts until ½ inch thick and slice in half crosswise. Pat chicken dry with paper towels, add to remaining spiced oil, and toss until evenly coated; set aside.

3   Trim outer leaves of cauliflower and cut stem flush with bottom. Cut head through core into 8 equal wedges so that core and florets remain intact. Add potatoes and cauliflower to large bowl with reserved spiced oil and toss gently to coat. Arrange vegetables cut sides down in single layer on aluminum foil–lined rimmed baking sheet. Roast until nearly tender, about 20 minutes. Using spatula, push vegetables to cover two-thirds of sheet (they will no longer be in single layer) and arrange chicken on now-empty side of sheet. Roast until breasts register 160 degrees and vegetables are softened and spotty brown, 10 to 12 minutes.

4   Transfer chicken and vegetables to serving platter and top with cucumber and pickled onions. Serve with yogurt sauce.

MAKE AHEAD • Cooked chicken and vegetables and prepared yogurt sauce can be refrigerated for up to 2 days.

MAKE IT DAIRY-FREE • Substitute plant-based yogurt for the dairy yogurt.

Green Mole with Chayote and Chicken

serves 4 • total time: 1¼ hours

why this recipe works • Mole verde, an herby green variety of mole, is highly popular in Mexico. Unlike mole poblano (perhaps more famous globally), which uses an assortment of dried chiles, fruit, and spices, green mole uses fresh chiles and tomatillos, sesame seeds, pepitas, and plenty of herbs. For our take, we used a pound of chicken thighs cut into pieces and then bulked up the meat with tender bites of nutrient-rich chayote. Though the meat is usually poached first (and the cooking liquid used as broth for the mole), we added the raw meat straight to the sauce; the chicken released rich juices into the sauce as it cooked. To make the mole sauce, we blended the aromatics and seeds into a smooth and luscious puree. You can substitute 1 drained 28-ounce can of tomatillos for fresh. If you can't find chayote, you can

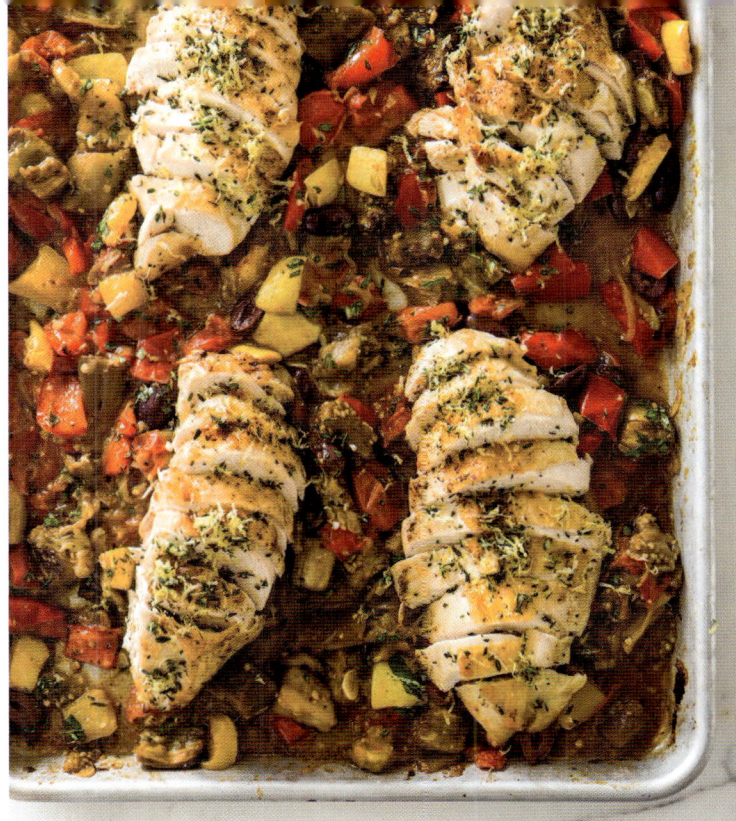

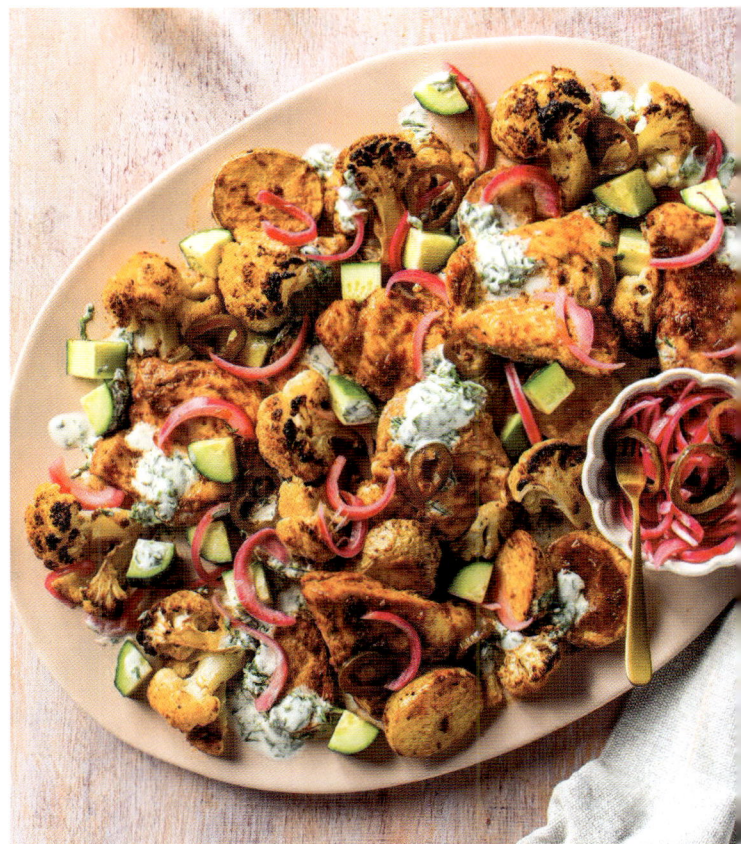

top	One-Pan Ratatouille with Chicken
bottom	Spiced Ginger Chicken with Potatoes, Cauliflower, and Pickled Onions

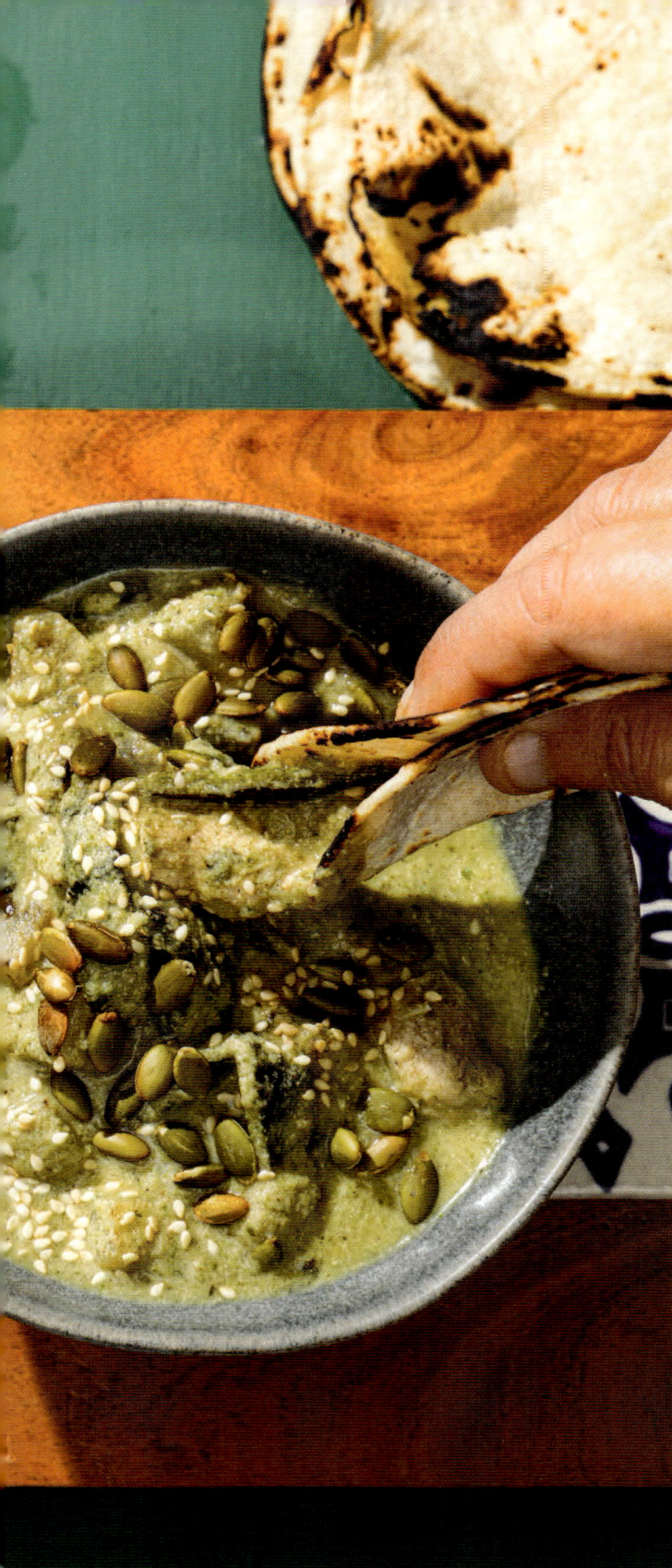

substitute 1½ pounds of zucchini, halved lengthwise and then sliced crosswise ¼ inch thick. After searing the zucchini in step 4, transfer it to a bowl and then stir it into the pot with the poblanos in step 6. Serve with rice or warm corn tortillas.

3	poblano chiles, stemmed, halved, and seeded
1	pound tomatillos, husks and stems removed, rinsed well and dried
1	serrano or jalapeño chile, stemmed, halved, and seeded
1	onion, chopped coarse
½	cup unsalted roasted pepitas, plus extra for serving
¼	cup sesame seeds, toasted, plus extra for serving
4	garlic cloves, chopped
1¼	teaspoons table salt, divided
1	teaspoon dried Mexican oregano
¾	teaspoon ground cumin
½	teaspoon ground allspice
1	tablespoon avocado oil
1½	pounds chayote, peeled, cored, and cut into ½-inch pieces
1	pound boneless, skinless chicken thighs, trimmed and cut into 1-inch pieces
1¾	cups unsalted chicken broth, divided, plus extra as needed
1	ounce fresh cilantro leaves and tender stems (about 2½ cups)

1   Adjust oven rack 3 to 4 inches from broiler element and heat broiler. Line rimmed baking sheet with aluminum foil. Arrange poblanos skin side up on prepared sheet and press to flatten. Broil until skin is puffed and most of surface is well charred, 5 to 10 minutes, rotating sheet halfway through broiling.

2   Using tongs, pile poblanos in center of foil. Gather foil over poblanos and crimp to form pouch. Let steam for 10 minutes. Open foil packet carefully and spread out poblanos. When cool enough to handle, peel poblanos (it's OK if some bits of skin remain intact) and discard skins. Slice crosswise into ½-inch-thick strips and set aside.

3   Meanwhile, combine tomatillos, serrano, onion, pepitas, sesame seeds, garlic, ¾ teaspoon salt, oregano, cumin, and allspice in blender and process until smooth, about 2 minutes.

Green Mole with Chayote and Chicken

4 Heat oil in Dutch oven over medium-high heat until just smoking. Add chayote and ¼ teaspoon salt and cook until well browned, 8 to 10 minutes. Off heat, carefully add tomatillo sauce (it will splatter). Cook over medium heat, stirring frequently, until slightly darkened and thickened, about 5 minutes.

5 Stir chicken, 1¼ cups broth, and remaining ¼ teaspoon salt into pot and bring to simmer. Cover, reduce heat to medium-low, and simmer gently until chicken is cooked through and chayote is tender, about 20 minutes.

6 Combine cilantro and remaining ½ cup broth in clean, dry blender jar and process until just smooth, 30 to 45 seconds (do not overprocess). Stir cilantro mixture and reserved poblanos into mole in pot and bring to simmer. Season with salt and pepper to taste, and thin mole with extra broth as needed. Sprinkle individual portions with extra pepitas and sesame seeds and serve.

MAKE AHEAD • Cooked chicken and mole can be prepared through step 5 and refrigerated for up to 2 days.

PREPPING CHAYOTE

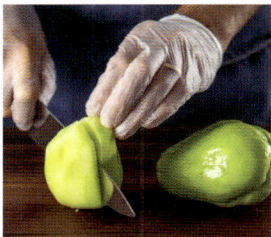

1 After peeling chayote, cut in half lengthwise. You can wear gloves to prevent getting sticky film on your hands.

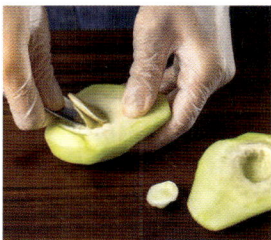

2 Using small spoon or your fingers, scoop out core and discard.

Chicken Mole with Cilantro-Lime Rice and Beans

serves 4 • total time: 1½ hours

why this recipe works • Rich sauces might scare those cooking for anti-inflammation, as they can be heavy with butter and cream, but a deeply flavored Mexican mole is both decadent and nourishing. The version here, decidedly quick but still complex, achieves richness from the fruity, nutty, and spicy flavors of chili powder, cocoa powder, tomato, and raisins. These all offer anti-inflammatory benefits, while a bit of peanut butter contributes more richness and helps thicken the sauce. The flavors of this sauce are imbued into boneless chicken thighs as they simmer to tenderness on the stovetop. We created a complete, fiberful meal by baking brown rice while the chicken and sauce simmered and then adding black beans to warm in the rice. Finally, we fluffed cilantro and lime into the rice and beans to complete our side. For an accurate measurement of boiling water, bring a full kettle of water to a boil and then measure out the desired amount. You will need a 12-inch skillet with a tight-fitting lid for this recipe.

2⅓ cups plus ¾ cup boiling water, divided
1½ cups long-grain brown rice, rinsed
4 teaspoons avocado oil, divided
½ teaspoon table salt, divided
3 tablespoons raisins
1 tablespoon chili powder
1 tablespoon unsweetened cocoa powder
1 tomato, cored and chopped
1 tablespoon creamy peanut butter
1 pound boneless, skinless chicken thighs, trimmed
1 (15-ounce) can no-salt-added black beans, rinsed
½ cup chopped fresh cilantro, divided
1 teaspoon grated lime zest and 1 tablespoon juice, plus lime wedges for serving

1 Adjust oven rack to middle position and heat oven to 375 degrees. Combine 2⅓ cups boiling water, rice, 2 teaspoons oil, and ¼ teaspoon salt in 8-inch square baking dish. Cover dish tightly with aluminum foil and bake until rice is tender and no water remains, about 1 hour.

2 Meanwhile, combine raisins, chili powder, cocoa, and remaining 2 teaspoons oil in small bowl. Microwave, stirring occasionally, until fragrant, 30 to 45 seconds. Process raisin mixture with tomato, peanut butter, remaining ¾ cup boiling water, and remaining ¼ teaspoon salt in blender until smooth, about 1 minute, scraping down sides of blender jar as needed. Transfer puree to 12-inch skillet.

3   Nestle chicken into sauce in skillet and bring to simmer over medium heat. Reduce heat to medium-low, cover, and cook until chicken registers at least 175 degrees, 20 to 25 minutes, flipping chicken halfway through cooking.

4   Transfer chicken to cutting board, tent with foil, and let rest while finishing sauce. Return sauce to simmer over medium heat and cook until thickened slightly, about 5 minutes. Whisk sauce to recombine and season with salt and pepper to taste.

5   Remove rice from oven and fluff with fork, scraping up any rice stuck to bottom of dish. Add beans in even layer over rice, cover, and let sit until beans are heated through, about 10 minutes. Add ¼ cup cilantro and lime zest and juice to rice and beans, fluff with fork to combine, and season with salt and pepper to taste. Slice chicken ½ inch thick and serve with rice and beans, sauce, lime wedges, and remaining ¼ cup cilantro.

MAKE AHEAD • Cooked chicken, rice and beans, and sauce can be refrigerated for up to 3 days.

Pulled Jackfruit and Chicken Sandwiches

serves 4 • total time: 50 minutes

why this recipe works • Ripe jackfruit tastes like a combination of papaya, pineapple, and mango, but immature jackfruit is entirely different: dense, vegetal, and fibrous. The latter, when cooked and shredded, has a tender, stringy texture remarkably reminiscent of pulled chicken or pork, so it's no surprise that the tropical ingredient—long beloved in many Asian cultures—is becoming a popular meat alternative all over the world. The fiber-rich fruit also has a knack for soaking up seasoning, so tossing it with shredded chicken smothered in a smoky-sweet sauce boosted the fiber content of our sandwich without sacrificing flavor. To prepare the jackfruit, we simmered it to slightly soften the texture before stirring it into our pulled chicken. In true pulled-meat-sandwich fashion, we included a tangy slaw of seasoned cabbage and carrot tossed with oil and vinegar. We layered the jackfruit-chicken mixture and slaw onto hamburger buns for a satisfyingly juicy handheld meal. Be sure to use young (unripe) jackfruit packed in water; do not use mature jackfruit packed in syrup. Jackfruit seeds are tender and edible; there is no need to remove them. To minimize added sugar and salt, we like to use our homemade Easy Barbecue Sauce, but you can use store-bought if you prefer. You can substitute 1¾ cups shredded coleslaw mix for the red cabbage and carrot.

1   (20-ounce) can young green jackfruit packed in water, drained
1   teaspoon avocado oil
4   scallions, white and green parts separated and sliced thin
2   garlic cloves, minced
¾   cup Easy Barbecue Sauce (recipe follows)
2   tablespoons low-sodium soy sauce
2   tablespoons water
12   ounces boneless skinless chicken thighs, trimmed
2   tablespoons cider vinegar
1   tablespoon extra-virgin olive oil
¼   teaspoon table salt
⅛   teaspoon pepper
1½   cups shredded red cabbage
1   carrot, peeled and shredded
4   hamburger buns, toasted
    Dill pickle chips (optional)

1   Place jackfruit in large saucepan, cover with water, and bring to boil over high heat. Reduce heat to medium and simmer for 10 minutes. Drain jackfruit in strainer, rinse well, and shake strainer to drain thoroughly. Transfer jackfruit to cutting board. Using potato masher, 2 forks, or your hands, shred jackfruit into bite-size pieces, then chop coarse with knife. Set aside.

2   Heat avocado oil in now-empty saucepan over medium heat until shimmering. Add scallion whites and garlic and cook, stirring occasionally, until scallions soften, about 2 minutes. Stir in barbecue sauce, soy sauce, and water, scraping up any browned bits. Nestle chicken into sauce, cover, and simmer until chicken registers 175 degrees, 8 to 12 minutes, flipping chicken halfway through cooking.

3   Remove saucepan from heat. Transfer chicken to plate and let cool slightly. Using 2 forks, shred chicken fine. Return shredded chicken and reserved shredded jackfruit to saucepan and stir to coat evenly in sauce. Cook over medium-low heat until chicken and jackfruit are heated through, 2 to 4 minutes, stirring occasionally.

4   Whisk vinegar, olive oil, salt, and pepper together in medium bowl. Add cabbage, carrot, and scallion greens and toss to coat. Divide chicken and jackfruit mixture among bun bottoms; top with slaw and bun tops. Top with pickles, if using, and serve.

MAKE AHEAD • Cooked and shredded chicken and jackfruit mixture can be refrigerated for up to 3 days.

MAKE IT GLUTEN-FREE • Substitute gluten-free hamburger buns for the hamburger buns and low-sodium tamari for low-sodium soy sauce.

Easy Barbecue Sauce

makes about 1¼ cups · **total time: 25 minutes**

- 1 tablespoon avocado oil
- ¼ cup grated onion
- ½ teaspoon garlic powder
- ½ teaspoon chili powder
- ⅛ teaspoon cayenne pepper
- ¾ cup ketchup
- 2 tablespoons molasses
- 2 tablespoons cider vinegar
- 1½ tablespoons Worcestershire sauce
- 1 tablespoon Dijon mustard
- ½ teaspoon hot sauce

1 Heat oil in small saucepan over medium heat until shimmering. Add onion and cook, stirring occasionally, until softened, about 5 minutes. Stir in garlic powder, chili powder, and cayenne and cook until fragrant, about 30 seconds.

2 Stir in ketchup, molasses, vinegar, Worcestershire, mustard, and hot sauce and bring to simmer. Reduce heat to low and cook until flavors meld, about 5 minutes. Let cool completely before serving. (Cooled sauce can be refrigerated for up to 1 week.)

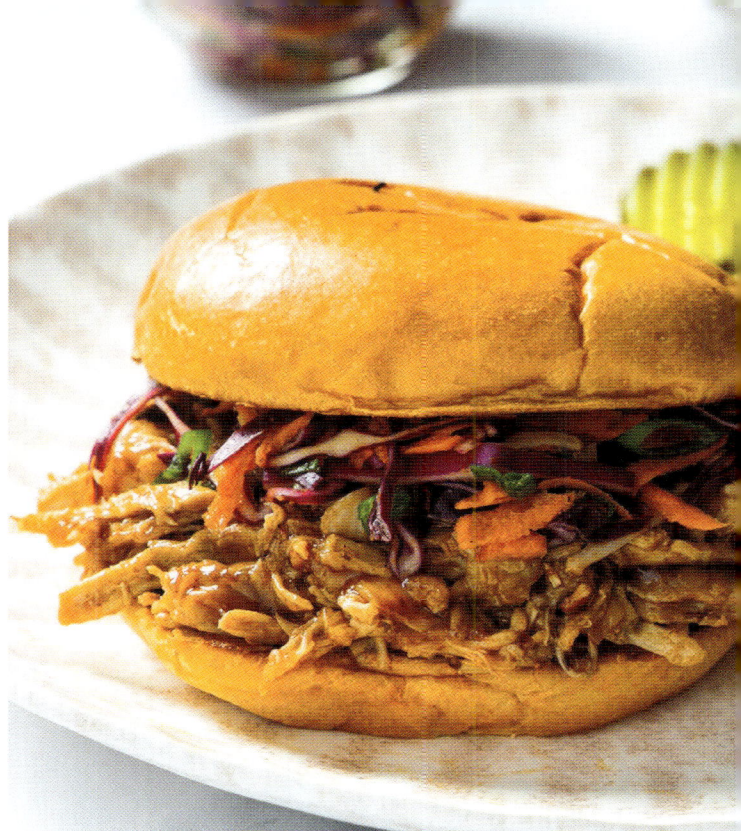

Cardamom-Spiced Chicken Curry with Tomatoes

serves 4 · **total time: 40 minutes** **FAST**

why this recipe works · Tomatoes, cardamom, ginger, and garlic are the highlights of this fragrant and antioxidant-filled chicken curry whose flavor payoff is far greater than what you might expect from such a simple dish. Chunks of boneless, skinless chicken thighs stayed moist and tender as they simmered in the flavorful curry sauce. The tomatoes added juiciness, texture, and sweet acidity as well as anti-inflammatory compounds. To give the dish body and creaminess (without the saturated fat from cream), we tempered ½ cup of tangy, gut-healthy yogurt with some of the sauce, then stirred it back into the dish (tempering helped prevent curdling). Serve with rice, other grains, or flatbread.

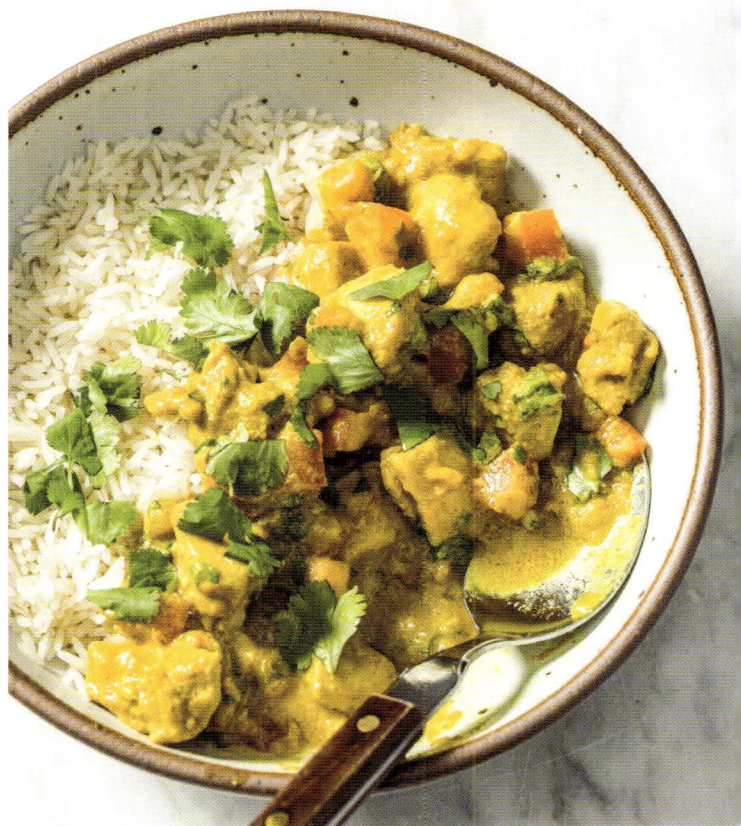

| top | Pulled Jackfruit and Chicken Sandwiches |
| bottom | Cardamom-Spiced Chicken Curry with Tomatoes |

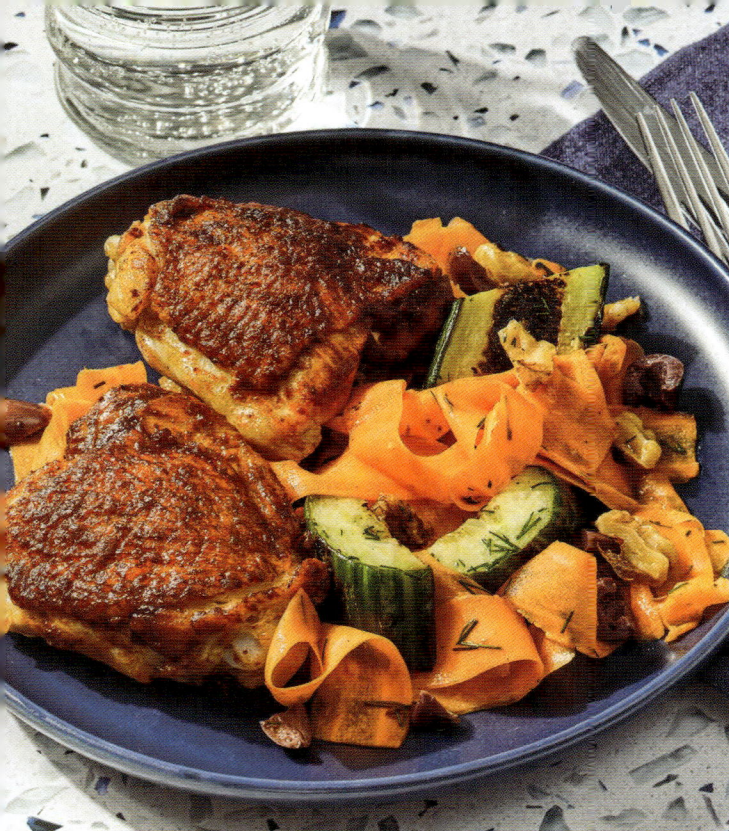

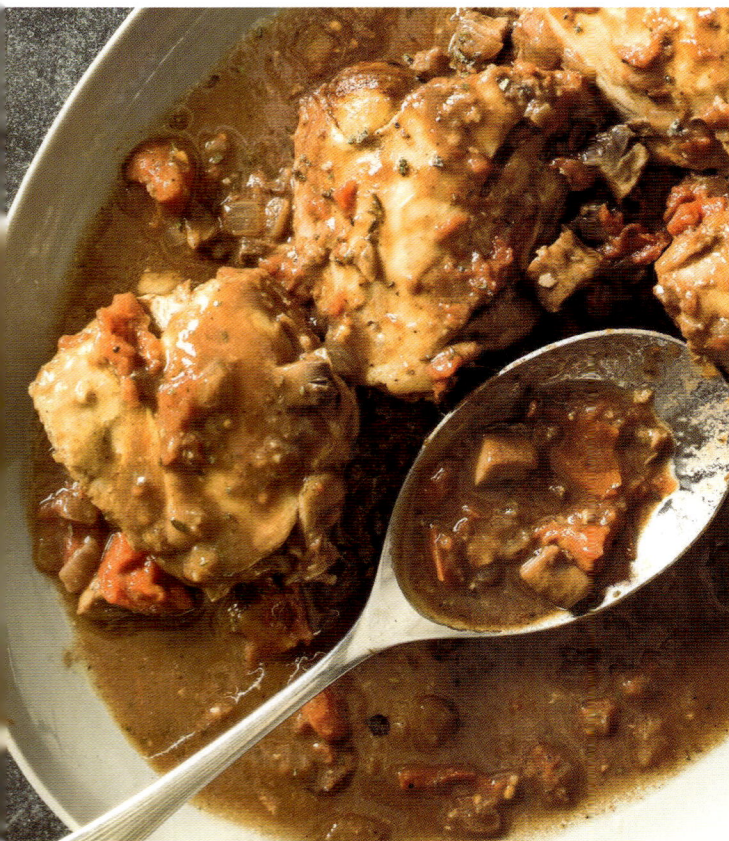

1½ pounds boneless, skinless chicken thighs, trimmed and cut into 1-inch pieces

1 tablespoon yellow curry powder, divided

1 teaspoon table salt, divided

¼ teaspoon pepper

2 tablespoons avocado oil

1 onion, chopped fine

4 garlic cloves, minced

2 teaspoons grated fresh ginger

1 teaspoon ground cardamom

¾ cup unsalted chicken broth

3 tomatoes, cored and chopped, divided

½ cup plain yogurt

2 tablespoons chopped fresh cilantro

1   Pat chicken dry with paper towels. Toss chicken with 2 teaspoons curry powder, ½ teaspoon salt, and pepper in bowl and set aside.

2   Heat oil in 12-inch skillet over medium heat until shimmering. Add onion and remaining ½ teaspoon salt and cook until softened, about 5 minutes. Add garlic, ginger, cardamom, and remaining 1 teaspoon curry powder and cook until fragrant, about 30 seconds. Stir in chicken and cook, stirring often, until lightly browned, about 3 minutes.

3   Stir in broth and half of tomatoes, scraping up any browned bits, and bring to boil over high heat. Reduce heat to medium-low and simmer until chicken is tender and sauce is slightly thickened and reduced by about half, 8 to 10 minutes.

4   Remove skillet from heat. In small bowl, whisk yogurt until smooth. Whisking constantly, slowly ladle about 1 cup hot liquid from skillet into yogurt and whisk until combined. Stir yogurt mixture back into skillet until combined. Stir in cilantro and remaining tomatoes, season with salt and pepper to taste, and serve.

Harissa-Rubbed Chicken Thighs with Charred Cucumber and Carrot Salad

serves 4 to 6 · total time: 1 hour

why this recipe works · We love the delicious simplicity of pan-roasted chicken thighs that emerge from the oven burnished a deep mahogany, with crispy skin. Here, a cast-iron skillet pulled double duty: first creating an unusual side dish of charred yet still tender cucumber chunks and then taking the chicken thighs from stovetop to oven in a classic pan-roasting technique. We brushed the chicken skin with harissa, but only after the initial sear, so the skin darkened beautifully in the oven and prevented the harissa from burning. To transform the humble cucumber, we cut it on the bias into large pieces and cooked it in the hot, preheated dry pan, preserving its interior cooling freshness while adding a light char. We also shaved carrots into thin ribbons, then softened their raw crunch in a concentrated, caraway-laced dressing. The acidity of the vinegar and the sweetness of the carrots and cucumber balanced the spicy richness of the chicken. Olives, toasted walnuts, and fresh dill added nutrients, texture, and flavors to complete this one-pan meal. If your chicken thighs are larger than 5 to 7 ounces each, use fewer of them to maintain a total weight of 2½ to 3½ pounds; adjust cooking time as needed. We prefer our homemade Harissa (page 106), but you can use store-bought if you prefer. A cast-iron skillet will achieve the best char on the cucumber, but a 12-inch stainless-steel skillet can also be used—before cooking the cucumber, heat 1 teaspoon avocado oil in the skillet over medium-high heat until just smoking.

2 tablespoons white wine vinegar
1 small shallot, minced
1 teaspoon caraway seeds, toasted and cracked
1 teaspoon Dijon mustard
1 teaspoon table salt, divided
¼ cup extra-virgin olive oil
1 pound carrots, peeled and shaved into ribbons using vegetable peeler
1 English cucumber, halved lengthwise and sliced crosswise 1 inch thick on bias
8 (5- to 7-ounce) bone-in chicken thighs, trimmed
1 tablespoon avocado oil
1 tablespoon harissa
½ cup pitted kalamata olives, chopped coarse
¼ cup walnuts, toasted and chopped
2 tablespoons chopped fresh dill

1 Adjust oven rack to middle position and heat oven to 400 degrees. Whisk vinegar, shallot, caraway seeds, mustard, and ¼ teaspoon salt together in large bowl. Whisking constantly, slowly drizzle in olive oil. Add carrots and toss until well coated; set aside.

2 Heat 12-inch cast-iron skillet over medium heat for 3 minutes. Increase heat to medium-high and arrange cucumber cut side down in skillet (skillet will be full). Cook, moving cucumber as little as possible, until charred on one side, 5 to 7 minutes. Flip cucumber and continue to cook until charred on second side, 3 to 5 minutes. Transfer to bowl with carrots and set aside.

3 Pat chicken dry with paper towels and sprinkle flesh side with remaining ¾ teaspoon salt. Heat avocado oil in now-empty skillet over medium-high heat until just smoking. Add chicken, skin side down, and cook until well browned, 6 to 8 minutes. Off heat, flip chicken and brush harissa evenly over skin. Transfer skillet to oven and roast until chicken registers 175 degrees, 10 to 15 minutes.

4 Transfer chicken to serving platter and let rest while finishing salad. Add olives, walnuts, and dill to bowl with carrots and cucumber and toss to combine. Season with salt and pepper to taste, and serve salad with chicken.

Braised Chicken with Mushrooms and Tomatoes

serves 4 to 6 · total time: 1½ hours

why this recipe works · Classic chicken cacciatore, an Italian stew that includes mushrooms, tomatoes, and red wine, should boast moist meat and a silken, robust sauce. But too often the chicken turns out dry and the sauce is greasy and heavy. Using bone-in chicken thighs and removing the skin after rendering some of the fat solved the problems of greasy sauce, dry meat, and soggy skin and created this delicious, Italian-inspired braise. Cooking the chicken in a combination of red wine, chicken broth, and diced tomatoes seasoned with fresh thyme yielded moist and deeply flavored chicken. Portobello mushrooms, a great source of anti-inflammatory benefits, gave the dish a meaty bite plus extra antioxidants, and fresh sage as a finisher highlighted our braise's woodsy notes. The Parmesan cheese rind is optional, but we highly recommend it for the rich, savory flavor it adds to the dish.

8 (5- to 7-ounce) bone-in chicken thighs, trimmed
1½ teaspoons table salt, divided
¼ teaspoon pepper
1 tablespoon avocado oil
1 onion, chopped
6 ounces portobello mushroom caps, cut into ¾-inch pieces
4 garlic cloves, minced
2 teaspoons minced fresh thyme
1½ tablespoons all-purpose flour
1½ cups dry red wine
½ cup unsalted chicken broth
1 (14.5-ounce) can no-salt-added diced tomatoes, drained
1 Parmesan cheese rind (optional)
2 teaspoons minced fresh sage

1 Adjust oven rack to middle position and heat oven to 300 degrees. Pat chicken dry with paper towels and sprinkle with 1 teaspoon salt and pepper. Heat oil in Dutch oven over medium-high heat until just smoking. Add chicken and cook until well browned, 8 to 10 minutes.

2 Transfer chicken to plate and discard skin. Pour off all but 1 tablespoon fat from pot. Add onion, mushrooms, and remaining ½ teaspoon salt to fat left in pot and cook, stirring occasionally, until softened and beginning to brown, 6 to 8 minutes. Stir in garlic and thyme and cook until fragrant, about 30 seconds. Stir in flour and cook for 1 minute. Slowly whisk in wine, scraping up any browned bits and smoothing out any lumps.

3 Stir in broth, tomatoes, and cheese rind, if using, and bring to simmer. Nestle thighs into pot, cover, and transfer to oven. Cook until chicken registers 195 degrees, 35 to 40 minutes.

4 Remove pot from oven and transfer chicken to serving platter. Discard cheese rind, if using. Stir sage into sauce and season with salt and pepper to taste. Spoon sauce over chicken and serve.

MAKE AHEAD • Chicken and sauce can be refrigerated for up to 2 days.

Chicken and Spiced Freekeh with Cilantro and Preserved Lemon

serves 4 to 6 • total time: 1½ hours   SUPERCHARGED

why this recipe works • We wanted to celebrate the dynamic duo that is freekeh and chicken, which appear together often in Middle Eastern cuisines, especially in Lebanon. Freekeh is an ancient grain that offers delectably nutty chewiness, plus loads of gut-friendly fiber. We turned to bone-in chicken thighs, which stay exceptionally juicy and tender while cooking. We browned them in a Dutch oven and then used the rendered fat to bloom an antioxidant-rich bevy of spices: smoked paprika, cardamom, and red pepper flakes. We deglazed the pan with broth and then used this richly seasoned liquid to cook the freekeh. After discarding the chicken skin, which would have turned soggy, we nestled the chicken thighs in with the grains so that the meat's juices could flavor the freekeh. Shredding the thighs into bite-size pieces before serving dispersed the meat throughout the dish. Chopped cilantro and toasted pistachios offered grassy notes along with a satisfying crunch, while preserved lemon brought tangy complexity. You can use store-bought preserved lemons or make our

Quick Preserved Lemon (recipe follows); you can also substitute 1 tablespoon lemon zest, though the flavor will be less complex. Look for cracked freekeh that is roughly the size of steel-cut oats. Avoid whole freekeh; it will not cook through in time. Freekeh is sometimes spelled frikeh or farik.

- 4 (5- to 7-ounce) bone-in chicken thighs, trimmed
- 1 teaspoon table salt, divided
- ¼ teaspoon pepper
- 1 tablespoon avocado oil, plus more for drizzling
- 1 onion, chopped fine
- 4 garlic cloves, minced
- 1½ teaspoons smoked paprika
- ¼ teaspoon ground cardamom
- ¼ teaspoon red pepper flakes
- 2¼ cups unsalted chicken broth
- 1½ cups cracked freekeh, rinsed
- ¼ cup plus 2 tablespoons chopped fresh cilantro, divided
- ½ cup shelled unsalted pistachios, toasted and chopped
- 2 tablespoons rinsed and minced preserved lemons

1 Adjust oven rack to lower-middle position and heat oven to 350 degrees. Pat chicken thighs dry with paper towels and sprinkle with ½ teaspoon salt and pepper. Heat oil in Dutch oven over medium-high heat until just smoking. Add chicken and cook until well browned, 8 to 10 minutes.

2 Transfer chicken to plate and discard skin. Add onion and remaining ½ teaspoon salt to fat left in pot and cook over medium heat until softened, about 5 minutes. Stir in garlic, paprika, cardamom, and pepper flakes and cook until fragrant, about 30 seconds. Stir in broth, scraping up any browned bits, then stir in freekeh.

3 Nestle chicken into freekeh mixture and add any accumulated juices. Cover, transfer pot to oven, and cook until freekeh is tender and chicken registers 195 degrees, 35 to 40 minutes.

4 Remove pot from oven. Transfer chicken to cutting board, let cool slightly, then shred into bite-size pieces using 2 forks; discard bones.

5 Meanwhile, gently fluff freekeh with fork. Lay clean dish towel over pot, replace lid, and let sit for 5 minutes. Stir in chicken, ¼ cup cilantro, pistachios, and preserved lemon. Season with salt and pepper to taste. Sprinkle with remaining 2 tablespoons cilantro, drizzle with extra oil, and serve.

MAKE AHEAD • Cooked chicken and freekeh can be refrigerated for up to 3 days.

Crispy Brown Rice with Soy Chicken and Shiitake Mushrooms

serves 4 to 6 • total time: 1¾ hours

why this recipe works • We love the comforting one-pot harmony of Chinese claypot chicken and rice—a dish known for its tender, soy-marinated chicken, umami-packed mushrooms, and most of all, the prized crispy rice layer that forms at the bottom of the pot. We wanted to take that formula and up the anti-inflammatory benefits, swapping in brown rice for the usual white rice for an extra dose of fiber. But replicating the signature texture with brown rice (which doesn't always crisp well) proved tricky. Our solution? We borrowed our baked brown rice method to ensure evenly cooked rice, serving the nutty grains with golden-browned chicken thighs and meaty shiitakes. We finished the dish with a brief stovetop sear to give the rice its signature irresistible crunch. To give our chicken thighs plenty of flavor, we seasoned them with scallion whites, soy sauce, Shaoxing wine, oyster sauce, ginger, and white pepper. We reserved some of this mixture to drizzle over the final dish, punching up the savory depth. The result: a deeply flavorful, fiber-rich twist on a beloved classic. We like brown jasmine rice in this dish, but any long-grain brown rice will work.

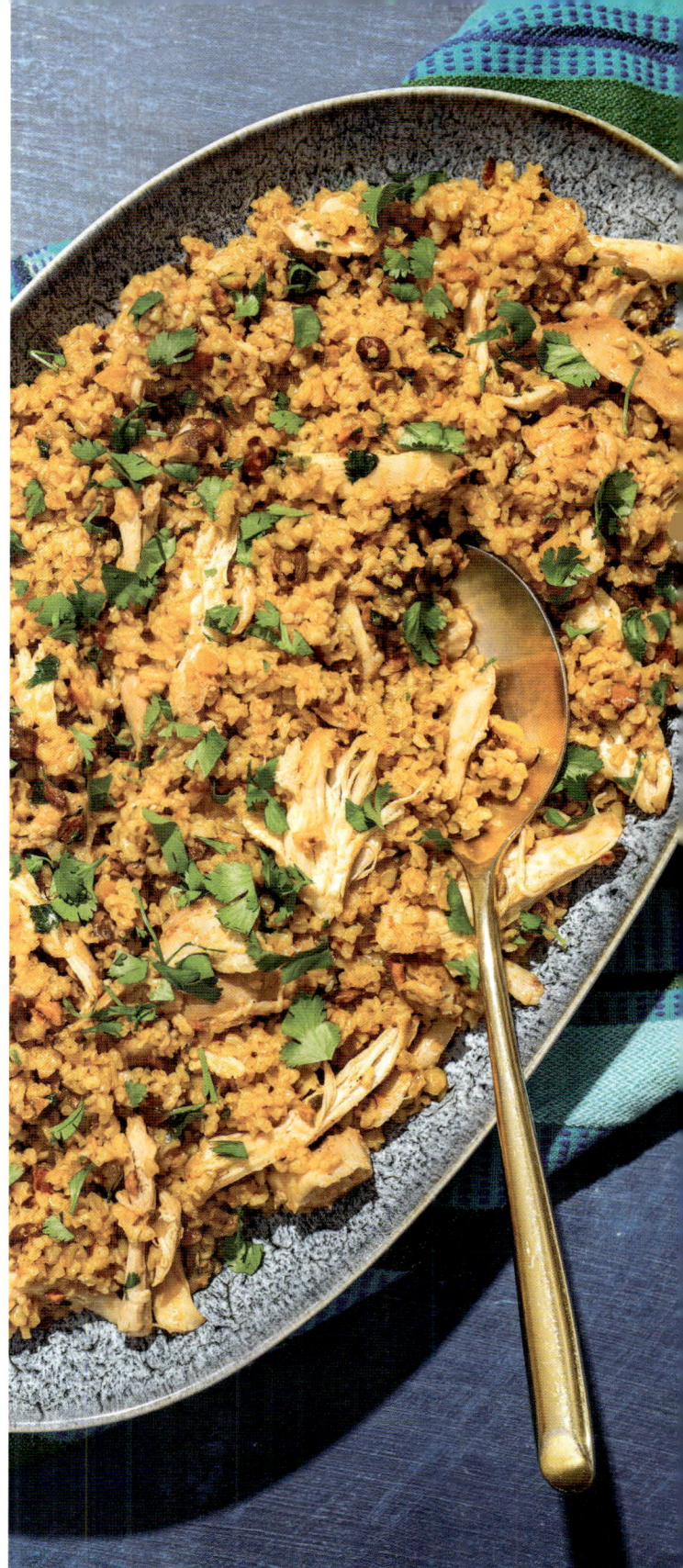

Chicken and Spiced Freekeh with Cilantro and Preserved Lemon

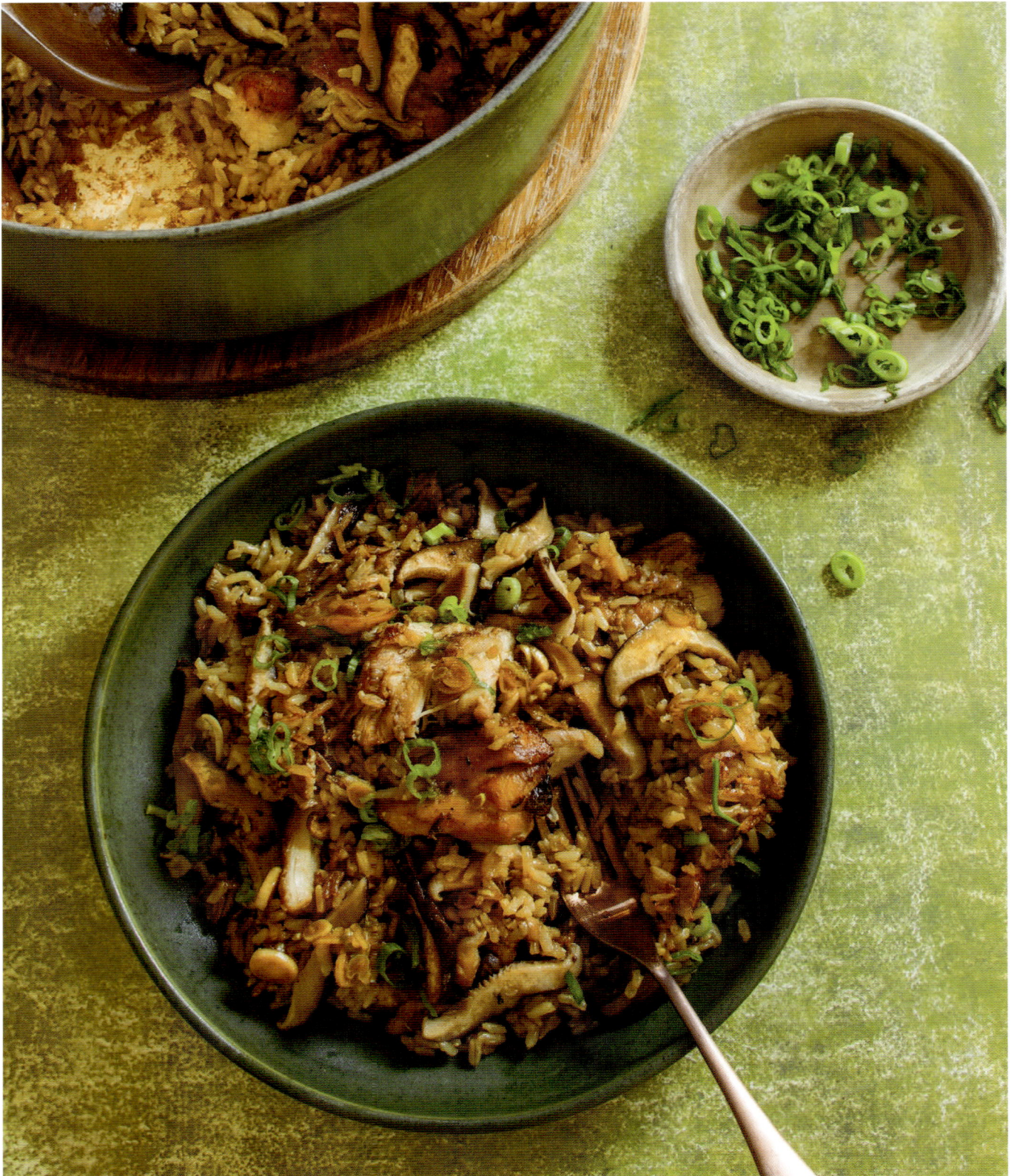

Crispy Brown Rice with Soy Chicken and Shiitake Mushrooms

1 pound boneless, skinless chicken thighs, trimmed, each piece halved

3 scallions, white and green parts separated and sliced thin

8 teaspoons low-sodium soy sauce

2 tablespoons Shaoxing wine or dry sherry

4 teaspoons oyster sauce

2 teaspoons grated fresh ginger

½ teaspoon white pepper

3 garlic cloves, minced

¼ cup avocado oil

2 cups water

1 cup unsalted chicken broth

1½ cups long-grain brown rice, rinsed

1 teaspoon table salt

8 ounces shiitake mushrooms, stems removed, sliced ¼ inch thick

1 Adjust oven rack to lowest position and heat oven to 375 degrees. Pat chicken dry with paper towels. Whisk scallion whites, soy sauce, Shaoxing wine, oyster sauce, ginger, and pepper together in large bowl. Measure out ¼ cup sauce and transfer to small bowl; set aside until ready to serve. Whisk garlic into remaining sauce in large bowl, then add chicken and toss to coat.

2 Heat oil in Dutch oven over medium-high heat until shimmering. Add chicken and cook until golden, 4 to 6 minutes, stirring occasionally; using slotted spoon, return chicken to bowl.

3 Add water and broth to fat left in pot, scraping up any browned bits. Cover pot and bring to boil over high heat. Off heat, stir in rice and salt, spread chicken and any accumulated juices in single layer over rice, then top with mushrooms. Cover, transfer pot to oven, and bake until rice is tender and top of rice is dry and beginning to brown, 60 to 70 minutes.

4 Remove pot from oven, place clean dish towel under lid, and cover pot tightly. Let rest for 10 minutes. Remove towel and lid from pot. Cook over medium-high heat until rice on bottom is crackling, about 2 minutes. Drizzle reserved sauce over chicken and sprinkle with scallion greens. Serve.

MAKE AHEAD • Cooked chicken and rice can be refrigerated for up to 3 days; crispy rice will soften over time.

MAKE IT GLUTEN-FREE • Substitute gluten-free low-sodium tamari for the low-sodium soy sauce and gluten-free oyster sauce for the oyster sauce.

Arroz con Pollo

serves 4 to 6 • **total time: 1¼ hours**

why this recipe works • It's easy to see why hearty, comforting arroz con pollo, or rice with chicken, is so beloved in Peru. The aromatic dish has complex layers of seasonings. This starts with an aderezo (Spanish for "seasoning"), the dish's aromatic base. This typically includes seasonings like ají amarillo (Peru's fruity, moderately hot yellow chile) paste, cumin, and oregano—all of which offer anti-inflammatory benefits. We bloomed the blend in a skillet alongside antioxidant-rich onion and bell pepper to invigorate the spices' aroma and coat the vegetables with flavor. We then deglazed the pan with some beer to amplify the impact of all the flavor-rich browned bits on the bottom of the pot. Using a food processor, we blitzed our aderezo with cilantro and spinach into a green herbaceous cooking liquid for the rice. Toasting the rice in the skillet before cooking enriched it with a nutty edge. Cooking the rice and chicken together allowed the grains to soak up the flavorful juices released by the meat. Any browned rice at the bottom of the pot adds to the overall experience of the dish, so be sure to include it when serving. For the beer, look for a brown ale or mild lager. Do not substitute other hot pepper pastes for ají amarillo. You will need a 12-inch nonstick skillet with a tight-fitting lid for this recipe. Serve with Sarza Criolla (page 212).

1 tablespoon extra-virgin olive oil, divided

1 red onion, halved and sliced into ½-inch-wide strips

1 red bell pepper, stemmed, seeded, and cut into ½-inch-wide strips, divided

1½ teaspoons table salt, divided

3 garlic cloves, smashed and peeled

1 tablespoon ají amarillo paste

1 teaspoon ground cumin

1 teaspoon dried oregano

½ teaspoon pepper, divided

1 cup beer

1½ cups fresh cilantro leaves and tender stems

1 cup baby spinach

¾ cup unsalted chicken broth, plus extra as needed

1½ cups long-grain white rice, rinsed

2 carrots, peeled, halved lengthwise, and sliced crosswise ½ inch thick

1 pound boneless, skinless chicken thighs, trimmed and cut into 1-inch strips

½ cup frozen peas

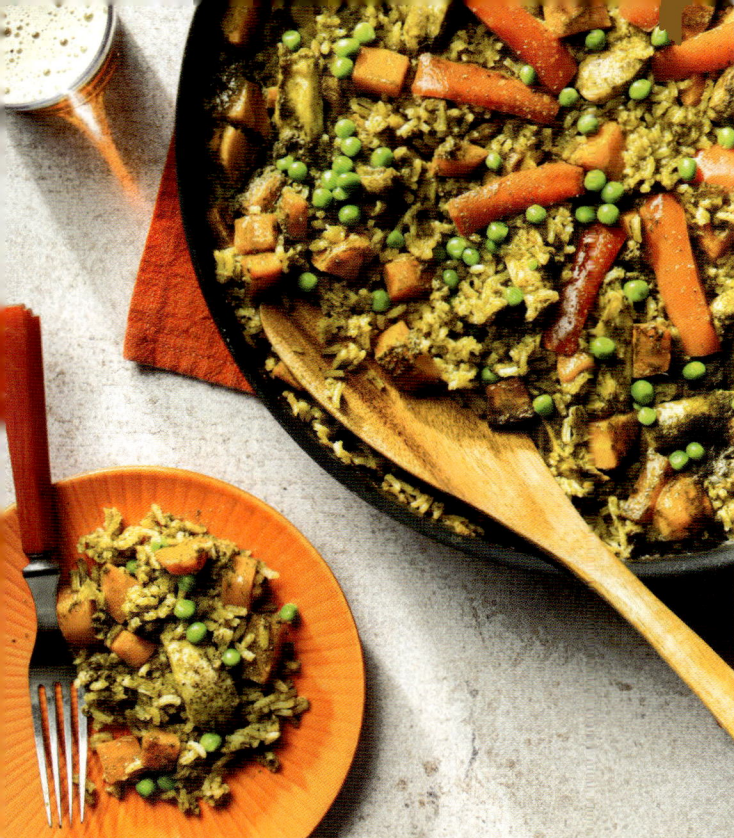

1   Heat 2 teaspoons oil in 12-inch nonstick skillet over medium-high heat until shimmering. Add onion, half of bell pepper, and 1 teaspoon salt and cook over medium heat until softened and lightly browned, about 5 minutes. Stir in garlic, ají amarillo paste, cumin, oregano, and ¼ teaspoon pepper and cook until fragrant, about 30 seconds. Stir in beer, scraping up any browned bits, and cook until liquid has reduced slightly, about 3 minutes.

2   Transfer vegetable mixture to blender. Add cilantro, spinach, broth, remaining ½ teaspoon salt, and remaining ¼ teaspoon pepper and process until smooth, about 1 minute, scraping down sides of blender jar as needed. Transfer puree to 4-cup liquid measuring cup. You should have 3½ cups; if necessary, spoon off excess or add extra broth so that volume equals 3½ cups.

3   Heat remaining 1 teaspoon oil in now-empty skillet over medium-high heat until shimmering. Add rice and carrots and cook until rice is lightly toasted and fragrant, about 2 minutes. Stir in pureed vegetable mixture and chicken and bring to simmer. Arrange remaining bell pepper strips attractively over top. Reduce heat to medium-low, cover, and cook until rice is tender, 25 to 30 minutes.

4   Off heat, scatter peas over top. Cover and let sit until heated through, about 10 minutes. Season with salt and pepper to taste, and serve.

MAKE AHEAD • Cooked chicken and rice can be refrigerated for up to 3 days.

MAKE IT GLUTEN-FREE • Substitute gluten-free beer for the beer.

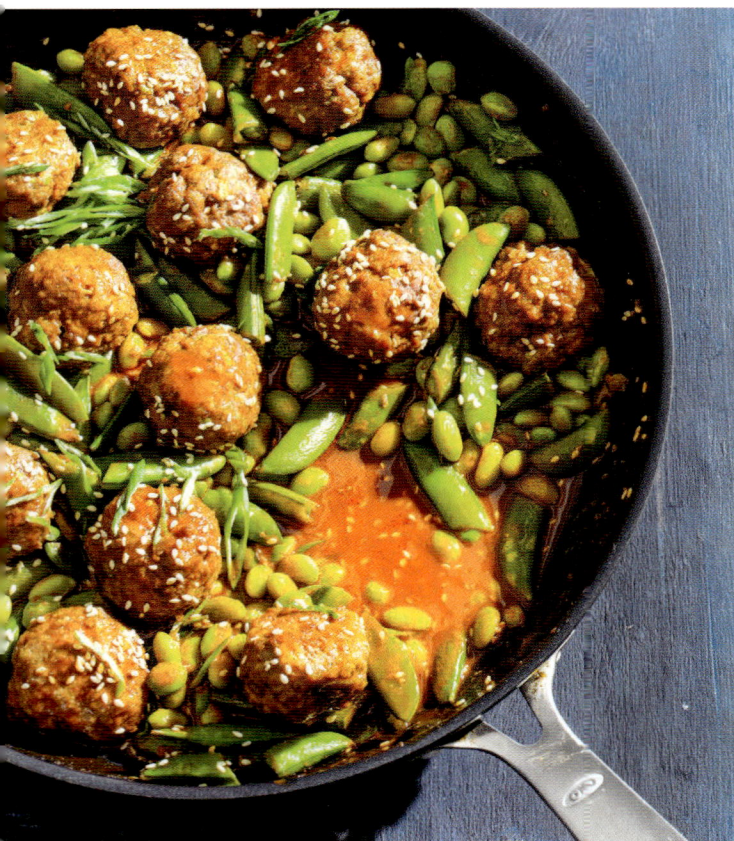

Sarza Criolla

makes ½ cup • total time: 15 minutes, plus 30 minutes chilling

- ½ red onion, sliced thin
- 1 tablespoon lime juice
- ¼ teaspoon table salt
-    Pinch pepper
- 2 tablespoons chopped fresh cilantro

Soak onion in ice water for 10 minutes. Drain well and pat dry with paper towels. Combine onion, lime juice, salt, and pepper in bowl. Cover with plastic wrap and refrigerate for at least 30 minutes. Stir in cilantro just before serving. (Sarza Criolla can be refrigerated for up to 2 days.)

top | *Arroz con Pollo*
bottom | *Gochujang Turkey Meatballs with Edamame and Sugar Snap Peas*

Gochujang Turkey Meatballs with Edamame and Sugar Snap Peas

serves 4 to 6 · total time: 45 minutes FAST

why this recipe works · We love frozen edamame—protein-packed soybeans harvested while still green—for their quick cooking time, bright color, and firm, hearty bite. Combined with fresh sugar snap peas, they served as a protein-rich side for gingery-garlicky meatballs, with everything tossed in a slightly spicy, sweet-savory sauce to create an easy and satisfying meal. Intensely flavored gochujang formed the backbone of our sauce, complemented by soy sauce and sesame oil with a bit of rice vinegar to balance all the flavors. Roasting the meatballs in the oven was quick. Just a few minutes in a hot skillet thawed the edamame and kept the snap peas snappy before we added the roasted meatballs and sauce and tossed everything together. Toasted sesame seeds and scallion greens made a fresh finish. Even after thorough cooking, the meatballs may retain some pink color; use a meat thermometer to ensure that they're cooked to temperature before serving. Do not thaw the edamame before adding them to the skillet in step 3.

¼ cup water
3 tablespoons gochujang
3 tablespoons low-sodium soy sauce
2 tablespoons toasted sesame oil
1 tablespoon unseasoned rice vinegar
3 garlic cloves, minced, divided
1¼ teaspoons grated fresh ginger, divided
1 pound ground turkey
½ cup panko bread crumbs
1 large egg, lightly beaten
3 scallions, white parts minced, green parts sliced thin on bias
1 teaspoon table salt
¼ teaspoon pepper
1 teaspoon avocado oil
8 ounces frozen shelled edamame (1½ cups)
8 ounces sugar snap peas, strings removed, halved crosswise on bias
2 tablespoons sesame seeds, toasted

1 Adjust oven rack to upper-middle position and heat oven to 400 degrees. Whisk water, gochujang, soy sauce, sesame oil, vinegar, one-third of garlic, and ¼ teaspoon ginger together in bowl; set aside.

2 Spray rimmed baking sheet with avocado oil spray. Combine turkey, panko, egg, scallion whites, salt, pepper, remaining garlic, and remaining 1 teaspoon ginger in bowl and mix with your hands until thoroughly combined. Divide mixture into 16 portions. Roll portions between your wet hands to form meatballs and arrange on prepared sheet. Transfer to oven and roast until meatballs register 160 degrees, 15 to 20 minutes.

3 Heat avocado oil in 12-inch nonstick skillet over medium-high heat until just smoking. Add edamame and snap peas and cook until snap peas are bright green, about 2 minutes. Reduce heat to medium-low and add meatballs and reserved gochujang mixture. Cook until sauce thickens, about 2 minutes, gently turning meatballs to coat. Sprinkle with scallion greens and sesame seeds and serve.

MAKE AHEAD · Shaped, uncooked meatballs can be refrigerated for up to 24 hours.

MAKE IT GLUTEN-FREE · Substitute low-sodium tamari for the low-sodium soy sauce and gluten-free panko for the panko. Not all gochujang is gluten-free; look for brands that are labeled gluten-free.

NOTES FROM THE TEST KITCHEN

Getting to Know Gochujang

Gochujang, a Korean spicy chile bean paste, also goes by gochu jang, kochujang, or kochu jang. It is a common topping for bibimbap, as well as for Korean salads, stews, soups, and marinades.

The fermented condiment has a smooth consistency, rich spicy flavor, and capsaicin for some anti-inflammatory benefits. It's made from glutinous rice powder (or sometimes regular short-grain rice, barley, pumpkin, or sweet potato) that's mixed with powdered fermented soybeans, red chili powder, and salt. For an anti-inflammatory eating pattern, look for no-sugar versions of gochujang and other condiments.

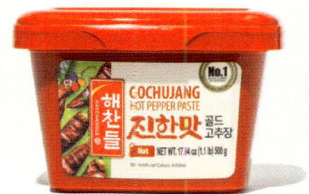

Turkey Meatballs with Lemony Brown Rice and Sun-Dried Tomatoes

serves 4 • total time: 1½ hours

why this recipe works • A skillet of meatballs and rice is a simple, hearty meal that's highly adaptable. In this version, we used lean ground turkey and nutty brown rice, both great choices for an anti-inflammatory diet. The addition of lemon, garlic, scallions, and parsley enlivened the pair, not to mention adding inflammation-fighting benefits. Cooking the brown rice in broth instead of water infused the grains with savory flavor. Sliced sun-dried tomatoes scattered atop the finished dish brought beautiful pops of red and a sweet, chewy bite. A quarter cup of Parmesan cheese was all we needed for a salty and funky finish. Be sure to use ground turkey, not ground turkey breast (also labeled 99 percent fat-free), in this recipe, as the latter will result in dry, tough, and less flavorful meatballs. You will need a 12-inch nonstick skillet with a tight-fitting lid for this recipe.

- 1 slice hearty sandwich bread, torn into 1-inch pieces
- 1 pound ground turkey
- 1 large egg
- 4 scallions, white and green parts separated and sliced thin, divided
- ¼ cup chopped fresh parsley, divided
- 2 teaspoons grated lemon zest, divided, plus 2 tablespoons juice
- ½ teaspoon table salt
- ½ teaspoon pepper
- 2 tablespoons extra-virgin olive oil
- 1 cup long-grain brown rice, rinsed
- 3 garlic cloves, minced
- 4 cups unsalted chicken broth
- ½ cup oil-packed sun-dried tomatoes, rinsed, patted dry, and sliced thin
- ¼ cup grated Parmesan cheese (optional)

1 Pulse bread in food processor to fine crumbs, 10 to 15 pulses; transfer to large bowl. Add turkey, egg, 3 tablespoons scallion greens, 2 tablespoons parsley, 1½ teaspoons lemon zest, salt, and pepper to bowl and, using your hands, gently knead mixture until combined. Divide mixture into 20 portions (about 1 heaping tablespoon each). Roll portions between your wet hands to form meatballs and transfer to rimmed baking sheet. Cover with greased plastic wrap and refrigerate for 15 minutes.

2 Heat oil in 12-inch nonstick skillet over medium-high heat until shimmering. Add meatballs and cook until well browned all over, 5 to 7 minutes. Transfer meatballs to paper towel–lined plate.

3 Return now-empty skillet to medium-high heat. Stir in rice and cook until edges of rice begin to turn translucent, about 1 minute. Add scallion whites and garlic and cook until fragrant, about 1 minute. Stir in broth and remaining ½ teaspoon lemon zest and juice and bring to boil.

4 Reduce heat to medium-low, cover, and cook for 15 minutes. Return meatballs to skillet, cover, and cook until rice is tender and meatballs are cooked through, about 15 minutes.

5 Off heat, scatter sun-dried tomatoes over rice and let sit, covered, for 5 minutes. Sprinkle with Parmesan, if using; remaining scallion greens; and remaining 2 tablespoons parsley. Serve.

MAKE AHEAD • Shaped, uncooked meatballs can be refrigerated for up to 24 hours.

MAKE IT GLUTEN-FREE • Substitute gluten-free sandwich bread for the sandwich bread.

Turkey Zucchini Burgers

serves 4 • total time: 30 minutes **FAST**

why this recipe works • These turkey burgers are tender and juicy, thanks to the shredded zucchini that's mixed in with the meat. The zucchini, a mild and moisture-rich source of fiber and phytonutrients, didn't require any precooking; simply squeezing it to eliminate excess moisture before kneading it into the ground turkey gave us succulent results. Poultry seasoning boosted the patties' savory flavor. Before cooking the patties, we pressed down on the center of each one with our fingertips; this divot prevented the center from bulging up when cooked. A scattering of peppery baby arugula made a bright finishing touch. Use the large holes of a box grater to shred the zucchini. Be sure to use ground turkey, not ground turkey breast (also labeled 99 percent fat-free), in this recipe, as the latter will result in dry, less flavorful burgers.

- 1 pound ground turkey
- 12 ounces zucchini, shredded (3 cups)
- 1½ teaspoons poultry seasoning
- ¾ teaspoon table salt
- ½ teaspoon pepper
- 1 tablespoon extra-virgin olive oil
- 4 thin slices sharp cheddar cheese (optional)
- 4 hamburger buns, toasted
- 2 ounces (2 cups) baby arugula or 4 leaves Boston or Bibb lettuce

1   Break ground turkey into small pieces in large bowl. Place shredded zucchini in dish towel. Gather dish towel ends together and twist tightly over sink to drain as much liquid as possible from zucchini. Add drained zucchini, poultry seasoning, salt, and pepper to turkey in bowl and knead gently with your hands until well combined. Divide turkey mixture into 4 equal portions, then gently shape each portion into ¾-inch-thick patty. Using your fingertips, press center of each patty down until about ½ inch thick, creating slight divot.

2   Heat oil in clean, dry, now-empty skillet over medium-low heat until shimmering. Transfer patties to skillet, divot side up, and cook until well browned on first side, 4 to 7 minutes. Flip patties and continue to cook until browned on second side and burgers register 160 degrees, 4 to 7 minutes; 1 minute before burgers finish cooking, top each burger with 1 slice cheese, if using. Transfer burgers to plate and let rest for 5 minutes. Transfer burgers to buns, top with arugula, and serve.

> **MAKE AHEAD** • Shaped, uncooked patties can be refrigerated for up to 24 hours.

> **MAKE IT GLUTEN-FREE** • Substitute gluten-free hamburger buns for the hamburger buns.

Turkey Shepherd's Pie

serves 4 • total time: 1½ hours, plus 10 minutes cooling

why this recipe works • We love how shepherd's pie features a meaty base bulked up by an assortment of vegetables. For a take that introduces even more fiber and antioxidants and cuts down on saturated fat, we swapped in cauliflower for potato and used turkey as a leaner option. Keeping the meat tender required us to refrain from browning it; instead, we browned mushrooms and onion first, which gave us a savory fond that we enhanced with tomato paste and garlic. The additions of carrots, thyme, and Worcestershire evoked the flavors we know and love in shepherd's pie. We simmered all this with chicken broth, making sure to scrape up the browned bits in the skillet. Only then did we add the meat, which we had tenderized with baking soda. Pinching off pieces of turkey by hand before incorporating them ensured craggy edges, which maximized the surface area to help the meat absorb flavor. Cauliflower, cooked and then pureed to a creamy consistency, made a highly satisfying topping. Be sure to use ground turkey, not ground turkey breast (also labeled 99 percent fat-free), in this recipe, as the latter will result in dry, tough, and less flavorful filling. You will need a 10-inch broiler-safe skillet for this recipe.

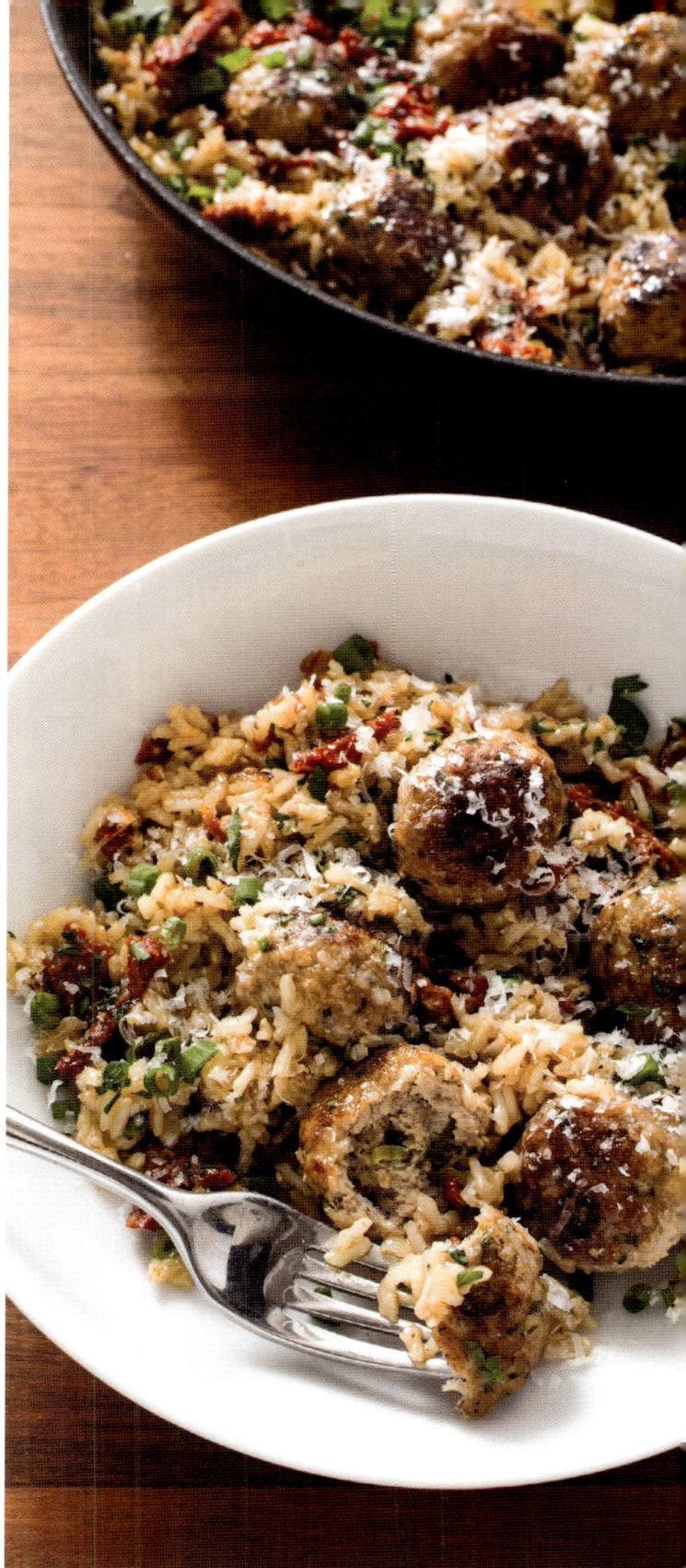

Turkey Meatballs with Lemony Brown Rice and Sun-Dried Tomatoes

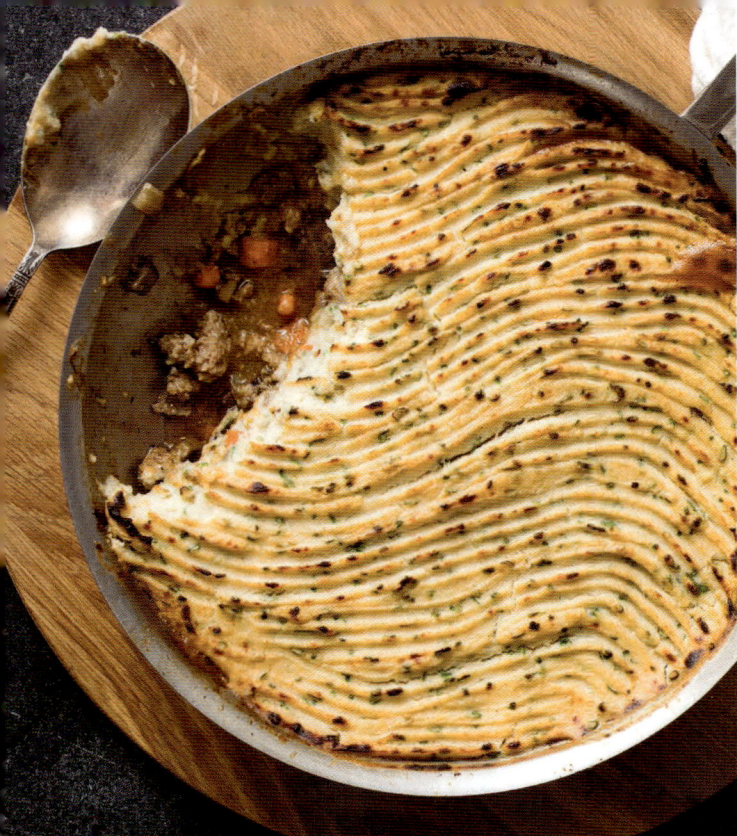

3 tablespoons extra-virgin olive oil, divided
1 large head cauliflower (3 pounds), cored and
   cut into ½-inch pieces
½ cup plus 2 tablespoons water, divided
1 teaspoon table salt, divided
1 large egg, lightly beaten
3 tablespoons minced fresh chives
1 pound ground turkey
¼ teaspoon pepper
¼ teaspoon baking soda
8 ounces cremini mushrooms, trimmed and chopped
1 onion, chopped
1 tablespoon no-salt-added tomato paste
2 garlic cloves, minced
¾ cup unsalted chicken broth
2 carrots, peeled and chopped
2 sprigs fresh thyme
1 tablespoon Worcestershire sauce
1 tablespoon cornstarch

1 Heat 2 tablespoons oil in Dutch oven over medium-low heat until shimmering. Add cauliflower and cook, stirring occasionally, until softened and beginning to brown, 10 to 12 minutes. Stir in ½ cup water and ¾ teaspoon salt, cover, and cook until cauliflower falls apart easily when poked with fork, about 10 minutes.

2 Transfer cauliflower and any remaining liquid to food processor and let cool for 5 minutes. Process until smooth, about 45 seconds. Transfer to large bowl and stir in beaten egg and chives; set aside.

3 Meanwhile, toss turkey, 1 tablespoon water, remaining ¼ teaspoon salt, pepper, and baking soda in bowl until thoroughly combined. Set aside for 20 minutes.

4 Heat remaining 1 tablespoon oil in 10-inch broiler-safe skillet over medium heat until shimmering. Add mushrooms and onion and cook, stirring occasionally, until liquid has evaporated and fond begins to form on bottom of skillet, 10 to 12 minutes. Stir in tomato paste and garlic and cook until bottom of skillet is dark brown, about 2 minutes.

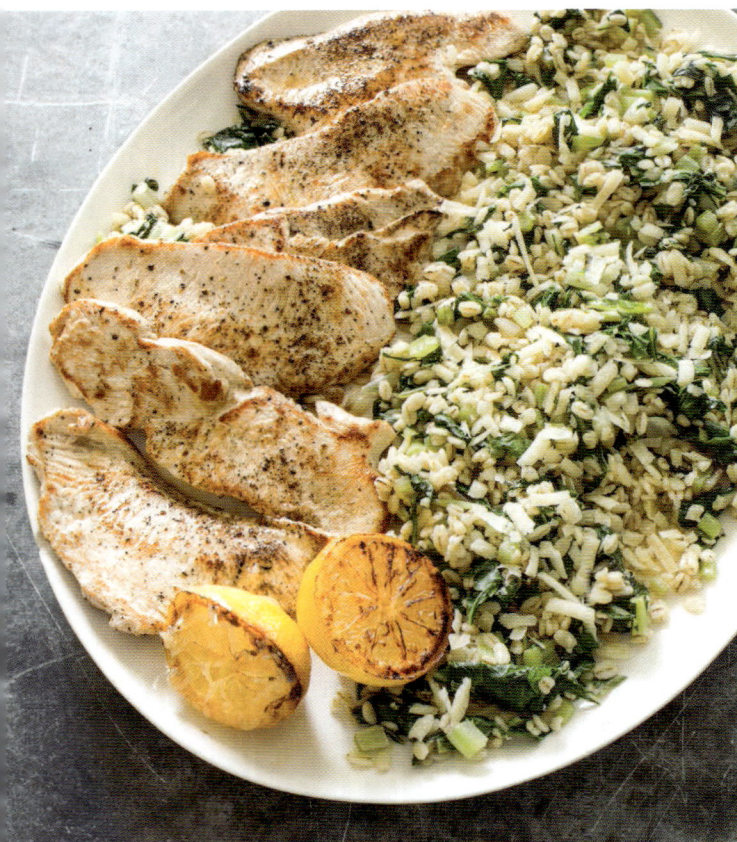

top | *Turkey Shepherd's Pie*
bottom | *Turkey Cutlets with Barley and Swiss Chard*

5 Add broth, carrots, thyme, and Worcestershire and bring to simmer, scraping up any browned bits. Reduce heat to medium-low. Pinch off turkey in ½-inch pieces and add to skillet, then bring to gentle simmer. Cover and cook until turkey is cooked through, 8 to 10 minutes, stirring and breaking up meat halfway through cooking.

6 Whisk cornstarch and remaining 1 tablespoon water together in small bowl, then stir mixture into filling and continue to simmer until thickened, about 1 minute. Discard thyme sprigs and season with salt and pepper to taste.

7 Adjust oven rack 5 inches from broiler element and heat broiler. Transfer cauliflower mixture to large zipper-lock bag. Using scissors, snip 1 inch off filled corner. Squeezing bag, pipe mixture in even layer over filling, making sure to cover entire surface. Smooth mixture with back of spoon, then use tines of fork to make ridges over surface. Place skillet on aluminum foil-lined rimmed baking sheet and broil until topping is golden brown and crusty and filling is bubbly, 10 to 15 minutes. Let cool for 10 minutes before serving.

Turkey Cutlets with Barley and Swiss Chard

serves 4 · total time: 1 hour

why this recipe works · Want to bring more whole grains into your weeknight routine? We updated the traditional chicken-and-rice formula by pairing quick-cooking turkey cutlets with rustic, fiber-packed barley and vitamin-rich Swiss chard. Since the cutlets cook so quickly, we prepared our barley first, simmering it with aromatics and chard stems before folding in the chard leaves. To give the turkey bright flavor, we employed a simple trick: We caramelized lemon halves in the cooking oil, infusing it (and thus the cutlets) with flavor. A hint of lemon zest in the barley matched the lemony oil. Finally, just ½ cup of Parmesan added salty richness, tying the dish together without going overboard on the saturated fat. Do not substitute hulled, hull-less, quick-cooking, or presteamed barley for the pearl barley in this recipe.

3 tablespoons extra-virgin olive oil, divided
¼ cup finely chopped onion
12 ounces Swiss chard, 1 cup chopped stems, leaves cut into 1-inch pieces
1½ cups pearl barley, rinsed
2 garlic cloves, minced
2½ cups unsalted chicken broth
1 teaspoon grated lemon zest, plus 1 lemon, halved
1 ounce Parmesan cheese, grated (½ cup), divided
6 (4-ounce) turkey cutlets, trimmed
½ teaspoon table salt
¼ teaspoon pepper

1 Heat 2 tablespoons oil in large saucepan over medium-high heat until shimmering. Add onion and chard stems and cook until softened, about 5 minutes. Stir in barley and garlic and cook until barley is lightly toasted and fragrant, about 3 minutes.

2 Stir in broth and bring to simmer. Reduce heat to low, cover, and simmer until barley is tender and broth is absorbed, 20 to 40 minutes.

3 Fold chard leaves and lemon zest into barley, increase heat to medium-high, and cook, uncovered and stirring gently, until chard is wilted, about 2 minutes. Off heat, stir in ¼ cup Parmesan and season with salt and pepper to taste. Cover to keep warm.

4 Pat cutlets dry with paper towels and sprinkle with salt and pepper. Heat 1 teaspoon oil in 12-inch nonstick skillet over medium-high heat until shimmering. Add lemon halves, cut side down, and cook until browned, about 2 minutes; set aside. Heat remaining 2 teaspoons oil in now-empty skillet until shimmering. Add cutlets to skillet and cook until well browned and tender, about 2 minutes per side. Off heat, squeeze lemon halves over cutlets. Serve cutlets with barley mixture, sprinkling individual portions with remaining ¼ cup Parmesan.

MAKE AHEAD · Barley, prepared through step 3, can be refrigerated for up to 3 days.

MAKE IT DAIRY-FREE · Substitute plant-based Parmesan cheese for the dairy Parmesan cheese.

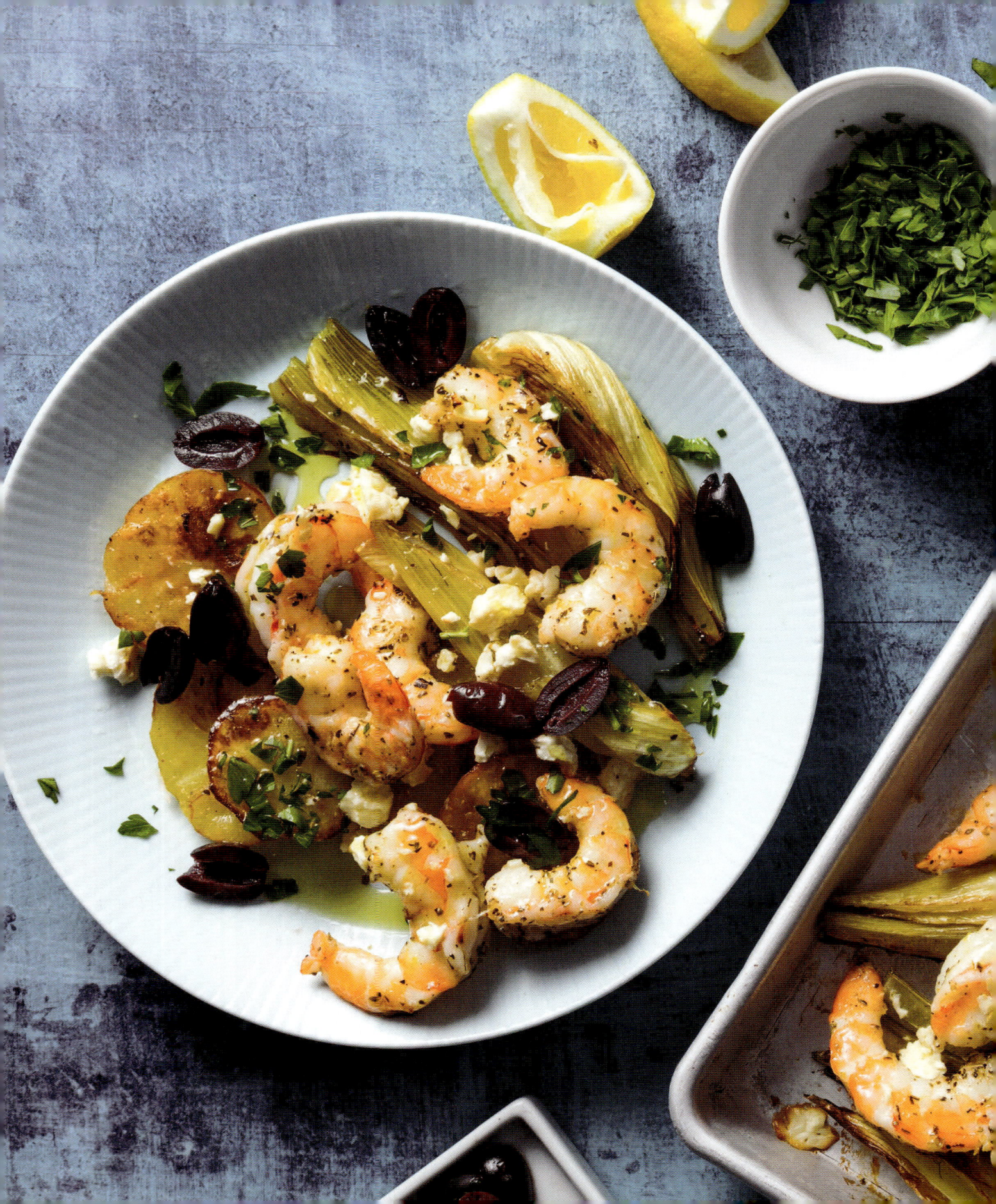

SEAFOOD

■ FAST   ■ SUPERCHARGED

Poached Salmon with Dijon-Herb Vinaigrette

serves 4 • total time: 40 minutes **FAST**

why this recipe works • It's no wonder salmon is so popular: Its flesh is flavorful and rich, with high levels of heart-healthy omega-3 fatty acids. A great way to ensure moist, tender salmon is to poach it; a vinaigrette packed with fresh herbs offers added nutritional value. Poaching the salmon in a small amount of water (and a dash of wine) ensured that we didn't lose flavor to the poaching liquid. However, the portion of the salmon that wasn't submerged needed to be steamed to cook through properly, and the low poaching cooking temperature didn't create enough steam. Replacing some of the water with more wine lowered the boiling point; the alcohol produced more vapor even at the lower temperature. To prevent the fillets from overcooking on the bottom, we placed them atop lemon slices. After poaching, we reduced the liquid and added olive oil for an easy vinaigrette-style sauce. To ensure uniform pieces that cook at the same rate, we prefer to purchase a whole 1½- to 2-pound center-cut salmon fillet and cut it into four equal pieces. If using wild salmon, cook it until it registers 120 degrees.

  1 lemon, sliced into ¼-inch-thick rounds, plus lemon wedges for serving
  2 tablespoons minced fresh parsley, stems reserved
  2 tablespoons minced fresh dill, stems reserved
  2 shallots, minced, divided
  ½ cup dry white wine
  ½ cup water
  4 (6- to 8-ounce) skinless salmon fillets, 1 inch thick
  ½ teaspoon table salt
  ⅛ teaspoon pepper
  1 tablespoon Dijon mustard
  1 tablespoon extra-virgin olive oil

1 Arrange lemon slices in single layer over bottom of 12-inch skillet. Scatter parsley stems, dill stems, and half of shallots over lemon slices, then add wine and water.

2 Pat salmon dry with paper towels and sprinkle with salt and pepper. Lay salmon skinned side down on top of lemons and herb sprigs. Set skillet over high heat and bring to simmer. Reduce heat to low, cover, and cook until centers of fillets are still translucent when checked with tip of paring knife and register 125 degrees (for medium-rare), 10 to 12 minutes.

3 Transfer salmon, herb sprigs, and lemon slices to paper towel–lined plate, cover with aluminum foil, and let drain while finishing sauce.

4 Return cooking liquid to medium-high heat and simmer until reduced to 1 tablespoon, 3 to 5 minutes. Combine remaining shallots, minced parsley, minced dill, mustard, and oil in bowl. Strain reduced cooking liquid through fine-mesh strainer into bowl, whisk to combine, and season with pepper to taste.

5 Gently transfer drained salmon to individual serving plates, discarding lemon slices and herb stems. Spoon vinaigrette evenly over tops and serve.

Salmon with Sweet Potatoes, Asparagus, and Yogurt

serves 4 • total time: 50 minutes

why this recipe works • We wanted an impressive salmon meal that was light, refreshing, and weeknight-friendly. To make this happen, we used a single baking sheet, staggering the cooking so that all the components would cook evenly. Sweet potatoes, tossed in oil and seasoned with salt and pepper, hit the sheet first for a head start. Next, we added asparagus as well as the salmon, the latter of which we brushed with a mixture of curry powder and cayenne that we had microwaved in oil to bloom. A drizzle of gut-friendly yogurt and some mint leaves added welcome cooling to balance out the salmon's heat. This recipe works best with thick asparagus spears that are between ½ and ¾ inch in diameter. To ensure uniform pieces that cook at the same rate, we prefer to purchase a whole 1½- to 2-pound center-cut salmon fillet and cut it into four equal pieces. If using wild salmon, cook it until it registers 120 degrees.

  1½ pounds sweet potatoes, unpeeled, cut into 1-inch-thick wedges
  2 tablespoons avocado oil, divided
  1 teaspoon table salt, divided
  ¾ teaspoon pepper, divided
  1 pound asparagus, trimmed
  2 teaspoons curry powder
  ½ teaspoon cayenne pepper
  4 (6- to 8-ounce) skinless salmon fillets, 1 inch thick
  ½ cup plain yogurt
  ½ cup torn fresh mint leaves

1 Adjust oven rack to lower-middle position and heat oven to 450 degrees. Toss potatoes, 1 tablespoon oil, ¼ teaspoon salt, and ¼ teaspoon pepper together in large bowl. Arrange potatoes skin side down in single layer on rimmed baking sheet, spaced evenly apart. Roast until potatoes begin to soften, about 25 minutes.

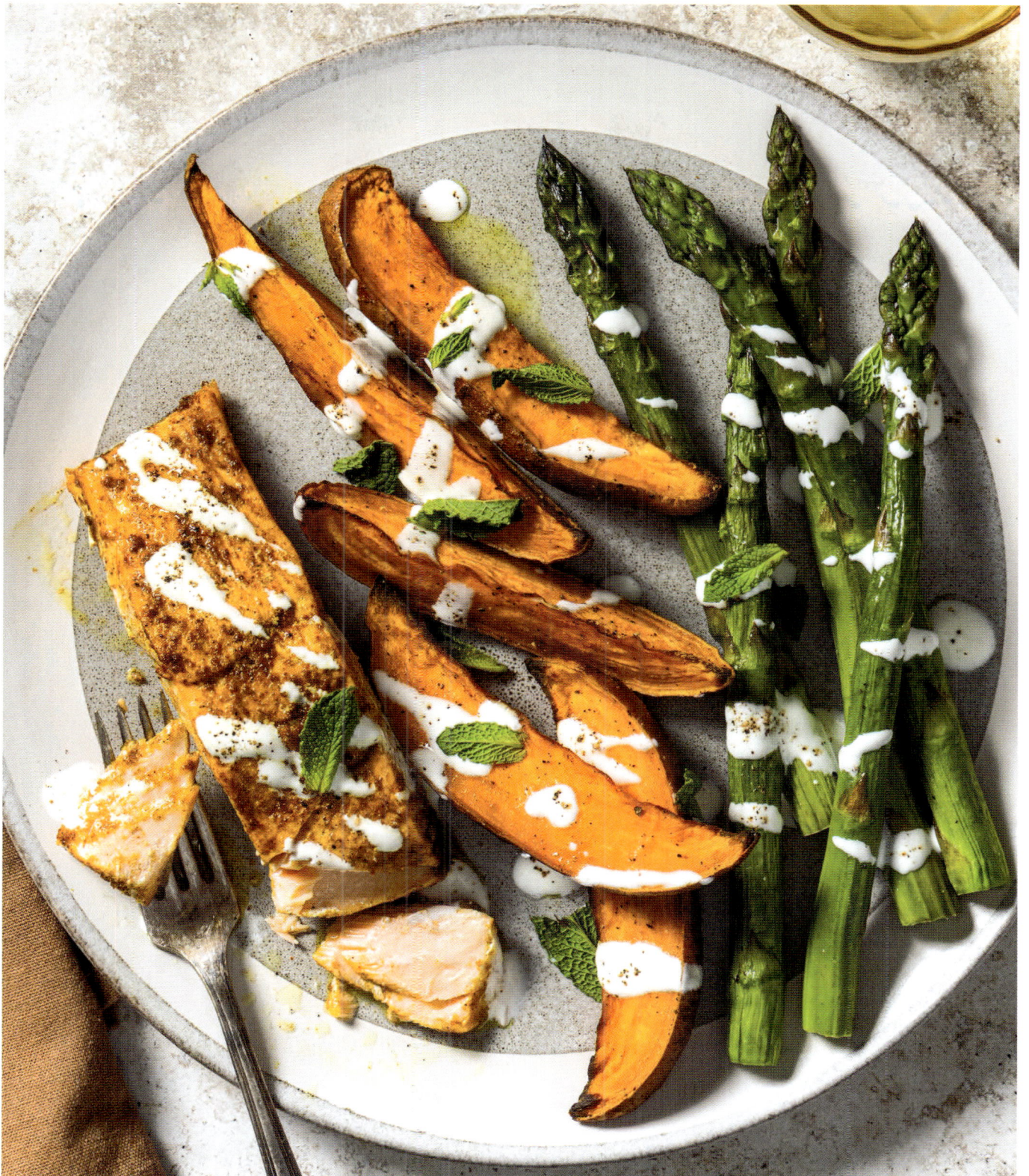

Salmon with Sweet Potatoes, Asparagus, and Yogurt

2   Meanwhile, toss asparagus with 1 teaspoon oil and ¼ teaspoon salt in now-empty bowl; set aside. Combine curry powder, cayenne, and remaining 2 teaspoons oil in separate bowl and microwave until bubbling and fragrant, about 1 minute. Pat salmon dry with paper towels, brush tops and sides of fillets with spice mixture, and sprinkle with remaining ½ teaspoon salt and remaining ½ teaspoon pepper.

3   Remove sheet from oven. Arrange potatoes in center of sheet in single column. Place salmon skinned side down on one empty side of sheet, spaced evenly apart. Arrange asparagus on remaining empty side of sheet. Roast until centers of fillets are still translucent when checked with tip of paring knife and register 125 degrees (for medium-rare), 8 to 10 minutes.

4   Serve salmon, sweet potatoes, and asparagus, drizzling individual portions with yogurt and sprinkling with mint.

MAKE IT DAIRY-FREE • Substitute plant-based yogurt for the dairy yogurt.

NOTES FROM THE TEST KITCHEN

All About Wild Salmon

Wild salmon are caught by fisherfolk in open waters, usually in the northern Pacific Ocean. **Farmed salmon**, usually a species called Atlantic salmon, are bred and raised in aquaculture systems which are like ocean farms. (Today, most Atlantic salmon is farmed due to overfishing in the 1900s.) Wild salmon typically has a higher ratio of anti-inflammatory omega-3 to omega-6 fatty acids, the latter of which can be pro-inflammatory in excess. Farmed salmon tends to have more fat in general and can be cooked to a slightly higher temperature (125 degrees versus 120 degrees for wild salmon).

Salmon Peperonata

serves 4 • total time: 55 minutes

why this recipe works • For a quick weeknight meal, we leaned on a quiet hero of Italian cuisine: peperonata. Made from sweet bell peppers, onion, garlic, and tomatoes stewed in oil until meltingly soft, this sauce can be served in myriad ways. We paired this mild, sweet vegetable mélange with rich, quick-cooking skinless salmon fillets. First, we sliced up two bell peppers and an onion, crushed six garlic cloves, and added them all to a skillet with avocado oil. We covered the skillet and cooked the mixture until the peppers and onion were soft. Next, we added a can of diced tomatoes along with some capers and red pepper flakes and cooked the mixture down until it melded together into a thick condiment. We nestled the salmon into our peperonata, covered the skillet, and let the magic happen. As the flavors of the peperonata and salmon mingled, the vegetables gained richness from the fish and the fish picked up a subtle sweetness from the vegetables. Lemon juice perked up the dish, a sprinkle of basil added freshness, and more pepper flakes brought on a little extra heat. To ensure uniform pieces that cook at the same rate, we prefer to purchase a whole 1½- to 2-pound center-cut salmon fillet and cut it into four equal pieces. If using wild salmon, cook it until it registers 120 degrees.

  4   (6- to 8-ounce) skinless salmon fillets, 1 inch thick
1¼   teaspoons table salt, divided
  1   teaspoon pepper
 ¼   cup avocado oil
  1   red bell pepper, stemmed, seeded, and cut into ¼-inch-wide strips
  1   yellow bell pepper, stemmed, seeded, and cut into ¼-inch-wide strips
  1   onion, halved and sliced ¼ inch thick
  6   garlic cloves, crushed and peeled
  1   (14.5-ounce) can no-salt-added diced tomatoes
  2   tablespoons capers, rinsed, plus 4 teaspoons brine
 ¼   teaspoon red pepper flakes, plus extra for sprinkling
1½   teaspoons lemon juice
 ¼   cup chopped fresh basil

1   Pat salmon dry with paper towels and sprinkle with ½ teaspoon salt and pepper. Heat oil in 12-inch nonstick skillet over medium-high heat until just smoking. Add bell peppers, onion, garlic, and remaining ¾ teaspoon salt. Cover and cook, stirring occasionally, until vegetables are soft, about 10 minutes.

2   Stir in tomatoes and their juice, capers and brine, and pepper flakes. Continue to cook, uncovered, until slightly thickened, about 5 minutes. Season with salt and pepper to taste. Reduce heat to medium-low. Nestle salmon into peperonata skinned side down. Cover and cook until centers of fillets are still translucent when checked with tip of paring knife and register 125 degrees (for medium-rare), 10 to 15 minutes.

3   Drizzle lemon juice over salmon. Sprinkle with basil and extra pepper flakes. Serve.

Buying and Storing Fish

What to Look For Fish is a great source of protein and fat for an anti-inflammatory diet. Always buy from a trusted source (ideally one with high volume to ensure freshness). All the fish should be on ice or refrigerated. Fillets and steaks should look shiny and firm, not dull or mushy. Whole fish should have moist, taut skin, clear eyes, and bright red gills.

What to Ask For It is always better to have your fishmonger slice steaks and fillets to order rather than buying precut pieces that may have been sitting around. Don't be afraid to be picky at the seafood counter; a ragged piece of fish is harder to cook properly. It is important to keep fish cold, so if you have a long ride home, ask for a bag of ice.

Buying Frozen Fish Firm fillets such as halibut, snapper, tilapia, and salmon are acceptable to buy frozen if you plan to cook them beyond medium-rare, but at a lower doneness they may have a dry, stringy texture. The fish should be frozen solid, with no signs of freezer burn, excessive crystallization, or blood in the package. The ingredient list should include only the name of the fish.

Defrosting Fish To defrost fish in the refrigerator overnight, remove the fish from its packaging, place it in a single layer on a rimmed plate or dish (to catch any water), and cover it with plastic wrap. You can also do a "quick thaw" by leaving the vacuum-sealed bags under cool running tap water for 30 minutes. Do not use a microwave to defrost fish; it will alter the texture of the fish or, worse, partially cook it. Dry the fish thoroughly with paper towels before seasoning and cooking it.

How to Store It If you're not using fish the day you buy it, unwrap it, pat it dry, put it in a zipper-lock bag, press out the air, and seal the bag. Set the fish on a bed of ice in a bowl or container (to hold the water once the ice melts), and place it in the back of the fridge, where it's coldest. If the ice melts before you use the fish, replenish it. The fish should keep for one day.

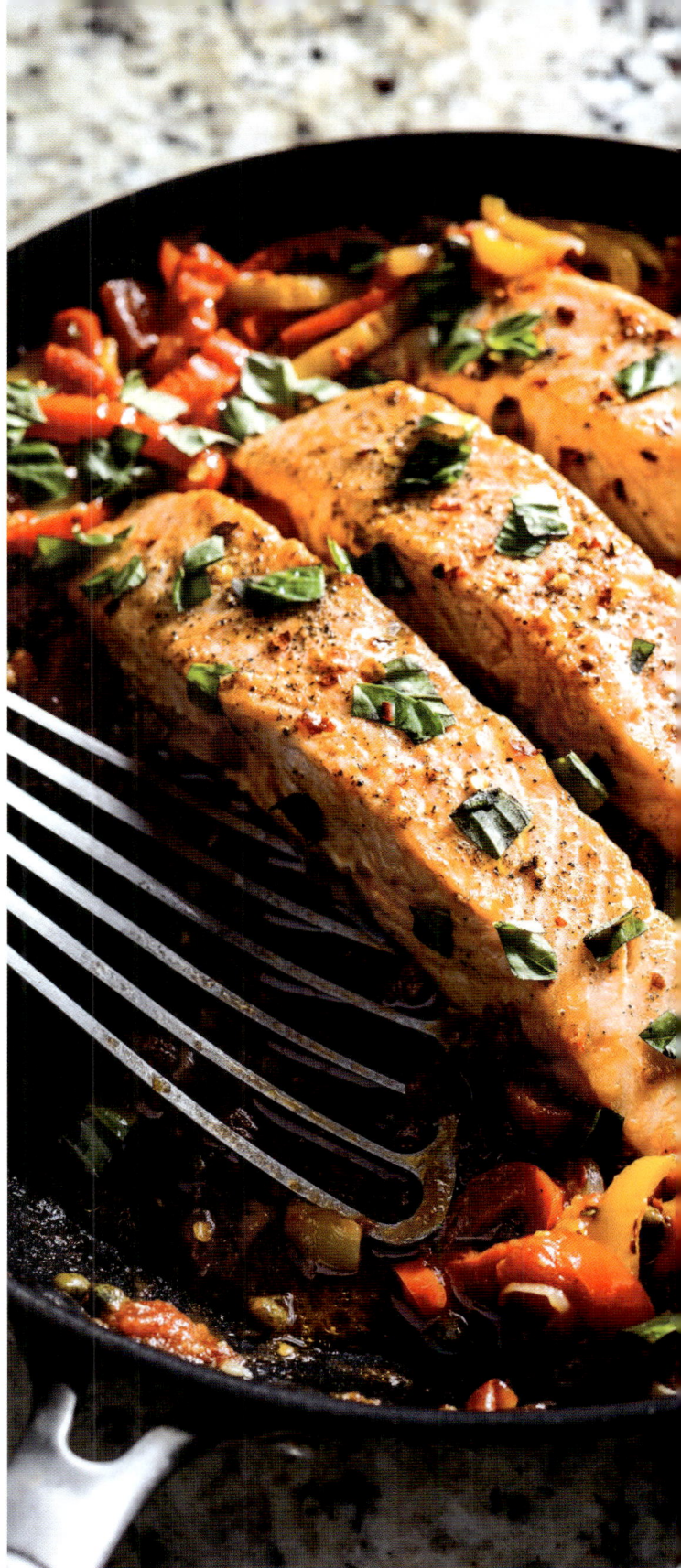

Salmon Peperonata

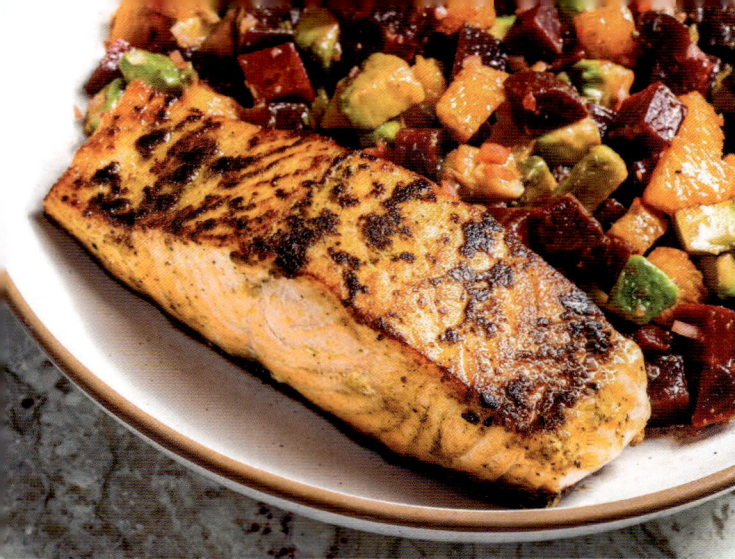

Coriander Salmon with Beets, Oranges, and Avocados

serves 4 • total time: 35 minutes   **FAST**   **SUPERCHARGED**

why this recipe works • Phyonutrient-rich beets, heart-healthy avocado, and vitamin C–rich oranges make a lovely anti-inflammatory trio for accompanying golden-seared, omega-3-rich salmon. We coated the salmon in a zingy combination of orange zest, coriander, salt, and pepper. Next, we tossed the orange slices, avocados, and beets together along with shallot and a little oil and vinegar for a bright and satisfying salad that beautifully complemented the salmon. We like to use vacuum-packed cooked beets in this recipe to cut down on prep; they are available in the produce section of many grocery stores. You can also use drained canned beets or leftover steamed or roasted beets, or you can cook your beets in the microwave: Peel and cut 1 pound of raw beets into ½-inch pieces and microwave in a covered bowl with ¼ cup water until tender, about 25 minutes. To ensure uniform pieces that cook at the same rate, we prefer to purchase a whole 1½- to 2-pound center-cut salmon fillet and cut it into four equal pieces. If using wild salmon, cook it until it registers 120 degrees.

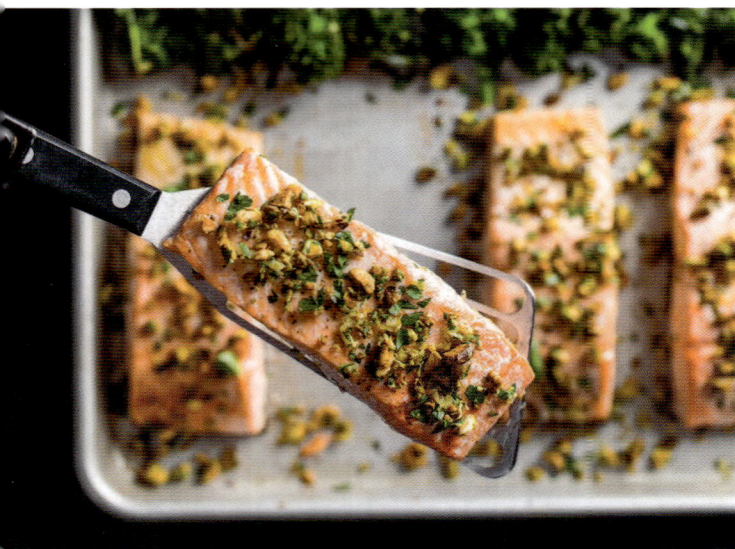

  2 oranges
1½ teaspoons table salt, divided
  1 teaspoon ground coriander
  ¾ teaspoon pepper, divided
  4 (6- to 8-ounce) skin-on salmon fillets, 1 inch thick
  3 tablespoons avocado oil, divided
  1 pound cooked beets, cut into ½-inch pieces
  2 avocados, halved, pitted, and cut into ½-inch pieces
  1 shallot, minced
  1 tablespoon cider vinegar

1 Grate 1 teaspoon zest from 1 orange. Combine zest with ½ teaspoon salt, coriander, and ½ teaspoon pepper in bowl, rubbing between your fingers to release oils from zest. Rub spice mixture over salmon flesh.

2 Heat 1 tablespoon oil in 12-inch nonstick skillet over medium-high heat until just smoking. Add salmon skin side up and cook until well browned, about 6 minutes. Flip and continue to cook until centers of fillets are still translucent when checked with tip of paring knife and register 125 degrees (for medium-rare), about 6 minutes. Transfer to platter.

3 Cut away peel and pith from oranges and cut into ½-inch pieces. Gently toss oranges and any released juices, beets, avocados, shallot, vinegar, remaining 2 tablespoons oil, remaining 1 teaspoon salt, and remaining ¼ teaspoon pepper together in bowl. Serve.

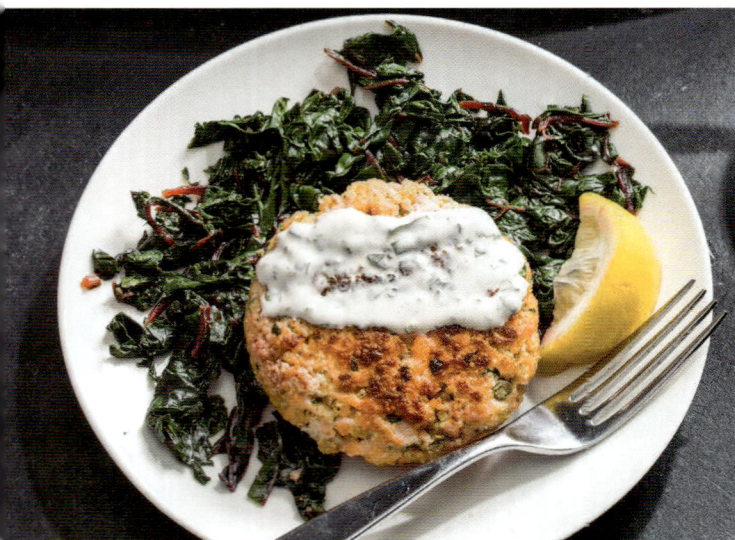

top	*Coriander Salmon with Beets, Oranges, and Avocados*
center	*Roasted Salmon and Broccoli Rabe with Pistachio Gremolata*
bottom	*Salmon Cakes with Sautéed Beet Greens and Lemon-Parsley Sauce*

The Benefits of Skin-On Fish

While we prefer skinless fish in many recipes, skin-on fish—as some of the recipes in this chapter use—can offer both a flavor and nutrient boost. Much of a fish's fat, which offers anti-inflammatory omega-3s, is found in or just beneath the skin. Searing the skin crisps it up while also locking in the moisture of the flesh, especially useful in leaner fillets such as halibut or snapper. As it cooks, collagen from the skin breaks down into gelatin, enriching the pan juices with subtle body.

Roasted Salmon and Broccoli Rabe with Pistachio Gremolata

serves 4 • total time: 30 minutes   **FAST**

why this recipe works • Quick-cooking fish is an appealing dinner choice for the busy cook who needs a healthful, one-pan dinner on the table fast. Salmon pairs well with many vegetables because it doesn't exude a lot of juices during cooking. We particularly like it with broccoli rabe; the pleasant bitterness of this green counterbalances the rich salmon. We accented the broccoli rabe with red pepper flakes and garlic for an antioxidant boost, and relegated it to one half of a baking sheet, placing the salmon on the other half for an easy sheet-pan meal. Roasted in a hot oven, the fillets cooked to a silky medium-rare in the same time it took the broccoli rabe to become tender. A nutty pistachio gremolata was a perfect finishing touch. Broccoli rabe is sometimes called rapini. To ensure uniform pieces that cook at the same rate, we prefer to purchase a whole 1½- to 2-pound center-cut salmon fillet and cut it into four equal pieces. If using wild salmon, cook it until it registers 120 degrees.

¼ cup shelled pistachios, toasted and chopped fine
2 tablespoons minced fresh parsley
2 garlic cloves, minced, divided
1 teaspoon grated lemon zest
1 pound broccoli rabe, trimmed and cut into 1½-inch pieces
2 tablespoons plus 2 teaspoons extra-virgin olive oil, divided
¾ teaspoon table salt, divided
½ teaspoon pepper, divided
   Pinch red pepper flakes
4 (6- to 8-ounce) skinless salmon fillets, 1 inch thick

1 Adjust oven rack to middle position and heat oven to 450 degrees. Combine pistachios, parsley, half of garlic, and lemon zest in small bowl; set gremolata aside until ready to serve.

2 Toss broccoli rabe, 2 tablespoons oil, ¼ teaspoon salt, ¼ teaspoon pepper, pepper flakes, and remaining garlic together in bowl. Arrange on half of rimmed baking sheet. Pat salmon dry with paper towels, rub with remaining 2 teaspoons oil, and sprinkle with remaining ½ teaspoon salt and remaining ¼ teaspoon pepper. Arrange salmon skinned side down on empty half of sheet.

3 Roast until center of fillets are still translucent when checked with tip of paring knife and register 125 degrees (for medium-rare) and broccoli rabe is tender, 4 to 12 minutes. Sprinkle salmon with gremolata and serve.

Salmon Cakes with Sautéed Beet Greens and Lemon-Parsley Sauce

serves 4 • total time: 35 minutes   **FAST**

why this recipe works • Fish cakes can be so much more than an appetizer—paired with a tasty vegetable and creamy sauce, they make a satisfying protein-rich main. We wanted to pair ultra-flavorful salmon cakes with a mild but hardy green, so we sautéed fiberful beet greens while the cakes kept warm in the oven after cooking. To make cakes with rich flavor and tender texture without using a lot of flavor-muting binders, we used a food processor to break up the salmon so that it wasn't overly dense. Parsley, mustard, and capers added tangy complexity, while yogurt ensured our patties stayed moist. Some of these ingredients then became part of a quick, bright, creamy sauce to drizzle over the cakes and greens. Don't overprocess the salmon in step 2 or the cakes will have a pasty texture. You can substitute Swiss chard for the beet greens.

¼ cup plain yogurt, divided
3 tablespoons minced fresh parsley, divided
2 tablespoons mayonnaise
2 teaspoons lemon juice, plus lemon wedges for serving
1 tablespoon Dijon mustard
2 teaspoons capers, rinsed and minced
¼ teaspoon table salt, divided
¼ teaspoon pepper, divided
1 pound skinless salmon, cut into 1-inch pieces
¾ cup panko bread crumbs
2 pounds beet greens, stemmed and chopped
5 teaspoons extra-virgin olive oil, divided

1   Combine 2 tablespoons yogurt, 1 tablespoon parsley, mayonnaise, and lemon juice in small bowl. Cover sauce and refrigerate until ready to serve. Whisk remaining 2 tablespoons yogurt, remaining 2 tablespoons parsley, mustard, capers, ⅛ teaspoon salt, and ⅛ teaspoon pepper together in large bowl

2   Working in 2 batches, pulse salmon in food processor until coarsely ground, about 4 pulses; transfer to large bowl with yogurt mixture. Gently fold in panko until well combined. Using your lightly moistened hands, divide salmon mixture into 4 equal portions, then gently shape each portion into 4-inch-wide cake.

3   Wash and drain beet greens, leaving greens slightly wet; set aside. Heat 2 teaspoons oil in 12-inch nonstick skillet over medium heat until shimmering. Cook cakes until well browned, 3 to 4 minutes per side. Transfer cakes to serving platter and tent with aluminum foil.

4   Heat remaining 1 tablespoon oil in now-empty skillet over medium-high heat until shimmering. Add drained greens, remaining ⅛ teaspoon salt, and remaining ⅛ teaspoon pepper. Cover and cook, stirring occasionally, until greens are wilted but still bright green, about 3 minutes. Increase heat to high and cook, uncovered, until liquid evaporates, 2 to 3 minutes. Serve salmon cakes with beet greens, lemon-parsley sauce, and lemon wedges.

MAKE AHEAD • Shaped salmon cakes can be refrigerated for up to 24 hours.

MAKE IT GLUTEN-FREE • Substitute gluten-free panko bread crumbs for the panko bread crumbs.

MAKE IT DAIRY-FREE • Substitute plant-based yogurt for the dairy yogurt.

Saumon aux Lentilles

serves 4 • total time: 1½ hours

why this recipe works • For our version of salmon with braised lentils, a classic French pairing and nutritionally vibrant duo, we started by building a flavorful foundation for our lentilles du Puy (also called French green lentils). This base came together by gently cooking onion, carrot, and celery in olive oil until soft; tomato paste and garlic added some antioxidants and even more depth before the lentils and water went in. When the lentils were fully softened and most of the moisture in the pot had either evaporated or been absorbed, we set them aside to focus on the

salmon, which we briefly brined in a saltwater solution to season the fish and to ensure that it retained plenty of moisture as it cooked. Unconventionally, we started the salmon skin side down in a cold nonstick skillet that had been sprinkled with salt and pepper. As the pan heated up, the salmon released some of the fat that lies just beneath the skin, crisping it and enabling us to cook the fish without any additional fat. Before serving, we stirred a bit of mustard and sherry vinegar into the lentils to brighten their flavor, making them an ideal pairing for the rich fish. To ensure uniform pieces, we prefer to purchase a whole 1½- to 2-pound center-cut salmon fillet and cut it into four equal pieces. Using skin-on salmon is important here, as this recipe relies on the fat underneath the skin as the cooking medium. If using wild salmon, cook it until it registers 120 degrees. Small, olive-green lentils du Puy are worth seeking out for their meaty texture, but if you can't find them, substitute another small green lentil. Do not use red or brown lentils.

Lentils
2   tablespoons extra-virgin olive oil, divided
1   large onion, chopped fine
1   celery rib, chopped fine
1   carrot, peeled and chopped fine
1½ teaspoons kosher salt
1   tablespoon minced garlic
1   tablespoon no-salt-added tomato paste
½   teaspoon dried thyme
½   teaspoon pepper
2½ cups water
1   cup dried lentilles du Puy (French green lentils), picked over and rinsed
1   tablespoon sherry vinegar, plus extra for seasoning
2   teaspoons Dijon mustard

Salmon
¼   cup kosher salt for brining
4   (6- to 8-ounce) skin-on salmon fillets, 1 inch thick
¾   teaspoon kosher salt, divided
¾   teaspoon pepper, divided

1   **For the lentils** Heat 1 tablespoon oil in medium saucepan over medium heat until shimmering. Add onion, celery, carrot, and salt and stir to coat vegetables. Cover and cook, stirring occasionally, until vegetables are softened but not browned, 8 to 10 minutes. Add garlic, tomato paste, thyme, and pepper and cook, stirring constantly, until fragrant, about 2 minutes. Stir in water and lentils. Increase heat and bring to boil. Adjust heat to simmer. Cover and cook, stirring occasionally, until lentils are tender but not mushy and have consistency of thick risotto, 40 to 50 minutes. Remove from heat and keep covered.

2 For the salmon While lentils are cooking, dissolve ¼ cup salt in 1 quart water in narrow container. Submerge salmon in brine and let stand for 15 minutes. Remove salmon from brine and pat dry with paper towels. Allow to stand while lentils finish cooking.

3 Sprinkle bottom of 12-inch nonstick skillet evenly with ½ teaspoon salt and ½ teaspoon pepper. Place salmon skin side down in skillet and sprinkle tops of fillets with remaining ¼ teaspoon salt and remaining ¼ teaspoon pepper. Heat skillet over medium-high heat and cook fillets, without moving them, until fat begins to render, skin begins to brown, and bottom ¼ inch of fillets turns opaque, 6 to 8 minutes.

4 Using tongs and thin spatula, flip fillets and continue to cook without moving them until centers are still translucent when checked with tip of paring knife and register 125 degrees (for medium-rare), 5 to 8 minutes. Transfer salmon skin side up to clean plate.

5 Warm lentils briefly if necessary. Stir in vinegar, mustard, and remaining 1 tablespoon oil. Season with salt, pepper, and vinegar to taste. Divide lentils among wide, shallow serving bowls. Arrange salmon skin side up on lentils and serve.

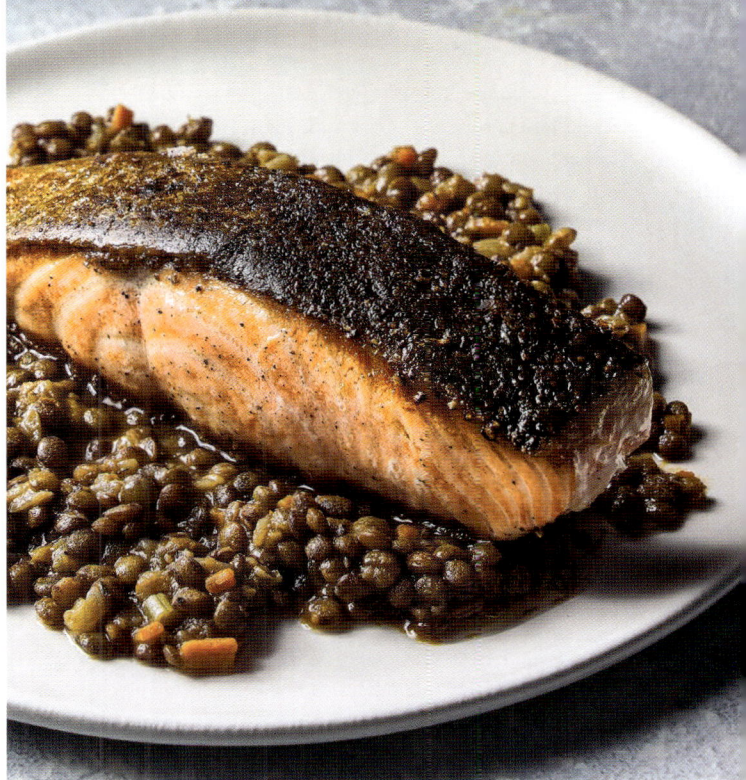

Glazed Salmon with Black-Eyed Peas, Walnuts, and Pomegranate

serves 4 · total time: 30 minutes **FAST** **SUPERCHARGED**

why this recipe works · Sweet-and-sour pomegranate molasses is the star of this nutrient-dense dish, in which it pulls double duty as both an enlivening glaze for roasted salmon and as the main ingredient in a bright vinaigrette for a hearty side salad. For perfect roasted salmon, we preheated the baking sheet in a 500-degree oven but then lowered the heat to 275 just before placing the fish on the sheet and into the oven; this firmed the exterior and rendered fat from the skin while cooking the salmon gently. Canned black-eyed peas, along with heart-healthy walnuts, punchy scallions, and tart pomegranate seeds, ably complemented the salmon with nutty, fresh, sweet, and acidic components. To ensure uniform pieces that cook at the same rate, we prefer to purchase a whole 1½- to 2-pound center-cut salmon fillet and cut it into four equal pieces. If using wild salmon, cook it until it registers 120 degrees.

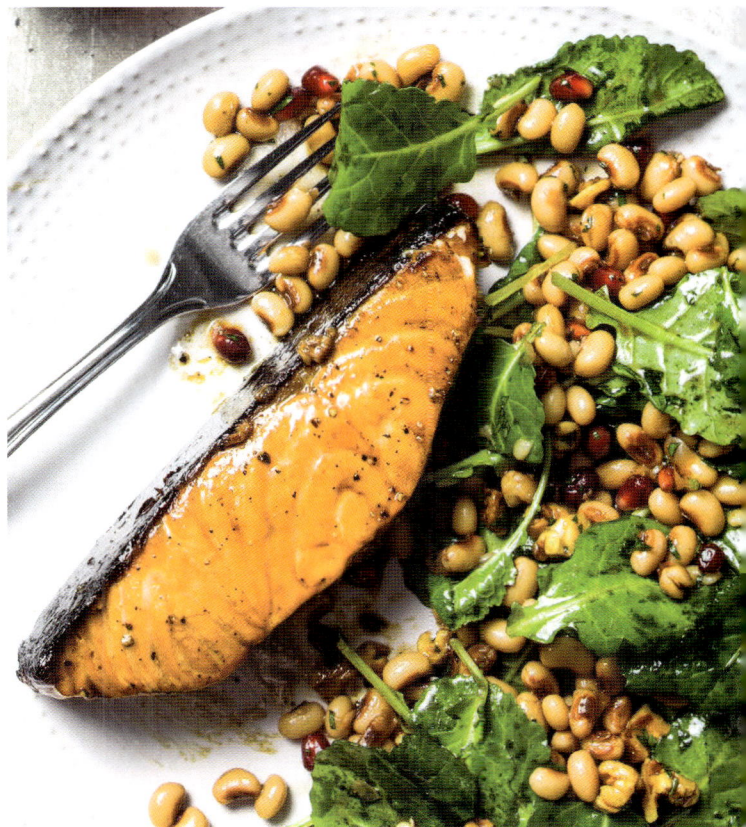

top	*Saumon aux Lentilles*
bottom	*Glazed Salmon with Black-Eyed Peas, Walnuts, and Pomegranate*

4 (6- to 8-ounce) skin-on salmon fillets, 1 inch thick

¼ cup pomegranate molasses, divided

¾ teaspoon table salt, divided

¼ teaspoon plus ⅛ teaspoon pepper, divided

3 tablespoons extra-virgin olive oil

2 tablespoons lemon juice

2 (15-ounce) cans no-salt-added black-eyed peas, rinsed

2 ounces (2 cups) baby kale

½ cup pomegranate seeds

½ cup walnuts, toasted and chopped

½ cup chopped fresh parsley

3 scallions, sliced thin

1 Adjust oven rack to lowest position, place rimmed baking sheet on rack, and heat oven to 500 degrees. Pat salmon dry with paper towels, brush with 1 tablespoon pomegranate molasses, and sprinkle with ½ teaspoon salt and ¼ teaspoon pepper.

2 Once oven reaches 500 degrees, reduce oven temperature to 275 degrees. Remove sheet from oven and carefully place salmon skin side down on hot sheet. Roast until centers of fillets are still translucent when checked with tip of paring knife and register 125 degrees (for medium-rare), 7 to 13 minutes.

3 Whisk oil, lemon juice, 2 tablespoons pomegranate molasses, remaining ¼ teaspoon salt, and remaining ⅛ teaspoon pepper in large bowl until combined. Add black-eyed peas, kale, pomegranate seeds, walnuts, parsley, and scallions and toss to combine. Season with salt and pepper to taste.

4 Remove sheet from oven and brush salmon with remaining 1 tablespoon pomegranate molasses. Slide fish spatula along underside of salmon and transfer to serving platter. Serve salmon with black-eyed-pea salad.

Roasted Salmon with White Beans, Fennel, and Tomatoes

serves 4 · total time: 45 minutes FAST

why this recipe works · For a flavorful salmon dinner with minimal fuss, we roasted it with a medley of vegetables on a single baking sheet—but not all at once. Subtly sweet fennel got a head start to soften and caramelize before we added creamy cannellini beans tossed with cherry tomatoes and garlic. Nestling the fillets atop the beans ensured that the fish cooked gently while the beans and vegetables absorbed the salmon's juices. Lemon juice and basil balanced the dish's savory depth. To ensure uniform pieces that cook at the same rate, we prefer to purchase a whole

1½- to 2-pound center-cut salmon fillet and cut it into four equal pieces. If using wild salmon, cook it until it registers 120 degrees.

2 pounds fennel bulbs, stalks discarded, bulbs halved, cored, and sliced ¼ inch thick

2 tablespoons extra-virgin olive oil, divided, plus extra for drizzling

1¼ teaspoons table salt, divided

¾ teaspoon pepper, divided

2 (15-ounce) cans no-salt-added cannellini beans, rinsed

10 ounces cherry tomatoes, halved

¼ cup dry white wine

2 garlic cloves, sliced thin

4 (6- to 8-ounce) skinless salmon fillets, 1 inch thick

2 tablespoons lemon juice, plus lemon wedges for serving

½ cup torn fresh basil or parsley, divided

1 Adjust oven rack to middle position and heat oven to 450 degrees. Toss fennel, 1 tablespoon oil, ¼ teaspoon salt, and ¼ teaspoon pepper together on rimmed baking sheet. Spread fennel into even layer and roast until beginning to brown around edges, about 15 minutes.

2 Meanwhile, toss beans, tomatoes, wine, garlic, ½ teaspoon salt, ¼ teaspoon pepper, and remaining 1 tablespoon oil together in bowl. Pat salmon dry with paper towels and sprinkle with remaining ½ teaspoon salt and remaining ¼ teaspoon pepper.

3 Remove sheet from oven. Add bean mixture to sheet with fennel, stir to combine, and spread into even layer. Arrange salmon on top of bean mixture, spaced evenly apart. Roast until centers of fillets are still translucent when checked with tip of paring knife and register 125 degrees (for medium-rare), 12 to 18 minutes.

4 Transfer salmon to serving platter. Stir lemon juice and ¼ cup torn basil into fennel and bean mixture. Season with salt and pepper to taste. Transfer fennel and bean mixture to platter with salmon. Drizzle with extra oil and sprinkle with remaining ¼ cup basil. Serve with lemon wedges.

Sautéed Tilapia with Grapefruit-Basil Relish

serves 4 · total time: 40 minutes FAST

why this recipe works · The flavor of tilapia may not be too far off from that of thicker white fish such cod or haddock. However, that doesn't mean it can be cooked the same way. Consider the anatomy of thin white fish: The thick half of a thin, wide fillet rests flat on the pan and browns nicely during sautéing, but the thin half tilts up, hardly making contact at all. The only way around this was to split them at their seams and cook the thick halves in one batch and the thin halves in a second. The result was uniform, evenly browned fish fillets. High heat turned the fish, both thick and thin pieces, beautifully golden-brown and evenly crisp on both sides. We paired the fillets with a complex relish of grapefruit and basil, which we seasoned with shallot and lemon juice—a medley of anti-inflammatory ingredients that also happened to create the ideal tangy foil for the mild fish. Flounder, sole, or catfish can be substituted for the tilapia.

Grapefruit-Basil Relish
- 2 red grapefruits
- 1 small shallot, minced
- 2 tablespoons chopped fresh basil
- 2 teaspoons lemon juice
- 2 teaspoons extra-virgin olive oil

Tilapia
- 4 (4- to 6-ounce) skinless tilapia fillets, halved lengthwise down natural seam
- ½ teaspoon table salt
- 2 tablespoons avocado oil

1 For the relish Cut away peel and pith from grapefruits. Cut grapefruits into 8 wedges, then slice crosswise into ½-inch-thick pieces. Place grapefruits in strainer set over bowl and let drain for 15 minutes; measure out and reserve 1 tablespoon drained juice. Combine reserved juice, shallot, basil, lemon juice, and oil in bowl. Stir in grapefruits and let sit for 15 minutes. Season with salt and pepper to taste.

2 For the tilapia Sprinkle tilapia with salt and let sit at room temperature for 15 minutes. Pat tilapia dry with paper towels.

3 Heat oil in 12-inch nonstick skillet over high heat until just smoking. Add thick halves of tilapia fillets to skillet and cook, tilting and gently shaking skillet occasionally to distribute oil, until golden brown and registering 130 to 135 degrees, 2 to 3 minutes per side. Transfer tilapia to serving platter.

4 Return skillet to high heat. When oil is just smoking, add thin halves of fillets and cook until golden brown, about 1 minute per side. Transfer tilapia to platter and serve with relish.

❙ **MAKE AHEAD** • Relish can be refrigerated for up to 2 days.

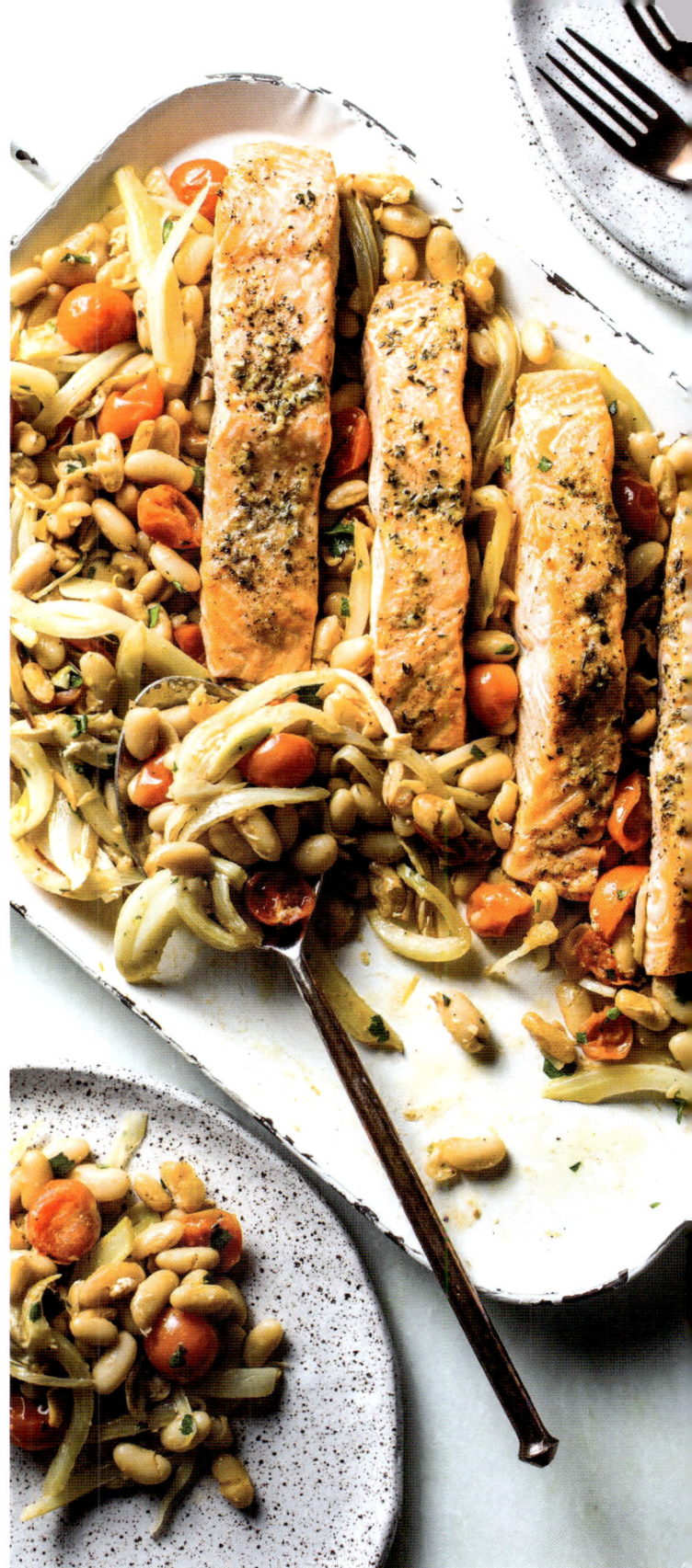

Roasted Salmon with White Beans, Fennel, and Tomatoes

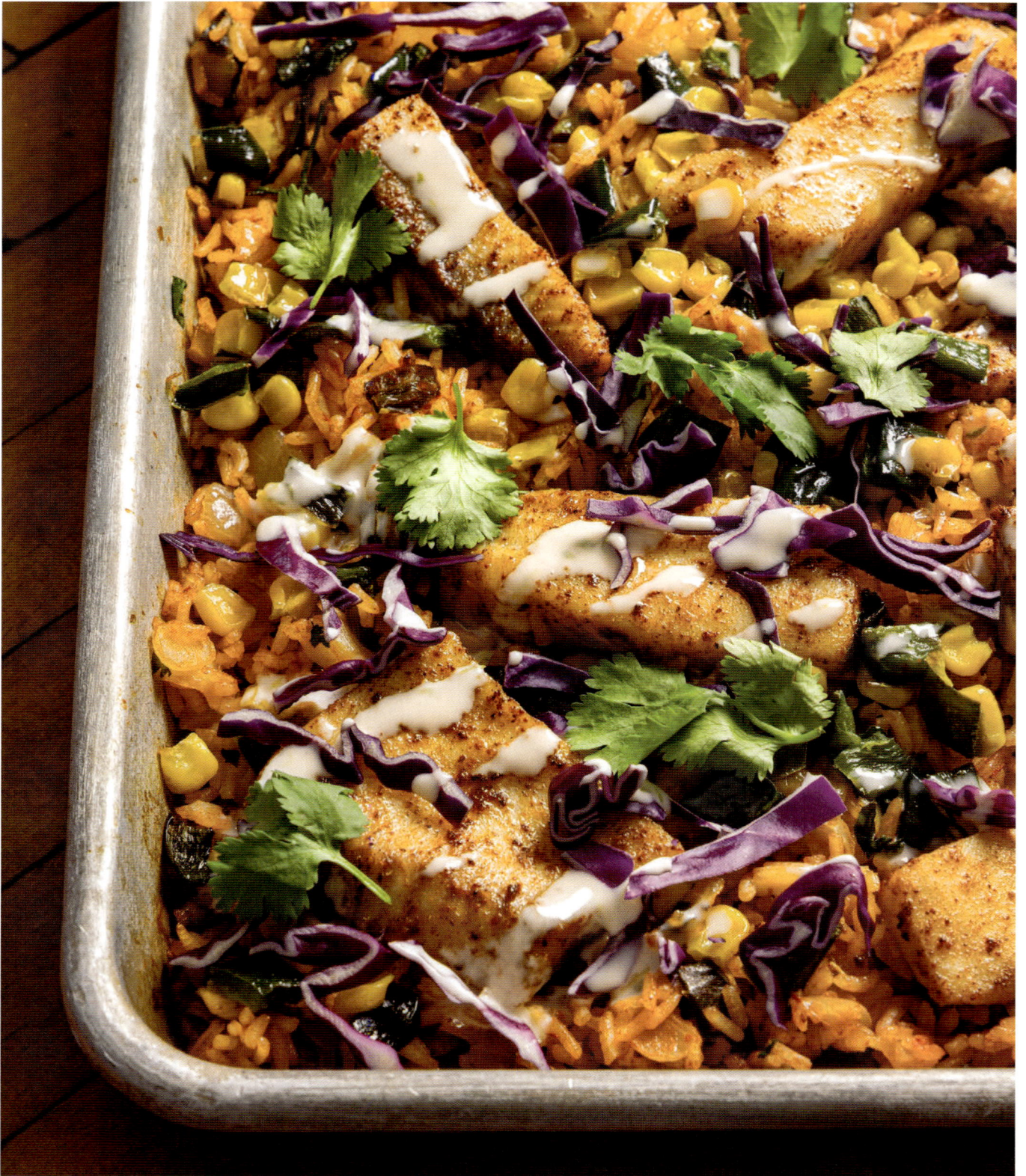

Sheet-Pan Mexican Rice with Tilapia

Sautéed Tilapia with Blistered Green Beans and Pepper Relish

serves 4 · total time: 45 minutes **FAST**

why this recipe works · Readily available and economical, tilapia has a lot going for it even before it hits your plate—the lean, firm fillets are easy to flip during sautéing, and this mild fish becomes golden and crispy on the outside but stays moist on the inside. Here, we pair it with a flavorful relish and vegetable side for a quick, healthy meal. We started by splitting the fish down the seams and separating the thick and thinner halves, so they cooked evenly. To accompany our tilapia we made a simple relish, which provided color, brightness, and contrasting texture. For our vegetable, we quickly steamed green beans until tender, letting them continue to cook uncovered, so they got some flavorful browning. Finally, we sautéed the tilapia in the same skillet until perfectly cooked. Flounder, sole, or catfish can be substituted for the tilapia.

- 4 (4- to 6-ounce) skinless tilapia fillets, halved lengthwise down natural seam
- 1¼ teaspoons table salt, divided
- 1 cup jarred roasted red peppers, patted dry and chopped fine
- ¼ cup whole almonds, toasted and chopped fine
- ¼ cup avocado oil, divided
- 1 tablespoon chopped fresh basil
- 1 teaspoon sherry vinegar
- ⅛ teaspoon plus ¼ teaspoon pepper, divided
- 1 pound green beans, trimmed
- ¼ cup water

1 Sprinkle tilapia with ½ teaspoon salt and let sit at room temperature for 15 minutes. Meanwhile, combine red peppers, almonds, 1 tablespoon oil, basil, vinegar, ⅛ teaspoon pepper, and ¼ teaspoon salt in bowl; set aside relish until ready to serve.

2 Combine green beans, water, 1 tablespoon oil, remaining ½ teaspoon salt, and remaining ¼ teaspoon pepper in 12-inch nonstick skillet. Cover and cook over medium-high heat, shaking pan occasionally, until water has evaporated, 6 to 8 minutes. Uncover and continue to cook until green beans are blistered and browned, about 2 minutes. Transfer to platter and tent with aluminum foil to keep warm.

3 Pat tilapia dry with paper towels. Heat remaining 2 tablespoons oil in now-empty skillet over high heat until just smoking. Add thick halves of tilapia fillets to skillet and cook, tilting and gently shaking skillet occasionally to distribute oil, until golden brown and registering 130 to 135 degrees, 2 to 3 minutes per side. Transfer to platter with green beans.

4 Return skillet to high heat. When oil is just smoking, add thin halves of fillets and cook until golden brown, about 1 minute per side. Transfer tilapia to platter with green beans. Serve with relish.

Sheet-Pan Mexican Rice with Tilapia

serves 4 to 6 · total time: 1¼ hours

why this recipe works · We wanted to combine all of our favorite elements of fish taco bowls—Mexican rice included—into one flavor-packed sheet-pan meal. For the fish, we decided to use flaky, widely available tilapia. First, we roasted vegetables on opposite ends of the sheet: onion and a portion of chopped poblano (to be combined with the rice later) on one end, and the rest of the chopped poblanos plus corn (to scatter atop the rice) on the other. We added big flavor to our rice by combining the uncooked grains with the roasted onion-poblano mixture, tomato paste, and garlic. We added boiling water to the mix before carefully transferring it to the now-empty sheet pan. Covering the pan tightly with foil allowed the rice to gently steam. Once the rice was tender, we took the sheet out of the oven, added the corn-poblano mixture back, nestled the spice-rubbed fish into the rice, and continued baking. After a few minutes, the fish was perfectly cooked. To finish, we scattered thinly sliced cabbage over top and drizzled everything with a lime crema. We like the color of purple cabbage in this recipe, but you can use green if you prefer. Flounder, sole, or catfish can be substituted for the tilapia.

- ½ cup Mexican crema or sour cream
- 2 teaspoons table salt, divided
- 1 teaspoon grated lime zest plus 2 tablespoons juice, plus lime wedges for serving
- 1 large onion, chopped
- 3 poblano chiles, stemmed, seeded, and chopped, divided
- ¼ cup avocado oil, divided
- 1 cup fresh or frozen corn
- 1½ cups long-grain white rice, rinsed
- 3 tablespoons no-salt-added tomato paste
- 1½ teaspoons garlic powder, divided
- 2½ cups boiling water
- 4 (4- to 6-ounce) skinless tilapia fillets, halved lengthwise down natural seam
- ¾ teaspoon ground cumin
- ½ teaspoon chipotle chile powder
- ⅓ cup chopped fresh cilantro leaves and tender stems, plus extra for serving
- 1 cup thinly sliced red cabbage

1   Adjust oven rack to middle position and heat to 400 degrees. Combine crema, ¼ teaspoon salt, and lime zest and juice in small bowl; set aside until ready to serve.

2   Combine onion, 1 cup chopped poblano, 1 tablespoon oil, and ¾ teaspoon salt in bowl, then transfer to rimmed baking sheet, spreading into even layer over half of sheet. Combine corn, remaining chopped poblano, 1 tablespoon oil, and ¼ teaspoon salt in now-empty bowl, then spread into even layer on other half of sheet, leaving some space between vegetables. Roast until vegetables are nearly tender, about 20 minutes.

3   Transfer roasted corn-poblano mixture to again-empty bowl; set aside. Transfer roasted onion-poblano mixture to large bowl; add rice, tomato paste, 1 tablespoon oil and 1 teaspoon garlic powder; and stir until rice is well coated. Stir in boiling water, then carefully pour rice mixture onto now-empty sheet. Using spatula, carefully spread rice into even layer over sheet. Cover sheet with aluminum foil, crimping edges tightly (using 2 sheets of foil and overlapping in center if necessary) and bake until rice is tender, about 25 minutes. Wipe bowl dry.

4   While rice cooks, pat tilapia dry with paper towels. Cut each thick piece in half crosswise, then in half again lengthwise. Cut each thin piece in half crosswise. Toss tilapia pieces with remaining 1 tablespoon oil, remaining ¾ teaspoon salt, cumin, chile powder, and remaining ½ teaspoon garlic powder in now-empty, dry bowl.

5   Once rice is tender (uncover one corner of sheet to test rice doneness), transfer sheet to wire rack and let rest, covered, for 5 minutes. Increase oven temperature to 450 degrees. Remove foil from sheet, sprinkle cilantro on top of rice, and fluff rice with fork. Spoon reserved corn-poblano mixture over rice, then nestle fish into rice spaced evenly around sheet. Return sheet to oven and roast until fish is opaque and thickest pieces register 130 to 135 degrees, 5 to 7 minutes.

6   Scatter cabbage over top and drizzle with lime crema. Serve with extra cilantro and lime wedges.

MAKE IT DAIRY-FREE • Substitute plant-based sour cream for the Mexican crema.

Pan-Seared Trout with Brussels Sprouts

serves 4 • total time: 40 minutes   FAST

why this recipe works • You don't often see hearty brussels sprouts in seafood recipes, but we love the heft, not to mention vitamins and minerals, they provide to an otherwise delicate dish— and trout has a presence and sturdiness that easily stands up to the sprouts. We microwaved the sprouts to soften them before finishing them on the stovetop; this ensured that the insides became tender while the outsides stayed pleasingly crisp. A little cornstarch on the trout helped it achieve crispy skin to complement the texture of the sprouts. We cooked the trout until it turned golden on both sides while the inside remained moist. Serve with lemon wedges.

- 1 pound brussels sprouts, trimmed and halved
- 1 teaspoon table salt, divided
- ½ teaspoon pepper, divided
- 5 tablespoons extra-virgin olive oil, divided
- 1 shallot, minced
- 2 garlic cloves, minced
- ½ teaspoon minced fresh thyme
- 3 tablespoons cornstarch
- 3 (8- to 10-ounce) boneless, butterflied whole trout, halved between fillets

1   Adjust oven rack to middle position and heat oven to 200 degrees. Combine brussels sprouts, 1 tablespoon water, ½ teaspoon salt, and ¼ teaspoon pepper in bowl. Microwave, covered, until sprouts are just tender, about 5 minutes; drain.

2   Meanwhile, heat 1 tablespoon oil in 12-inch nonstick skillet over medium heat until shimmering. Add shallot and cook until softened, about 2 minutes. Stir in garlic and thyme and cook until fragrant, about 30 seconds. Add drained sprouts and cook until lightly browned, about 3 minutes; transfer to ovensafe platter and keep warm in oven.

3   Spread cornstarch in shallow dish. Pat trout dry with paper towels, sprinkle with remaining ½ teaspoon salt and remaining ¼ teaspoon pepper, then dredge in cornstarch, pressing gently to adhere. Wipe out now-empty skillet with paper towels, add 2 tablespoons oil, and heat over high heat until shimmering. Lay 3 pieces trout skin side down in skillet and reduce heat to medium-high. Cook until golden on both sides and fish flakes apart when gently prodded with paring knife, about 4 minutes per side; transfer to platter with sprouts and keep warm in oven.

4   Wipe out now-empty skillet with paper towels and repeat with remaining 2 tablespoons oil and remaining 3 trout pieces. Serve with brussels sprouts.

Reheating Fish

Fish is an excellent source of protein and healthy fats, but it can be notoriously susceptible to overcooking, so reheating previously cooked fillets can be dicey. Firm, meaty white fish cuts, however, are ideal candidates for reheating. They retain their moisture well, with no detectable change in flavor. Use this gentle approach: Place the fillets or steaks on a wire rack set in a rimmed baking sheet; cover with aluminum foil (to prevent the exteriors from drying out); and heat in a 275-degree oven until the fish registers 125 to 130 degrees, about 15 minutes for 1-inch-thick fish (timing varies according to fish size).

For other fish that don't fare as well, such as thin fish, we recommend serving them in cold applications like salads. Salmon reheats well, but be aware that doing so brings out a bit more of the fish's pungent aroma.

Moroccan Fish and Couscous Packets

serves 4 · total time: 55 minutes

why this recipe works · Moroccan chermoula is a spice and herb mixture that's at once bright, herbaceous, and earthy, packing a punch of flavor wherever it's used. Pairing it with quick-cooking tilapia and couscous and baking it all in foil makes for an effortless yet incredibly flavorful, fragrant meal. We placed mounds of fluffy, lemony couscous on the foil and then topped them with chermoula-slathered tilapia fillets before sealing the packets. For an accurate measurement of boiling water, bring a full kettle of water to a boil and then measure out the desired amount. To test for doneness without opening the foil packets, use a permanent marker to mark an "X" on the outside of the foil where the fish fillet is the thickest and then insert an instant-read thermometer through the "X" into the fish to measure its internal temperature. Flounder, sole, or catfish can be substituted for the tilapia; you may need to tuck the tapered ends under to achieve a more uniform thickness for even cooking. For catfish, start checking for doneness at 26 minutes; for flounder, start checking for doneness at 16 minutes; for sole, start checking for doneness at 23 minutes.

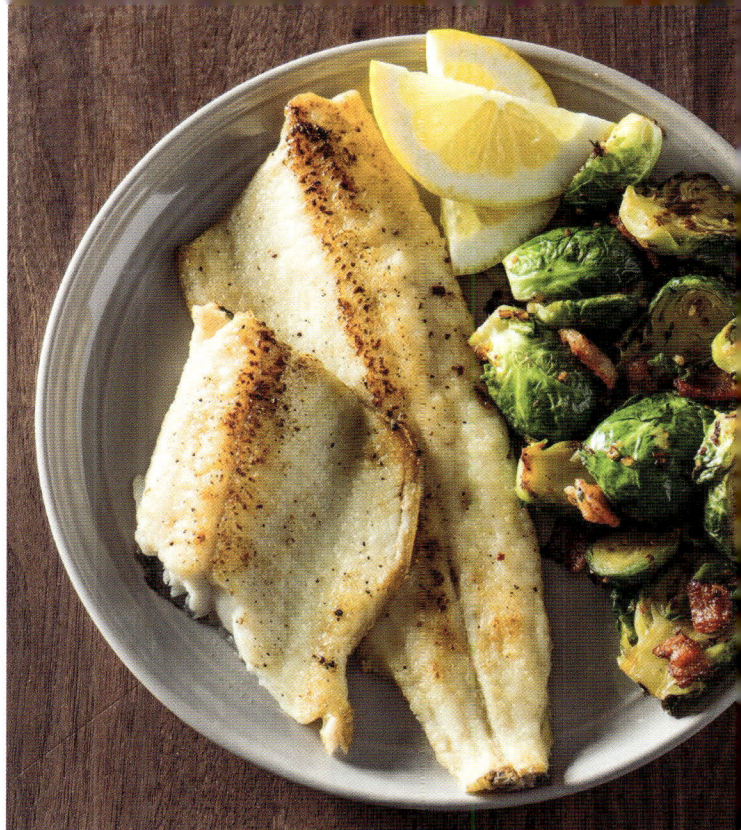

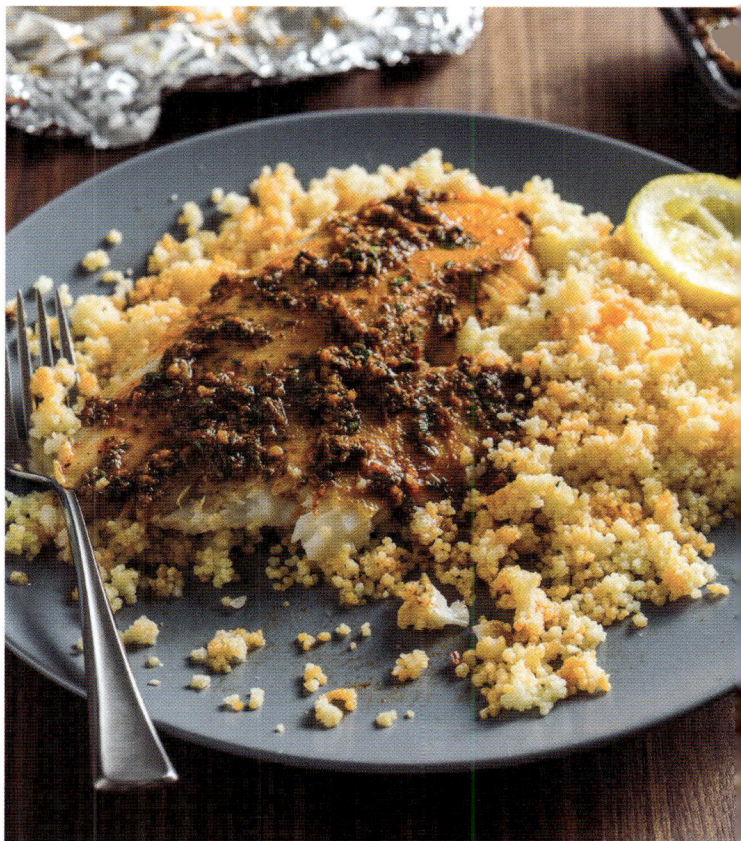

| top | Pan-Seared Trout with Brussels Sprouts |
| bottom | Moroccan Fish and Couscous Packets |

½ cup minced fresh cilantro, divided

¼ cup extra-virgin olive oil

2 tablespoons grated fresh ginger

4 teaspoons smoked paprika

4 garlic cloves, minced

4 teaspoons grated lemon zest, divided, plus 2 tablespoons juice

2 teaspoons ground cumin

1½ teaspoons table salt, divided

½ teaspoon pepper, divided

½ teaspoon brown sugar

¼ teaspoon red pepper flakes

1½ cups couscous

2 cups boiling water

4 (4- to 6-ounce) skinless tilapia fillets, ¾ inch thick

1 Adjust oven rack to middle position and heat oven to 400 degrees. Combine 6 tablespoons cilantro, oil, ginger, paprika, garlic, 1 tablespoon lemon zest, lemon juice, cumin, ½ teaspoon salt, ¼ teaspoon pepper, sugar, and pepper flakes in bowl; set chermoula aside.

2 Combine couscous, ½ teaspoon salt, and boiling water in bowl; cover; and let sit until liquid is absorbed and couscous is tender, about 5 minutes. Fluff couscous with fork, stir in remaining 1 teaspoon lemon zest, and season with salt and pepper to taste.

3 Lay four 16 by 12-inch rectangles of aluminum foil on counter with short sides parallel to counter edge. Divide couscous evenly among foil rectangles, arranging in center of lower half of each foil sheet. Pat tilapia dry with paper towels and sprinkle with remaining ½ teaspoon salt and remaining ¼ teaspoon pepper. Place tilapia on top of couscous and spoon 1 tablespoon chermoula over top of each fillet; reserve remaining chermoula for serving. Fold top half of foil over fish and couscous, then tightly crimp edges into rough 9 by 6-inch packets.

4 Place packets on rimmed baking sheet (they may overlap slightly) and bake until fish registers 130 to 135 degrees, 20 to 24 minutes. Carefully open packets, allowing steam to escape away from you. Using thin metal spatula, gently slice couscous and tilapia onto individual plates, then sprinkle with remaining 2 tablespoons cilantro. Serve with remaining chermoula.

Thai Curry Rice with Mahi-Mahi

serves 4 · total time: 1 hour

why this recipe works · Mahi-mahi is meaty, lean, and mild, perfect for pairing with the rich and aromatic flavors of Thai curry. To create an entire Thai-inspired meal without lots of prep and multiple pans, we layered the components of both the fish curry and rice all in one skillet and timed everything just right for maximum flavor with minimum effort. The rice became a canvas for anti-inflammatory add-ins when we sautéed it with meaty mushrooms, crunchy bamboo shoots, spicy ginger, and fresh scallions. After adding water to the skillet and giving the rice a 10-minute head start, we placed the mahi-mahi fillets on top of the simmering rice and drizzled everything with a simple mixture of coconut milk and Thai curry paste. The fish finished cooking at the same time that the rice became irresistibly crispy on the bottom. All we needed was a sprinkle of scallions, a few more spoonfuls of sauce, and a squeeze of lime to get this impressive dinner on the table. Halibut, red snapper, striped bass, or swordfish can be substituted for the mahi-mahi.

1 tablespoon avocado oil

1½ cups long-grain white rice, rinsed

8 ounces white mushrooms, trimmed and sliced thin

1 (8-ounce) can sliced bamboo shoots, rinsed

2 teaspoons grated fresh ginger

3 scallions, white and green parts separated and sliced thin on bias

2¼ cups water

½ teaspoon table salt, divided

¾ cup canned low-fat coconut milk

3 tablespoons red curry paste

4 (6- to 8-ounce) skinless mahi-mahi fillets, 1 inch thick

¼ teaspoon pepper

Lime wedges

1 Heat oil in 12-inch nonstick skillet over medium heat until shimmering. Add rice, mushrooms, bamboo shoots, ginger, and scallion whites. Cook, stirring often, until edges of rice begin to turn translucent, about 2 minutes. Add water and ¼ teaspoon salt and bring to boil. Cover, reduce heat to low, and simmer for 10 minutes.

2 Meanwhile, whisk coconut milk and curry paste together in bowl. Pat mahi-mahi dry with paper towels and sprinkle with remaining ¼ teaspoon salt and pepper. Lay fillets skinned side down on top of rice mixture in skillet and drizzle with one-third of coconut-curry sauce. Cover skillet and cook until liquid is absorbed, rice is tender, and fish flakes apart when gently prodded with paring knife and registers 130 degrees, 10 to 12 minutes. Remove from heat and let sit, covered, for 10 minutes.

3 Microwave remaining coconut-curry sauce mixture until warm, about 1 minute. Drizzle remaining coconut-curry sauce over fish and rice mixture and sprinkle with scallion greens. Serve with lime wedges.

Seared Tilapia with Olive Vinaigrette and Warm Chickpea Salad

serves 4 · total time: 40 minutes **FAST**

why this recipe works · This tilapia dinner is a powerhouse of anti-inflammatory ingredients—and as a bonus it's also fast enough for a busy weeknight. Tilapia, a lean white fish, paired perfectly with chickpeas, which provided filling fiber and plant-based protein. Olive oil and Castelvetrano olives contributed heart-healthy fats and polyphenols, while red bell pepper and red onion added vitamins and antioxidants. Tilapia fillets naturally have a thick side and a thin side; separating them allowed us to achieve perfectly cooked portions with a golden-brown exterior. We prefer mild, buttery Castelvetrano olives here; if you use a more robust type, reduce the amount to 2 tablespoons. Flounder, sole, or catfish can be substituted for the tilapia.

   4 (4- to 6-ounce) skinless tilapia fillets, halved lengthwise down natural seam
2½ teaspoons kosher salt, divided
   1 red bell pepper, stemmed, seeded, and chopped fine
   1 small red onion, chopped fine
   2 tablespoons red wine vinegar, divided
  ¾ teaspoon pepper, divided
   2 (15-ounce) cans no-salt-added chickpeas, rinsed
  ½ cup extra-virgin olive oil, divided
   1 tablespoon chopped fresh oregano
  ¼ cup pitted Castelvetrano olives, chopped coarse

1 Sprinkle tilapia all over with ½ teaspoon salt and let sit for 15 minutes. Combine bell pepper, onion, 1 tablespoon vinegar, ½ teaspoon pepper, and 1¾ teaspoons salt in large bowl. Heat chickpeas and ¼ cup oil in 12-inch nonstick skillet over medium heat until warmed through, about 3 minutes, coarsely mashing about one-quarter of them. Stir chickpeas into vegetable mixture.

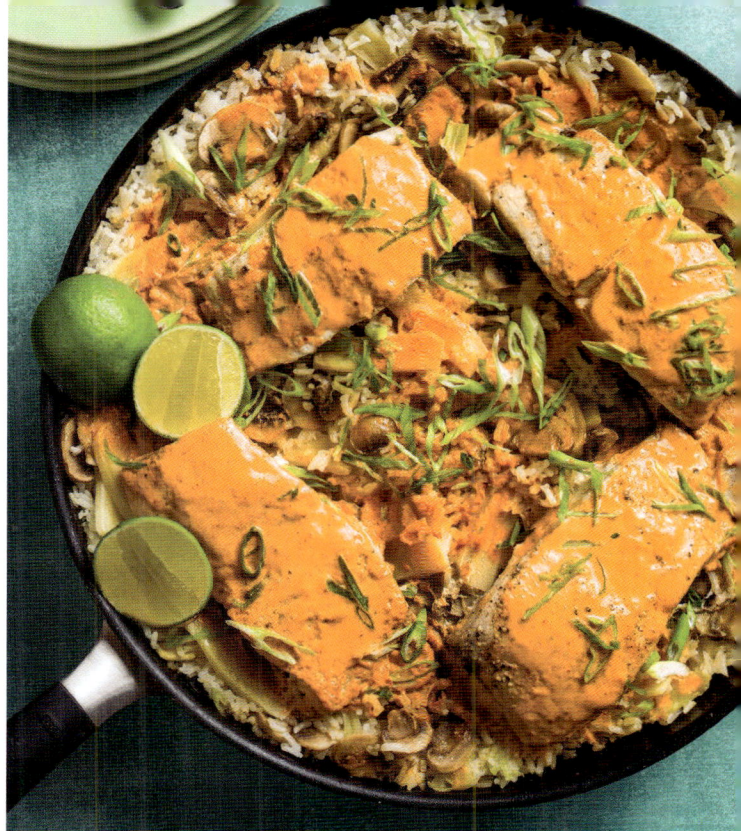

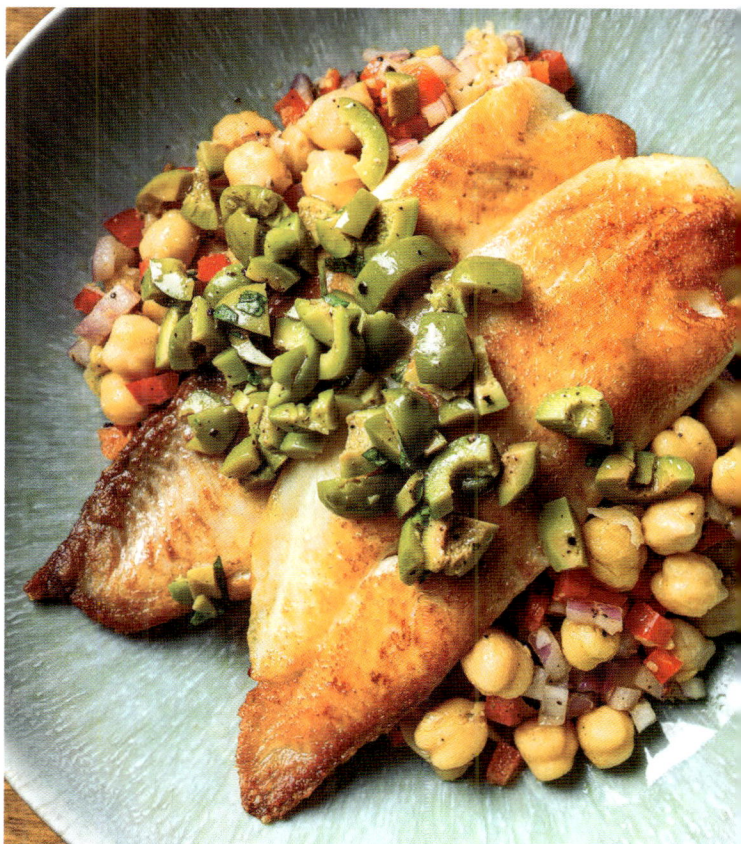

top | *Thai Curry Rice with Mahi-Mahi*
bottom | *Seared Tilapia with Olive Vinaigrette and Warm Chickpea Salad*

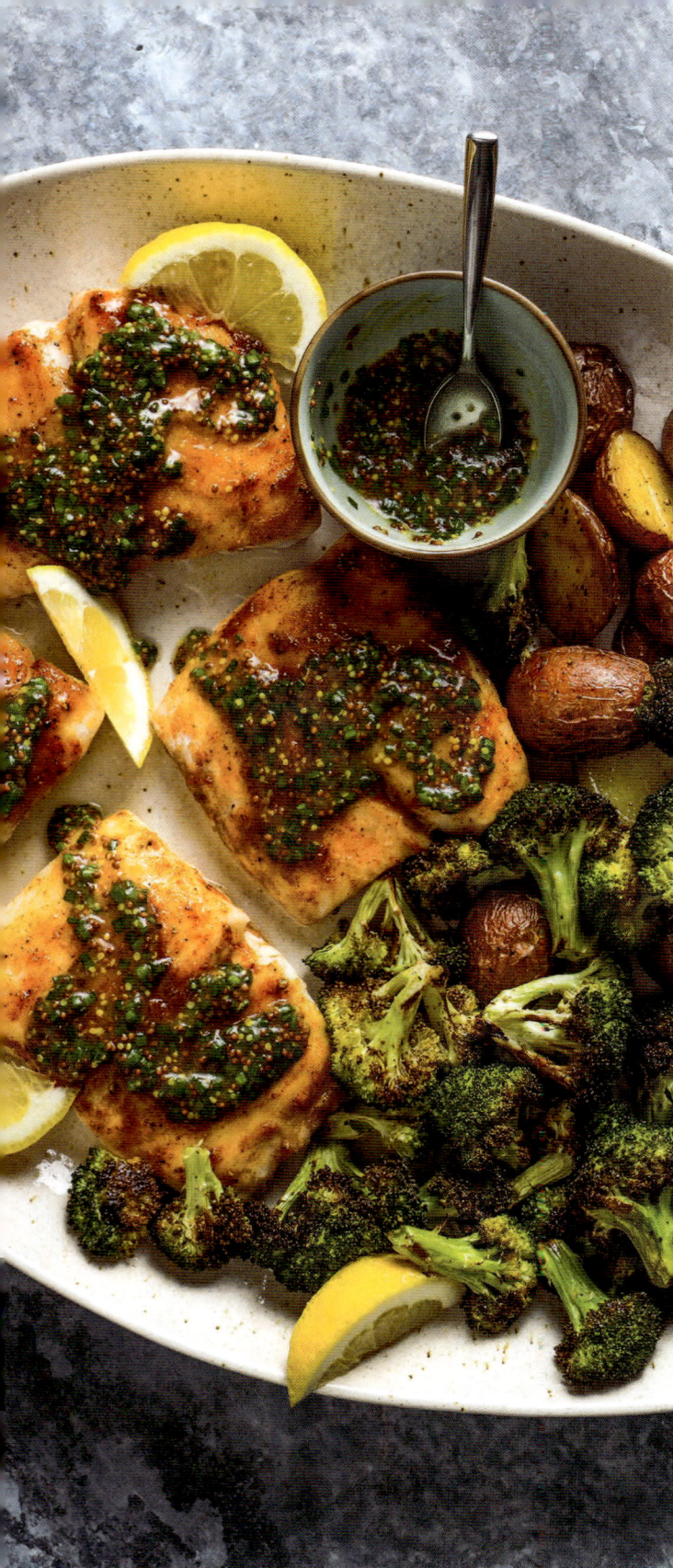

2 Pat tilapia dry with paper towels. Heat 2 tablespoons oil in now-empty skillet over high heat until just smoking. Add thick halves of tilapia fillets to skillet and cook, tilting and gently shaking skillet occasionally to distribute oil, until golden brown and registering 130 to 135 degrees, 2 to 3 minutes per side. Transfer to plate. Return skillet to high heat. When oil is just smoking, add thin halves of fillets and cook until golden brown, about 1 minute per side. Transfer to plate.

3 Combine oregano and remaining ¼ teaspoon salt, remaining 1 tablespoon vinegar, and remaining ¼ teaspoon pepper in bowl. Slowly whisk in remaining 2 tablespoons oil until emulsified. Stir in olives. Serve with tilapia and chickpea salad.

Roasted Snapper and Vegetables with Mustard Sauce

serves 4 • **total time: 1 hour**

why this recipe works • Looking for a seafood version of the classic meat-and-potatoes dinner? Try this easy one-pan meal of hearty red snapper, golden-brown potatoes, and gently charred broccoli. We started by tossing halved red potatoes and broccoli florets with oil, salt, and pepper separately and placing each on one side of a baking sheet to roast in a hot oven. We removed the broccoli once it was spotty brown and added our red snapper fillets to the free side of the sheet, dropping the oven temperature to allow the fish to cook more gently and the potatoes to continue cooking through. A simple mix of lemon zest, paprika, and honey brushed on before roasting the fillets added just enough flavor and color to the fish, and paired beautifully with a bright sauce of chives and mustard. Use small red potatoes measuring 1 to 2 inches in diameter. Halibut, mahi-mahi, striped bass, or swordfish can be substituted for the red snapper. Serve with lemon wedges.

6 tablespoons plus 2 teaspoons extra-virgin olive oil, divided
¼ cup minced fresh chives
2 tablespoons whole-grain mustard
1 tablespoon honey, divided
1 teaspoon grated lemon zest plus 2 teaspoons juice
   Pinch plus 1 teaspoon table salt, divided
   Pinch plus ¾ teaspoon pepper, divided
1 pound small red potatoes, unpeeled, halved
1 pound broccoli florets, cut into 2-inch pieces
½ teaspoon paprika
4 (6- to 8-ounce) skinless red snapper fillets, 1 inch thick

1 Adjust oven rack to lowest position and heat oven to 500 degrees. Combine 2 tablespoons oil, chives, mustard, 1 teaspoon honey, lemon juice, pinch salt, and pinch pepper in bowl; set mustard sauce aside until ready to serve. Brush rimmed baking sheet with 1 tablespoon oil.

2 Toss potatoes with 1 tablespoon oil, ¼ teaspoon salt, and ¼ teaspoon pepper in bowl. Place potatoes, cut sides down, on half of sheet. In now-empty bowl, toss broccoli with 2 tablespoons oil, ¼ teaspoon salt, and ¼ teaspoon pepper, then place on empty side of sheet. Roast until potatoes are golden brown and broccoli is spotty brown and tender, 12 to 14 minutes, rotating sheet halfway through roasting.

3 While potatoes and broccoli roast, combine 1 teaspoon oil, lemon zest, paprika, remaining 2 teaspoons honey, remaining ½ teaspoon salt, and remaining ¼ teaspoon pepper in small bowl; microwave until bubbling and fragrant, 10 to 15 seconds. Pat red snapper dry with paper towels, brush skinned sides of fillets with remaining 1 teaspoon oil, then brush tops of fillets with honey mixture.

4 Remove sheet from oven and reduce oven temperature to 275 degrees. Transfer broccoli to platter and tent with aluminum foil to keep warm. Place red snapper skinned side down on now-empty side of sheet. Continue to roast until fish flakes apart when gently prodded with paring knife and registers 130 degrees, 6 to 8 minutes, rotating sheet halfway through roasting.

5 Transfer potatoes and red snapper to platter with broccoli. Tent with foil and let sit for 10 minutes. Serve with mustard sauce.

Pan-Roasted Cod with Cilantro Chimichurri

serves 4 · **total time: 45 minutes** `FAST`

why this recipe works · We love a moist white fish fillet with a chestnut-brown crust almost as much as we love its quick cooking time. But lean cod is also easy to overcook at home. So for a cooking method that reliably turned out delicious, flaky white fish fillets, we used a common technique borrowed from professional kitchens: Sear the fillets in a hot skillet, flip, and transfer the skillet to the oven to continue cooking rather than finishing on the stove. A well-browned crust appeared in around a minute, giving the interior time to turn succulent in the oven. A cilantro chimichurri brought lovely herbaceous flavor to the dish and was easy to make by simply stirring the ingredients together. Black sea bass, haddock, hake, or pollock can be substituted for the cod.

Cilantro Chimichurri
- 2 tablespoons hot water
- 2 tablespoons red wine vinegar
- 1 teaspoon dried oregano
- ½ cup minced fresh parsley
- ¼ cup minced fresh cilantro
- 3 garlic cloves, minced
- ½ teaspoon table salt
- ¼ teaspoon red pepper flakes
- ¼ cup extra-virgin olive oil

Cod
- 4 (6- to 8-ounce) skinless cod fillets, 1 inch thick
- ½ teaspoon table salt
- ¼ teaspoon pepper
- 1 tablespoon avocado oil

1 **For the cilantro chimichurri** Combine hot water, vinegar, and oregano in bowl; let stand for 5 minutes. Add parsley, cilantro, garlic, salt, and pepper flakes and stir to combine. Whisk in oil until incorporated.

2 **For the cod** Adjust oven rack to middle position and heat oven to 425 degrees. Pat cod dry with paper towels and sprinkle with salt and pepper.

3 Heat oil in 12-inch ovensafe nonstick skillet over medium-high heat until just smoking. Lay fillets in skillet and, using spatula, lightly press fillets for 20 to 30 seconds to ensure even contact with skillet. Cook until browned on first side, 1 to 2 minutes.

4 Using 2 spatulas, flip fillets, then transfer skillet to oven. Roast until fish flakes apart when gently prodded with paring knife and registers 135 degrees, 7 to 10 minutes. Transfer cod to platter and serve with chimichurri.

MAKE AHEAD · Chimichurri can be refrigerated for up to 2 days.

Nut-Crusted Cod Fillets with Broiled Broccoli Rabe

serves **4** · **total time: 1 hour**

why this recipe works · Whether roasted or sautéed, we like to dress up cod because it takes well to just about any flavoring. Here we coated it with pistachios and paired it with fiberful broccoli rabe. To get everything just right, we used two cooking methods. The cod got a low-and-slow roast on a wire rack, which kept it tender and flaky. Once the cod was finished cooking, we cranked up the heat to broil the broccoli rabe, caramelizing it and rendering it irresistibly crispy in minutes. But perhaps the real star of the show was the nutty, golden pistachio crust. The ground pistachios brought crunch, color, and a hint of sweetness, and we combined them with panko, shallot, and garlic for added depth. A quick zap in the microwave pre-toasted the mix, giving it a head start before it even hit the fish. To ensure the coating stayed put, we brushed the fillets with a zippy combo of egg yolk, mustard, and lemon zest before pressing on the nut mixture. A gentle roast locked in moisture while crisping the crust to perfection. With the cod resting, the broccoli rabe went straight onto the sheet pan and under the broiler, where it took on a beautiful light char. Since slicing the florets can unlock bitterness, we kept the leafy tops whole and trimmed only the stems for even cooking. The result? A flavor-packed sheet-pan dinner with crispy fish and smoky greens—all without breaking a sweat. Black sea bass, haddock, hake, or pollock can be substituted for the cod. We like to use pistachios for the fish coating, but any nut will work.

- ¼   cup shelled pistachios
- ¼   cup panko bread crumbs
- 1   shallot, minced
- ¼   cup avocado oil, divided
- 2   garlic cloves, minced, divided
- 1   teaspoon minced fresh thyme or ¼ teaspoon dried
- 1⅛ teaspoons table salt, divided
-     Pinch plus ¼ teaspoon pepper, divided
- 1   tablespoon minced fresh parsley
- 1   large egg yolk
- 1   teaspoon Dijon mustard
- ½   teaspoon grated lemon zest, plus lemon wedges for serving
- 4   (6- to 8-ounce) skinless cod fillets, 1 inch thick
- 1   pound broccoli rabe
- ¼   teaspoon red pepper flakes

1   Adjust one oven rack to middle position and second oven rack 4 inches from broiler element. Heat oven to 300 degrees. Set wire rack in rimmed baking sheet and spray with avocado oil spray. Process pistachios in food processor until finely chopped, 20 to 30 seconds. Toss pistachios, panko, shallot, 1 tablespoon oil, half of garlic, thyme, ⅛ teaspoon salt, and pinch pepper together in bowl. Microwave, stirring frequently, until panko is light golden brown, 2 to 4 minutes. Let cool for 10 minutes, then stir in parsley.

2   Whisk egg yolk, mustard, and lemon zest together in bowl. Pat cod dry with paper towels and sprinkle with ½ teaspoon salt and remaining ¼ teaspoon pepper. Brush tops of fillets evenly with yolk mixture. Working with 1 fillet at a time, dredge coated side in nut mixture, pressing gently to adhere.

3   Transfer cod, crumb side up, to prepared wire rack and bake on lower rack until fish flakes apart when gently prodded with paring knife and registers 135 degrees, 25 to 30 minutes, rotating sheet halfway through baking.

4   While cod roasts, trim and discard bottom 1 inch of broccoli rabe stems. Wash broccoli rabe with cold water, then dry with clean dish towel. Cut tops (leaves and florets) from stems, then cut stems into 1-inch pieces (keep tops whole). Drizzle 1 tablespoon oil over second clean sheet, then arrange broccoli rabe in even layer over sheet. Combine remaining 2 tablespoons oil, garlic, remaining ½ teaspoon salt, and pepper flakes in bowl, then drizzle evenly over broccoli rabe on sheet and toss to combine; set aside.

5   Remove cod from oven, transfer to serving platter nut side up, and set aside while broiling broccoli rabe. Heat broiler. Broil broccoli rabe on upper rack until exposed half of leaves are well browned, 2 to 2½ minutes. Using tongs, toss to expose unbrowned leaves. Return sheet to oven and continue to broil until most leaves are lightly charred and stalks are crisp-tender, 2 to 2½ minutes. Transfer to serving platter with cod. Serve with lemon wedges.

MAKE IT GLUTEN-FREE · Substitute gluten-free panko bread crumbs for the panko bread crumbs.

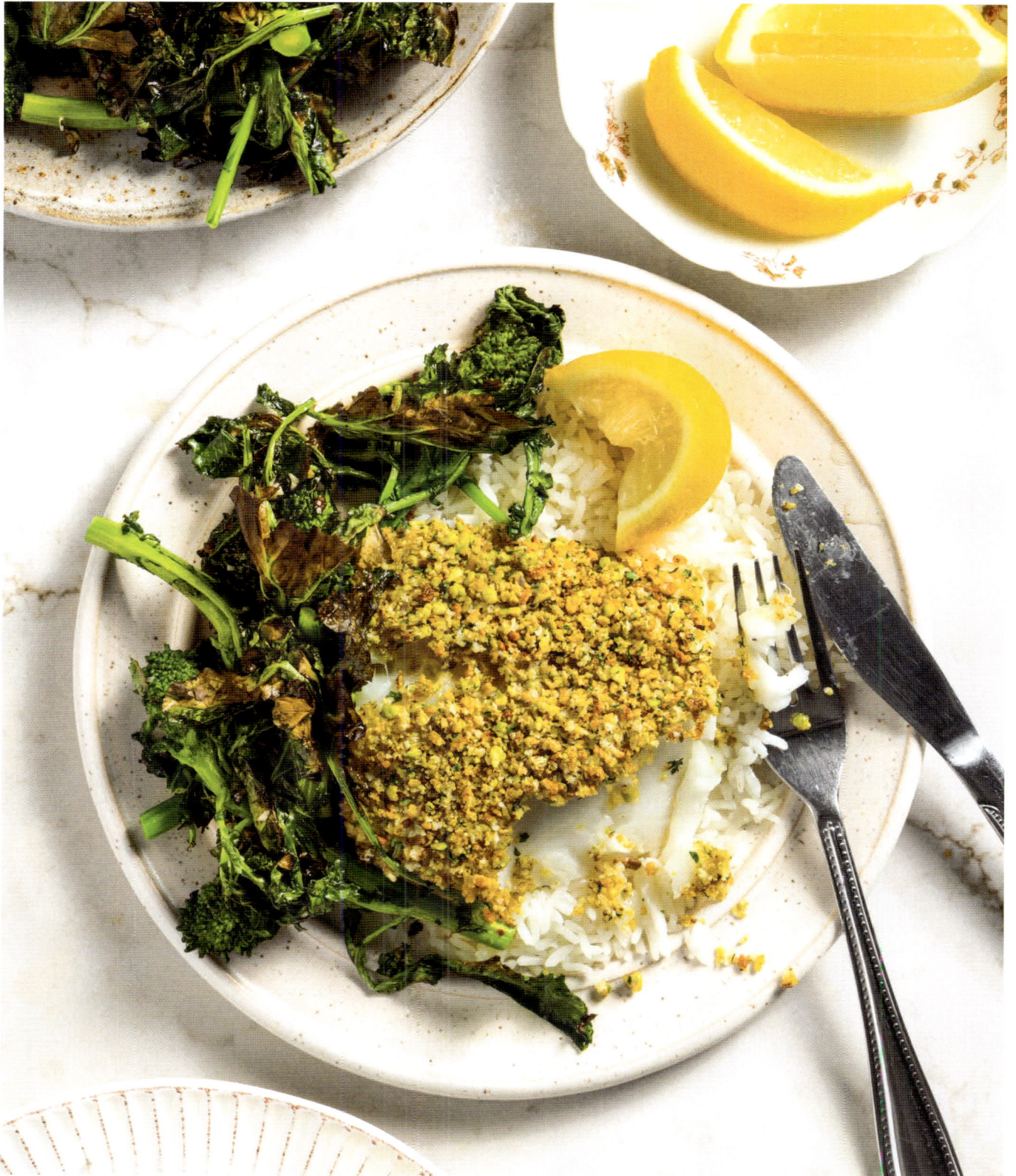

Nut-Crusted Cod Fillets with Broiled Broccoli Rabe

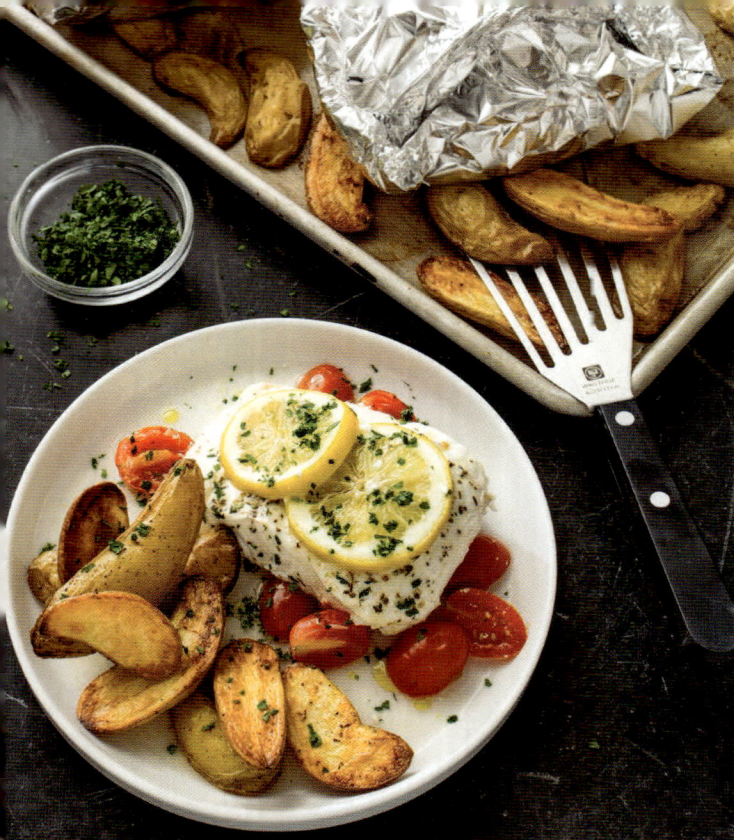

Lemon-Poached Halibut with Roasted Fingerling Potatoes

serves 4 • total time: 50 minutes

why this recipe works • We like roasting halibut wrapped in foil because the method ensures the lean, meaty fish will stay moist while absorbing flavor. We paired the fish with starchy potatoes that we cooked on the same baking sheet, roasting the tubers until they turned crisp on the outside and creamy on the inside. Placing the foil-wrapped fish on top of the potatoes gave the halibut less direct heat, helping it cook more gently. Adding tomatoes brought savory-sweet flavor and antioxidants. Use potatoes measuring 1 inch in diameter. To test for doneness without opening the foil packets, use a permanent marker to mark an "X" on the outside of the foil where the fish fillet is the thickest and then insert an instant-read thermometer through the "X" into the fish to measure its internal temperature. Mahi-mahi, red snapper, striped bass, or swordfish can be substituted for the halibut.

1½   pounds fingerling potatoes, halved lengthwise
2   tablespoons extra-virgin olive oil, divided
½   teaspoon table salt
½   teaspoon pepper
8   ounces cherry tomatoes, halved
4   (6-ounce) skinless halibut fillets, 1 inch thick
½   teaspoon dried oregano
8   thin lemon slices
2   tablespoons minced fresh parsley

1   Adjust oven rack to lower-middle position and heat oven to 450 degrees. Toss potatoes with 2 teaspoons oil, ½ teaspoon salt, and ½ teaspoon pepper. Arrange potatoes on rimmed baking sheet, cut side down, in even layer. Roast until cut sides are starting to brown, about 10 minutes.

2   Meanwhile, lay four 12-inch-long pieces of foil on counter. Place one-quarter of tomatoes in center of each piece of foil, then place 1 fillet on each tomato pile. Sprinkle each fillet with ⅛ teaspoon oregano and season with salt and pepper, then top each with 2 lemon slices and 1 teaspoon oil. Pull edges of foil up around fish and tomatoes and crimp to form packet.

3   Place packets on top of potatoes and bake until fish is just cooked through, about 15 minutes. Divide potatoes among 4 bowls. Open 1 packet over each bowl, slide fish and tomatoes onto potatoes, then pour broth (accumulated juices) over top. Sprinkle with parsley and serve.

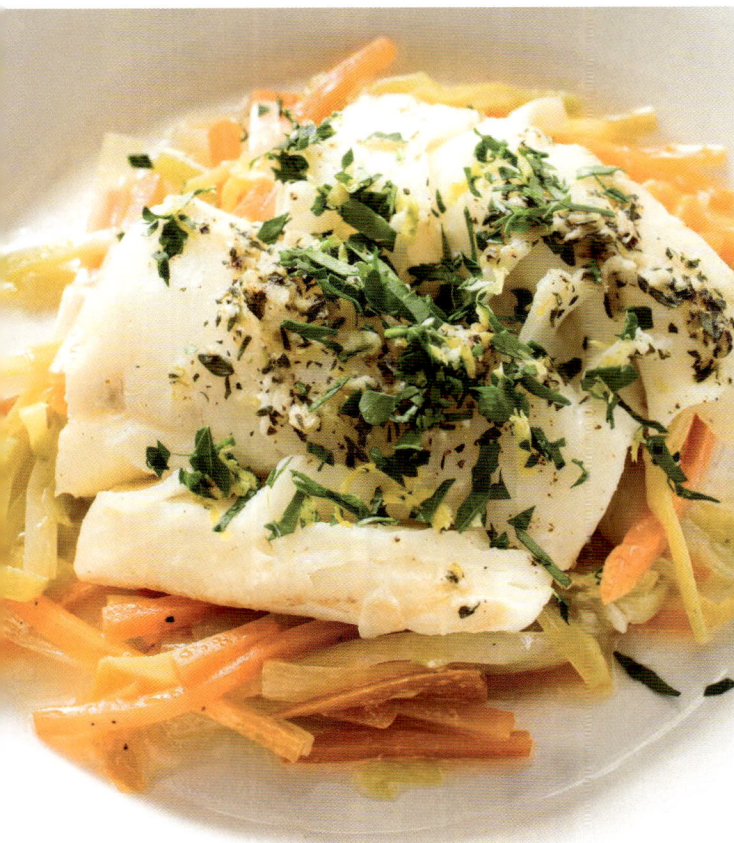

top | *Lemon-Poached Halibut with Roasted Fingerling Potatoes*
bottom | *Cod Baked in Foil with Leeks and Carrots*

Pan-Roasted Sea Bass with Wild Mushrooms

serves 4 • total time: 45 minutes   FAST

why this recipe works • This flavorful recipe is a great way to pack mushrooms—a rich source of B vitamins and minerals—into your diet. Dried mushrooms, which are in the mix here as well, contain a concentrated amount of those nutrients. For a sea bass and mushroom dinner, we liked a combination of full-flavored cremini and portobellos, with a small amount of dried porcini for a deep, woodsy flavor. We first tried sautéing the mushrooms and fish separately, but the result lacked unity. We decided to add the fish to the sautéed mushrooms in the hot skillet and then slide the pan into the oven; this allowed the flavors of the fish and mushrooms to meld together, and the porcini liquid reduced to a light, flavorful sauce. Cod, haddock, hake, or pollock can be substituted for the sea bass.

½   cup water
⅓   ounce dried porcini mushrooms, rinsed
 4   (6- to 8-ounce) skinless black sea bass fillets, 1 inch thick
¼   cup extra-virgin olive oil, divided
¾   teaspoon table salt, divided
⅛   teaspoon pepper
 1   sprig fresh rosemary
 1   pound cremini mushrooms, trimmed and halved if small or quartered if large
12   ounces portobello mushroom caps, halved and sliced ½ inch thick
 1   red onion, halved and sliced thin
 2   garlic cloves, minced
 1   tablespoon minced fresh parsley
     Lemon wedges

1 Adjust oven rack to lower-middle position and heat oven to 475 degrees. Microwave water and porcini mushrooms in covered bowl until steaming, about 1 minute. Let sit until softened, about 5 minutes. Drain porcini mushrooms in fine-mesh strainer lined with coffee filter, reserving liquid, and finely chop porcini.

2 Pat sea bass dry with paper towels, rub with 2 tablespoons oil, and sprinkle with ¼ teaspoon salt and pepper.

3 Heat remaining 2 tablespoons oil and rosemary in 12-inch ovensafe skillet over medium-high heat until shimmering Add cremini mushrooms, portobello mushrooms, onion, and remaining ½ teaspoon salt. Cook, stirring occasionally, until mushrooms

have released their liquid and are beginning to brown, 8 to 10 minutes. Stir in garlic and minced porcini mushrooms and cook until fragrant, about 30 seconds.

4 Off heat, stir in reserved porcini liquid. Nestle sea bass skinned side down into skillet, transfer to oven, and roast until sea bass flakes apart when gently prodded with paring knife and registers 135 degrees, 10 to 12 minutes. Discard rosemary sprig, sprinkle with parsley, and serve with lemon wedges.

Cod Baked in Foil with Leeks and Carrots

serves 4 • total time: 45 minutes   FAST

why this recipe works • Cooking fish en papillote, or folded in a pouch, is a classic French technique that, in addition to being incredibly easy (and virtually cleanup-free), allows the fish to steam in its own juices and emerge moist and flavorful. We found that foil was easier to work with than parchment and created a leakproof seal. Placing the packets on the lower-middle rack of the oven, close to the heat source, concentrated the exuded liquid in the packets and deepened its flavor. Vegetable selection was important: Hardy vegetables such as potatoes and squash failed to cook evenly in the packets, while water-absorbing vegetables like eggplant turned to mush when enclosed. Carrots and leeks, cut into elegant matchsticks, cooked at the same rate as the fish plus packed in some welcome antioxidants. Open each packet promptly after baking to prevent overcooking. To test for doneness without opening the foil packets, use a permanent marker to mark an "X" on the outside of the foil where the fish fillet is the thickest and then insert an instant-read thermometer through the "X" into the fish to measure its internal temperature. Black sea bass, haddock, hake, or pollock can be substituted for the cod.

¼   cup extra-virgin olive oil
 1   teaspoon minced fresh thyme
 2   garlic cloves, minced, divided
1¼   teaspoons grated lemon zest, divided, plus lemon wedges for serving
 1   teaspoon table salt, divided
½   teaspoon pepper, divided
 2   tablespoons minced fresh parsley
 2   carrots, peeled and cut into matchsticks
 1   pound leeks, white and light green parts only, halved lengthwise, washed thoroughly, and cut into matchsticks
¼   cup dry white wine
 4   (6- to 8-ounce) skinless cod fillets, 1 inch thick

1 Adjust oven rack to lower-middle position and heat oven to 450 degrees. Whisk oil, thyme, half of garlic, ¼ teaspoon lemon zest, ¼ teaspoon salt, and ⅛ teaspoon pepper in bowl. Combine parsley, remaining garlic, and remaining 1 teaspoon lemon zest in second bowl. Combine carrots, leeks, ¼ teaspoon salt, and ⅛ teaspoon pepper in third bowl.

2 Lay four 16 by 12-inch rectangles of aluminum foil on counter with short sides parallel to counter edge. Divide vegetable mixture evenly among foil rectangles, arranging in center of lower half of each sheet of foil. Mound vegetables slightly and sprinkle with wine. Pat cod dry with paper towels, sprinkle with remaining ½ teaspoon salt and remaining ¼ teaspoon pepper, and place on top of vegetables. Whisk oil mixture to recombine, then pour evenly over fillets. Fold top half of foil over fish, then tightly crimp edges into rough 9 by 6-inch packets.

3 Place packets on rimmed baking sheet (they may overlap slightly) and bake until cod registers 135 degrees, about 15 minutes. Carefully open packets, allowing steam to escape away from you. Using thin metal spatula, gently slide cod and vegetables onto individual plates and top with any accumulated juices. Sprinkle with parsley mixture and serve with lemon wedges.

Cod with Cilantro Rice

serves 4 • total Time: 40 minutes **FAST**

why this recipe works • Cilantro is a delicious way of jazzing up rice while incorporating some antioxidants. For this recipe, we tossed still-warm rice with a garlic and cilantro vinaigrette, so the grains drank up all of the sauce's tart, herbal flavors. It's critical to have uniform grains of rice, so we cooked it like pasta—we simply dumped the rice into a pot of boiling water (no need for finicky ratios) and drained it when it was done. While all that was happening, we seared cod fillets in a piping-hot skillet to achieve a gorgeous crust before gently finishing them in the oven. Once everything was ready, we drizzled some of the reserved cilantro sauce over the top to tie it all together. Black sea bass, haddock, hake, or pollock can be substituted for the cod.

3 cups fresh cilantro leaves and stems, chopped coarse
2 tablespoons red wine vinegar
2 garlic cloves, smashed and peeled
¾ teaspoon table salt, divided, plus salt for cooking rice
½ teaspoon pepper, divided
½ cup extra-virgin olive oil

1 cup long-grain white rice
4 (6- to 8-ounce) skinless cod fillets, 1 inch thick
1 tablespoon avocado oil

1 Adjust oven rack to middle position and heat oven to 425 degrees. Pulse cilantro, vinegar, garlic, ¼ teaspoon salt, and ¼ teaspoon pepper in food processor until finely chopped, about 12 pulses, scraping down sides of bowl as needed. Transfer to bowl, whisk in extra-virgin olive oil, and set aside.

2 Bring 2 quarts water to boil in large saucepan. Stir in rice and 1 teaspoon salt and cook until rice is tender, about 12 minutes. Drain rice well, return to saucepan, and stir in ¼ cup reserved cilantro sauce; season with salt and pepper to taste. Cover and set aside until ready to serve.

3 Meanwhile, pat cod dry with paper towels and sprinkle with remaining ½ teaspoon salt and remaining ¼ teaspoon pepper. Heat avocado oil in 12-inch ovensafe nonstick skillet over medium-high heat until just smoking. Lay fillets in skillet and, using spatula, lightly press fillets for 20 to 30 seconds to ensure even contact with skillet. Cook until golden brown on first side, 1 to 2 minutes.

4 Using 2 spatulas, flip fillets, then transfer skillet to oven. Roast until fish flakes apart when gently prodded with paring knife and registers 135 degrees, 7 to 10 minutes. Transfer cod to platter, drizzle with remaining reserved cilantro sauce, and serve with reserved rice.

MAKE AHEAD • Cooked white rice can be refrigerated for up to 3 days.

Baked Halibut with Cherry Tomatoes and Chickpeas

serves 4 • total time: 1 hour

why this recipe works • We wanted to infuse mild halibut with robust flavors and bake it with a savory side dish for a quick, complete dinner. An anti-inflammatory, olive oil–based rub infused with coriander and paprika provided aromatic flavor, and a little bit of cayenne added just the right amount of subtle heat. We tried many accompaniments to pair with this spiced fish, but our favorite turned out to be a mix of chickpeas and cherry tomatoes. We flavored the vegetables with more coriander and paprika, plus shallots, garlic, and lemon for a bright dimension. We nestled the halibut fillets into the chickpea-tomato mixture before baking it all in the oven. The chickpeas soaked up the broth and some of the tomatoes broke down, creating a bright sauce that complemented the halibut beautifully. Mahi-mahi, red snapper, swordfish, or striped bass can be substituted for the halibut.

2 (15-ounce) cans no-salt-added chickpeas, rinsed
12 ounces cherry tomatoes, halved
2 shallots, minced
5 tablespoons avocado oil, divided
¼ cup unsalted chicken or vegetable broth
5 garlic cloves, minced
1 tablespoon grated lemon zest plus 1 tablespoon juice
2 teaspoons ground coriander, divided
2 teaspoons paprika, divided
1 teaspoon table salt, divided
½ teaspoon pepper
4 (6- to 8-ounce) skinless halibut fillets, 1 inch thick
⅛ teaspoon cayenne pepper
2 tablespoons chopped fresh cilantro

1 Adjust oven rack to middle position and heat oven to 400 degrees. Combine chickpeas, tomatoes, shallots, 1 tablespoon oil, broth, garlic, lemon zest and juice, 1 teaspoon coriander, 1 teaspoon paprika, ½ teaspoon salt, and pepper in 13 by 9-inch baking dish.

2 Pat halibut dry with paper towels. Combine 2 tablespoons oil, remaining 1 teaspoon coriander, remaining 1 teaspoon paprika, remaining ½ teaspoon salt, and cayenne in bowl. Add halibut and gently turn to coat. Nestle halibut into chickpea mixture in dish and bake until fish flakes apart when gently prodded with paring knife and registers 130 degrees, 20 to 30 minutes. Remove baking dish from oven, tent with aluminum foil, and let rest for 10 minutes.

3 Drizzle with remaining 2 tablespoons oil and sprinkle with cilantro. Serve.

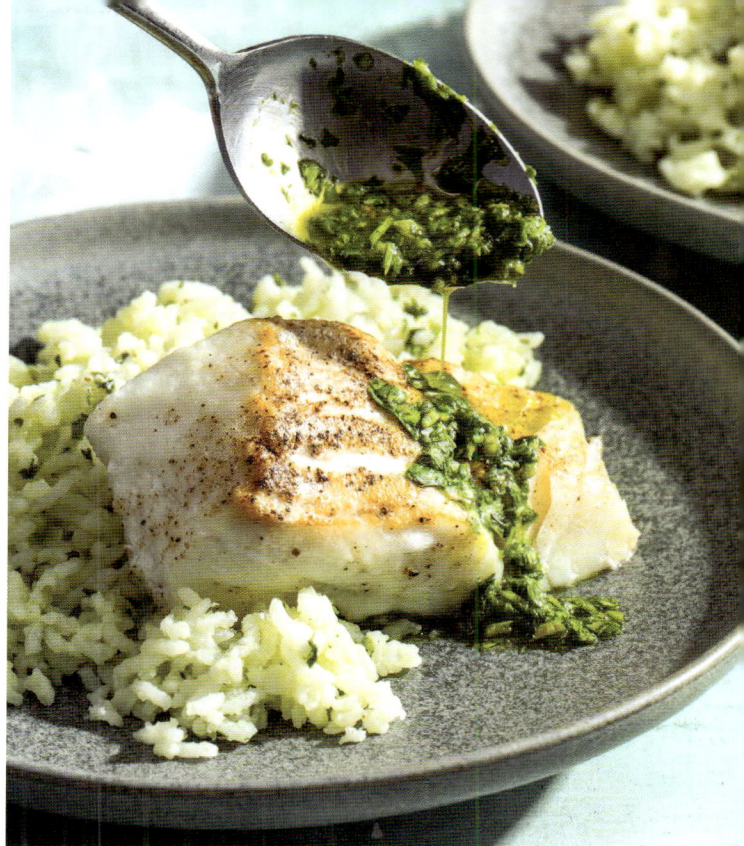

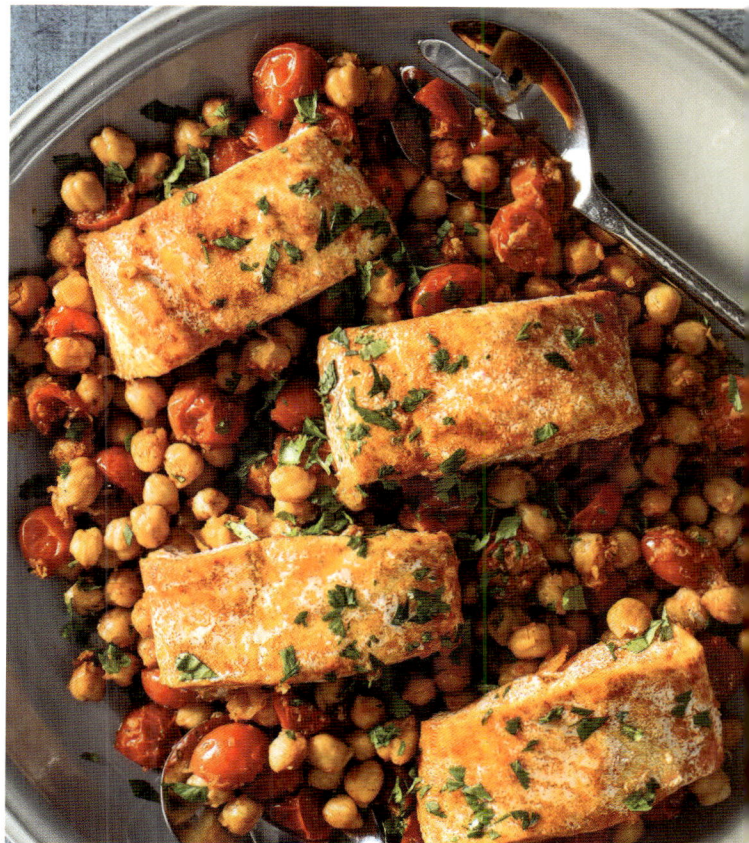

Tabil Couscous with Sardines

serves 4 · total time: 1 hour

why this recipe works · Couscous is airy and mild, the perfect canvas for bold flavors that turn the pasta into a centerpiece meal. We seasoned it with tabil, a spice blend used across Tunisia. The simple mix—which typically includes seasonings such as coriander, cumin, and caraway seeds—offered antioxidants and paired

| top | Cod with Cilantro Rice |
| bottom | Baked Halibut with Cherry Tomatoes and Chickpeas |

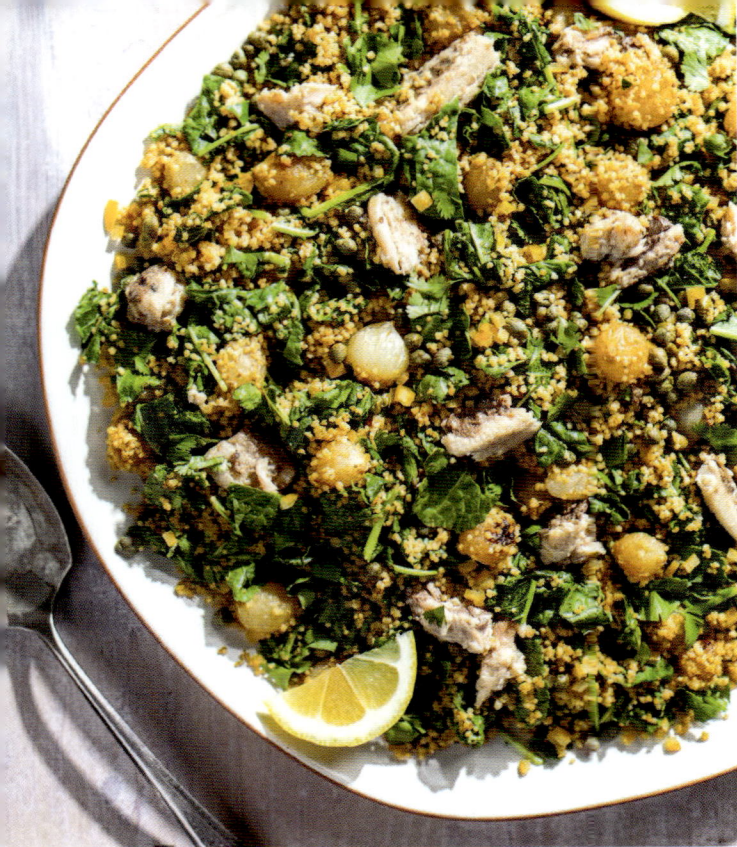

well with bright preserved lemon, while pearl onions brought out the seasoning blend's sweeter side. Frozen pearl onions cut down on prep; when browned, they added caramelized flavor to our finished dish. We also incorporated capers and canned sardines, the latter of which is an excellent source of protein and heart-healthy fats. Be sure to pick through the sardines and discard any lingering skin and bones before flaking. Inexpensive sardines can be overly fishy-tasting; for the best flavor, use high-quality sardines. You can use store-bought preserved lemons or make our Quick Preserved Lemon (page 209); you can also substitute 1 tablespoon of lemon zest, using half in step 2 and half in step 3, though the flavor will be less complex.

3 tablespoons extra-virgin olive oil, divided, plus extra for drizzling

1½ cups couscous

2 cups frozen pearl onions, thawed

2 tablespoons Tabil (recipe follows)

4 garlic cloves, minced

½ teaspoon table salt

¼ teaspoon red pepper flakes

2 tablespoons rinsed and minced preserved lemons, divided

2¼ cups unsalted chicken or vegetable broth, divided

5 ounces (5 cups) baby kale, chopped

½ cup chopped fresh cilantro

6 ounces canned sardines packed in oil, drained, patted dry, and flaked into 1-inch pieces

2 tablespoons capers, rinsed
Lemon wedges

1 Heat 2 tablespoons oil in 12-inch skillet over medium-high heat until just smoking. Add couscous and cook, stirring frequently, until grains are just beginning to brown, about 5 minutes. Transfer to bowl and wipe skillet clean with paper towels.

2 Heat remaining 1 tablespoon oil in now-empty skillet over medium heat until shimmering. Add onions and cook until beginning to brown, 6 to 8 minutes. Stir in tabil, garlic, salt, pepper flakes, and 1 tablespoon preserved lemon and cook until fragrant, about 30 seconds. Stir in ½ cup broth and bring to simmer. Cover, reduce heat to medium-low, and simmer until onions are tender, 12 to 15 minutes.

3 Stir in toasted couscous, kale, and remaining 1¾ cups broth and bring to simmer. Cover, remove skillet from heat, and let sit until couscous is tender, about 7 minutes. Off heat, add cilantro and fluff couscous and cilantro together with fork to combine. Season with salt and pepper to taste. Top with sardines, capers, and remaining 1 tablespoon preserved lemon. Drizzle with extra oil and serve with lemon wedges.

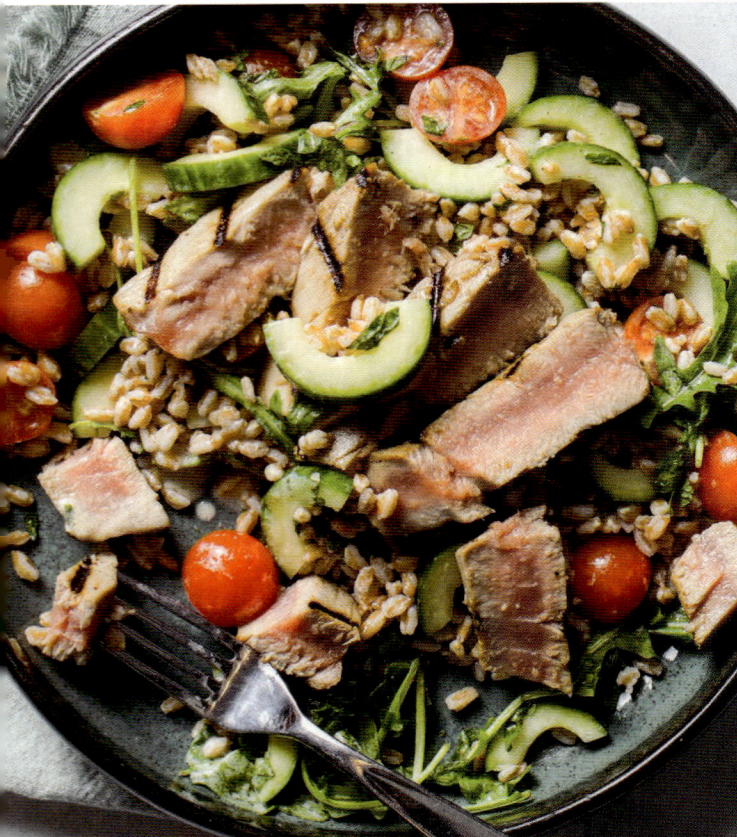

top | *Tabil Couscous with Sardines*
bottom | *Seared Tuna Steaks with Cucumber-Mint Farro Salad*

Tabil

makes about ½ cup · total time: 5 minutes

3½ tablespoons coriander seeds
 2 tablespoons plus 2 teaspoons caraway seeds
 1 tablespoon plus 2 teaspoons cumin seeds

Combine all ingredients in bowl. (Tabil can be stored in airtight container at room temperature for up to 1 year.)

Seared Tuna Steaks with Cucumber-Mint Farro Salad

serves 4 · total time: 1 hour

**why this recipe works · ** This recipe combines high-protein tuna with fiber-rich farro for a meal that's as nutritious as it is filling and satisfying. Farro, an ancient grain packed with prebiotic fiber, supports healthy digestion while providing a nutty, chewy base for the salad. We balanced its hearty texture with cooling cucumbers as well as arugula, which added a peppery bite along with a dose of glucosinolates. For a dressing, we opted for a creamy, lemony yogurt sauce, which not only brightened the dish but also introduced vitamin C and probiotics. As for the tuna—a good source of omega-3 fatty acids—we seared it quickly over high heat to develop a crust while maintaining a rare center. Cutting the steaks in half crosswise before cooking ensured even searing without overcooking. We prefer the flavor and texture of whole farro; pearled farro can be used, but the texture may be softer. Do not use quick-cooking or presteamed farro. The cooking time for farro can vary greatly across brands, so we recommend beginning to check for doneness after 10 minutes. We prefer our tuna served rare or medium-rare. If you like your tuna cooked medium, observe the timing for medium-rare, then tent the steaks with foil for 5 minutes.

1½ cups whole farro
 1 teaspoon table salt, divided, plus salt for cooking farro
 ¼ cup avocado oil, divided
 2 tablespoons lemon juice
 2 tablespoons plain Greek yogurt
 ¼ teaspoon pepper, divided
 1 English cucumber, halved lengthwise, seeded, and cut into ¼-inch pieces
 6 ounces cherry tomatoes, halved
 2 ounces (2 cups) baby arugula
 3 tablespoons chopped fresh mint
 2 (8- to 12-ounce) skinless tuna steaks, 1 inch thick, halved crosswise

1 Bring 4 quarts water to boil in Dutch oven. Add farro and 1 tablespoon salt and cook until grains are tender with slight chew, 15 to 30 minutes. Drain farro, spread evenly on rimmed baking sheet, and let cool completely, about 15 minutes.

2 Whisk 3 tablespoons oil, lemon juice, yogurt, ½ teaspoon salt, and ⅛ teaspoon pepper together in large bowl. Add drained farro, cucumber, tomatoes, arugula, and mint and toss gently to combine. Season with salt and pepper to taste; set aside. Pat tuna dry with paper towels and sprinkle with remaining ½ teaspoon salt and remaining ⅛ teaspoon pepper.

3 Heat remaining 1 tablespoon oil in now-empty skillet over medium-high heat until just smoking. Place steaks in skillet and cook, flipping every 1 to 2 minutes, until center is translucent red when checked with tip of paring knife and registers 110 degrees (for rare), 2 to 4 minutes or until opaque at perimeter and reddish pink at center and registers 125 degrees (for medium-rare), 3 to 5 minutes. Serve tuna with farro salad.

**MAKE AHEAD · ** Cooked farro can be refrigerated for up to 3 days.

**MAKE IT GLUTEN-FREE · ** Substitute brown rice or oat berries for the farro.

**MAKE IT DAIRY-FREE · ** Substitute plant-based Greek yogurt for the dairy Greek yogurt.

Pan-Seared Shrimp with Tangy Soy-Citrus Sauce

serves 4 • total time: 25 minutes   **FAST**

why this recipe works • Shrimp are a great source of omega-3 fatty acids and are especially appealing when pan-seared: The exterior becomes caramelized while the interior remains tender and moist. But achieving this ideal with quick-cooking shellfish requires just the right technique. To start, we peeled the shrimp and then seasoned them simply with salt and pepper, which brought out their natural sweetness and aided in browning. After quickly browning one side of the shrimp in a piping-hot skillet, we removed the pan from the heat, flipped the shrimp, and allowed the residual heat to gently finish cooking them through. The result was shrimp that were golden-brown on the outside, juicy on the inside. A dressing of soy sauce, citrus, and ginger complemented the sweet, oceanic flavor of the shrimp. We prefer untreated shrimp, but if your shrimp are treated with salt or additives such as sodium tripolyphosphate (STPP), do not add the salt. Serve with rice.

Soy-Citrus Sauce
- ¼ cup low-sodium soy sauce
- 1½ teaspoons lemon juice
- 1½ teaspoons lime juice
- 1 scallion, sliced thin
- ½ teaspoon grated fresh ginger

Shrimp
- 1½ pounds extra-large shrimp (21 to 25 per pound), peeled and deveined
- ¼ teaspoon table salt
- ¼ teaspoon pepper
- 2 tablespoons avocado oil

1 For the soy-citrus sauce Combine all ingredients in bowl.

2 For the shrimp Pat shrimp dry with paper towels, then toss with salt and pepper in bowl. Heat 1 tablespoon oil in 12-inch skillet over high heat until just smoking. Add half of shrimp in single layer and cook until spotty brown and edges begin to turn pink, about 1 minute. Off heat, flip shrimp and cook second side using residual heat of skillet until all but center is opaque, about 30 seconds; transfer to bowl. Repeat with remaining 1 tablespoon oil and remaining shrimp. Return all shrimp to skillet, cover, and cook until shrimp are opaque throughout, 1 to 2 minutes. Transfer shrimp to platter. Serve immediately with sauce.

MAKE IT GLUTEN-FREE • Substitute low-sodium tamari for the low-sodium soy sauce.

Salmon Tacos with Super Slaw

serves 4 • total time: 30 minutes   **FAST**

why this recipe works • California-style fish tacos generally star deep-fried fish, a tangy slaw, and a creamy sauce. We wanted to boost the nutrition of each element for a supernourishing take. We opted for salmon, which is richer than the more typical white fish even without frying. Sturdy collards—combined with radishes, jicama, onion, cilantro, and lime—made a salad that perfectly complemented the fish. Two cups thinly sliced purple cabbage can be substituted for the collards, or use a combination. Serve with chopped mango and lime wedges, if desired. To ensure uniform pieces, we prefer to purchase a whole 1½- to 2-pound center-cut salmon fillet and cut it into four equal pieces. If using wild salmon, cook it until it registers 120 degrees.

- ¼ teaspoon grated lime zest plus 2 tablespoons juice, plus lime wedges for serving
- 1 teaspoon table salt, divided
- 4 ounces collard greens, stemmed and sliced thin (2 cups)
- 4 ounces jicama, peeled and cut into 2-inch-long matchsticks
- 4 radishes, trimmed and cut into 1-inch-long matchsticks
- ½ small red onion, halved and sliced thin
- ¼ cup fresh cilantro leaves
- 1½ teaspoons chili powder
- ¼ teaspoon pepper
- 4 (6- to 8-ounce) skin-on salmon fillets, 1 inch thick
- 1 tablespoon avocado oil
- 1 avocado, halved, pitted, and cut into ½-inch pieces
- 12 (6-inch) corn tortillas, warmed
  Hot sauce

1 Whisk lime zest and juice and ¼ teaspoon salt together in large bowl. Add collard greens, jicama, radishes, onion, and cilantro and toss to combine.

2 Combine chili powder, remaining ¾ teaspoon salt, and pepper in small bowl. Pat salmon dry with paper towels and sprinkle evenly with spice mixture. Heat oil in 12-inch nonstick skillet over medium-high heat until shimmering. Cook salmon skin side up until well browned, 3 to 5 minutes. Gently flip salmon using 2 spatulas and continue to cook until salmon is still translucent when checked with tip of paring knife and registers 125 degrees (for medium-rare), 3 to 5 minutes. Transfer salmon to plate and let cool slightly, about 2 minutes. Using 2 forks, flake fish into 2-inch pieces, discarding skin.

3 Divide fish, collard slaw, and avocado evenly among tortillas, and drizzle with hot sauce to taste. Serve with lime wedges.

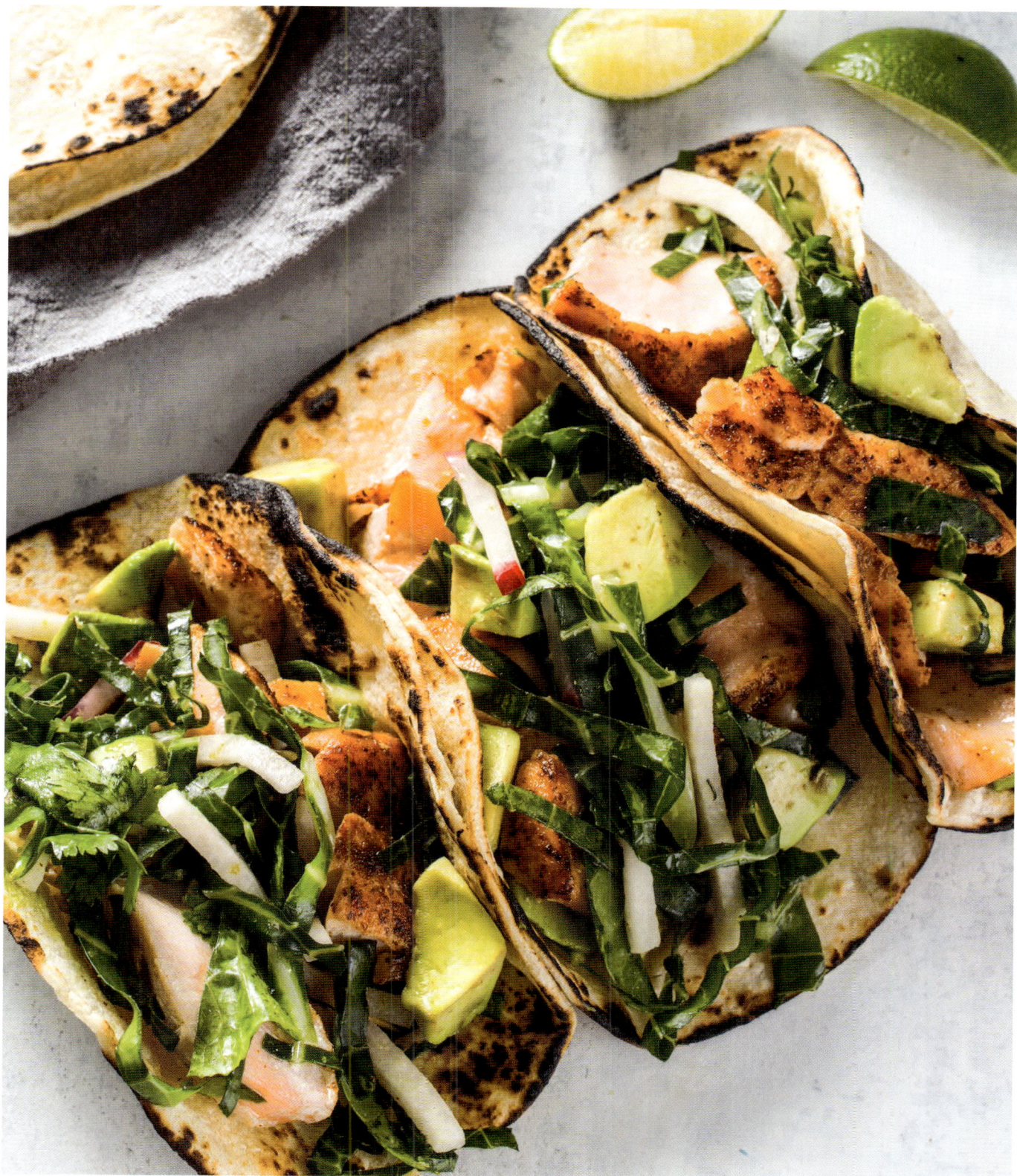

Salmon Tacos with Super Slaw

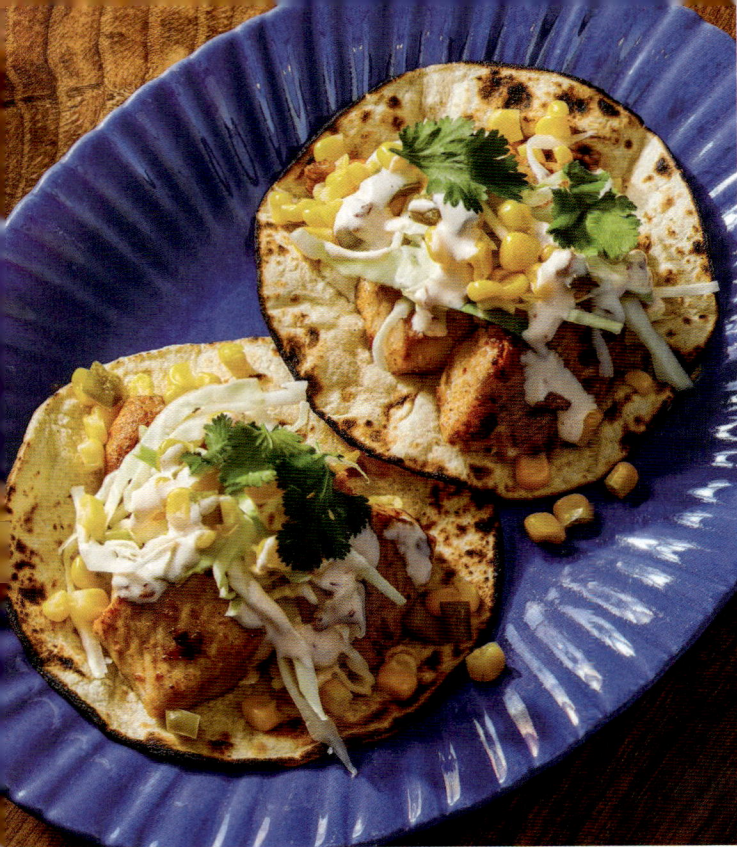

Tilapia Tacos with Quick Corn Relish

serves 4 • total time: 45 minutes **FAST**

why this recipe works • These bright, flavorful tacos deliver big taste with minimal effort. Tilapia's mild flavor made it the perfect blank canvas for our spicy-sweet corn relish, while its quick cooking time kept this meal weeknight-friendly. To ensure that the fish cooked evenly and stayed moist, we salted it first (enhancing both texture and flavor) and then cut each fillet into uniform pieces. This guaranteed that every bite was perfectly cooked—golden on the outside, flaky inside—without any dry or underdone spots. For the corn relish, we skipped fresh corn in favor of frozen kernels, which were just as sweet and tender but required no shucking. A quick sauté with cider vinegar, jalapeño, and a little sugar balanced the relish with tangy, spicy, and sweet notes. A chipotle-spiked crema tied everything together, adding cooling richness and a boost of heat. These tacos are delicious as is, but you can also top them with finely shredded cabbage and cilantro and serve them with rice and/or beans. Flounder, sole, or catfish can be substituted for the tilapia.

- 4 (4- to 6-ounce) skinless tilapia fillets, halved lengthwise down natural seam
- 1¼ teaspoons table salt, divided
- ½ cup Mexican crema
- 2 tablespoons minced canned chipotle chile in adobo sauce, divided
- 1½ cups frozen corn
- ⅓ cup cider vinegar
- 1 jalapeño chile, stemmed, seeded, and chopped
- 1 tablespoon sugar
- 1 teaspoon ground cumin
- 2 tablespoons avocado oil
- 12 (6-inch) corn tortillas, warmed

1 Sprinkle tilapia all over with ½ teaspoon salt and let sit for 15 minutes. Combine crema, 1 tablespoon chipotle, and ¼ teaspoon salt in bowl; set aside. Cook corn, vinegar, jalapeño, sugar, and remaining ½ teaspoon salt in small saucepan over medium-high heat, stirring occasionally, until softened, about 4 minutes. Transfer to bowl and refrigerate until cool.

2 Pat tilapia dry with paper towels. Cut each thick piece in half crosswise, then in half again lengthwise, and cut each thin piece in half crosswise. Toss all pieces with cumin and remaining 1 tablespoon chipotle until coated.

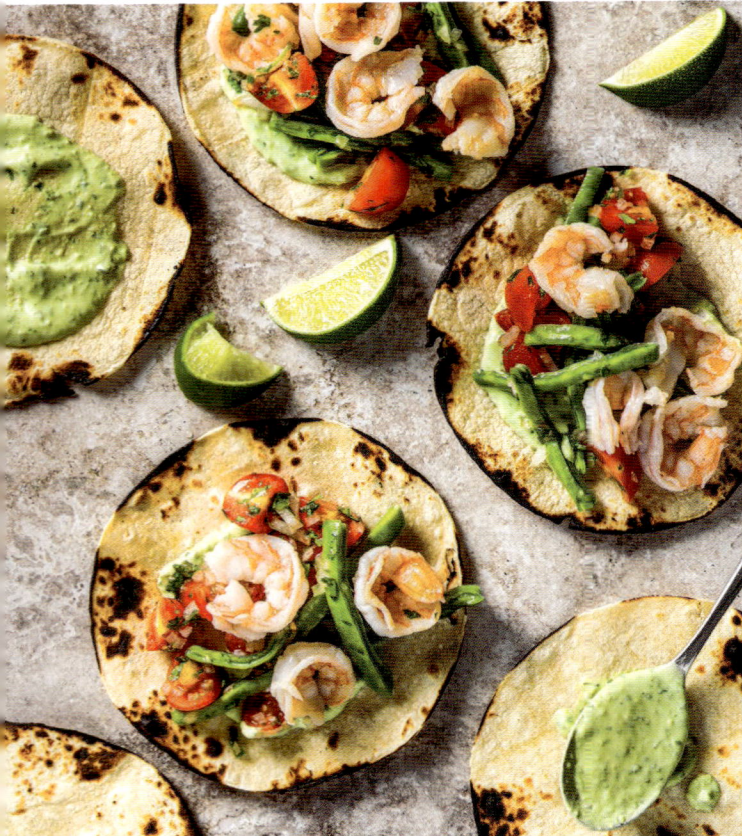

top	Tilapia Tacos with Quick Corn Relish
bottom	Nopales and Shrimp Tacos

3 Heat oil in 12-inch nonstick skillet over medium-high heat until just smoking. Add tilapia to skillet and cook, stirring and flipping occasionally, until golden brown all over and thickest pieces register 130 to 135 degrees, about 4 minutes. Drain corn mixture. Divide fish, crema, and corn mixture evenly among tortillas. Serve.

> **MAKE IT DAIRY-FREE** • Substitute plant-based sour cream for the Mexican crema.

Spicy Shrimp Lettuce Wraps

serves 4 • total time: 25 minutes **FAST**

why this recipe works • Lettuce wraps are a nice alternative to tortillas for a hands-on eating experience. Pairing sweet shrimp with spice is a winning path to a creative meal; quickly cooking chili powder–coated shrimp and topping them with a jalapeño-enhanced mango salsa made the perfect filling combination for the wraps. Cutting the shrimp into bite-size pieces before cooking made them easy to pile into the delicate lettuce and eat. Bibb lettuce's crisp spines, tender leaves, and mild flavor made them an ideal wrapper for the shrimp and salsa. We prefer untreated shrimp, but if your shrimp are treated with salt or additives such as sodium tripolyphosphate (STPP), do not add the salt in step 2.

Mango Salsa

½ ripe mango, peeled and cut into ¼-inch pieces
½ red onion, chopped fine
¼ cup chopped fresh cilantro
1 jalapeño chile, stemmed, seeded, and minced
2 tablespoons lime juice
1 tablespoon extra-virgin olive oil
½ teaspoon table salt
¼ teaspoon pepper

Shrimp

1 pound extra-large shrimp (21 to 25 per pound), peeled, deveined, and tails removed, cut into ½-inch pieces
2 teaspoons chili powder
¼ teaspoon table salt
¼ teaspoon pepper
2 tablespoons avocado oil
1 head Bibb lettuce (8 ounces), leaves separated

1 **For the mango salsa** Combine all ingredients in bowl; set aside until ready to serve.

2 **For the shrimp** Pat shrimp dry with paper towels, then sprinkle with chili powder, salt, and pepper. Heat oil in 12-inch nonstick skillet over medium-high heat until just smoking. Add shrimp and cook, stirring occasionally, until spotty brown and opaque throughout, about 4 minutes; transfer to serving bowl. Serve shrimp in lettuce leaves, topped with mango salsa.

Nopales and Shrimp Tacos

serves 4 • total time: 1 hour

why this recipe works • Nopales, or fresh cactus paddles, are beloved in Mexico, where cooks add them to stews, tacos, and more. The fiberful vegetable has a tender yet slightly snappy texture like green beans or asparagus, and citrus notes reminiscent of sorrel or purslane. Salting the nopales released some of their mucilage, which we rinsed off before adding the cactus to the other ingredients. We paired the cactus with sautéed shrimp seasoned with lime zest and garlic, plus a cooling avocado-based sauce. Look for fresh cactus paddles at Mexican and Latino grocery stores; you might also find them at some well-stocked supermarkets. We prefer untreated shrimp, but if your shrimp are treated with salt or additives such as sodium tripolyphosphate (STPP), do not add the salt in step 4. The nopales will continue to release mucilage if left to sit; add the nopales to the salad last and serve immediately.

1 pound nopales (4 to 5 paddles)
¼ teaspoon plus ⅛ teaspoon table salt, divided, plus salt for salting vegetables
6 ounces grape tomatoes, quartered
⅓ cup finely chopped white onion
¼ cup fresh chopped fresh cilantro
4 teaspoons extra-virgin olive oil, divided
1 teaspoon grated lime zest plus 2 teaspoons juice, plus lime wedges for serving
½ serrano chile, seeded and minced
1 pound extra-large shrimp (21 to 25 per pound), peeled, deveined, and tails removed, halved lengthwise
1 garlic clove, minced
1 recipe Avocado Crema (page 250)
12 (6-inch) corn tortillas, warmed

1 Working with 1 cactus paddle at a time, place flat on cutting board and grasp thick end with tongs or dish towel. Place knife blade parallel to paddle, then slide knife away from you across surface to remove any thorns and small raised bumps. Repeat process on second side. Trim outer ¼ inch of paddle, then trim bottom ½ inch of thick end of paddle; discard trimmings. Rinse paddles well and clean cutting board.

2   Line rimmed baking sheet with dish towel; set aside. Cut paddles into ¼-inch-wide by 3-inch-long matchsticks. Combine nopales and 1 tablespoon salt in bowl, stirring until nopales are well coated and begin to release a viscous liquid, about 1 minute. Let nopales sit for 10 minutes, stirring occasionally. Transfer nopales to colander and rinse under cold running water, agitating vigorously with your hands to remove all viscous liquid. Drain well, then transfer to prepared baking sheet in even layer to dry; set aside.

3   Combine tomatoes, onion, cilantro, 2 teaspoons oil, lime juice, serrano, and ¼ teaspoon salt, in large bowl. Set aside.

4   Heat remaining 2 teaspoons oil in 12-inch nonstick skillet over medium-high heat until shimmering. Pat shrimp dry with paper towels and sprinkle with remaining ⅛ teaspoon salt. Add shrimp to skillet in even layer and cook, stirring frequently, until just opaque, about 2 minutes. Off heat, stir in garlic and lime zest.

5   Add reserved nopales (nopales may not be completely dry) to tomato mixture and toss to combine. Divide avocado crema evenly among tortillas, then top with nopales mixture and shrimp. Serve immediately with lime wedges.

Avocado Crema

makes about ⅔ cup • total time: 10 minutes

- ½ avocado, chopped
- ½ cup chopped fresh cilantro
- ¼ cup dairy sour cream or plant-based sour cream
- ¼ cup water
- ½ serrano chile, seeded and minced
- 1 teaspoon lime juice
- ¼ teaspoon table salt

Process avocado, cilantro, sour cream, water, serrano, lime juice, and salt in food processor until smooth, about 1 minute, scraping down sides of bowl as needed. Season with salt and pepper to taste. (Crema can be refrigerated with plastic wrap pressed directly onto surface of sauce for up to 3 days.)

PREPARING NOPALES

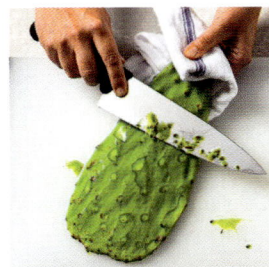

1   Grasp thick end of cactus paddle with tongs or dish towel and slide knife away from you across surface to remove any thorns and small raised bumps. Repeat on second side.

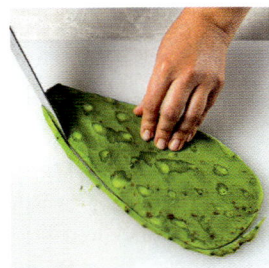

2   Trim outer ¼ inch of paddle, then trim bottom ½ inch of thick end of paddle; discard trimmings.

Braised Halibut with Carrots and Coriander

serves 4 • total time: 40 minutes   **FAST**

why this recipe works • When it comes to methods for cooking fish, braising is often overlooked. But the approach, which requires cooking the fish in a small amount of liquid so that it gently simmers and steams, has a lot going for it. As a moist-heat cooking method, braising is gentle, which makes it forgiving, all but guaranteeing perfectly moist and tender fish. We chose halibut for its delicate flavor and firm texture, which made for easier handling. Because the portion of the fillets submerged in liquid cooked more quickly than the upper half that cooked in the steam, we cooked the fillets for a few minutes in the pan on just one side and then braised them parcooked-side-up to even out the cooking. For the cooking liquid, wine plus the juices released by the fish delivered a sauce with balanced flavor and just the right amount of brightness. Mahi-mahi, red snapper, striped bass, or swordfish can be substituted for the halibut. You will need a 12-inch skillet with a tight-fitting lid for this recipe.

- 4 (6- to 8-ounce) skinless halibut fillets, 1 inch thick
- ½ teaspoon plus ⅛ teaspoon table salt, divided
- ¼ cup avocado oil
- 1 pound carrots, peeled and shaved
- 4 shallots, halved and sliced thin

½ teaspoon ground coriander

¾ cup dry white wine

1½ teaspoons lemon juice, plus lemon wedges for serving

1 tablespoon minced fresh cilantro

1 Pat halibut dry with paper towels and sprinkle with ½ teaspoon salt. Heat oil in 12-inch skillet over medium heat until warm, about 15 seconds. Place halibut skinned side up in skillet and cook until bottom half of halibut begins to turn opaque (halibut should not brown), about 4 minutes. Using 2 spatulas, carefully transfer halibut raw side down to large plate.

2 Add carrots, shallots, coriander, and remaining ⅛ teaspoon salt to oil left in skillet and cook over medium heat, stirring frequently, until softened, 10 to 12 minutes. Stir in wine and bring to simmer. Place halibut raw side down on top of vegetables. Reduce heat to medium-low, cover, and simmer gently until halibut flakes apart when gently prodded with paring knife and registers 130 degrees, 6 to 10 minutes. Carefully transfer halibut to serving platter, tent loosely with aluminum foil, and let rest while finishing vegetables.

3 Return vegetables to high heat and simmer briskly until mixture is thickened slightly, 2 to 4 minutes. Stir lemon juice into vegetables and season with pepper to taste. Arrange vegetable mixture around halibut and sprinkle with cilantro. Serve with lemon wedges.

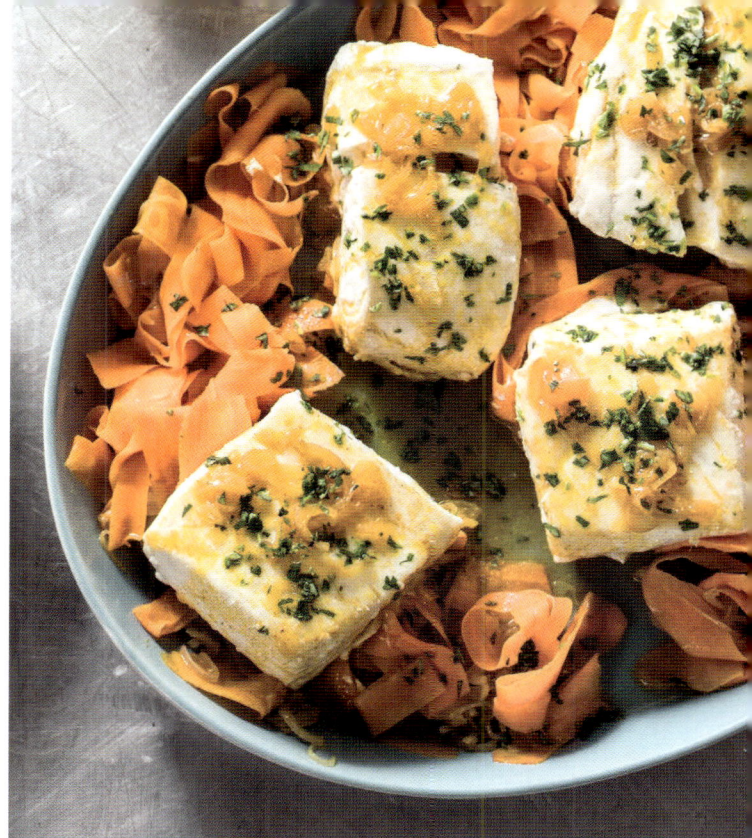

Swordfish en Cocotte with Shallots, Cucumber, and Mint

serves 4 • total time: 1¼ hours   **SUPERCHARGED**

why this recipe works • The premise behind the French method of cooking en cocotte (or casserole roasting) is to slow down the cooking process in order to concentrate flavor. Although fish cooked for an extended period of time often winds up dry, a combination of low oven temperature, moist-heat environment, and the right cut of fish allows it to remain juicy and tender. We found that meaty swordfish steaks were particularly well suited to cooking en cocotte. The fresh and vitamin-rich Mediterranean flavors of mint, parsley, lemon, and garlic easily combined with sliced cucumber to provide an insulating layer on which to cook the fish; we then turned the cucumber mixture into a complementary flavorful topping for serving. It is important to choose steaks that are similar in size and thickness to ensure that each piece cooks at the same rate. Halibut, mahi-mahi, red snapper, or striped bass can be substituted for the swordfish.

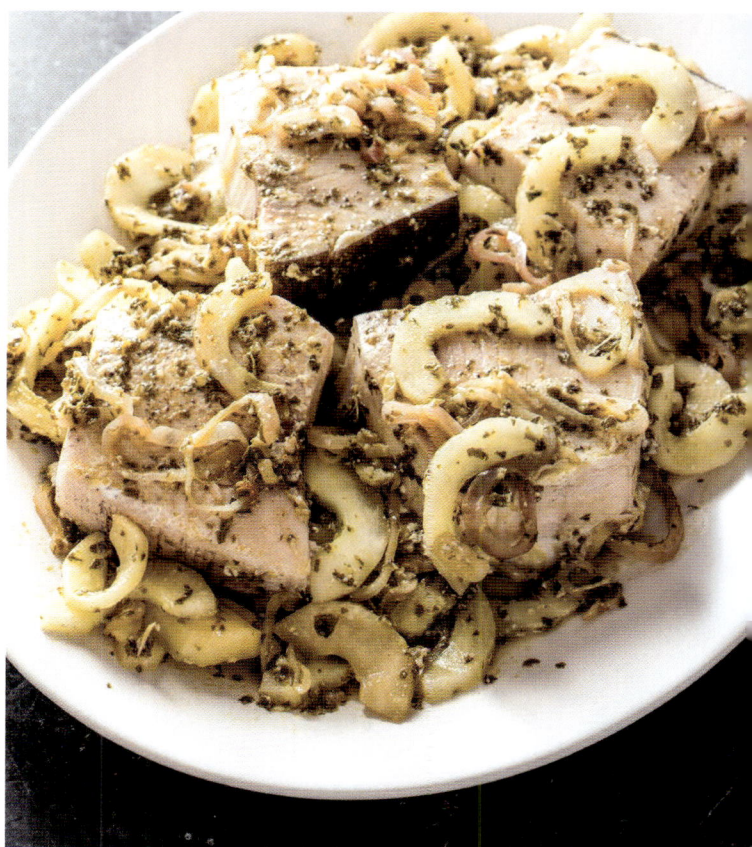

top	*Braised Halibut with Carrots and Coriander*
bottom	*Swordfish en Cocotte with Shallots, Cucumber, and Mint*

¾ cup fresh mint leaves

¼ cup fresh parsley leaves

5 tablespoons extra-virgin olive oil, divided

2 tablespoons lemon juice

4 garlic cloves, minced

1 teaspoon ground cumin

¼ teaspoon cayenne pepper

⅛ teaspoon plus ½ teaspoon table salt, divided

3 shallots, sliced thin

1 cucumber, peeled, seeded, and sliced thin

4 (6- to 8-ounce) skin-on swordfish steaks, 1 inch thick

⅛ teaspoon pepper

1 Adjust oven rack to lowest position and heat oven to 250 degrees. Process mint, parsley, 3 tablespoons oil, lemon juice, garlic, cumin, cayenne, and ⅛ teaspoon salt in food processor until smooth, about 20 seconds, scraping down sides of bowl as needed.

2 Heat remaining 2 tablespoons oil in Dutch oven over medium-low heat until shimmering. Add shallots, cover, and cook, stirring occasionally, until softened, about 5 minutes. Off heat, stir in processed mint mixture and cucumber.

3 Pat swordfish dry with paper towels and sprinkle with remaining ½ teaspoon salt and pepper. Place swordfish on top of cucumber-mint mixture. Place large sheet of aluminum foil over pot and press to seal, then cover with lid. Transfer pot to oven and cook until swordfish flakes apart when gently prodded with paring knife and registers 130 degrees, 35 to 40 minutes.

4 Transfer swordfish to serving platter. Season cucumber-mint mixture with pepper to taste, then spoon evenly over swordfish. Serve.

Nutritional Knowledge This swordfish recipe combines powerful anti-inflammatory ingredients, each offering unique health benefits. Mint and parsley are packed with antioxidants such as rosmarinic acid and flavonoids, while garlic and cumin bring sulfur compounds and polyphenols that support immune health. Shallots add quercetin to help reduce inflammation, and cayenne pepper's capsaicin boosts circulation and inhibits inflammatory pathways. Swordfish contributes omega-3s and selenium, supporting heart and brain health (though it's best enjoyed in moderation due to its higher mercury content). —*Alicia*

Chraime

serves 4 • total time: 1 hour `SUPERCHARGED`

why this recipe works • This spicy, garlicky, saucy, and aromatic tomato-based fish stew was brought to Israel by Libyan and Moroccan Jewish immigrants and commonly appears on Shabbat, Rosh Hashanah, and Passover tables. Libyan versions typically consist of a fiery sauce of tomato paste, hot peppers, and spices—primarily cumin, caraway and paprika—while Moroccan versions include more fresh vegetables (tomatoes and bell peppers) along with generous amounts of herbs. Our take pays homage to both: Grassy fresh jalapeño and bright Aleppo pepper brought varied heat, while tomato paste and bell pepper provided balancing sweetness. Cherry tomatoes, added with the haddock toward the end of cooking, added fresh pops of sweet acidity. The Tunisian spice blend tabil added a range of flavors from earthy muskiness to bright citrus notes (plus beneficial antioxidants). A finishing handful of cilantro and a squeeze of lemon balanced all the flavors. Black sea bass, cod, hake, or pollock can be substituted for the haddock. Thin tail-end fillets can be folded to achieve proper thickness. This dish is typically spicy; for a milder dish, reduce the amount of Aleppo pepper to 1 or 2 teaspoons. Serve with challah. You will need a 12-inch skillet with a tight-fitting lid for this recipe.

3 tablespoons extra-virgin olive oil, plus extra for drizzling

1 onion, chopped fine

1 red bell pepper, stemmed, seeded, and chopped

1 jalapeño chile, stemmed, seeded, and minced

¾ teaspoon table salt

¼ cup no-salt-added tomato paste

6 garlic cloves, minced

1 tablespoon Tabil (page 245)

1 tablespoon ground dried Aleppo pepper

2 teaspoons paprika

¼ teaspoon pepper

1½ cups water

1½ pounds skinless haddock fillets, ½ to ¾ inch thick, cut into 3-inch pieces

10 ounces cherry tomatoes

½ cup chopped fresh cilantro

Lemon wedges

1 Heat oil in 12-inch skillet over medium heat until shimmering. Add onion, bell pepper, jalapeño, and salt and cook until vegetables are softened, 5 to 7 minutes. Stir in tomato paste, garlic, tabil, Aleppo pepper, paprika, and pepper and cook until fragrant, about 30 seconds. Stir in water, scraping up any browned bits, and bring to simmer. Reduce heat to low, cover, and cook until flavors meld, about 15 minutes.

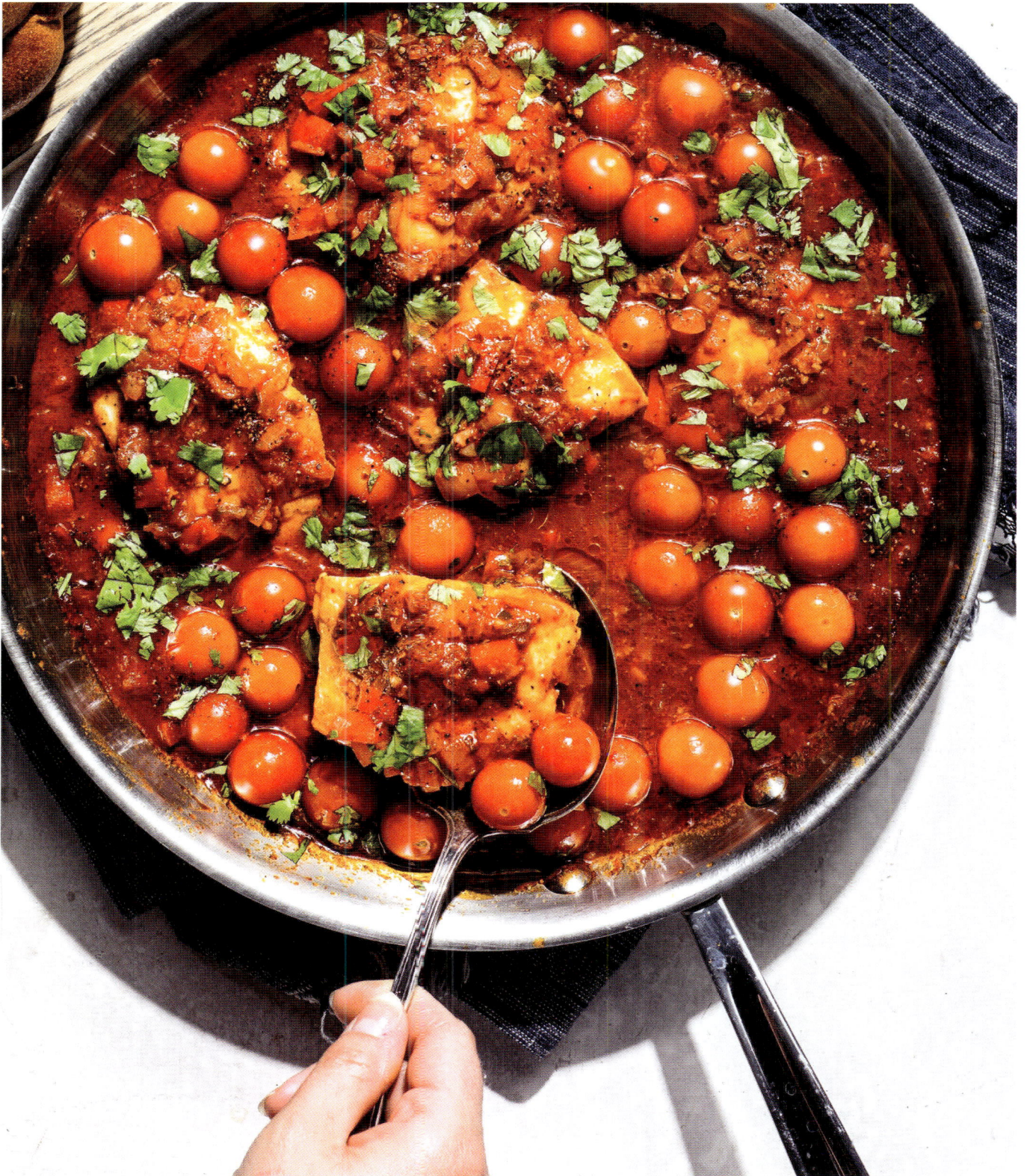

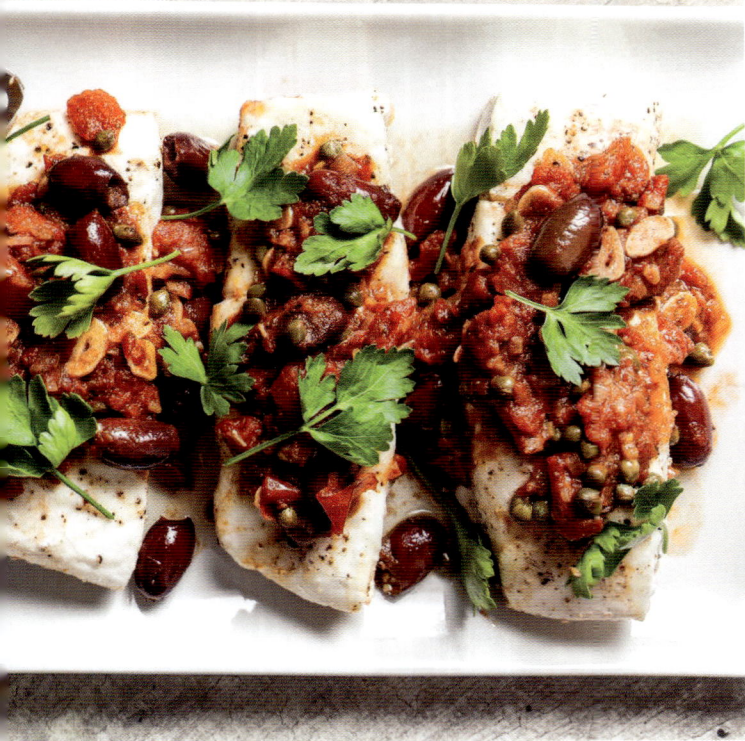

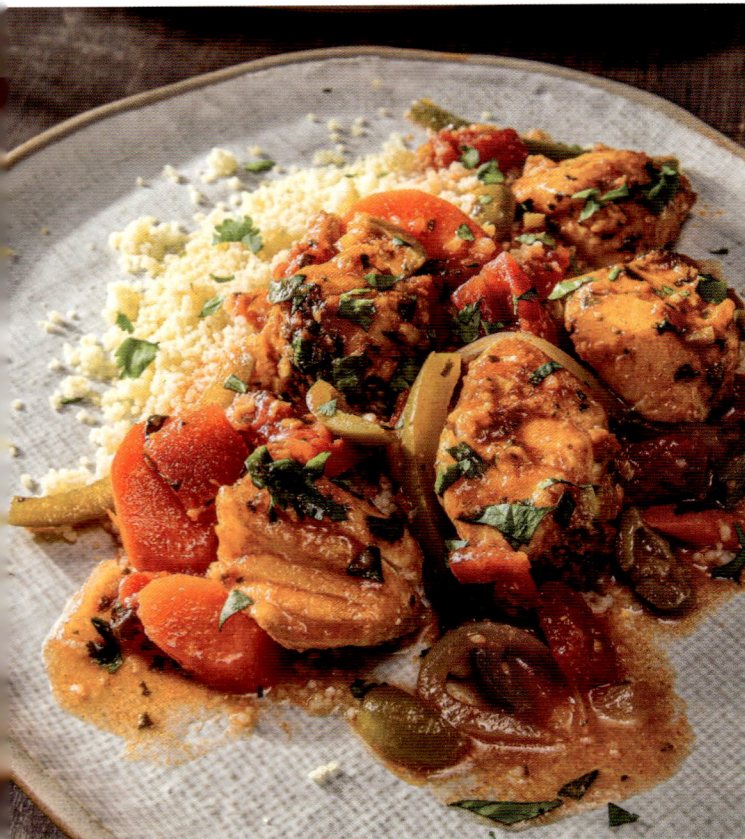

2 Nestle haddock into sauce and spoon some of sauce over fish. Sprinkle tomatoes around haddock and return to simmer. Reduce heat to low, cover, and cook until fish flakes apart when gently prodded with paring knife and registers 135 degrees, 5 to 7 minutes. Season with salt and pepper to taste. Sprinkle with cilantro and drizzle with extra oil. Serve with lemon wedges.

Halibut Puttanesca

serves 4 • total time: 35 minutes   **FAST**

why this recipe works • Halibut puttanesca—a dish of mild fish simmered in a puttanesca-inspired tomato sauce—delivers bold flavor in a flash. We sautéed a punchy and antioxidant-dense mixture of shallot, garlic, anchovies, oregano, and pepper flakes before adding canned tomatoes; then we nestled the halibut fillets into the sauce, which we cooked gently in the oven. The tomato sauce slowly reduced as it cooked, concentrating its flavor. A mixture of kalamata olives and capers added pops of savory saltiness to the sauce. Using six anchovies may sound like a lot, but the anchovies mellowed in the sauce and gave it incredible depth of flavor. A shower of parsley before serving added freshness and color to this bold, simple supper. Mahi-mahi, red snapper, striped bass, or swordfish can be substituted for the halibut.

- 4 (6- to 8-ounce) skinless halibut fillets, 1 inch thick
- ½ teaspoon table salt
- ½ teaspoon pepper
- ¼ cup extra-virgin olive oil, plus extra for drizzling
- 1 shallot, minced
- 5 garlic cloves, sliced thin
- 6 anchovy fillets, patted dry and chopped
- 2 teaspoons dried oregano
- ½ teaspoon red pepper flakes
- 1 (14.5-ounce) can no-salt-added diced tomatoes
- ½ cup pitted kalamata olives
- ¼ cup capers, rinsed
- ¼ cup fresh parsley leaves

1 Adjust oven rack to middle position and heat oven to 375 degrees. Sprinkle halibut with salt and pepper; set aside. Add oil, shallot, garlic, anchovies, oregano, and pepper flakes to 12-inch ovensafe nonstick skillet and cook over medium-low heat until fragrant and shallot softens, about 4 minutes.

2 Stir in tomatoes and their juice, olives, and capers. Nestle halibut into sauce and bring to simmer over medium-high heat. Transfer skillet to oven and bake until fish flakes apart when gently prodded with paring knife and registers 130 degrees, 10 to 15 minutes.

3 Using spatula, transfer halibut to serving platter. Stir sauce to recombine, then spoon over halibut. Sprinkle with parsley and drizzle with extra oil. Serve.

Fish Tagine

serves 4 · total time: 45 minutes   **FAST**   **SUPERCHARGED**

why this recipe works · This Moroccan-inspired fish tagine delivers anti-inflammatory benefits through a strategic combination of spices, healthy fats, and phytonutrient-rich vegetables. We started with cod, a lean white fish. The cod received a dose of vibrant flavor from chermoula, a flavorful paste made with cilantro, garlic, and spices such as cumin and paprika. To build a nutrient-rich base, we sautéed onion, bell pepper, and carrot in olive oil. Adding preserved lemon and green olives provided a bright, briny contrast while contributing anti-inflammatory compounds. Gentle cooking was key: By arranging the fish over the vegetables and letting it steam in its own juices, we preserved the cod's delicate texture while allowing the flavors to meld. A sprinkle of fresh cilantro added a burst of freshness and additional antioxidants. Black sea bass, haddock, hake, or pollock can be substituted for the cod. Picholine or Cerignola olives work well in this recipe. You can use store-bought preserved lemons or make our Quick Preserved Lemon (page 209); you can also substitute 1 tablespoon of lemon zest, but the flavor will be less complex.

- 1½ pounds skinless cod fillets, 1 inch thick, cut into 1½- to 2-inch pieces
- ¾ teaspoon table salt, divided
- ½ cup fresh cilantro leaves, plus ¼ cup chopped
- 4 garlic cloves, peeled
- 1¼ teaspoons ground cumin
- 1¼ teaspoons paprika
- ¼ teaspoon cayenne pepper
- 1½ tablespoons lemon juice
- 6 tablespoons extra-virgin olive oil, divided
- 1 onion, halved and sliced through root end ¼ inch thick
- 1 green bell pepper, stemmed, seeded, and cut into ¼-inch-wide strips
- 1 carrot, peeled and sliced on bias ¼ inch thick
- 1 (14.5-ounce) can no-salt-added diced tomatoes
- ⅓ cup pitted brine-cured green olives, quartered lengthwise
- 2 tablespoons rinsed and minced preserved lemons

1 Place cod in bowl and toss with ½ teaspoon salt; set aside. Pulse cilantro leaves, garlic, cumin, paprika, and cayenne in food processor until cilantro and garlic are finely chopped, about 12 pulses, scraping down sides of bowl as needed. Add lemon juice and pulse briefly to combine. Transfer mixture to small bowl and stir in 2 tablespoons oil; set aside.

2 Heat remaining ¼ cup oil in Dutch oven over medium heat until shimmering. Add onion, bell pepper, carrot, and remaining ¼ teaspoon salt and cook, stirring frequently, until softened, 5 to 7 minutes. Stir in tomatoes and their juice, olives, and preserved lemon. Spread mixture in even layer on bottom of pot.

3 Toss cod with cilantro mixture until evenly coated, then arrange cod over vegetables in single layer. Cover and cook until cod starts to turn opaque and juices released from cod are simmering vigorously, 3 to 5 minutes. Remove pot from heat and let sit, covered, until cod flakes apart when gently prodded with paring knife and registers 135 degrees, 3 to 5 minutes. Season with salt and pepper to taste. Sprinkle with chopped cilantro and serve.

Baked Shrimp with Fennel, Potatoes, and Olives

serves 4 to 6 · total time: 1 hour

why this recipe works · In this baked shrimp dish, the bold flavors of oregano and lemon infuse quick-cooking sweet shrimp with big flavor, and adding vegetables to the pan easily turns the dish into a complete sheet-pan meal with little fuss and lots of nutrients. Since shrimp cook so quickly, we first roasted our vegetables—potatoes and fennel—in the oven before scattering the shrimp over the top to roast while the vegetables finished. Complementary choices of briny kalamata olives and salty feta cheese gave this simple dish a savory bite, and lemon zest brought it all to life. Don't core the fennel before cutting it into wedges; the core helps hold the wedges together during cooking. We prefer untreated shrimp, but if your shrimp are treated with salt or additives such as sodium tripolyphosphate (STPP), do not add the salt in step 2.

- 1½ pounds Yukon Gold potatoes, peeled and sliced ½ inch thick
- 2 fennel bulbs, stalks discarded, bulbs halved and cut into 1-inch-thick wedges
- 3 tablespoons extra-virgin olive oil, divided, plus extra for drizzling
- 1¼ teaspoons table salt, divided

½ teaspoon pepper, divided

2 pounds jumbo shrimp (16 to 20 per pound), peeled, deveined, and tails removed

2 teaspoons dried oregano

1 teaspoon grated lemon zest, plus lemon wedges for serving

4 ounces feta cheese, crumbled (1 cup)

½ cup pitted kalamata olives, halved

2 tablespoons chopped fresh parsley

1 Adjust oven rack to lower-middle position and heat oven to 450 degrees. Toss potatoes and fennel with 2 tablespoons oil, ¾ teaspoon salt, and ¼ teaspoon pepper in bowl. Spread vegetables in single layer on rimmed baking sheet and roast until just tender, about 25 minutes.

2 Pat shrimp dry with paper towels. Toss shrimp with oregano, lemon zest, remaining 1 tablespoon oil, remaining ½ teaspoon salt, and remaining ¼ teaspoon pepper in now-empty bowl.

3 Using spatula, flip potatoes and fennel so browned sides are facing up. Scatter shrimp and feta over top. Return to oven and roast until shrimp are cooked through, 6 to 8 minutes. Sprinkle olives and parsley over top and drizzle with extra oil. Serve with lemon wedges.

| **MAKE IT DAIRY-FREE** • Omit the feta cheese or substitute plant-based feta cheese for the dairy feta cheese.

Seared Shrimp with Tomato, Avocado, and Lime Quinoa

serves 4 • total time: 55 minutes

why this recipe works • For an easy main-course quinoa and seafood dish, we paired the fiber-rich grain with seared shrimp and flavorful Southwestern-inspired ingredients such as chipotle chile powder, avocado, and cilantro. Cooking the shrimp in two batches ensured that they browned rather than steamed. Toasting the quinoa prior to cooking enhanced its nuttiness A quick, fresh tomato sauce pulled together the juicy, smoky shrimp and quinoa. We like the convenience of prewashed quinoa; rinsing removes the quinoa's bitter protective coating (called saponin). If you buy unwashed quinoa, rinse it and then spread it out on a clean dish towel to dry for 15 minutes. We prefer untreated shrimp, but if your shrimp are treated with salt or additives such as sodium tripolyphosphate (STPP), do not add the salt in step 2.

1½ cups prewashed white quinoa

1¾ cups water

½ teaspoon table salt, divided

¼ teaspoon grated lime zest plus 2 tablespoons juice, divided, plus lime wedges for serving

½ cup chopped fresh cilantro, divided

1½ pounds extra-large shrimp (21 to 25 per pound), peeled and deveined

½ teaspoon chipotle chile powder

¼ teaspoon pepper

2 tablespoons avocado oil, divided

1 pound tomatoes, cored and cut into ½-inch pieces

3 scallions, sliced thin, white and green parts separated

3 garlic cloves, minced

1 avocado, halved, pitted, and cut into ½-inch pieces

1 Toast quinoa in medium saucepan over medium-high heat, stirring frequently, until quinoa is very fragrant and makes continuous popping sound, 5 to 7 minutes. Stir in water and ⅛ teaspoon salt and bring to simmer. Cover, reduce heat to low, and simmer until quinoa is tender and liquid is absorbed, 18 to 22 minutes, stirring once halfway through cooking. Remove quinoa from heat and let sit, covered, for 10 minutes. Fluff quinoa with fork; stir in lime zest, 1 tablespoon lime juice, and ¼ cup cilantro; and cover to keep warm.

2 While quinoa cooks, pat shrimp dry with paper towels, then toss with chile powder, pepper, and ¼ teaspoon salt. Heat 1 tablespoon oil in 12-inch nonstick skillet over medium-high heat until just smoking. Add half of shrimp in single layer and cook, without stirring, until spotty brown and edges turn pink on bottom side, about 1 minute. Flip shrimp and continue to cook until all but very center is opaque, about 30 seconds. Transfer shrimp to clean large plate. Repeat with remaining 1 tablespoon oil and remaining shrimp.

3 Return now-empty skillet to medium-high heat. Add tomatoes, scallion whites, garlic, remaining ⅛ teaspoon salt, remaining 1 tablespoon lime juice, and remaining ¼ cup cilantro. Cook until tomatoes soften slightly, about 1 minute. Stir in shrimp and cook until shrimp are opaque throughout, about 1 minute. Transfer to platter, sprinkle with scallion greens and top with avocado. Serve with quinoa and lime wedges.

Farrotto Primavera with Shrimp

serves 4 • total time: 1¾ hours **SUPERCHARGED**

why this recipe works • This spring-inspired farrotto turns wholesome ingredients into an anti-inflammatory one-pot meal. We maximized flavor by first creating an aromatic shrimp stock with the shrimp shells—a technique that added depth without extra salt. The nutty farro, which we lightly pulsed before simmering to help the grains cook faster, absorbed the rich stock while retaining their satisfying chew. For vibrant, nutrient-packed additions, we chose asparagus and fava beans, both excellent sources of vitamins and antioxidants. A quick sear preserved the shrimp's delicate texture and enlivened their natural sweetness. The finishing touch was a bright blend of parsley, tarragon, and fennel fronds, which added freshness and herbaceous aroma, while toasted walnuts contributed crunch and beneficial fats. If your fennel bulb doesn't have fronds, you can increase the amount of parsley or tarragon by 2 tablespoons. We prefer untreated shrimp, but if your shrimp are treated with salt or additives such as sodium tripolyphosphate (STPP), do not add the salt in step 1. Serve with lemon wedges.

1 pound extra-large shrimp (21 to 25 per pound), peeled, deveined, and tails removed, shells reserved

1¼ teaspoons table salt, divided

5 tablespoons extra-virgin olive oil, divided

6 cups water

1 fennel bulb, 2 tablespoons fronds minced, stalks reserved, bulb halved, cored, and chopped fine

¼ teaspoon black peppercorns

2 bay leaves

1½ cups whole farro

1 onion, chopped fine

½ cup coarsely chopped fresh parsley

¼ cup coarsely chopped fresh tarragon

¼ cup walnuts, toasted and chopped

1 teaspoon grated lemon zest plus 1 tablespoon juice

12 ounces asparagus, trimmed and sliced ½ inch thick on bias

1 cup frozen fava beans, thawed

1 garlic clove, minced

1 Pat shrimp dry with paper towels and sprinkle with ¼ teaspoon salt; set aside. Heat 1 tablespoon oil in large saucepan over medium-high heat until shimmering. Add reserved shrimp shells and cook, stirring frequently, until shells begin to turn spotty brown, 2 to 4 minutes. Add water, reserved fennel stalks, peppercorns, and bay leaves and bring to boil. Reduce heat to low and simmer for 5 minutes. Strain stock through fine-mesh strainer set over large bowl, pressing on solids to extract as much liquid as possible; discard solids.

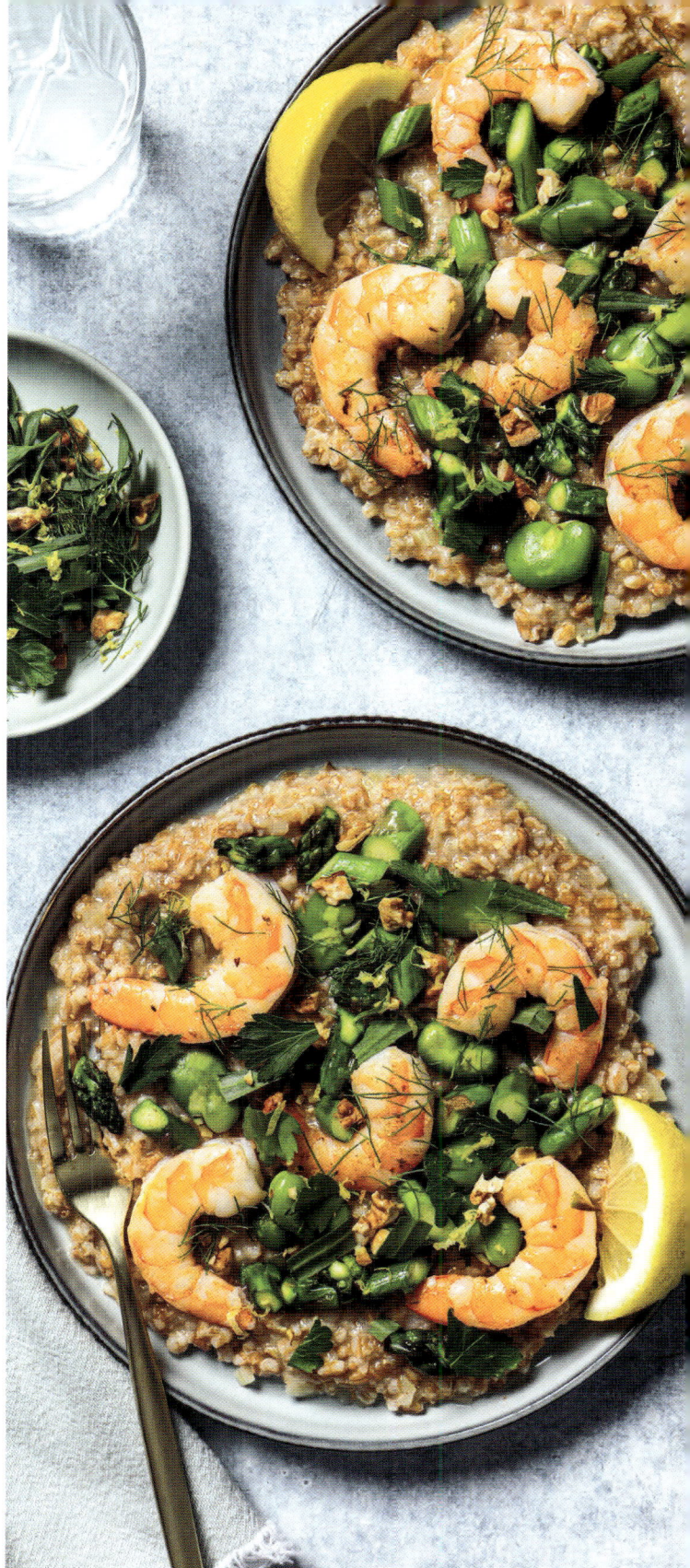

Farrotto Primavera with Shrimp

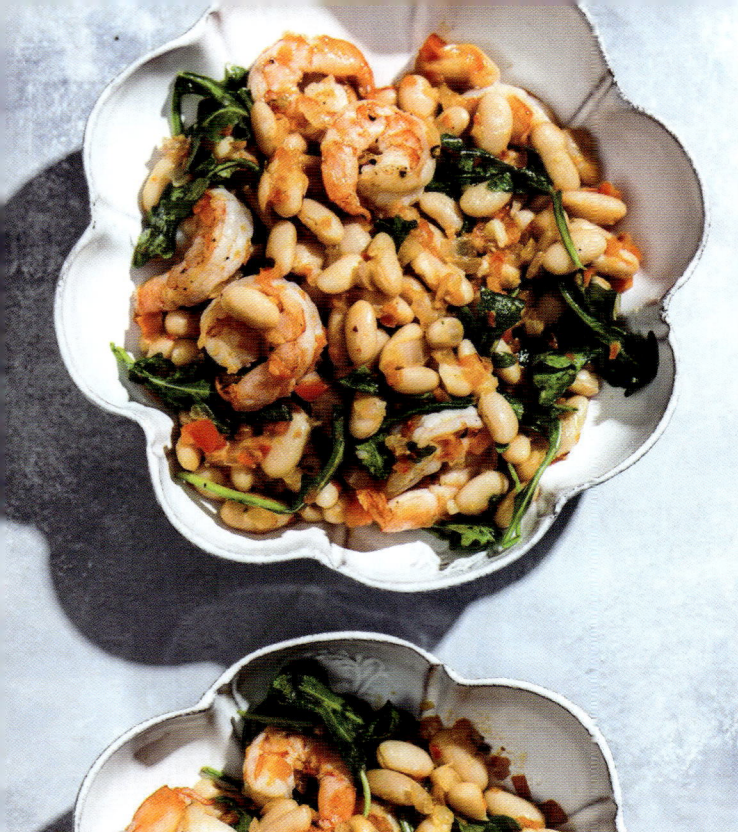

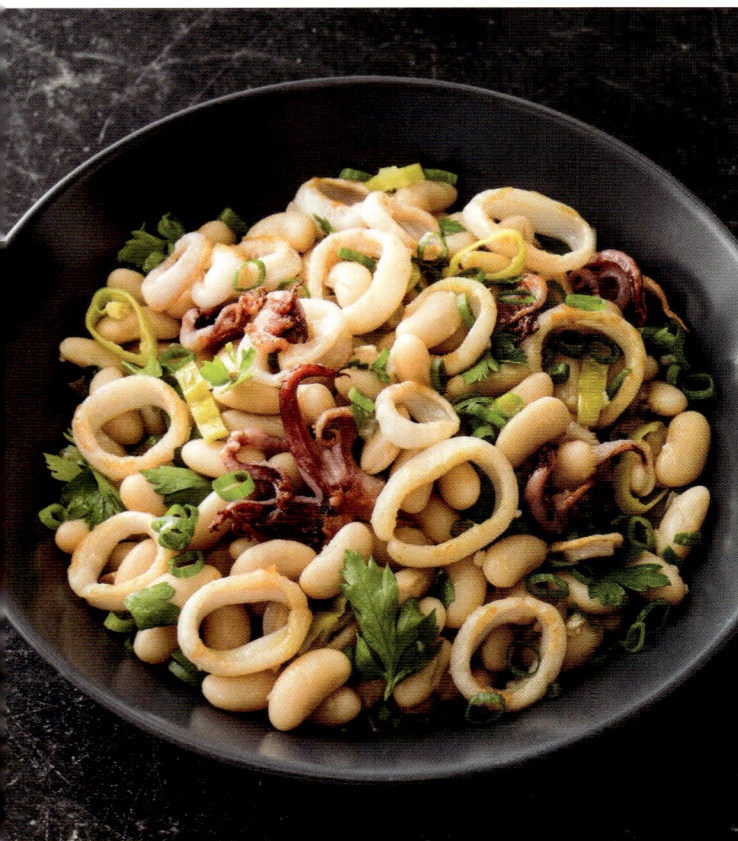

2   Pulse farro in blender until about half of grains are broken into smaller pieces, about 6 pulses.

3   Heat 2 tablespoons oil in now-empty saucepan over medium heat until shimmering. Add chopped fennel bulb, onion, and remaining 1 teaspoon salt and cook, stirring frequently, until vegetables are softened but not browned, 8 to 10 minutes. Add farro and cook, stirring frequently, until grains are lightly toasted, about 3 minutes.

4   Stir 4 cups stock into farro, reduce heat to medium-low, cover, and cook until almost all liquid has been absorbed and farro is just al dente, about 25 minutes, stirring twice during cooking. Uncover and continue to cook, stirring frequently, until creamy, about 10 minutes.

5   Meanwhile, combine parsley, tarragon, walnuts, lemon zest, and fennel fronds in bowl; set aside. Heat remaining 2 tablespoons oil in 12-inch skillet over medium-high heat until shimmering. Add shrimp in even layer and cook until edges turn pink, about 2 minutes. Flip shrimp and continue to cook until opaque throughout, about 1 minute; transfer to plate. Add asparagus and fava beans to fat left in skillet and cook over medium-high heat until tender and slightly blistered, about 4 minutes; transfer to plate with shrimp.

6   Adjust consistency of farrotto as needed with remaining stock. Stir in lemon juice and garlic and season with salt and pepper to taste. Transfer farrotto to serving platter, top with shrimp and vegetables, and sprinkle with parsley mixture. Serve.

Nutritional Knowledge   I love that this farrotto highlights the anti-inflammatory benefits of some of nature's most nourishing ingredients. Shrimp, which offer omega-3 fatty acids, help reduce inflammation and support heart health. Fennel, with its antioxidants and fiber, promotes digestive health and combats oxidative stress. Fresh parsley and tarragon, packed with vitamin C and flavonoids, help boost immunity, while asparagus offers essential vitamins A, C, and K. Farro and walnuts contribute fiber, magnesium, and omega-3s, all of which enhance cardiovascular health and reduce inflammatory responses.   —*Alicia*

top	*Shrimp and White Bean Salad*
bottom	*Warm White Bean Salad with Sautéed Squid and Pepperoncini*

Shrimp and White Bean Salad

serves 4 • total time: 35 minutes **FAST**

why this recipe works • Northern Italians combine their beloved cannellini beans with a wide array of ingredients. Inspired by this versatility, we combined these beans with tender shrimp to create a hearty salad with Italian flair. We sautéed the shrimp, which kept them juicy while crisping their exteriors. We also briefly cooked red onion and bell pepper, which kept their flavors fresh and their textures appealingly crunchy. The sweetness of the mild, creamy beans was the perfect foil for the briny, tender shrimp. The peppery bite of arugula tied all the flavors together to make a delectable one-dish meal. We prefer untreated shrimp, but if your shrimp are treated with salt or additives such as sodium tripolyphosphate (STPP), do not add the salt in step 1.

Shrimp
- 1 pound extra-large shrimp (21 to 25 per pound), peeled, deveined, and tails removed
- ¼ teaspoon table salt
- ¼ teaspoon pepper
- 1 tablespoon avocado oil

Salad
- ¼ cup extra-virgin olive oil
- 1 red, orange, or yellow bell pepper, stemmed, seeded, and chopped fine
- 1 small red onion, chopped fine
- ½ teaspoon table salt
- 2 garlic cloves, minced
- ¼ teaspoon red pepper flakes
- 2 (15-ounce) cans no-salt-added cannellini beans, rinsed
- 2 ounces (2 cups) baby arugula or baby spinach
- 2 tablespoons lemon juice

1 For the shrimp Pat shrimp dry with paper towels and sprinkle with salt and pepper. Heat oil in 12-inch nonstick skillet over medium-high heat until just smoking. Add shrimp in single layer and cook, without stirring, until spotty brown and edges turn pink on bottom, about 1 minute. Flip shrimp and continue to cook until all but very center is opaque, about 30 seconds; transfer shrimp to plate and let cool slightly.

2 For the salad Heat oil in now-empty skillet over medium heat until shimmering. Add bell pepper, onion, and salt and cook until softened, about 5 minutes. Stir in garlic and pepper flakes and cook until fragrant, about 30 seconds. Stir in beans and cook until heated through, about 5 minutes.

3 Add arugula and reserved shrimp along with any accumulated juices and toss gently until arugula is wilted, about 1 minute. Stir in lemon juice and season with salt and pepper to taste. Serve.

Warm White Bean Salad with Sautéed Squid and Pepperoncini

serves 4 • total time: 45 minutes plus, 15 minutes brining

why this recipe works • Recipes that pair savory white beans with lean, mild squid are common in Italy, and it's easy to understand why: The delicate flavor of the beans complements but doesn't overpower the subtle seafood flavor of the squid. We used a baking soda brine to tenderize the squid, which made it less likely to overcook. Cooking the squid in two batches encouraged more even browning. Using canned beans kept the overall cooking time short, and simmering them in an aromatic liquid infused them with flavor. Sherry vinegar and pepperoncini were winning additions that added tang to the complex flavor profile of this dish; to bring out more of the pepperoncini flavor, we also added some of the brine. Scallions and parsley leaves provided a finishing touch of freshness plus a boost of vitamins. Be sure to use small squid (with bodies 3 to 4 inches in length); they cook more quickly and are more tender than larger squid.

- 1 tablespoon baking soda
- 1 tablespoon table salt for brining
- 1 pound squid, bodies sliced crosswise into ½-inch-thick rings, tentacles halved
- 6 tablespoons extra-virgin olive oil, divided
- 1 red onion, chopped fine
- ½ teaspoon table salt
- 3 garlic cloves, minced
- 2 (15-ounce) cans no-salt-added cannellini beans, rinsed
- ⅓ cup pepperoncini, stemmed and sliced into ¼-inch-thick rings, plus 2 tablespoons brine
- 2 tablespoons sherry vinegar
- ½ cup fresh parsley leaves
- 3 scallions, green parts only, sliced thin

1 Dissolve baking soda and 1 tablespoon salt in 3 cups cold water in medium container. Add squid, cover, and refrigerate for 15 minutes. Dry squid thoroughly with paper towels and toss with 1 tablespoon oil.

2   Heat 1 tablespoon oil in medium saucepan over medium heat until shimmering. Add onion and salt and cook, stirring occasionally, until softened and lightly browned, 5 to 7 minutes. Stir in garlic and cook until fragrant, about 30 seconds. Stir in beans and ¼ cup water and bring to simmer. Reduce heat to low, cover, and continue to simmer, stirring occasionally, for 2 to 3 minutes; set aside.

3   Heat 1 tablespoon oil in 12-inch nonstick skillet over high heat until just smoking. Add half of squid in single layer and cook, without moving, until golden brown, about 3 minutes. Flip squid and continue to cook, without moving, until golden brown on second side, about 2 minutes; transfer to bowl. Wipe skillet clean with paper towels and repeat with 1 tablespoon oil and remaining squid.

4   Whisk remaining 2 tablespoons oil, pepperoncini brine, and vinegar together in large bowl. Add beans and any remaining cooking liquid, squid, parsley, scallions, and pepperoncini and toss to combine. Season with salt and pepper to taste. Serve.

Shaved Salad with Seared Scallops

serves 4 · total time: 45 minutes `FAST`

why this recipe works · Serving scallops on a salad is a healthful way to enjoy the delectable seafood. The ingredients in our salad call to mind Mexican antojitos (snacks) of refreshing produce such as sweet mango, crisp cucumber, crunchy jicama, peppery radish, and spicy jalapeño, all showered with chile limon. We shaved into ribbons or thinly sliced these ingredients and tossed them with mesclun. Lime dressing, cilantro, and roasted pepitas pulled this main course seafood salad together. We recommend buying "dry" scallops, which don't have chemical additives and taste better than "wet." Dry scallops will look ivory or pinkish; wet scallops are bright white. Use a sharp Y-shaped vegetable peeler or mandoline to shave the jicama and cucumbers. For more spice, reserve, mince, and add the ribs and seeds from the jalapeño.

1¼   pounds large sea scallops, tendons removed
1   pound jicama, peeled and shaved into ribbons
1   mango, peeled, pitted, and sliced thin
3   Persian cucumbers or 8 ounces English cucumber, shaved lengthwise into ribbons
4   ounces (4 cups) mesclun
2   radishes, trimmed and sliced thin
1   shallot, sliced thin
1   jalapeño or serrano chile, stemmed, halved, seeded, and sliced thin crosswise

¾   teaspoon table salt, divided
¼   teaspoon pepper
6   tablespoons extra-virgin olive oil, divided
1   tablespoon honey
2   teaspoons grated lime zest plus ¼ cup juice (2 limes)
¼   cup fresh cilantro or parsley leaves
3   tablespoons roasted pepitas or sunflower seeds

1   Place scallops on clean dish towel, then top with second clean dish towel and gently press to dry. Let scallops sit between towels at room temperature for 10 minutes.

2   Meanwhile, gently toss jicama, mango, cucumbers, mesclun, radishes, shallot, and jalapeño in large bowl, then arrange attractively on individual plates.

3   Line large plate with double layer of paper towels. Sprinkle scallops with ½ teaspoon salt and pepper. Heat 1 tablespoon oil in 12-inch nonstick skillet over medium-high heat until just smoking. Add half of scallops in single layer, flat side down, and cook, without moving them, until well browned, 1½ to 2 minutes. Using tongs, flip scallops and continue to cook until sides of scallops are firm and centers are opaque, 30 to 90 seconds. Transfer scallops to prepared plate. Wipe out skillet with paper towels and repeat with 1 tablespoon oil and remaining scallops.

4   Divide scallops evenly among salad on prepared plates. Whisk honey, lime zest and juice, and remaining ¼ teaspoon salt together in bowl. Whisking constantly, slowly drizzle in remaining ¼ cup oil until emulsified. Drizzle salad and scallops with dressing, then sprinkle with cilantro and pepitas. Serve.

Seared Scallops with Watermelon, Cucumber, and Jicama Salad

serves 4 · total time: 40 minutes `FAST`

why this recipe works · This dish combines restaurant-quality seared scallops with a salad that oozes summery vibes—for a light yet satisfying meal. The key to ensuring the scallops turned crisp on the outside but didn't overcook was thoroughly drying them before cooking them in a hot skillet; a good sear created a pleasing golden crust while preserving the scallops' tender interior. But what took this meal over the top was the salad we partnered with the scallops. Watermelon and cucumber, tossed with sugar and salt to season them and draw out some excess moisture, stayed refreshingly crisp; their brightness and crunch perfectly complemented the rich scallops. Jicama added a satisfying crunch and gut-friendly fiber, while avocado brought creamy richness plus healthy fats. A spicy-sweet lime-chile dressing tied all the elements together. A sprinkling of pepitas and cilantro provided a final flourish. We recommend buying "dry" scallops, which don't have chemical additives and taste better than "wet." Dry scallops will look ivory or pinkish; wet scallops are bright white.

 4 cups (¾-inch) seedless watermelon pieces
 ½ English cucumber, halved lengthwise and sliced thin crosswise
 1 tablespoon sugar, divided
 ⅛ teaspoon plus ¾ teaspoon table salt, divided
 6 tablespoons extra-virgin olive oil, divided
 ½ teaspoon grated lime zest plus 2 tablespoons juice
 ½ teaspoon chipotle chile powder, plus extra for seasoning
 1¼ pounds large sea scallops, tendons removed
 4 ounces jicama, peeled and cut into 2-inch-long matchsticks (1 cup)
 1 avocado, halved, pitted, and cut into ½-inch pieces
 2 tablespoons roasted pepitas
 2 tablespoons fresh cilantro leaves

1 Toss watermelon and cucumber with 2 teaspoons sugar and ⅛ teaspoon salt in colander set over bowl or in sink; set aside for 20 minutes. Whisk ¼ cup oil, lime zest and juice, chile powder, remaining 1 teaspoon sugar, and ¼ teaspoon salt together in large bowl; set aside.

2 Place scallops on clean dish towel, then top with second clean dish towel and gently press to dry. Let scallops sit between towels at room temperature for 10 minutes. Line large plate with double layer of paper towels. Sprinkle scallops with remaining ½ teaspoon salt. Heat 1 tablespoon oil in 12-inch nonstick skillet over medium-high heat until just smoking. Add half of scallops in single layer, flat side down, and cook, without moving them, until well browned, 1½ to 2 minutes. Using tongs, flip scallops and continue to cook until sides of scallops are firm and centers are opaque, 30 to 90 seconds. Transfer scallops to prepared plate. Wipe out skillet with paper towels and repeat with remaining 1 tablespoon oil and remaining scallops.

3 Drizzle 1 tablespoon dressing over scallops. Add jicama, watermelon, and cucumber to remaining dressing and toss to combine. Gently fold in avocado. Season with salt and extra chile powder to taste. Sprinkle with pepitas and cilantro. Serve scallops with salad.

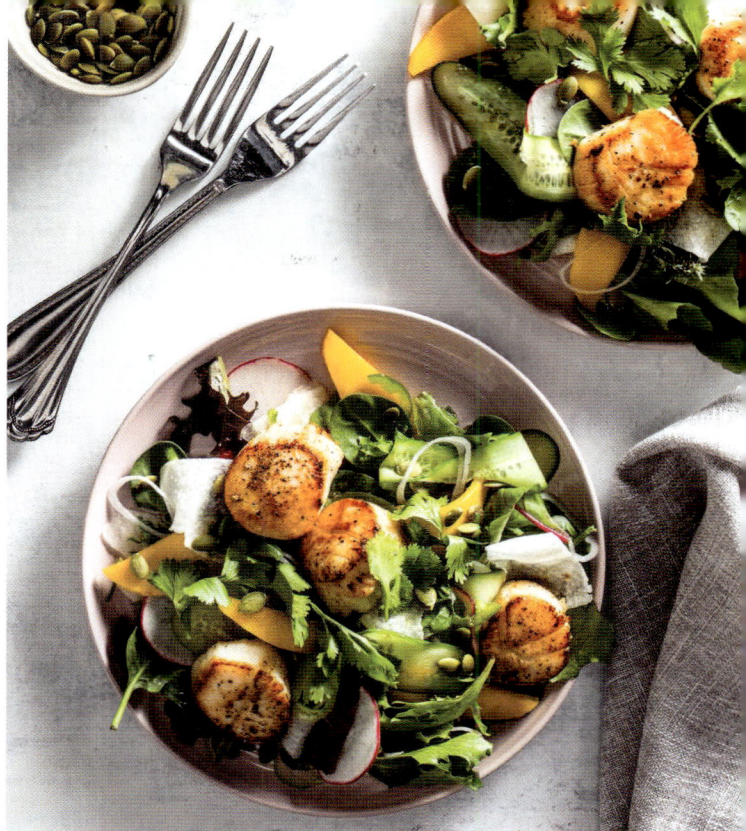

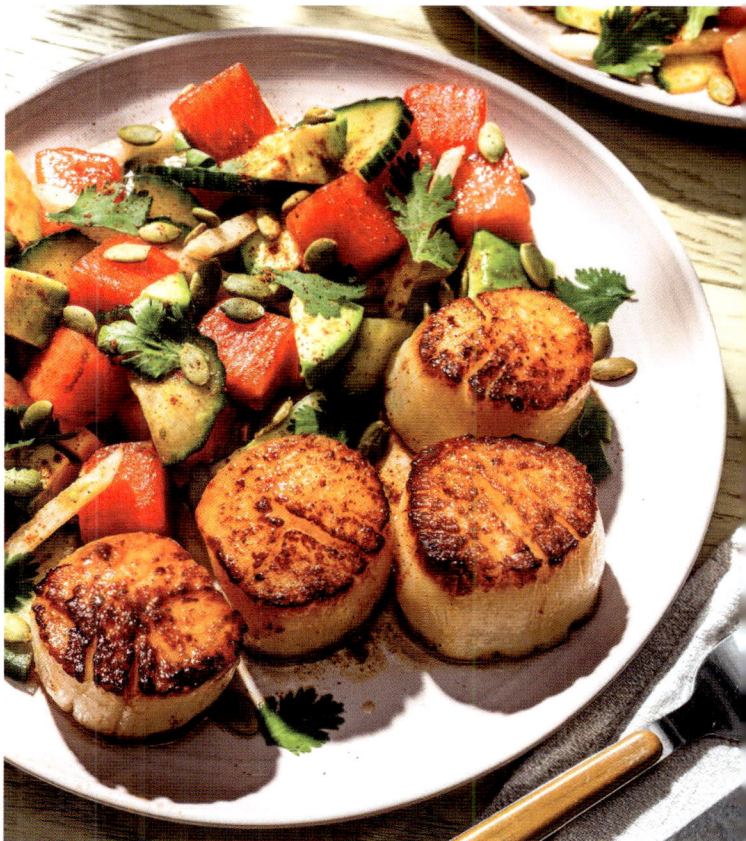

| top | *Shaved Salad with Seared Scallops* |
| **bottom** | *Seared Scallops with Watermelon, Cucumber, and Jicama Salad* |

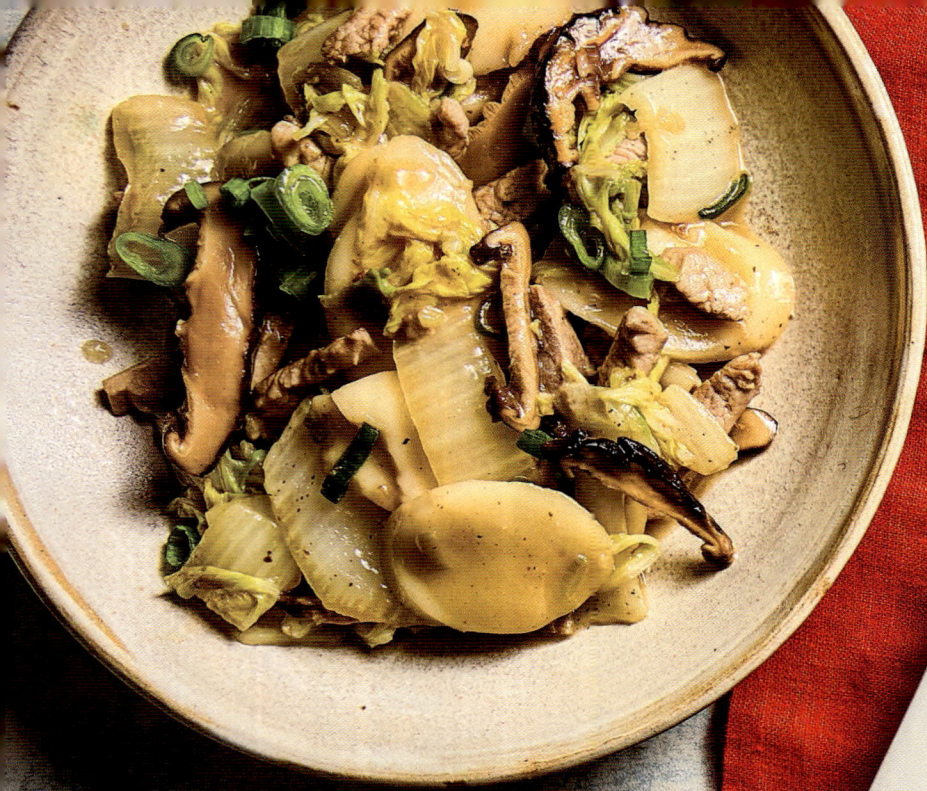

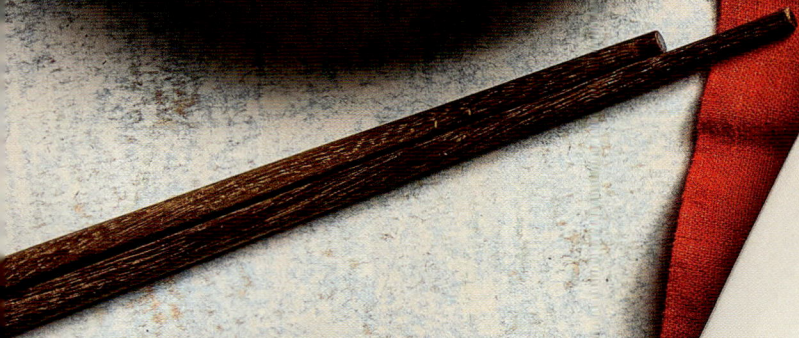

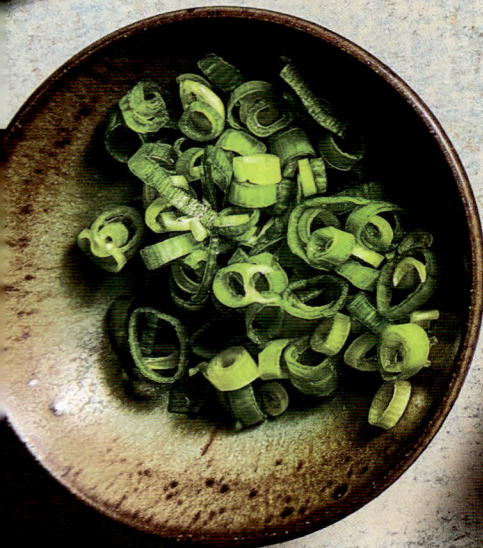

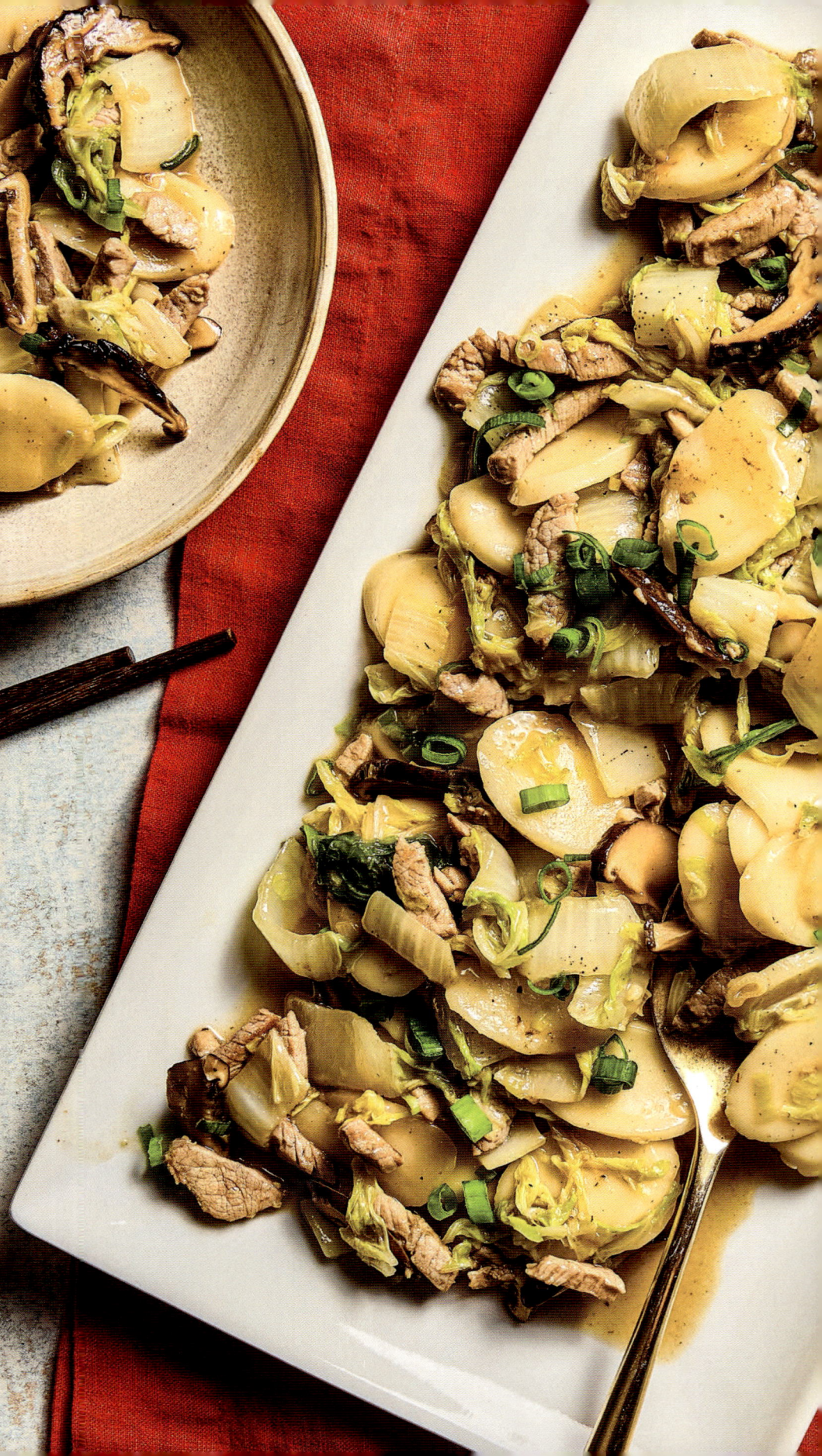

LEAN PORK & BEEF

■ FAST   ■ SUPERCHARGED

Perfect Pan-Seared Pork Tenderloin Steaks with Orange, Jicama, and Pepita Relish

serves 4 • total time: 1¼ hours

why this recipe works • Pork tenderloin steaks are relatively lean and packed with protein. They also have ample surface area for browning, so we wanted to make sure to sear them right. After seasoning them with salt and pepper, we applied the reverse searing technique, first cooking the steaks gently in the oven at a relatively low temperature, so the meat cooked evenly from edge to edge and was moist and tender. We then finished them by searing in a hot skillet until well browned on both sides. We plated the meat with a zesty, savory relish packed with texturally diverse anti-inflammatory ingredients—jicama, orange, pepitas, and more. We tossed the ingredients in a mixture of jalapeños, shallots, garlic, and oil, which came together quickly with the help of the microwave. Choose tenderloins that are equal in size to ensure that all the pork cooks at the same rate. Open the oven as infrequently as possible in step 1. If the meat is not yet up to temperature, wait at least 5 minutes before taking its temperature again

Pork
- 2 (1-pound) pork tenderloins, trimmed
- ½ teaspoon table salt
- ¼ teaspoon pepper
- 2 tablespoons avocado oil

Relish
- 1 orange
- ¼ cup extra-virgin olive oil, divided
- 2 jalapeño chiles, stemmed, seeded, and sliced into thin rings
- 3 shallots, sliced thin
- 6 garlic cloves, sliced thin
- 14 ounces jicama, peeled and cut into ¼-inch pieces (2 cups)
- ¼ cup roasted pepitas
- 3 tablespoons chopped fresh cilantro
- 3 tablespoons lime juice (2 limes)
- 1 teaspoon sugar
- ¾ teaspoon table salt
- ½ teaspoon pepper

1 For the pork Adjust oven rack to middle position and heat oven to 275 degrees. Set wire rack in rimmed baking sheet and lightly spray rack with avocado oil spray. Pound tenderloins to 1-inch thickness, then halve each tenderloin crosswise. Sprinkle steaks with salt and pepper. Place steaks on prepared rack and transfer to oven. Cook until meat registers 135 degrees, 25 to 35 minutes.

2 For the relish Meanwhile, cut away peel and pith from orange. Quarter orange, then slice crosswise into ¼-inch-thick pieces. Microwave 2 tablespoons olive oil, jalapeños, shallots, and garlic in medium bowl, stirring occasionally, until vegetables are softened, about 5 minutes. Stir in orange pieces, remaining 2 tablespoons olive oil, jicama, pepitas, cilantro, lime juice, sugar, salt, and pepper; set aside until ready to serve.

3 Move steaks to 1 side of rack. Line cleared side with double layer of paper towels. Transfer steaks to paper towels, cover with another double layer of paper towels, and let stand for 10 minutes.

4 Pat steaks until surfaces are very dry. Heat avocado oil in 12-inch skillet over medium-high heat until just smoking. Increase heat to high, place steaks in skillet, and sear until well browned on both sides, 1 to 2 minutes per side. Transfer to cutting board and let rest for 5 minutes. Slice steaks against grain ½ inch thick and transfer to serving platter. Serve with relish.

❙ MAKE AHEAD • Relish can be refrigerated for up to 24 hours.

Pan-Seared Pork Cutlets with Tomato Chutney

serves 4 • total time: 35 minutes **FAST**

why this recipe works • For a quick, weeknight-friendly pork recipe, we opted for thin cutlets that sear in minutes and develop a crisp crust while staying tender inside. We paired the meat with a show-stealing sweet-tangy tomato chutney: Microwaving intensified the tomatoes' natural umami, while just a tablespoon of sugar helped the chutney thicken so that it clung to the juicy, golden pork cutlets. Scallion greens and cilantro, stirred into the chutney, added freshness. The chutney's vibrant acidity made the perfect counterpoint to the pork's richness.

- ¾ cup canned no-salt-added diced tomatoes, drained and patted dry
- 1 tablespoon packed light brown sugar
- 2 teaspoons cider vinegar
- ¾ teaspoon table salt, divided
- ⅛ teaspoon plus ¼ teaspoon pepper, divided
- 2 scallions, green parts only, sliced thin
- 1 tablespoon chopped fresh cilantro
- 8 (3-ounce) boneless pork cutlets, ¼ inch thick, trimmed
- 1 tablespoon avocado oil

1   Microwave tomatoes, sugar, vinegar, ¼ teaspoon salt, and ⅛ teaspoon pepper in bowl until mixture is thickened, about 8 minutes, stirring halfway through microwaving. Let chutney cool completely, then stir in scallion greens and cilantro. Season with salt and pepper to taste; set aside for serving.

2   Pat cutlets dry with paper towels and sprinkle with remaining ½ teaspoon salt and remaining ¼ teaspoon pepper. Heat oil in 12-inch skillet over medium-high heat until just smoking. Add cutlets and cook until golden brown and cooked through, about 2 minutes per side. Transfer to plate, tent with aluminum foil, and let rest 5 minutes. Serve cutlets with chutney.

MAKE AHEAD • The chutney can be refrigerated for up to 3 days.

Seared Pork Chops with Couscous and Celery Salad

serves 4 • total time: 45 minutes   **FAST**

why this recipe works • Pork chops are quick to cook on a busy weeknight, so we wanted to pair them with a starch and vitamin-rich vegetable for an easy, well-rounded anti-inflammatory meal. We chose hearty, easy-to-make couscous (all it needs is a soak in boiling water for 10 minutes) and enhanced it with bites of dried fruit (currants or raisins offered an ideal balance of sweet and tangy) and fiberful celery. Sliced thin, celery brought refreshing crunch, counterbalancing the fluffy couscous. Use celery ribs with leaves, if available, and include the whole leaves in the salad. For an accurate measurement of boiling water, bring a kettle of water to a boil and then measure out the desired amount.

1½ cups boiling water
1½ cups couscous
1¼ teaspoons table salt, divided
 3 tablespoons extra-virgin olive oil
 2 tablespoons lemon juice, plus lemon wedges for serving
 ¼ cup chopped fresh parsley, divided
 1 large garlic clove, minced
 ½ teaspoon pepper, divided
 8 celery ribs, sliced thin on bias
 ¼ cup dried currants or raisins
 4 (6- to 8-ounce) boneless pork chops, ¾ to 1 inch thick, trimmed
 1 tablespoon avocado oil

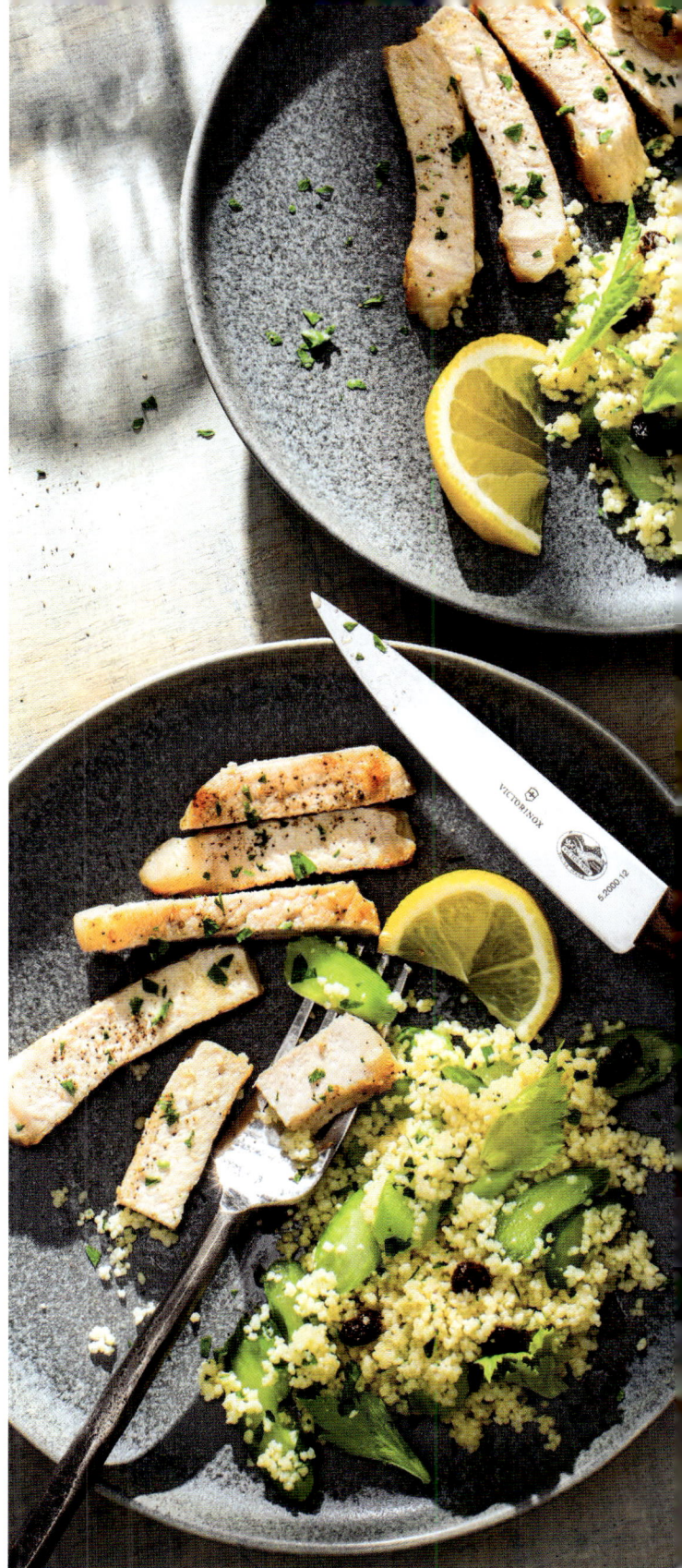

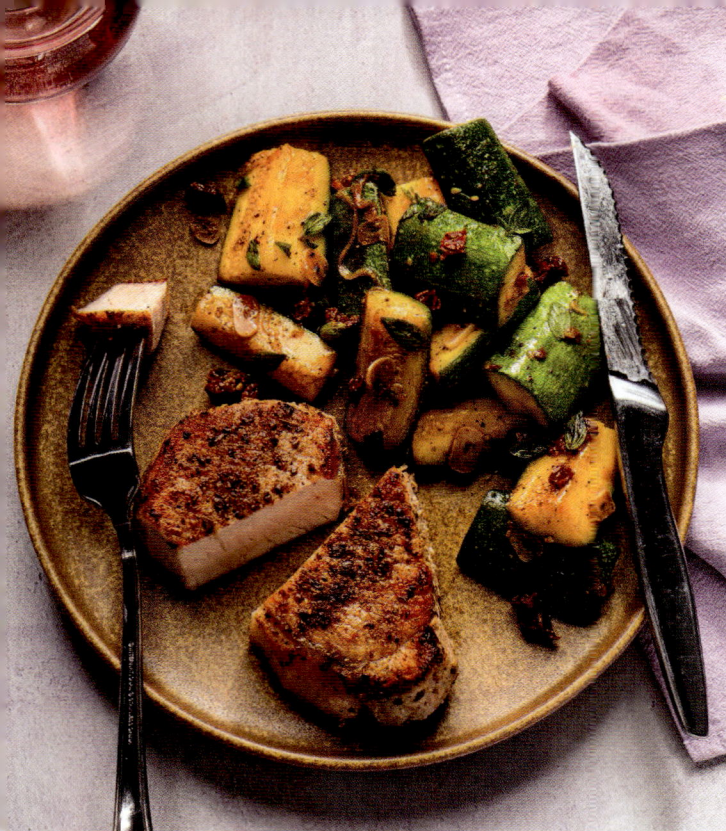

1   Combine boiling water, couscous, and ½ teaspoon salt in large bowl. Cover and let sit for 10 minutes. Fluff couscous with fork. Whisk olive oil, lemon juice, 2 tablespoons parsley, garlic, ¼ teaspoon salt, and ¼ teaspoon pepper together in bowl. Add dressing to couscous, along with celery and currants and toss to combine; set salad aside.

2   Pat pork dry with paper towels and sprinkle with remaining ½ teaspoon salt and remaining ¼ teaspoon pepper. Heat avocado oil in 12-inch nonstick skillet over medium heat until just smoking. Add pork and cook, flipping every 2 minutes, until well browned and meat registers 135 degrees, 8 to 10 minutes. Transfer pork to cutting board, tent with aluminum foil, and let rest for 5 minutes.

3   Sprinkle pork with remaining 2 tablespoons parsley and serve with couscous salad and lemon wedges.

Greek-Spiced Pork Chops with Warm Zucchini Salad

serves 4 • total time: 40 minutes   **FAST**

why this recipe works • When developing a pork chop dinner that channeled Greek flavors, our goal was a dish that felt vibrant and sun-drenched, calling to mind a summer evening by the Aegean. To start, we cooked zucchini, seasoned with the oil from sun-dried tomatoes, until it was tender and lightly browned. This ensured that the zucchini retained a hint of bite (rather than turning mushy). We then seasoned boneless pork chops with a tangy-earthy combination of lemon zest and dried oregano and put them in a hot skillet. Flipping the chops every 2 minutes ensured that the spice rub didn't burn. We mixed the zucchini with sun-dried tomatoes, lemon juice, and oregano to give our warm salad a savory-tangy depth. Stirring the fresh oregano into the salad just before serving ensured that the leaves stayed bright and verdant and gave us the herbaceous flavor we were after.

4 zucchini (8 ounces each), quartered lengthwise and cut crosswise into 2-inch pieces
¼ cup oil-packed sun-dried tomatoes, drained and chopped, plus 1 tablespoon sun-dried tomato oil, divided
1 shallot, sliced thin
2 garlic cloves, sliced thin
1 teaspoon table salt, divided
1¼ teaspoons pepper, divided

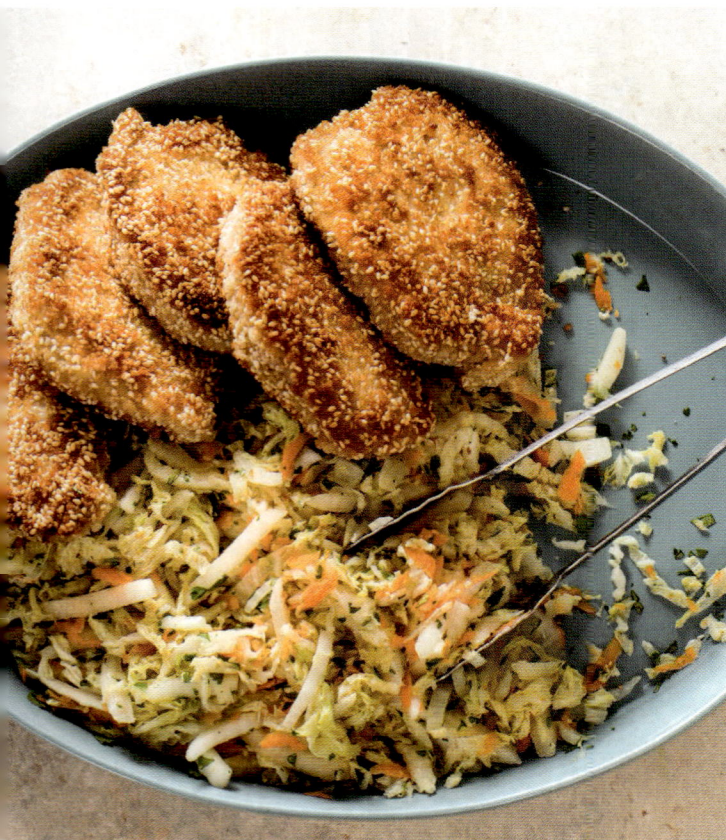

top | *Greek-Spiced Pork Chops with Warm Zucchini Salad*
bottom | *Sesame Pork Cutlets with Wilted Napa Cabbage Salad*

4 (6- to 8-ounce) boneless pork chops, ¾ to 1 inch thick, trimmed

2 teaspoons grated lemon zest plus 1 teaspoon juice

2 teaspoons dried oregano

1 tablespoon avocado oil

2 tablespoons fresh oregano leaves

1 Cook zucchini, tomato oil, shallot, garlic, ½ teaspoon salt, and ¼ teaspoon pepper in 12-inch nonstick skillet over medium-high heat until zucchini is just tender and lightly browned, 10 to 12 minutes. Transfer to serving bowl and set aside.

2 Pat pork dry with paper towels and sprinkle with lemon zest, dried oregano, remaining ½ teaspoon salt, and remaining 1 teaspoon pepper, pressing to adhere. Heat avocado oil in now-empty skillet over medium-high heat until just smoking. Add pork and cook, flipping every 2 minutes, until well browned and meat registers 135 degrees, 8 to 10 minutes. Transfer to cutting board, tent with aluminum foil, and let rest for 5 minutes.

3 Add fresh oregano, sun-dried tomatoes, and lemon juice to zucchini mixture and stir to combine. Serve pork with zucchini.

Sesame Pork Cutlets with Wilted Napa Cabbage Salad

serves 4 · total time: 45 minutes **FAST**

why this recipe works · A crisp coating on pork cutlets enlivens them with a bit of richness. Bread crumb coatings can turn out mushy and soggy, so we updated the traditional flour, egg, and bread crumb formula with a less traditional take: a combo of sesame seeds and panko. Using a whopping ⅔ cup of seeds ensured that the crust had ample sesame flavor and turned out extra-crisp, while giving our dish a dose of beneficial fats and lignans. Once the pork was seared and crisp, we reused the skillet to make a salad to complement the sesame chops. We browned garlic and ginger in sesame oil (to amplify that sesame flavor) and then added cabbage and carrot, cooking them until the cabbage leaves wilted slightly. Matchsticks of Asian pear contributed crunch and a touch of sweetness, a perfect contrast to the savory pork cutlets. We like using Asian pear in this recipe for its bright crispness, but Bosc or Anjou pears will also work. You will need a 12-inch nonstick skillet with a tight-fitting lid for this recipe.

2 (1-pound) pork tenderloins, trimmed

1 teaspoon table salt, divided

½ teaspoon pepper, divided

2 large eggs

1 cup panko bread crumbs

⅔ cup sesame seeds

½ cup avocado oil for frying, divided

1 tablespoon toasted sesame oil

2 garlic cloves, minced

1 teaspoon grated fresh ginger

1 small head napa cabbage (1½ pounds), cored and sliced thin

1 carrot, peeled and shredded

1 Asian pear, peeled, halved, cored, and cut into 2-inch matchsticks

¼ cup fresh cilantro leaves

3 tablespoons unseasoned rice vinegar

1 Cut each tenderloin on bias into 4 equal pieces. Working with 1 piece at a time, place pork cut side down between 2 sheets of parchment paper or plastic wrap and pound to even ½-inch thickness. Pat pork dry with paper towels and sprinkle with ½ teaspoon salt and ¼ teaspoon pepper.

2 Beat eggs, remaining ½ teaspoon salt, and remaining ¼ teaspoon pepper in shallow dish. Combine panko and sesame seeds in second shallow dish. Working with 1 cutlet at a time, dredge in egg mixture, allowing excess to drip off, then coat with sesame-panko mixture, pressing gently to adhere; transfer to platter.

3 Heat ¼ cup avocado oil and small pinch panko mixture in 12-inch nonstick skillet over medium-high heat. When panko has turned golden brown, place 4 cutlets in skillet. Cook, without moving cutlets, until bottoms are deep golden brown, 2 to 3 minutes. Using tongs, carefully flip cutlets and cook on second side until deep golden brown, 2 to 3 minutes. Transfer to paper towel–lined plate. Wipe skillet clean with paper towels. Repeat with remaining ¼ cup avocado oil and remaining 4 cutlets; transfer to platter.

4 Wipe skillet clean with paper towels. Cook sesame oil, garlic, and ginger in now-empty skillet over medium heat until fragrant, about 30 seconds. Add cabbage and carrot, cover, and cook, stirring occasionally, until the cabbage is just wilted, about 5 minutes. Off heat, add pear, cilantro, and vinegar and toss to combine. Season with salt and pepper to taste, and serve with pork.

MAKE IT GLUTEN-FREE · Substitute gluten-free panko bread crumbs for the panko bread crumbs.

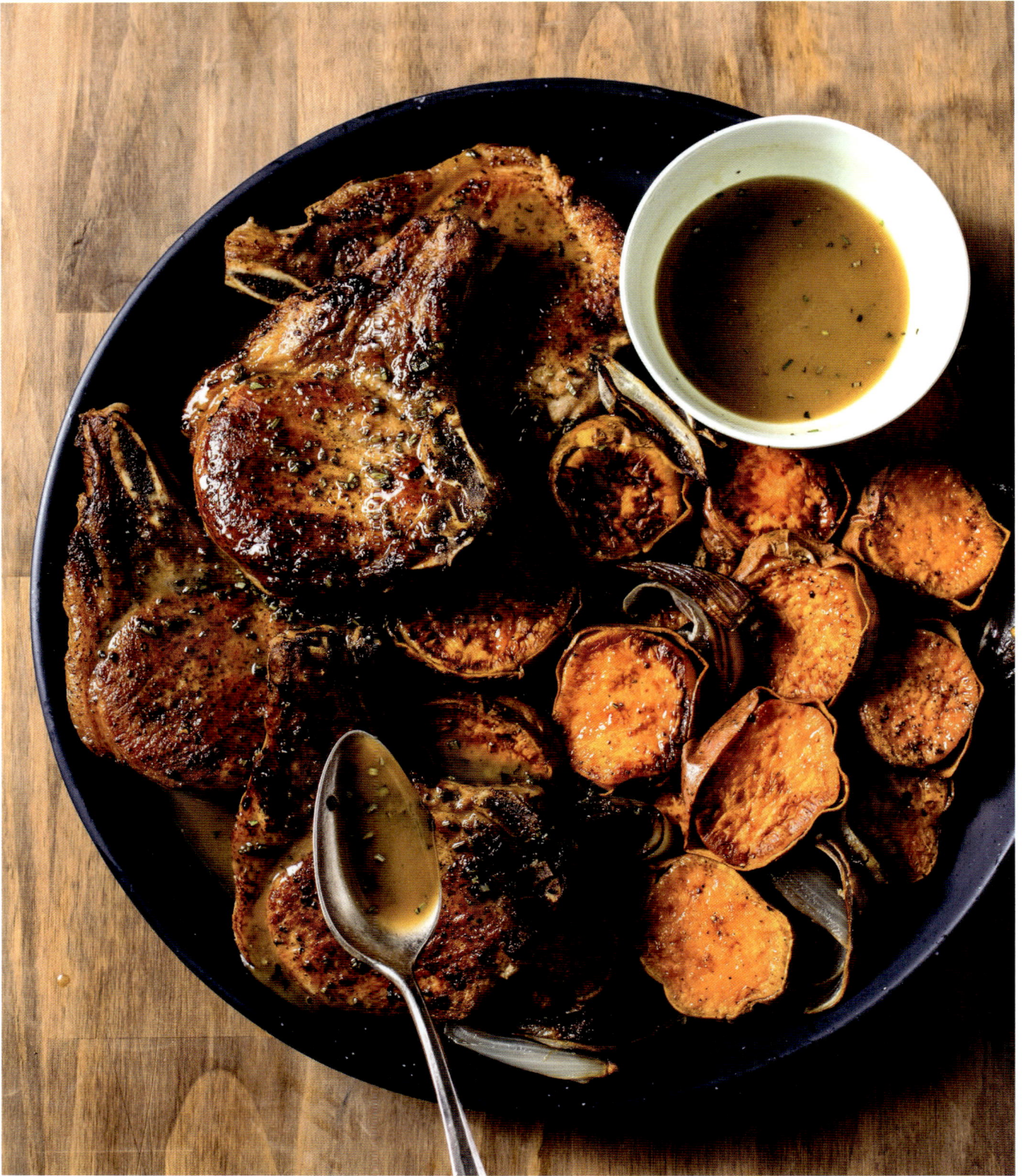

Pork Chops with Sweet Potatoes and Rosemary-Maple Sauce

Pork Chops with Sweet Potatoes and Rosemary-Maple Sauce

serves 4 • total time: 50 minutes

why this recipe works • This flavor-packed dinner pairs savory pork chops with fiberful sweet potatoes that are drizzled with a rosemary-maple sauce. We first roasted the potatoes with red onion until they turned tender. Meanwhile, we browned the chops in a skillet, where cayenne added gentle heat. We let them rest while we built a sauce in the same pan, adding broth and rosemary to the juices, along with maple syrup for subtle sweetness. After a brief simmer, we had a sauce that captured all the flavor of the pork and minimized cleanup. Served together, the pork and potatoes created a comforting meal that was satiating and nutritious.

- 2 pounds sweet potatoes, unpeeled, cut into ¾-inch-thick rounds
- 1 red onion, cut into ¾-inch-thick slices
- 2 tablespoons avocado oil, divided
- 1 teaspoon table salt, divided
- 1 teaspoon pepper, divided
- 4 (8- to 10-ounce) bone-in pork rib chops, ¾ to 1 inch thick, trimmed
- ½ teaspoon cayenne pepper
- 1 cup unsalted chicken broth
- 1 tablespoon maple syrup
- 1 tablespoon minced fresh rosemary
- 2 tablespoons minced fresh chives

1 Adjust oven rack to upper-middle position and heat oven to 450 degrees. Toss potatoes, onion, 1 tablespoon oil, ½ teaspoon salt, and ½ teaspoon pepper together on rimmed baking sheet. Arrange onions around perimeter of sheet and potatoes in single layer, cut side down, in center of sheet. Roast until onions are browned and potatoes are very tender, about 30 minutes.

2 Meanwhile, pat pork dry with paper towels. Combine cayenne, remaining ½ teaspoon pepper, and remaining ½ teaspoon salt in bowl, then sprinkle evenly over pork. Heat remaining 1 tablespoon oil in 12-inch nonstick skillet over medium-high heat until just smoking. Add pork and cook until well browned and meat registers 140 degrees, about 6 minutes per side. Transfer pork to platter, tent with aluminum foil, and let rest while vegetables finish cooking.

3 Add broth, maple syrup, and rosemary to now-empty skillet and bring to boil over medium-high heat, scraping up any browned bits. Cook until reduced by half, about 4 minutes. Transfer vegetables to platter with pork chops, drizzle with sauce, and sprinkle with chives. Serve.

Pork Chops with Spicy Tomato-Braised Escarole

serves 4 • total time: 35 minutes **FAST**

why this recipe works • Escarole, a mildly bitter green in the chicory family, is prized in Italian kitchens, where it is often simmered into soups or sautéed with garlic and olive oil. The fiberful green turns soft and buttery when cooked, so we emphasize this quality by braising them. The greens' bitter edge was tamed by adding tomatoes and red wine vinegar. We paired the vegetable with lean pork chops, which we browned on one side and then finished cooking (browned side up) atop the escarole. We prefer cutting up canned whole peeled tomatoes in this recipe, as they break down more readily than canned diced tomatoes. Use kitchen shears to cut up the tomatoes with no mess by snipping them directly in the can. Serve with crusty bread.

- 4 (8- to 10-ounce) bone-in pork rib chops, ¾ to 1 inch thick, trimmed
- 1 teaspoon table salt, divided
- ¾ teaspoon pepper
- 1 tablespoon extra-virgin olive oil
- 4 garlic cloves, sliced thin
- 2 anchovy fillets, rinsed, patted dry, and minced
- ½ teaspoon red pepper flakes
- 2 pounds escarole, trimmed and cut into rough 1-inch pieces
- 1 (28-ounce) can no-salt-added whole peeled tomatoes, drained with juice reserved, cut into 1-inch pieces
- 1 tablespoon chopped fresh oregano
- 1 tablespoon red wine vinegar

1 Cut 2 slits about 2 inches apart through fat on edges of each pork chop. Pat chops dry with paper towels and sprinkle with ½ teaspoon salt and pepper. Heat oil in Dutch oven over medium-high heat until shimmering. Add pork and cook until well browned on 1 side, about 5 minutes. Transfer pork, browned side up, to plate.

2 Add garlic, anchovies, and pepper flakes to fat left in pot and cook until fragrant, about 1 minute. Stir in escarole, tomatoes and their juice, oregano, and remaining ½ teaspoon salt. Cook until escarole is wilted, about 3 minutes, stirring occasionally.

3 Arrange pork, browned side up, in pot and add any accumulated juices. Reduce heat to medium-low, cover, and simmer until pork registers 140 degrees, 5 to 10 minutes. Transfer chops to cutting board, carve meat from bone, and slice ½ inch thick. Stir vinegar into escarole, season with salt and pepper to taste, and serve alongside pork.

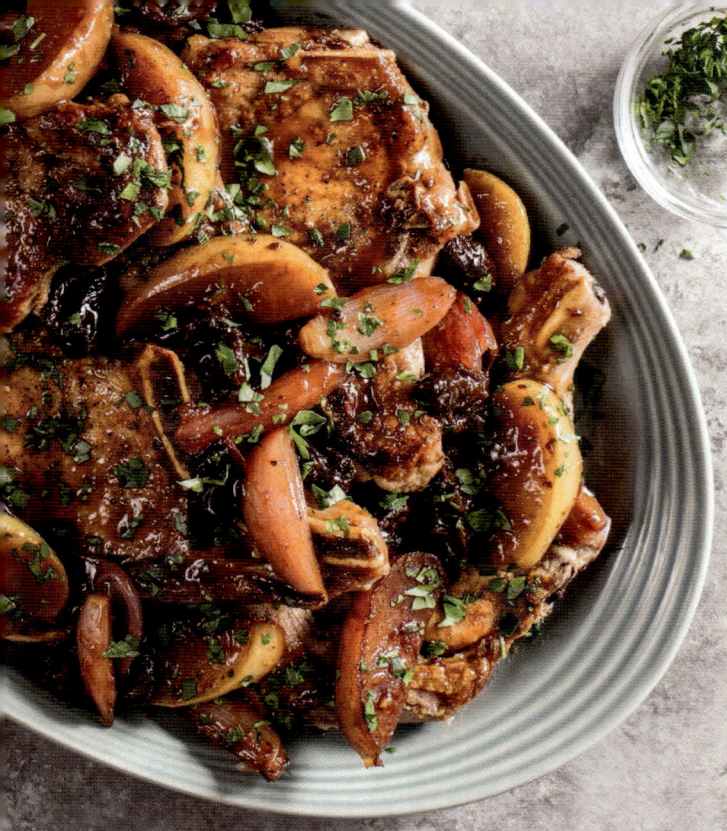

Fennel-Crusted Pork Chops with Apples, Shallots, and Prunes

serves 4 • total time: 40 minutes   **FAST**

why this recipe works • Fennel seeds—known to be protective against inflammation—add a distinctive anise-like flavor, plus antioxidants, to this nutritious take on a classic skillet dinner. Pork and apples are a match made in heaven, but adding shallots and prunes to the pan turned it into a party. Not only did this combination create a medley of contrasting flavors, but it also amped up the fiber and vitamins in the dish. The same skillet was used to cook both the pork and the fruit, the latter of which soaked up all the savory juices left behind by the meat. A mixture of chicken broth and cider vinegar made a complex braising liquid that became a flavorful concentrated sauce for the chops. You will need a 12-inch skillet with a tight-fitting lid for this recipe. You can substitute a Honeycrisp or Fuji apple for the Braeburn apple, if desired. Try to avoid using shallots heavier than 1 ounce each as they may not cook through before the apple turns mushy. Serve with rice.

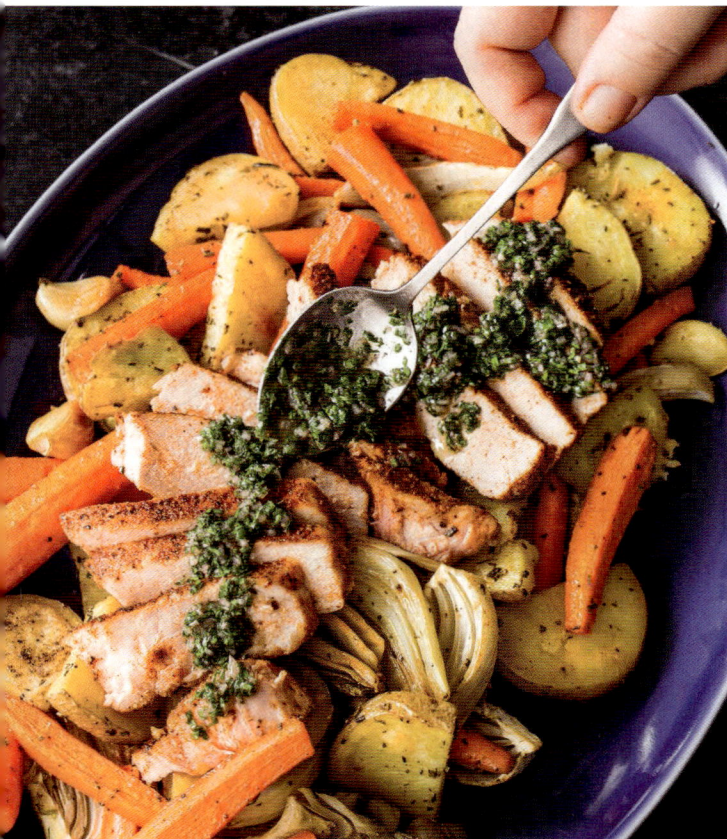

- 1 tablespoon ground fennel seeds, divided
- 1¼ teaspoons table salt, divided
- ¼ teaspoon pepper
- 4 (8- to 10-ounce) bone-in pork rib chops, ¾ to 1 inch thick, trimmed
- 2 tablespoons avocado oil, divided
- 6 small shallots, peeled and halved through root end
- 1 Braeburn apple, peeled, cored, and sliced into ¾-inch-thick wedges
- 1 cup unsalted chicken broth
- ½ cup cider vinegar
- ½ cup prunes, halved
- 1 teaspoon grated orange zest plus ½ cup juice
- 2 tablespoons chopped fresh parsley

1   Combine 2 teaspoons fennel, ½ teaspoon salt, and pepper in bowl. Cut 2 slits about 2 inches apart through fat on edges of each pork chop. Pat chops with paper towels and season with fennel mixture. Heat 1 tablespoon oil in 12-inch skillet over medium-high heat until just smoking. Add pork and cook until well browned and meat registers 140 degrees, 3 to 5 minutes per side. Transfer to platter, tent with aluminum foil, and let rest for 5 minutes.

2   While chops rest, heat remaining 1 tablespoon oil in now-empty skillet over medium-high heat until shimmering. Add shallots and apple cut side down and cook, without moving, until well browned, 2 to 4 minutes. Stir in broth and vinegar, scraping up any browned bits, then stir in prunes, orange zest and juice, remaining 1 teaspoon fennel, and remaining ¾ teaspoon salt. Bring to boil, reduce heat to medium-low, cover, and simmer for 5 minutes.

3 Uncover, stir in any accumulated pork juices, and continue to simmer until shallots are tender and sauce has thickened, 7 to 10 minutes. Off heat, stir in parsley and season with salt and pepper to taste. Pour sauce over pork and serve.

One-Pan Roasted Pork Chops and Vegetables with Parsley Vinaigrette

serves 4 · total time: 1 hour   **SUPERCHARGED**

why this recipe works · Bone-in center-cut pork chops deliver the succulence of a larger roast but cook more quickly, making them perfect for weeknights. They are high in protein and stand up to bold flavors, so it was natural to pair them with starchy, fiberful root vegetables and to season everything generously (adding an antioxidant boost). We opted for a hearty, vitamin-rich mix of thick-sliced Yukon Gold potatoes, carrot sticks, and fennel wedges. To add base notes of flavor, we first tossed them with fresh rosemary and peeled whole garlic, which turned creamy after a roast. Once the vegetables softened, we added our chops, which we had seasoned with paprika and coriander for a flavorful crust. The chops roasted atop the veggies, distributing their juices throughout the dish. An olive oil–parsley vinaigrette finished the pork on an herby note with healthy fats.

  1 pound Yukon Gold potatoes, unpeeled, halved lengthwise and sliced ½ inch thick
  1 pound carrots, peeled and cut into 3-inch lengths, thick ends quartered lengthwise
  1 fennel bulb, stalks discarded, bulb halved, cored, and cut into ½-inch-thick wedges
 10 garlic cloves, peeled
  3 tablespoons plus 1 teaspoon extra-virgin olive oil, divided
  2 teaspoons minced fresh rosemary or ¾ teaspoon dried
  1 teaspoon table salt, divided
1½ teaspoons pepper, divided
  1 teaspoon paprika
  1 teaspoon ground coriander
  4 (8- to 10-ounce) bone-in center-cut pork chops, 1 inch thick, trimmed
  4 teaspoons red wine vinegar
  2 tablespoons minced fresh parsley
  1 small shallot, minced

1 Adjust oven rack to upper-middle position and heat oven to 450 degrees. Toss potatoes, carrots, fennel, garlic, 1 tablespoon oil, rosemary, ¼ teaspoon salt, and ¼ teaspoon pepper together in bowl. Spread vegetables into single layer on rimmed baking sheet. Roast until beginning to soften, about 25 minutes.

2 Combine 1 teaspoon oil, paprika, coriander, ½ teaspoon salt, and 1 teaspoon pepper in bowl. Pat pork dry with paper towels, then rub with spice mixture. Lay chops on top of vegetables and continue to roast until pork register 135 degrees and vegetables are tender, 10 to 15 minutes, rotating sheet halfway through.

3 Remove sheet from oven, tent with aluminum foil, and let rest for 5 minutes. Whisk remaining 2 tablespoons oil, vinegar, parsley, shallot, remaining ¼ teaspoon salt, and remaining ¼ teaspoon pepper together in bowl. Transfer chops to cutting board, carve meat from bone, and slice ½ inch thick. Drizzle vinaigrette over pork before serving with vegetables.

Fried Brown Rice with Pork and Shrimp

serves 6 · total time: 1¼ hours

why this recipe works · For an anti-inflammatory fried rice, we wanted to swap out the typical white rice for a more fiberful alternative: brown rice. Because of its bran, brown rice digests more slowly—minimizing blood sugar spikes—and offers a pleasing chew. It also turned out to be perfect for making fried rice: While freshly cooked white rice tends to be too soft and sticky for fried rice, the bran layer prevented the freshly cooked brown rice from clumping, so we could use the grains fresh without having to refrigerate them before cooking (like we do with white rice). Additionally, the bran acted as a nonstick coating on each grain, so the grains separated nicely when cooking. To balance the nuttier flavor of brown rice, we used more ginger, garlic, and soy sauce than we do for white-rice fried rice. The addition of a quick version of Chinese barbecue pork, along with shrimp and scrambled eggs, made this dish hearty and protein-rich enough to serve as a main course. Do not use leftover rice here, and do not use a rice cooker to cook the brown rice. The stir-frying portion of this recipe moves quickly, so be sure to have all your ingredients in place before starting. We prefer untreated shrimp, but if your shrimp are treated with salt or additives such as sodium tripolyphosphate (STPP), reduce salt by half in steps 2 and 3.

2 cups short-grain brown rice

¾ teaspoon table salt, divided, plus salt for cooking rice

10 ounces boneless country-style pork ribs, trimmed

1 tablespoon hoisin sauce

⅛ teaspoon five-spice powder

  Pinch cayenne pepper

4 teaspoons avocado oil, divided

8 ounces large shrimp (26 to 30 per pound), peeled, deveined, tails removed, and cut into ½-inch pieces

3 eggs, lightly beaten

1 tablespoon toasted sesame oil

6 scallions, white and green parts separated, sliced thin on bias

2 garlic cloves, minced

1½ teaspoons grated fresh ginger

2 tablespoons low-sodium soy sauce

1 cup frozen peas

1 Bring 2 quarts water to boil in large pot. Add rice and 1 teaspoon salt. Cook, stirring occasionally, until rice is tender, about 35 minutes. Drain well and return to pot. Cover and set aside.

2 While rice cooks, cut pork into 1-inch pieces and slice each piece against grain ¼ inch thick. Toss pork with hoisin, five-spice powder, cayenne, and ½ teaspoon salt in bowl; set aside.

3 Heat 1 teaspoon avocado oil in 12-inch nonstick skillet over medium-high heat until shimmering. Add shrimp in even layer and cook without moving until browned, about 90 seconds. Stir and cook until just cooked through, about 90 seconds longer. Push shrimp to 1 side of skillet. Add 1 teaspoon avocado oil to cleared side of skillet. Add eggs to clearing and sprinkle with remaining ¼ teaspoon salt. Using silicone spatula, stir eggs gently until set but still wet, about 30 seconds. Stir eggs into shrimp and continue to cook, breaking up large pieces of egg, until eggs are fully cooked, about 30 seconds. Transfer shrimp-egg mixture to clean bowl.

4 Heat remaining 2 teaspoons avocado oil in now-empty skillet over medium-high heat until shimmering. Add pork in even layer and cook, without moving, until well browned, 2 to 3 minutes per side. Transfer to bowl with shrimp-egg mixture.

5 Heat sesame oil in now-empty skillet over medium-high heat until shimmering. Add scallion whites and cook, stirring frequently, until softened and starting to brown, about 1 minute. Add garlic and ginger and cook, stirring frequently, until fragrant and beginning to brown, 30 to 60 seconds. Add soy sauce and half of

rice and stir until all ingredients are fully incorporated, making sure to break up clumps of ginger and garlic. Reduce heat to medium-low and add remaining rice, shrimp-pork mixture, and peas. Stir until all ingredients are evenly incorporated and heated through, 2 to 4 minutes. Remove from heat and stir in scallion greens. Transfer to warmed platter and serve.

MAKE AHEAD • Pork can be trimmed and sliced and shrimp can be peeled and cut and then refrigerated separately for up to 24 hours.

MAKE IT GLUTEN-FREE • Substitute gluten-free hoisin and low-sodium tamari for the hoisin and low-sodium soy sauce.

Chorizo and Potato Tacos

serves 6 • total time: 1 hour

why this recipe works • Juicy, super-savory Mexican chorizo makes for hearty tacos, so we wanted a quick method for making our own chorizo that moderated the saturated fat and sodium. We started by blooming ancho chile powder, paprika, coriander, oregano, and cinnamon—a bevy of antioxidant-rich spices—in oil to intensify their flavors and then we mixed ground pork into the spiced oil along with some vinegar. We cooked the mixture in a skillet, adding parboiled diced potatoes to absorb the flavorful juices from the meat. Mashing some of the potatoes and mixing them into the filling made the entire mixture more cohesive. A bright, creamy, antioxidant-rich puree of tomatillos, avocado, cilantro, and jalapeños complemented the richness of the filling.

Filling

1 pound Yukon Gold potatoes, peeled and cut into ½-inch pieces

3 tablespoons extra-virgin olive oil

1 tablespoon ancho chile powder

1 tablespoon paprika

1½ teaspoons ground coriander

1½ teaspoons dried oregano

¼ teaspoon ground cinnamon

  Pinch cayenne pepper

  Pinch ground allspice

2 teaspoons table salt, divided

½ teaspoon pepper

2 tablespoons cider vinegar

1 garlic clove, minced

8 ounces ground pork

Sauce

- 4 ounces tomatillos, husks and stems removed, rinsed well, dried, and cut into 1-inch pieces
- ½ avocado, halved, pitted, and cut into 1-inch pieces
- 1 jalapeño chile, stemmed, seeded, and chopped
- 2 tablespoons chopped fresh cilantro leaves and tender stems
- 1½ teaspoons lime juice
- 1 garlic clove, minced
- ½ teaspoon table salt

Tacos

- 12 (6-inch) corn tortillas, warmed
  Finely chopped white onion
  Fresh cilantro leaves
  Lime wedges

1 For the filling Add potatoes to medium saucepan, add water to cover by 1 inch, and bring to boil over high heat. Reduce heat to medium and boil until potatoes are tender, 6 to 8 minutes. Drain potatoes and set aside.

2 Meanwhile, combine oil, chile powder, paprika, coriander, oregano, cinnamon, cayenne, allspice, 1 teaspoon salt, and pepper in 12-inch nonstick skillet. Cook over medium heat, stirring constantly, until mixture is bubbling and fragrant, about 2 minutes. Off heat, carefully stir in vinegar and garlic (mixture will sputter). Let stand until steam subsides and skillet cools slightly, about 5 minutes. Add pork to skillet. Mash and mix with silicone spatula until spice mixture is evenly incorporated into pork.

3 Return skillet to medium-high heat and cook, mashing and stirring, until pork has broken into fine crumbles and juices are bubbling, about 3 minutes.

4 Stir in potatoes, cover, and reduce heat to low. Cook until potatoes are fully softened and have soaked up most of pork juices, 6 to 8 minutes, stirring halfway through cooking. Off heat, using spatula, mash approximately one-eighth of potatoes. Stir mixture until mashed potatoes are evenly distributed. Cover and keep warm.

5 For the sauce Blend all ingredients in blender until smooth, about 1 minute, scraping down sides of blender jar as needed. Transfer to serving bowl.

6 For the tacos Spoon filling into center of each tortilla and serve, passing sauce, onion, cilantro, and lime wedges separately.

MAKE AHEAD • Sauce can be refrigerated in an airtight container for up to 3 days.

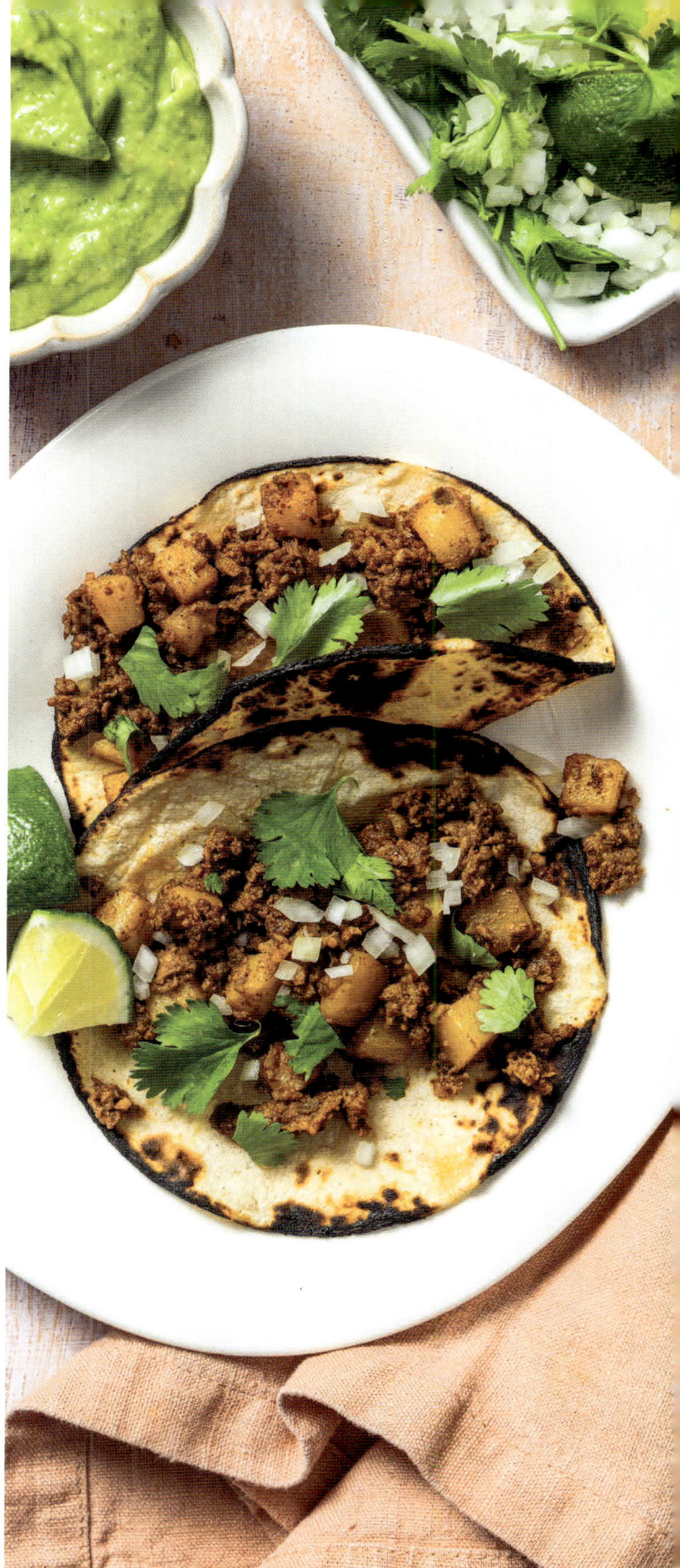

Chorizo and Potato Tacos

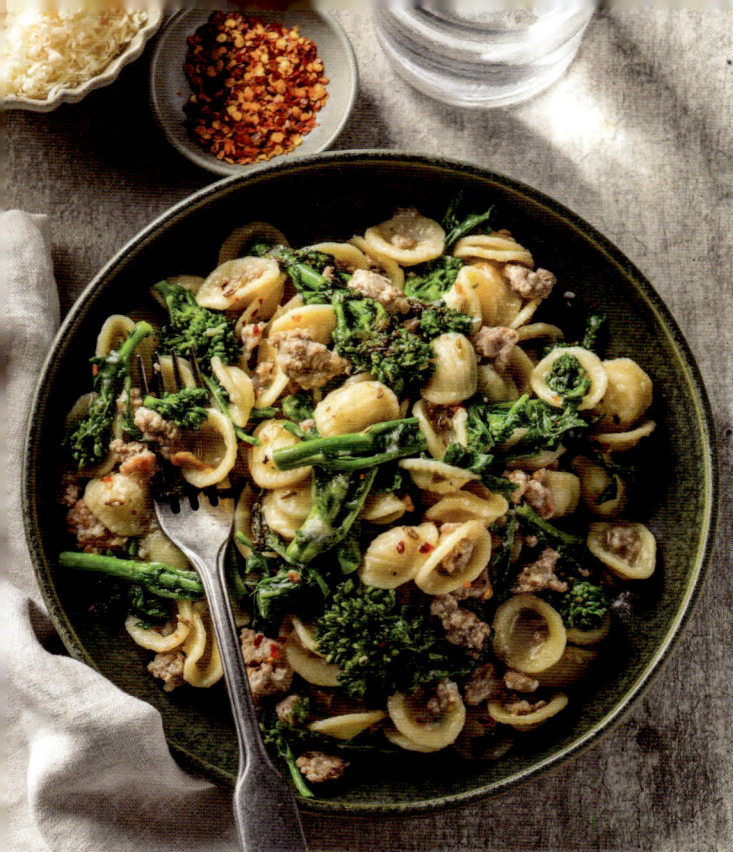

Orecchiette with Broccoli Rabe, Fennel, and Spiced Pork

serves 4 to 6 • total time: 30 minutes **FAST**

why this recipe works • Orecchiette is a small, bowl-shaped pasta that's perfect for catching sauce. It's ideal for cradling chunky ingredients such as broccoli rabe and sausage, an iconic southern Italian preparation. For our version, we swapped out the sausage for ground pork to moderate the saturated fat and keep an eye on sodium. We cooked broccoli rabe in a skillet just long enough for it to soften but retain its crisp-tender bite. We then cooked ground pork with garlic, fennel seeds, oregano and pepper flakes. Tossing the pork, broccoli rabe, and Parmesan with the pasta and a bit of the pasta cooking water melded the flavors. For a spicier dish, use the larger amount of pepper flakes.

  2 tablespoons extra-virgin olive oil, divided
  1 pound broccoli rabe, trimmed and cut into 1½-inch pieces
  1 teaspoon table salt, divided, plus salt for cooking pasta
  8 ounces ground pork
  8 garlic cloves, minced
  1 teaspoon fennel seeds, cracked
  1 teaspoon dried oregano
¼–½ teaspoon red pepper flakes
  ¼ cup dry white wine
  1 pound orecchiette
  2 ounces Parmesan cheese, grated (1 cup), plus extra for serving

1   Heat 1 tablespoon oil in 12-inch nonstick skillet over medium heat until shimmering. Add broccoli rabe and ¼ teaspoon salt, cover, and cook, stirring occasionally, until softened, 3 to 5 minutes. Using slotted spoon, transfer broccoli rabe to bowl and set aside.

2   Add pork, remaining ¾ teaspoon salt, and remaining 1 tablespoon oil to now-empty skillet and cook over medium-high heat, breaking up meat with wooden spoon, until lightly browned, about 5 minutes. Stir in garlic, fennel seeds, oregano, and pepper flakes and cook until fragrant, about 1 minute. Stir in wine, scraping up any browned bits. Set aside off heat.

3   Meanwhile, bring 2 quarts water to boil in large pot. Add pasta and ½ tablespoon salt and cook, stirring often, until al dente. Reserve 1 cup cooking water, then drain pasta and return it to pot.

4   Add reserved pork mixture, reserved broccoli rabe, Parmesan, and ½ cup pasta cooking water to pasta in pot and toss to combine. Adjust consistency with remaining reserved cooking water as needed. Serve with extra Parmesan.

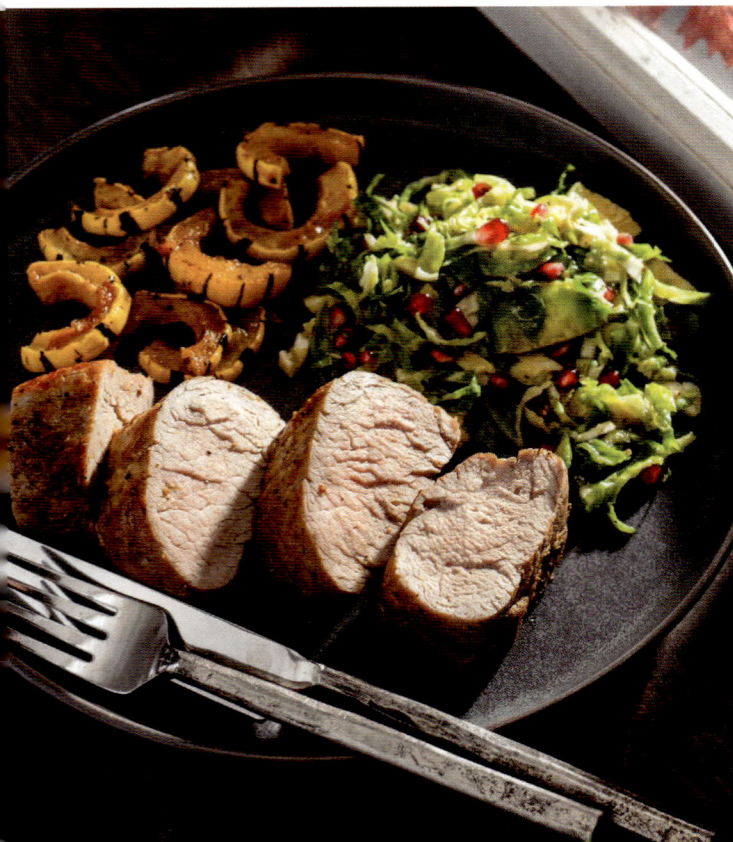

top | Orecchiette with Broccoli Rabe, Fennel, and Spiced Pork
bottom | Miso-Glazed Pork with Squash and Brussels Sprouts

MAKE IT GLUTEN-FREE • Substitute gluten-free pasta for the pasta.

MAKE IT DAIRY-FREE • Substitute plant-based Parmesan for the dairy Parmesan.

Pork Tenderloin with Black Bean, Orange, and Quinoa Salad

serves 4 to 6 • total time: 1 hour   **SUPERCHARGED**

why this recipe works • This well-rounded dinner pairs lean pork with fiberful quinoa, hearty black beans, and tangy oranges. To start, we toasted the quinoa to deepen its nutty flavor, then combined it with fiberful black beans and vitamin C–rich oranges for a nourishing salad. A citrus-shallot vinaigrette brightened the vegetables and echoed the orangey tang. Pork tenderloin gave this recipe a star source of lean protein. We gave the meat a rub with cumin before searing in a skillet (for a flavorful crust) and then roasting in the oven to juicy perfection. We like the convenience of prewashed quinoa (rinsing removes the quinoa's bitter protective coating, called saponin).

1½ cups prewashed white quinoa
2¼ cups water
1¾ teaspoons table salt, divided
2 (1-pound) pork tenderloins, trimmed
¾ teaspoon ground cumin
¼ teaspoon pepper
1 tablespoon avocado oil
2 oranges
¼ cup extra-virgin olive oil
¼ cup lime juice (2 limes), plus lime wedges for serving
1 shallot, minced
1 jalapeño chile, stemmed, seeded, and minced
1 red bell pepper, stemmed, seeded, and cut into ½-inch pieces
1 (15-ounce) can no-salt-added black beans, rinsed
1 avocado, halved, pitted, and cut into ¾-inch pieces
½ cup chopped fresh cilantro, divided

1 Adjust oven rack to middle position and heat oven to 400 degrees. Toast quinoa in large saucepan over medium-high heat, stirring often, until quinoa is very fragrant and makes continuous popping sound, 5 to 7 minutes. Stir in water and ½ teaspoon salt and bring to simmer. Cover, reduce heat to low, and simmer gently until most of water has been absorbed and quinoa is nearly tender, about 15 minutes. Spread quinoa on rimmed baking sheet and let cool completely, about 15 minutes; set aside.

2 Meanwhile, pat tenderloins dry with paper towels and sprinkle with cumin, ½ teaspoon salt, and pepper. Heat avocado oil in 12-inch skillet over medium-high heat until just smoking. Add tenderloins and cook until well browned all over, about 5 minutes. Transfer to rimmed baking sheet and roast until tenderloins register 135 degrees, 10 to 15 minutes. Transfer to cutting board and let rest for 5 minutes.

3 Cut away peel and pith from oranges. Quarter oranges, then slice crosswise ¼ inch thick. Whisk olive oil, lime juice, shallot, jalapeño, and remaining ¾ teaspoon salt together in large bowl. Add cooled quinoa, orange slices, bell pepper, black beans, avocado, and ¼ cup cilantro and toss to combine. Sprinkle remaining ¼ cup cilantro over top.

4 Slice pork against grain ½ inch thick and serve with salad and lime wedges.

MAKE AHEAD • Cooked quinoa can be refrigerated for up to 3 days.

Nutritional Knowledge   I love the starring cast in this pork tenderloin dinner. Quinoa and black beans support gut health with fiber and polyphenols, while avocado adds creamy texture and inflammation-fighting monounsaturated fats. Bright citrus and red bell pepper bring a punch of vitamin C and beta-carotene, and the heat from shallots and jalapeño adds quercetin and capsaicin to help calm inflammation. Tender, gently roasted pork tenderloin provides lean protein without the inflammatory byproducts of high-heat cooking.

—*Alicia*

Miso-Glazed Pork with Squash and Brussels Sprouts

serves 4 • total time: 40 minutes   **FAST**

why this recipe works • Dense, hearty pork tenderloins make an excellent canvas for a funky-savory glaze of miso and maple syrup. The savory-sweet concoction did double duty for the overall flavor profile: It added depth to both seared pork and roasted squash, and it also flavored the dressing for a hearty shaved brussels sprout salad. The tender chewiness of the squash perfectly complemented the crunchy bite of the sprouts. Delicata squash has a thin, edible skin that needn't be removed.

1 delicata squash (1 pound), ends trimmed, halved lengthwise, seeded, and sliced crosswise ½ inch thick

5 tablespoons avocado oil, divided

1 teaspoon table salt, divided

1 teaspoon pepper, divided

2 (1-pound) pork tenderloins, trimmed

2 tablespoons maple syrup

2 tablespoons white miso

1 tablespoon cider vinegar

12 ounces brussels sprouts, trimmed, halved, and sliced very thin

½ cup pomegranate seeds

1 Adjust oven rack to middle position and heat oven to 450 degrees. Toss squash, 1 tablespoon oil, ¼ teaspoon salt, and ¼ teaspoon pepper together on rimmed baking sheet. Roast until lightly browned, 8 to 10 minutes.

2 Meanwhile, pat tenderloins dry with paper towels and sprinkle with ½ teaspoon salt and ½ teaspoon pepper. Heat 1 tablespoon oil in 12-inch nonstick skillet over medium-high heat until just smoking. Add pork and cook until well browned on all sides, about 7 minutes. Whisk maple syrup and miso together in small bowl.

3 Remove sheet from oven, flip squash, and push to 1 half of sheet. Place pork on now-empty side of sheet. Brush pork and squash with 3 tablespoons maple syrup mixture. Return sheet to oven and roast until pork registers 135 degrees and squash is tender, 12 to 15 minutes. Transfer pork to cutting board, tent with aluminum foil, and let rest for 5 minutes. Transfer squash to serving platter and cover with foil to keep warm.

4 Whisk remaining 3 tablespoons oil, vinegar, remaining ¼ teaspoon salt, remaining ¼ teaspoon pepper, and remaining 1 tablespoon maple mixture together in large bowl. Add brussels sprouts and pomegranate seeds and toss to combine. Slice pork against grain ½ inch thick and serve with squash and brussels sprouts.

Pork Tenderloin with White Beans and Mustard Greens

serves 4 · total time: 1 hours

why this recipe works · The South of France is known for its rich stews that combine creamy white beans, fresh greens, and tender pork. For a melange of these ingredients that was more plated dinner than stew, we turned to tender, quick-cooking pork tenderloins. We first browned the pork and then set it aside while we built a flavorful base in the Dutch oven using abundant aromatics: onion, garlic, thyme, and wine. Next, we stirred in fiberful mustard greens, wilting them only slightly; then protein-rich white beans entered the pot. Resting the pork on top of the greens lifted the lean cut of meat out of the braising liquid, which allowed it to cook through gently by way of the surrounding heat within the pot. While all that baked in the oven, we used that time to microwave bread crumbs with olive oil and season them with lemon to sprinkle over the finished dish. Finally, a crumble of tangy goat cheese added pleasant richness and a bit of funk.

2 (1-pound) pork tenderloins, trimmed and halved crosswise

1 teaspoon table salt, divided

¼ teaspoon pepper

2 tablespoons extra-virgin olive oil, divided

1 onion, chopped fine

1 tablespoon minced fresh thyme or 1 teaspoon dried

2 garlic cloves, minced

¾ cup unsalted chicken broth

¼ cup dry white wine

1 pound mustard greens, stemmed and cut into 2-inch pieces

2 (15-ounce) cans no-salt-added navy beans, rinsed

½ cup panko bread crumbs

2 tablespoons chopped fresh parsley

½ teaspoon grated lemon zest plus 1 teaspoon juice

2 ounces goat cheese, crumbled (½ cup)

1 Adjust oven rack to middle position and heat oven to 450 degrees. Pat tenderloins dry with paper towels and sprinkle with ½ teaspoon salt and pepper. Heat 1 tablespoon oil in Dutch oven over medium-high heat until just smoking. Add pork and cook until browned on all sides, 5 to 7 minutes; transfer to large plate.

2 Add onion and remaining ½ teaspoon salt to fat left in pot and cook over medium heat until softened, about 5 minutes. Stir in thyme and garlic and cook until fragrant, about 30 seconds. Stir in broth and wine, scraping up any browned bits. Add mustard greens, 1 handful at a time, and cook, stirring constantly, until beginning to wilt, 2 to 3 minutes.

3 Stir in beans, then nestle pork on top. Transfer pot to oven and cook until pork registers 135 degrees and greens are tender, about 15 minutes.

4 Meanwhile, toss panko with remaining 1 tablespoon oil in bowl until evenly coated. Microwave, stirring every 30 seconds, until light golden brown, 2 to 5 minutes. Let cool slightly, then stir in parsley and lemon zest.

5 Remove pot from oven. Transfer pork to cutting board, tent with aluminum foil, and let rest for 5 minutes. Stir lemon juice into mustard greens mixture and season with salt and pepper to taste. Slice pork against grain ½ inch thick and serve with mustard greens mixture, sprinkling individual portions with bread crumbs and goat cheese.

MAKE IT GLUTEN-FREE • Substitute gluten-free panko bread crumbs for the panko bread crumbs.

MAKE IT DAIRY-FREE • Substitute plant-based goat cheese for the dairy goat cheese, or omit it.

Spice-Rubbed Pork Tenderloin with Fennel, Tomatoes, Artichokes, and Olives

serves 4 • total time: 1 hour

why this recipe works • The fine-grained, buttery-smooth texture of pork tenderloin makes an absorbent canvas for bold seasonings. We wondered if a dry rub might allow us to skip the step of browning, adding both flavor and color to our tenderloin without the extra work. We looked for a distinct flavor profile and reasoned that herbes de Provence would give a distinctly Mediterranean flavor to our pork. A little of this spice went a long way; a mere 2 teaspoons were sufficient to flavor and coat the tenderloins. For a vegetable that would complement both the rub and the pork, we thought of sweet, mild fennel and supplemented it with artichokes and kalamata olives. After jump-starting the fennel in the microwave, we combined it with the other vegetables and roasted the tenderloin on top of them in the oven so that the savory juices could imbue them with meaty flavor. In just an hour, we were transported to Provence with a weeknight dinner that required minimal fuss but delivered maximum flavor.

- 2 large fennel bulbs, stalks discarded, bulbs halved, cored, and sliced ½ inch thick
- 12 ounces frozen artichoke hearts, thawed and patted dry
- ½ cup pitted kalamata olives, halved
- ¼ cup extra-virgin olive oil, divided
- 2 teaspoons herbes de Provence
- 1 teaspoon table salt
- ½ teaspoon pepper
- 2 (1-pound) pork tenderloins, trimmed
- 1 pound cherry tomatoes, halved
- 1 tablespoon grated lemon zest
- 2 tablespoons minced fresh parsley

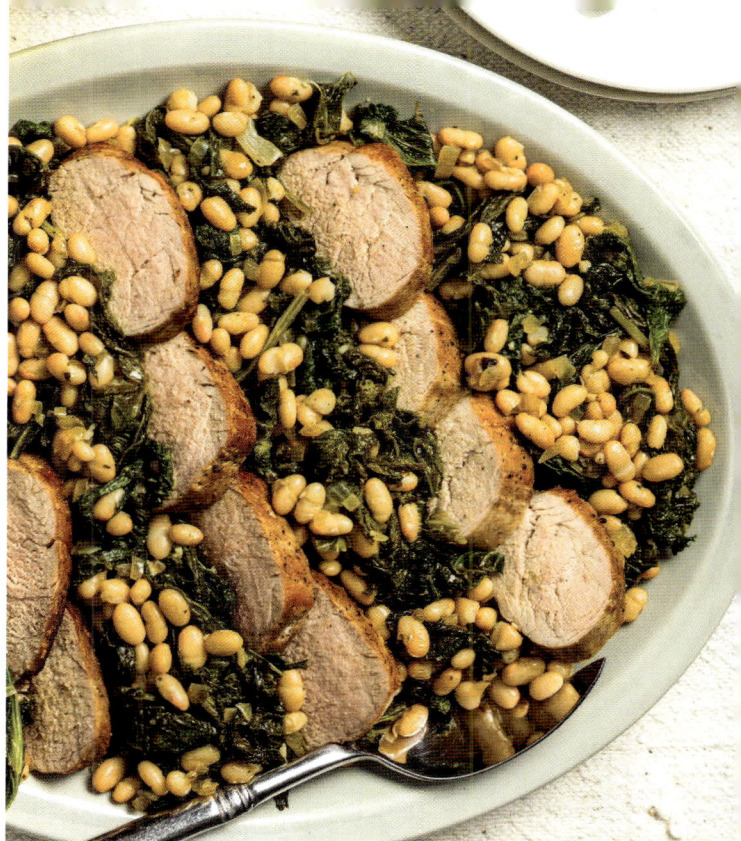

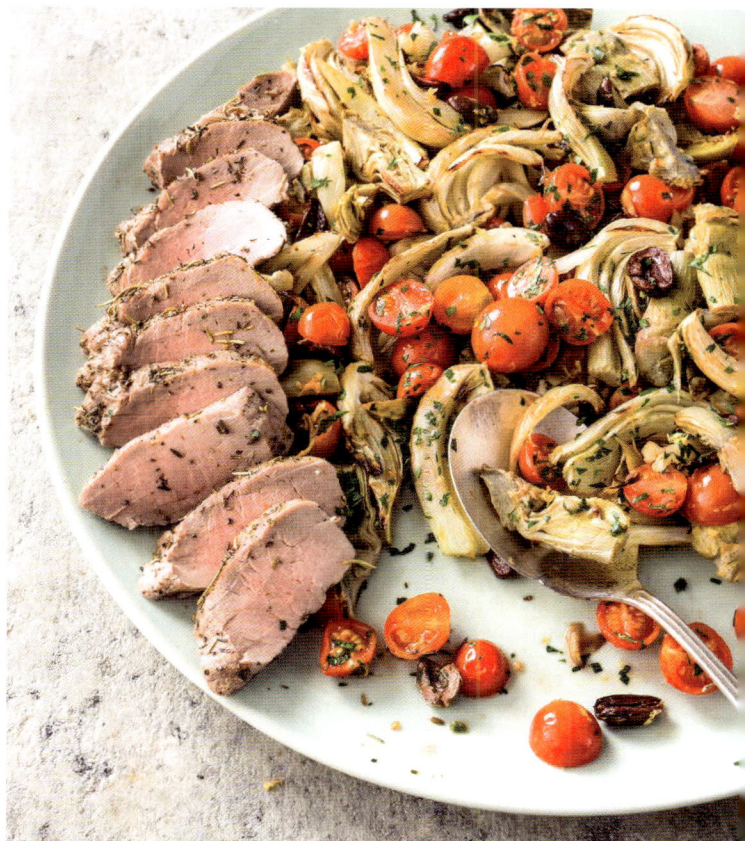

top | *Pork Tenderloin with White Beans and Mustard Greens*
bottom | *Spice-Rubbed Pork Tenderloin with Fennel, Tomatoes, Artichokes, and Olives*

1 Adjust oven rack to lower-middle position and heat oven to 450 degrees. Microwave fennel and 2 tablespoons water in covered bowl until softened, about 5 minutes. Drain fennel well, then toss with artichoke hearts, olives, and 2 tablespoons oil.

2 Combine herbes de Provence, salt, and pepper in bowl. Pat pork dry with paper towels, then rub with remaining 2 tablespoons oil and sprinkle with herb mixture. Spread vegetables into even layer on rimmed baking sheet, then lay pork on top. Roast until pork registers 135 degrees, 25 to 30 minutes, rotating sheet halfway through roasting.

3 Remove sheet from oven. Transfer pork to cutting board, tent with aluminum foil, and let rest while vegetables finish cooking. Stir tomatoes and lemon zest into vegetables and continue to roast until fennel is tender and tomatoes have softened, about 10 minutes. Stir in parsley and season with salt and pepper to taste. Slice pork against grain ½ inch thick and serve with vegetables.

One-Pan Pork Tenderloin and Panzanella Salad

serves 4 to 6 • total time: 50 minutes

why this recipe works • Panzanella is a hearty salad of summer vegetables with toasted bread that soaks up a piquant dressing and becomes just a little chewy in the process. We built an easy one-pan meal around the salad by adding roast pork tenderloin and a mix of fresh and roasted vegetables for complexity and lots of phytonutrients. First, we placed pork tenderloins on a rimmed baking sheet and brushed them with a mixture of balsamic vinegar and whole-grain mustard that complemented the savory pork and gave it some color. A bit of cornstarch ensured that the glaze stuck. Then, we surrounded the tenderloins with summer squash, red onion, bell pepper, and pieces of baguette and roasted it all until the pork was rosy in the center, the vegetables were tender, and the bread was toasted and crunchy. While the tenderloins rested, we tossed the bread and vegetables with fresh cucumber, cherry tomatoes, and basil for their refreshing crunch, fiber, and anti-inflammatory nutrients. To dress our salad, we whisked up a mustard-scented balsamic vinaigrette, adding salty capers along with a splash of their brine for a kick. Any rustic bread can be used in place of the baguette.

3 tablespoons balsamic vinegar, divided
2 tablespoons whole-grain mustard, divided
1 teaspoon cornstarch

2 (1-pound) pork tenderloins, trimmed
1⅛ teaspoons table salt, divided
¾ teaspoon plus ⅛ teaspoon pepper, divided
1 (12-inch) baguette, cut into 1-inch pieces
1 red onion, cut into 1-inch pieces
1 red bell pepper, stemmed, seeded, and cut into ½-inch-wide strips
1 yellow summer squash, quartered lengthwise and cut into 1-inch pieces
½ cup extra-virgin olive oil, divided
1 tablespoon capers plus 1 tablespoon brine
1 garlic clove, minced
½ English cucumber, quartered lengthwise and cut into ½-inch pieces
6 ounces cherry tomatoes, halved
½ cup chopped fresh basil

1 Adjust oven rack to middle position and heat oven to 450 degrees. Whisk 1 tablespoon vinegar, 1 tablespoon mustard, and cornstarch together in bowl until no lumps of cornstarch remain. Pat tenderloins dry with paper towels and sprinkle with ½ teaspoon salt and ¼ teaspoon pepper. Place tenderloins in center of rimmed baking sheet (it's OK if they touch) and brush tops and sides with all of vinegar mixture.

2 Toss baguette, onion, bell pepper, squash, ¼ cup oil, ½ teaspoon salt, and ½ teaspoon pepper in large bowl until baguette and vegetables are well coated with oil. Distribute vegetable mixture around tenderloins on sheet. Roast until pork registers 135 degrees, about 20 minutes, stirring vegetable mixture halfway through roasting.

3 Meanwhile, whisk remaining ¼ cup oil, remaining 2 tablespoons vinegar, remaining 1 tablespoon mustard, capers and brine, garlic, remaining ⅛ teaspoon salt, and remaining ⅛ teaspoon pepper together in now-empty bowl.

4 Transfer tenderloins to cutting board, tent with aluminum foil, and let rest for 5 minutes. While tenderloins rest, add cucumber, tomatoes, 6 tablespoons basil, and vegetable mixture to bowl with caper dressing and toss to combine.

5 Transfer salad to serving platter. Slice pork against grain ½ inch thick and arrange over salad. Sprinkle with remaining 2 tablespoons basil and serve.

MAKE IT GLUTEN-FREE • Substitute gluten-free baguette for the baguette.

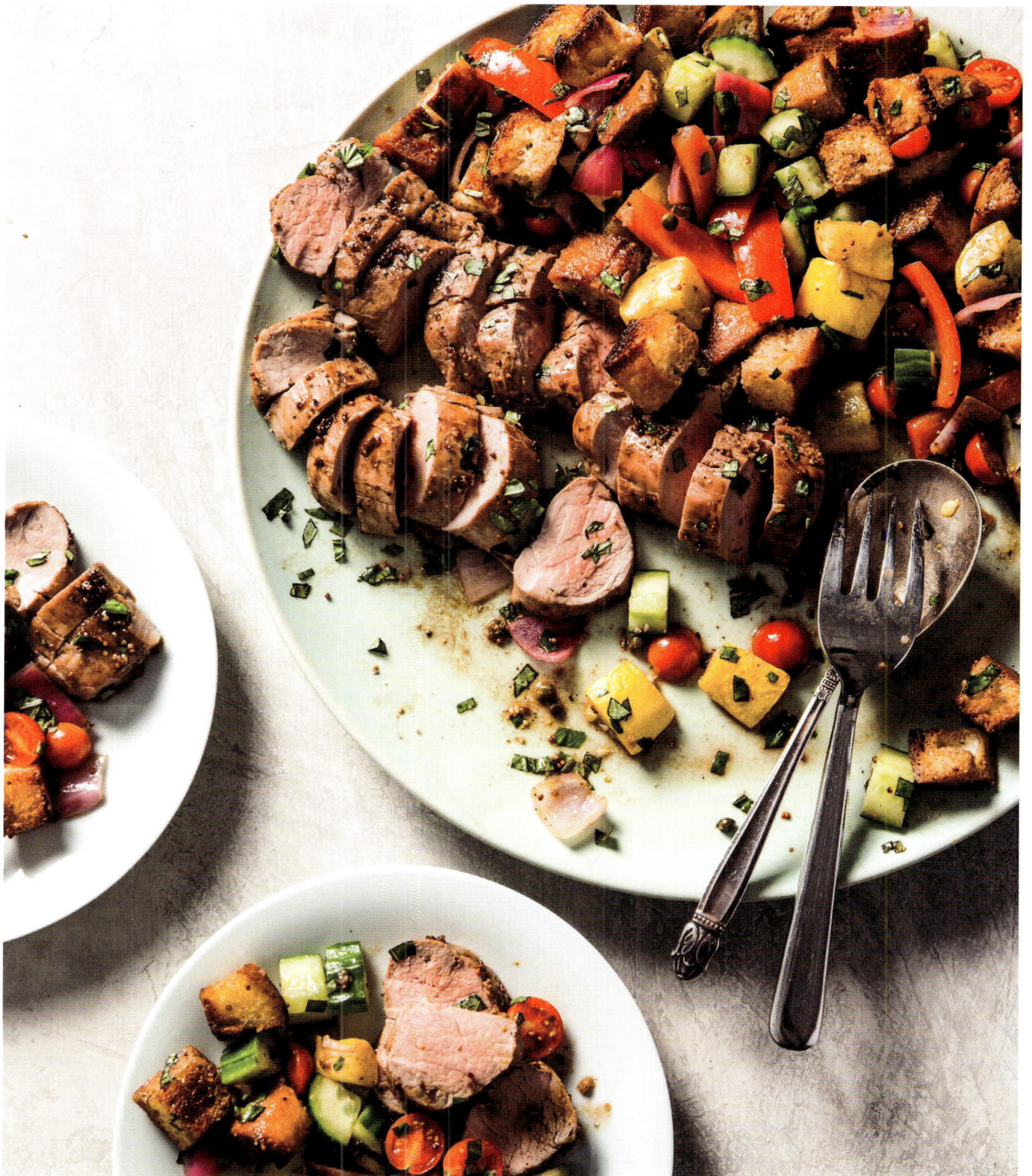

One-Pan Pork Tenderloin and Panzanella Salad

Chao Nian Gao

serves 4 to 6 • **total time: 35 minutes, plus 30 minutes marinating**

why this recipe works • Chao nian gao, the beloved Shanghainese stir-fry of sliced nian gao (rice cakes), protein (usually pork), and vegetables (often fiberful napa cabbage) glossed with an umami-rich sauce, is a weeknight-friendly one-pot meal perfect for busy cooks. Soaking strips of pork tenderloin in a mixture of Shaoxing wine, soy and oyster sauces, white pepper, avocado and sesame oils, and a touch of cornstarch served a dual purpose: The highly seasoned liquid flavored the meat and helped it retain moisture during cooking, while the oils and cornstarch helped the mixture tenderize. Rinsing the rice cakes rid them of excess surface starch that would otherwise cause them to stick together, and spreading them evenly over the pork and vegetables in the skillet and briefly steaming them (lid-on) ensured that they turned delightfully chewy but tender. We needed only 8 ounces of pork, yet every bite of the chao nian gao was savory and packed with flavor. To save time, prepare the other ingredients while the pork marinates. You will need a 12-inch nonstick skillet with a tight-fitting lid for this recipe. Look for sliced rice cakes, refrigerated or frozen, in a Chinese grocer or online. If using frozen rice cakes, defrost them before cooking. Rinse the rice cakes just before cooking; if they sit with moisture clinging to them, they will stick together. The cooking moves quickly, so have all your ingredients ready before you start cooking in step 4.

- 2 tablespoons plus 1 teaspoon avocado oil, divided
- 5 teaspoons Shaoxing wine or dry sherry, divided
- 1 tablespoon oyster sauce, divided
- 1 tablespoon low-sodium soy sauce
- 1¼ teaspoons cornstarch
- 1 teaspoon toasted sesame oil
- ½ teaspoon white pepper, divided
- 8 ounces pork tenderloin, trimmed
- 1⅓ ounces dried shiitake mushrooms
- 1 pound sliced rice cakes
- 1 (½-inch) piece ginger, peeled and sliced into ¼-inch-thick rounds
- 4 scallions, white and green parts separated, sliced thin
- 4 garlic cloves, minced
- ½ small head napa cabbage, cored and sliced crosswise ½ inch thick (10 cups)
- ⅔ cup unsalted chicken broth
- ¾ teaspoon table salt

1 Whisk 1 teaspoon avocado oil, 2 teaspoons Shaoxing wine, 1 teaspoon oyster sauce, soy sauce, cornstarch, sesame oil, and ¼ teaspoon white pepper together in medium bowl. Slice pork crosswise ¼ inch thick, then cut each slice into ¼-inch-wide strips. Add pork to marinade and stir well to combine. Cover and refrigerate for 30 minutes. Combine remaining 1 tablespoon Shaoxing wine and remaining 2 teaspoons oyster sauce in small bowl and set aside.

2 Meanwhile, microwave 2 cups hot water and mushrooms in covered bowl until steaming, about 1 minute. Let sit until softened, about 15 minutes. Drain mushrooms, pressing to extract all liquid. Discard liquid and slice mushrooms thin; set aside.

3 Place rice cakes in medium bowl, separating any that are stuck together. Cover with cold water and, using your hands, agitate cakes to remove excess starch. Drain and set aside.

4 Heat remaining 2 tablespoons avocado oil in 12-inch nonstick skillet over medium-high heat until just smoking. Add ginger and cook, stirring constantly, for 30 seconds. Add scallion whites and garlic and cook, stirring constantly, for 15 seconds. Add pork and cook, stirring occasionally, for 1 minute. Add mushrooms and continue to cook, stirring occasionally, until pork is no longer pink, about 1 minute.

5 Add half of cabbage and cook, stirring constantly to incorporate pork, until cabbage has wilted to half its volume, about 2 minutes. Stir in remaining cabbage and continue to cook until cabbage has wilted to half its volume, about 1 minute. Stir in Shaoxing wine mixture. Spread cabbage into even layer, pour broth over cabbage, and add rice cakes on top in single layer. Increase heat to high, cover, and cook for 2 minutes. Uncover, add salt and remaining ¼ teaspoon white pepper, and continue to cook, stirring frequently, until sauce has thickened slightly and rice cakes are tender but still chewy, 1 to 2 minutes. Remove ginger, if desired. Garnish with scallion greens and serve immediately.

MAKE AHEAD • Pork can be refrigerated in marinade for up to 2 hours.

MAKE IT GLUTEN-FREE • Substitute gluten-free oyster sauce and low-sodium tamari for the oyster sauce and low-sodium soy sauce.

Maple-Ginger Roasted Pork Tenderloin with Swiss Chard and Carrots

serves 4 · total time: 55 minutes

why this recipe works · Pork tenderloin is the leanest part of the pig, so it cooks much more quickly than other pork roasts and makes a great protein source that doesn't overdo the saturated fat. Its leanness also means it benefits from a hearty side—think the hearty, fiberful chew of Swiss chard and carrots. We pan-seared the tenderloin in a skillet and then moved the pan to a hot oven to roast. When the pork was done, we sautéed a colorful medley of sweet carrots and earthy Swiss chard in the same pan, making use of the flavorful fond. And we didn't just use the chard leaves: We found that we can quickly boost fiber by using the stems too. So we sliced them thin on a bias and sautéed them first with the carrots over relatively high heat to achieve the ideal tender-crisp texture. The lightly caramelized stems acted as a foil to the tender leaves, which we added later in separate handfuls. What made the complete dish extra-special was a whisk-together glaze of maple syrup, soy sauce, and ginger: We tossed a portion into the vegetable side and poured the remainder elegantly over the slices of perfectly cooked pork. You will need a 12-inch ovensafe skillet for this recipe.

- 3 tablespoons maple syrup
- 3 tablespoons avocado oil, divided
- 1 tablespoon low-sodium soy sauce
- 1 tablespoon unseasoned rice vinegar
- 2 teaspoons grated fresh ginger
- 1 garlic clove, minced
- 1 teaspoon toasted sesame oil
- 2 (1-pound) pork tenderloins, trimmed
- ¼ teaspoon pepper
- 2 pounds Swiss chard, stems sliced ¼ inch thick on bias, leaves chopped
- 4 carrots, peeled and sliced ¼ inch thick on bias
- 1 tablespoon sesame seeds, toasted

1 Adjust oven rack to middle position and heat oven to 400 degrees. Whisk maple syrup, 2 tablespoons avocado oil, soy sauce, vinegar, ginger, garlic, and sesame oil in bowl until smooth; set glaze aside.

2 Pat tenderloins dry with paper towels and sprinkle with pepper. Heat remaining 1 tablespoon avocado oil in 12-inch ovensafe skillet over medium-high heat until just smoking. Add pork and cook until browned on all sides, 5 to 7 minutes. Transfer skillet to oven and roast until pork registers 135 degrees, 10 to 15 minutes, flipping pork halfway through roasting.

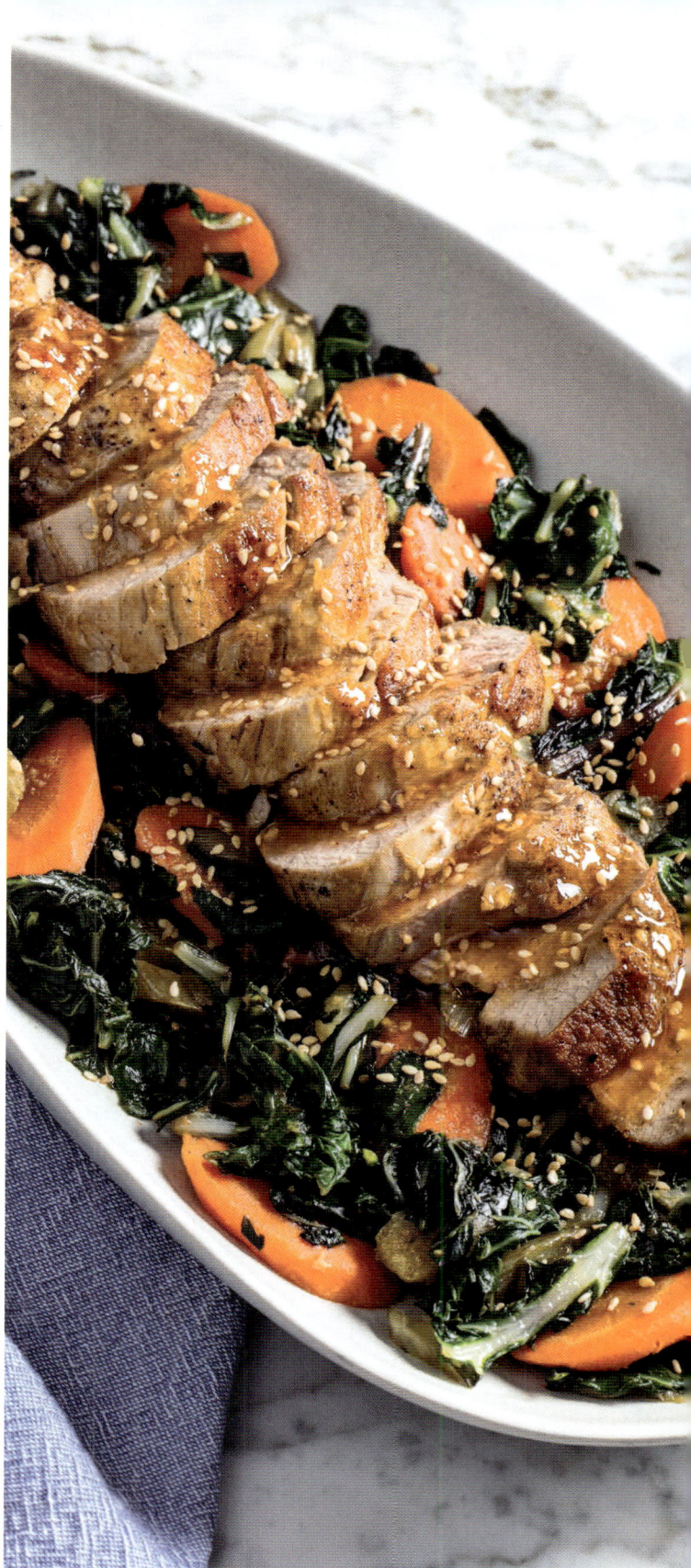

Maple-Ginger Roasted Pork Tenderloin with Swiss Chard and Carrots

3 Remove skillet from oven, being careful of hot skillet handle. Transfer pork to cutting board, tent with aluminum foil, and let rest while preparing vegetables.

4 Being careful of hot skillet handle, add chard stems and carrots to fat left in skillet and cook over medium-high heat, stirring occasionally, until crisp-tender, 8 to 10 minutes. Add chard leaves, one handful at a time, and cook until tender, about 5 minutes. Increase heat to high and cook until liquid has evaporated, about 5 minutes. Off heat, add half of maple mixture and stir until vegetables are well coated, then transfer to serving platter.

5 Slice pork against grain ½ inch thick and add to platter with vegetables. Drizzle remaining maple glaze over pork, sprinkle with sesame seeds, and serve.

> **MAKE IT GLUTEN-FREE** • Substitute low-sodium tamari for the low-sodium soy sauce.

Caraway-Crusted Pork Tenderloin with Sauerkraut and Apples

serves 4 • total time: 40 minutes **FAST**

why this recipe works • In this recipe, we packed pork and cabbage—a winning combo—with elevated punches that happen to be great for fighting inflammation. First, the cabbage we chose was sauerkraut, giving us an opportunity to cook with the fermented vegetable that we always keep around for its beneficial probiotics. Pairing it with apples in a sweet-tart side dish gave the cabbage a complementary counterpart. A caraway crust on the pork added crunchy texture and aromatic flavor to the lean meat. We softened the apples and sauerkraut in the same skillet used to brown the tenderloins—we couldn't let the savory fond go to waste—and then finished roasting the tenderloins on top of the mixture in the oven to meld all the flavors. We prefer red-skinned Fujis or Galas to give the dish more color, but any sweet apple will do.

2 (1-pound) pork tenderloins, trimmed
1 tablespoon caraway seeds
½ teaspoon table salt
½ teaspoon plus ⅛ teaspoon pepper, divided
2 tablespoons avocado oil, divided
3 apples, cored, halved, and cut into ¼-inch-thick slices
1 pound sauerkraut, rinsed and squeezed dry
2 tablespoons packed light brown sugar
2 tablespoons minced fresh dill

1 Adjust oven rack to middle position and heat oven to 400 degrees. Pat tenderloins dry with paper towels and sprinkle with caraway seeds, salt, and ½ teaspoon pepper, pressing lightly to adhere. Heat 1 tablespoon oil in 12-inch ovensafe skillet over medium-high heat until just smoking. Brown tenderloins on all sides, 5 to 7 minutes; transfer to large plate.

2 Add remaining 1 tablespoon oil, apples, and remaining ⅛ teaspoon pepper to now-empty skillet and cook over medium heat until softened, about 5 minutes, scraping up any browned bits. Stir in sauerkraut and sugar then place tenderloins on top. Transfer skillet to oven and roast until pork registers 135 degrees, 10 to 15 minutes.

3 Being careful of hot skillet handle, remove skillet from oven. Transfer tenderloins to cutting board, tent with aluminum foil, and let rest for 5 minutes. Slice pork against grain ½ inch thick. Stir dill into sauerkraut mixture and serve with pork.

Greek-Style Braised Pork with Leeks

serves 4 • total time: 1½ hours

why this recipe works • Pork braised with a hearty amount of leeks in white wine is a classic Greek preparation. Taking inspiration from this style, we started by browning pieces of pork butt to seal in the juices and add depth of flavor. Because leeks are a milder aromatic, we used a full 2 pounds to ensure that we got a ton of flavor—which also meant a big dose of anti-inflammatory benefits. After sautéing the leeks in the fat left from searing the pork, we built our aromatic base by adding diced tomatoes and garlic. We then stirred in white wine, chicken broth, and a bay leaf and put it all in the oven to cook low and slow until the pork was meltingly tender and the leeks were soft. A sprinkle of fresh oregano added pleasant earthy and minty notes, plus more antioxidants. Pork butt roast is often labeled "Boston butt" in the supermarket. You will need a Dutch oven with a tight-fitting lid for this recipe.

1½ pounds boneless pork butt roast, trimmed and cut into 1-inch pieces
1 teaspoon table salt, divided
¾ teaspoon pepper, divided
2 tablespoons extra-virgin olive oil, divided
2 pounds leeks, white and light green parts only, halved lengthwise, sliced 1 inch thick, and washed thoroughly
2 garlic cloves, minced
½ teaspoon grated lemon zest
1 (14.5-ounce) can no-salt-added diced tomatoes

1 cup dry white wine
½ cup unsalted chicken broth
1 bay leaf
2 teaspoons chopped fresh oregano

1 Adjust oven rack to lower-middle position and heat oven to 325 degrees. Pat pork dry with paper towels and sprinkle with ½ teaspoon salt and ¼ teaspoon pepper. Heat 1 tablespoon oil in Dutch oven over medium-high heat until just smoking. Brown pork on all sides, about 8 minutes; transfer to bowl.

2 Add leeks, remaining 1 tablespoon oil, remaining ½ teaspoon salt, and remaining ½ teaspoon pepper to fat left in pot and cook over medium heat until softened and lightly browned, 5 to 7 minutes. Stir in garlic and lemon zest and cook until fragrant, about 30 seconds. Stir in tomatoes and their juice, scraping up any browned bits, and cook until tomato liquid is nearly evaporated, 10 to 12 minutes.

3 Stir in wine, broth, bay leaf, and pork along with any accumulated juices and bring to simmer. Cover, transfer pot to oven, and cook until pork is tender, 1 to 1½ hours. Discard bay leaf. Stir in oregano, season with salt and pepper to taste, and serve.

MAKE AHEAD • Braised pork and vegetables can be refrigerated for up to 3 days.

Mexican Pork and Rice

serves 6 • total time: 2¼ hours

why this recipe works • Spiced with chipotle chiles and bathed in a tomatoey sauce, this Mexican-inspired pork and rice dish is a luxury to eat. Rather than spooning braised pork and sauce onto tortillas or tostadas, we used brown rice to absorb the sauce's flavors and make a simple one-pot meal. The challenge lay in maintaining the dish's bold essence while achieving perfectly tender pork and well-cooked rice, all in the same pot. We built a rich fond by cooking onions, garlic, herbs, and chipotle chile to pack in both flavor and antioxidants. The chipotle lent the dish a subtle heat, as well as smokiness and depth. We deglazed with broth and tomato sauce before cooking the pork in the flavorful liquid. Next, we stirred in brown rice and pinto beans for more fiber and heft. The starches cooked while absorbing the flavors of the savory meat. Finally, we finished our dish with a sprinkling of peas and fresh chopped scallions and cilantro, along with a splash of lime juice. The result was a one-pot meal brimming with flavor. Pork butt roast is often labeled "Boston butt" in the supermarket. You will need a Dutch oven with a tight-fitting lid for this recipe.

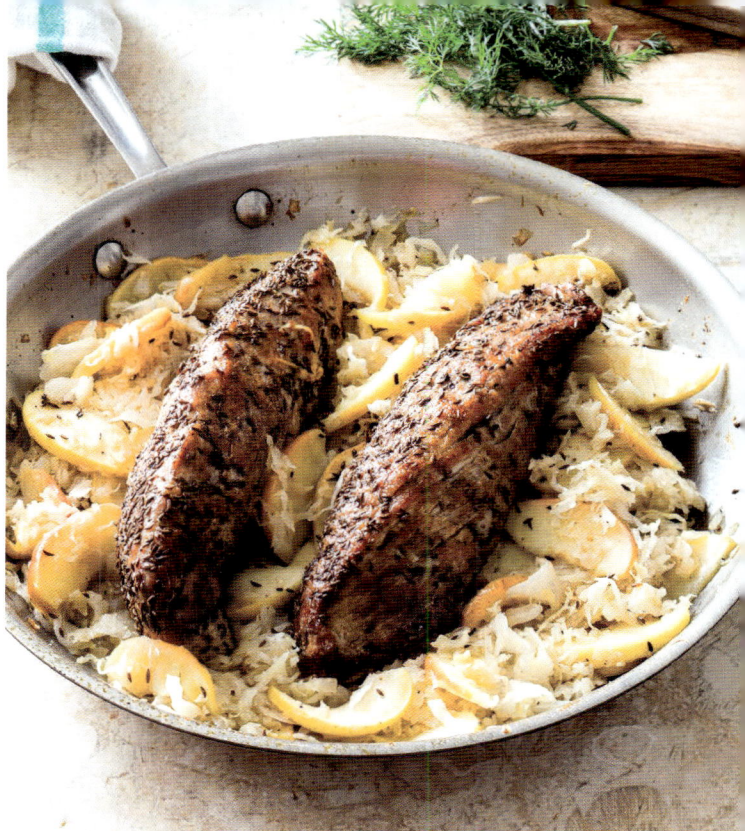

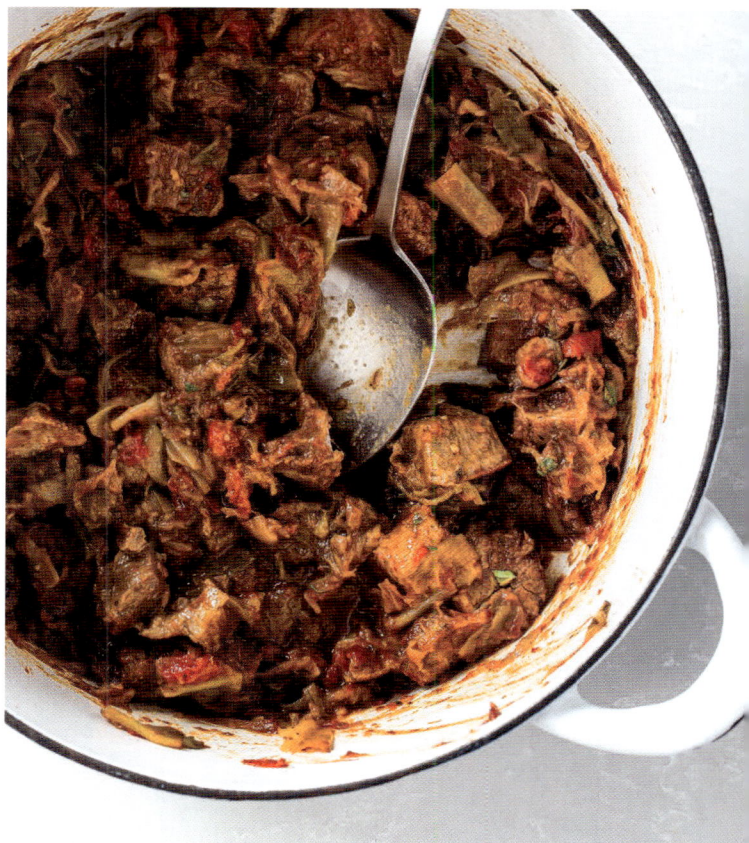

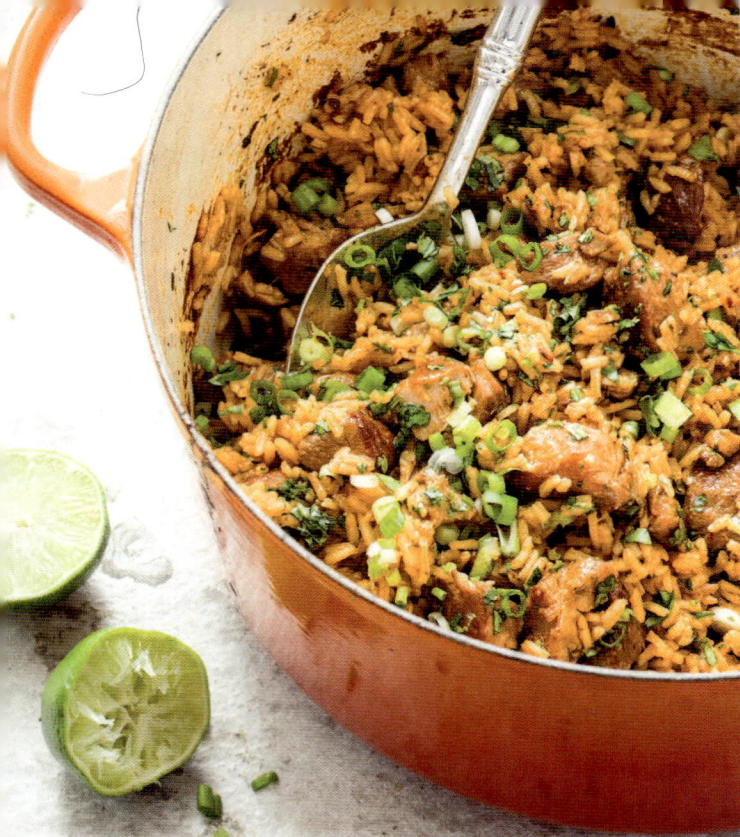

1 tablespoon extra-virgin olive oil

2 onions, chopped fine

1 teaspoon table salt, divided

5 garlic cloves, minced

1 tablespoon minced canned chipotle chile in adobo sauce

2 teaspoons minced fresh oregano or ½ teaspoon dried

1 teaspoon minced fresh thyme or ¼ teaspoon dried

2 cups unsalted chicken broth

1 (8-ounce) can no-salt-added tomato sauce

1½ pounds boneless pork butt roast, trimmed and cut into 1-inch pieces

1 cup long-grain brown rice, rinsed

2 (15-ounce) cans no-salt-added pinto beans, rinsed

1 cup frozen peas

½ cup minced fresh cilantro, divided

3 scallions, sliced thin

1 tablespoon lime juice, plus lime wedges for serving

1 Adjust oven rack to lower-middle position and heat oven to 300 degrees. Heat oil in Dutch oven over medium heat until shimmering. Add onions and ½ teaspoon salt and cook until softened, about 5 minutes. Stir in garlic, chipotle, oregano, and thyme and cook until fragrant, about 30 seconds. Stir in broth and tomato sauce, scraping up any browned bits, and bring to simmer. Stir in pork, cover, and transfer pot to oven. Cook until pork is tender, 1 to 1½ hours.

2 Remove pot from oven and increase oven temperature to 350 degrees. Stir in rice, beans, and remaining ½ teaspoon salt, cover, and return pot to oven. Cook until rice is tender and all liquid has been absorbed, 40 to 50 minutes, gently stirring rice from bottom of pot halfway through cooking.

3 Remove pot from oven. Sprinkle peas over rice mixture, cover, and let sit until heated through, about 5 minutes. Add ¼ cup cilantro, scallions, and lime juice and gently fluff with fork to combine. Season with pepper to taste. Sprinkle with remaining ¼ cup cilantro and serve with lime wedges.

MAKE AHEAD • Cooked Mexican pork and rice can be refrigerated for up to 3 days.

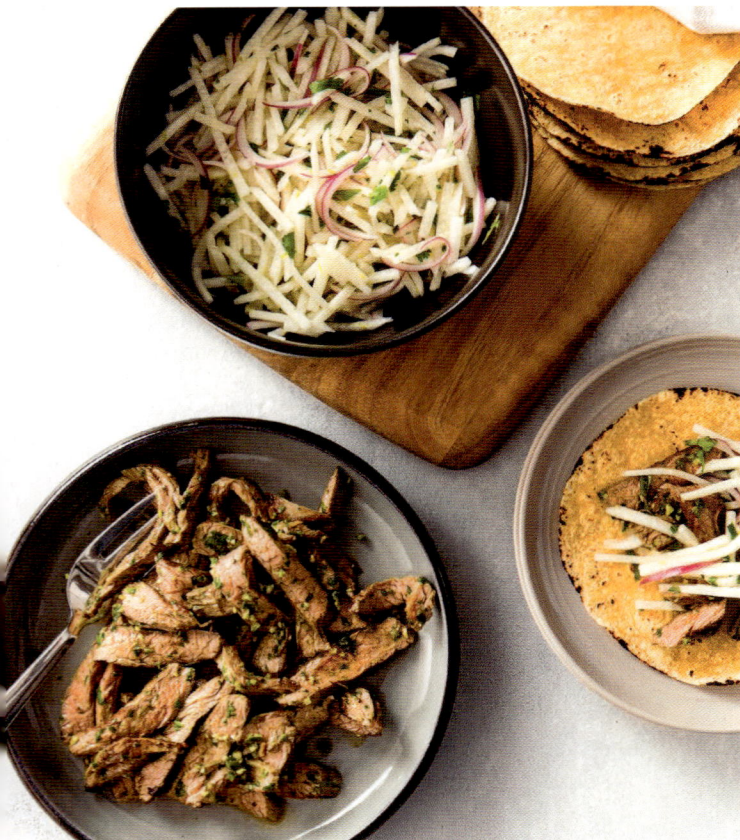

top | *Mexican Pork and Rice*

bottom | *Steak Tacos with Jicama Slaw*

Steak Tacos with Jicama Slaw

serves 6 · total time: 50 minutes plus, 30 minutes marinating

why this recipe works · To create indoor steak tacos as tender, juicy, and rich-tasting as grilled, we chose flank steak, searing it to achieve the browned exterior and crisp, brittle edges characteristic of grilled meat—without going overboard and pushing the meat into charred territory (inflammation alert). A puree of cilantro, scallions, garlic, and jalapeño gave our steak a flavor boost while packing in some antioxidants. A bright jicama slaw seasoned with red onion, cilantro, and lime made the perfect crunchy, zesty accompaniment to the rich meat. We served them together on warm corn tortillas for a flavor-packed handheld meal. To make this dish spicier, include the seeds from the chile.

Slaw

- 1 pound jicama, peeled and cut into 3-inch-long matchsticks
- ¼ cup thinly sliced red onion
- 3 tablespoons chopped fresh cilantro
- 1 tablespoon extra-virgin olive oil
- 1 teaspoon grated lime zest plus 2 tablespoons juice
- ¼ teaspoon table salt

Tacos

- ½ cup fresh cilantro leaves
- 3 scallions, chopped
- 3 garlic cloves, peeled
- 1 jalapeño chile, stemmed, seeded, and chopped
- ½ teaspoon ground cumin
- 2 tablespoons avocado oil, divided
- 1 tablespoon lime juice
- 1 (1-pound) flank steak, trimmed and cut lengthwise into 3 equal pieces
- ½ teaspoon table salt
- 12 (6-inch) corn tortillas, warmed

1 For the slaw Combine all ingredients in bowl. Cover and refrigerate until ready to serve.

2 For the tacos Pulse cilantro, scallions, garlic, jalapeño, cumin, and 4 teaspoons oil in food processor to paste, 10 to 12 pulses, scraping down sides of bowl as needed. Transfer 2 tablespoons herb paste to bowl, whisk in lime juice, and set aside for serving.

3 Using fork, poke each piece of steak 10 to 12 times on each side. Pat dry with paper towels then sprinkle steaks with salt and place in 13 by 9-inch baking dish. Coat steaks thoroughly with remaining herb paste, cover dish, and marinate in refrigerator for at least 30 minutes.

4 Scrape herb paste off steaks and pat dry with paper towels. Heat remaining 2 teaspoons oil in 12-inch nonstick skillet over medium-high heat until just smoking. Add steaks and cook until well browned and meat registers 120 to 125 degrees (for medium-rare) or 130 to 135 degrees (for medium), 5 to 7 minutes per side, adjusting heat as needed to prevent scorching. Transfer steaks to cutting board, tent with aluminum foil, and let rest for 5 minutes.

5 Slice steaks thin against grain on bias and transfer to large bowl. Toss steak with reserved herb mixture and season with salt and pepper to taste. Divide steak evenly among tortillas, top with slaw, and serve.

❙ MAKE AHEAD · Steaks can be marinated for up to 1 hour.

Orange-Sesame Beef and Vegetable Stir-Fry

serves 4 · total time: 35 minutes **FAST**

why this recipe works · Beef and broccoli is a classic combination for an American Chinese stir-fry. Flank steak is the perfect choice for the beef, as it is lean but packs loads of savory flavor. We needed only 12 ounces for a beefy, hearty stir-fry. For more phytonutrient punch and to up the fiber quotient, we added two red bell peppers. A simple, flavor-packed sauce with orange juice and chicken broth as its base was easy to whisk together and set aside while we prepared the other ingredients. To ensure even cooking, we first steamed our vegetables until they were perfectly crisp and tender. Next, we sautéed the thinly sliced beef and then the aromatics in heart-healthy avocado oil before adding the vegetables and sauce to heat through quickly. To make slicing the steak easier, freeze it for 15 minutes. You will need a 12-inch nonstick skillet with a tight-fitting lid for this recipe.

Sauce

- ½ cup unsalted chicken broth
- ½ cup orange juice
- 3 tablespoons low-sodium soy sauce
- 2 tablespoons toasted sesame oil
- 1½ tablespoons cornstarch

Stir-Fry

- 3 scallions, minced
- 3 garlic cloves, minced
- 1 tablespoon grated fresh ginger
- ⅛ teaspoon red pepper flakes
- 1 tablespoon avocado oil, divided
- 12 ounces flank steak, trimmed
- 1 pound broccoli, florets cut into 1-inch pieces, stalks peeled and sliced thin
- 2 red bell peppers, stemmed, seeded, and cut into 2-inch-long matchsticks
- ½ teaspoon toasted sesame oil
- Pinch table salt
- 1 tablespoon toasted sesame seeds

1 For the sauce Whisk all ingredients together in bowl and set aside.

2 For the stir-fry Combine scallions, garlic, ginger, pepper flakes, and 1 teaspoon avocado oil in small bowl; set aside. Cut beef with grain into 2½- to 3-inch-wide strips, then slice each strip against grain into ⅛-inch-thick slices.

3 Cook broccoli and ⅓ cup water in covered 12-inch nonstick skillet over high heat until water is boiling and broccoli is green and beginning to soften, about 2 minutes. Uncover, add bell peppers, and cook until vegetables are crisp-tender, about 3 minutes; transfer to colander and drain.

4 Heat 1 teaspoon avocado oil in now-empty skillet over high heat until just smoking. Add half of beef in single layer and cook without stirring for 1 minute. Continue to cook, stirring occasionally, until spotty brown on both sides, about 1 minute; transfer to clean bowl. Repeat with remaining beef and 1 teaspoon avocado oil; transfer to bowl.

5 Add scallion mixture to again-empty skillet and cook over high heat, mashing mixture into skillet, until fragrant, about 30 seconds. Stir in beef and cooked vegetables. Whisk sauce to recombine, then add to skillet and cook, stirring constantly, until sauce has thickened, about 30 seconds. Stir in sesame oil and salt, sprinkle with sesame seeds, and serve immediately.

> **MAKE AHEAD** • Prepped vegetables and steak can be refrigerated separately for up to 24 hours.

> **MAKE IT GLUTEN-FREE** • Substitute low-sodium tamari for the low-sodium soy sauce.

Stir-Fried Beef with Gai Lan and Oyster Sauce

serves 4 • **total time: 45 minutes** FAST

why this recipe works • For a different take on the ever-evolving Chinese American standard of stir-frying beef with a leafy green, we chose gai lan, also known as Chinese broccoli, and flank steak. The vegetable delivers two textures in one: firm and crunchy stalks, tender and silky leaves. To up the nutritional value, we increased the typical ratio of gai lan to beef for a more fiber-rich, vegetable-forward stir-fry. To ensure properly cooked gai lan, we first blanched it, staggering the cooking time of the stalks and the florets and leaves, so they were perfectly crisp-tender. Quarter gai lan stalks that are thicker than 1 inch at base. If you can't find gai lan, broccolini is a good substitute; halve stalks that are thicker than ½ inch. To make slicing the steak easier, freeze for 15 minutes. Serve with rice.

- ¼ teaspoon baking soda
- 1 pound flank steak, trimmed
- 3 tablespoons oyster sauce, divided
- 2 teaspoons cornstarch, divided
- 1½ tablespoons low-sodium soy sauce
- 1 tablespoon packed brown sugar
- 1 tablespoon toasted sesame oil
- 2 pounds gai lan, trimmed, florets and leaves chopped, stalks cut into 3-inch lengths and halved lengthwise
- Table salt for blanching gai lan
- 3 tablespoons avocado oil, divided
- 1 tablespoon grated fresh ginger
- 2 garlic cloves, minced
- 6 scallions, green parts only, cut into 1-inch lengths

1 Combine 1 tablespoon water and baking soda in bowl. Cut beef with grain into 2½- to 3-inch-wide strips, then slice each strip against grain into ⅛-inch-thick slices. Add beef to baking soda mixture and toss to coat; let sit for 5 minutes. Add 1 tablespoon oyster sauce and ½ teaspoon cornstarch and toss until well combined; let sit for 15 minutes.

2 Meanwhile, whisk 3 tablespoons water, remaining 2 tablespoons oyster sauce, soy sauce, sugar, sesame oil, and remaining 1½ teaspoons cornstarch in small bowl until sugar and cornstarch are dissolved; set aside. Bring 4 quarts water to boil in large pot. Add gai lan stalks and 1 tablespoon table salt and cook, stirring often, until crisp-tender, about 3 minutes. Stir in gai lan florets and leaves and cook until wilted, about 1 minute. Drain well and transfer to paper towel–lined plate; set aside.

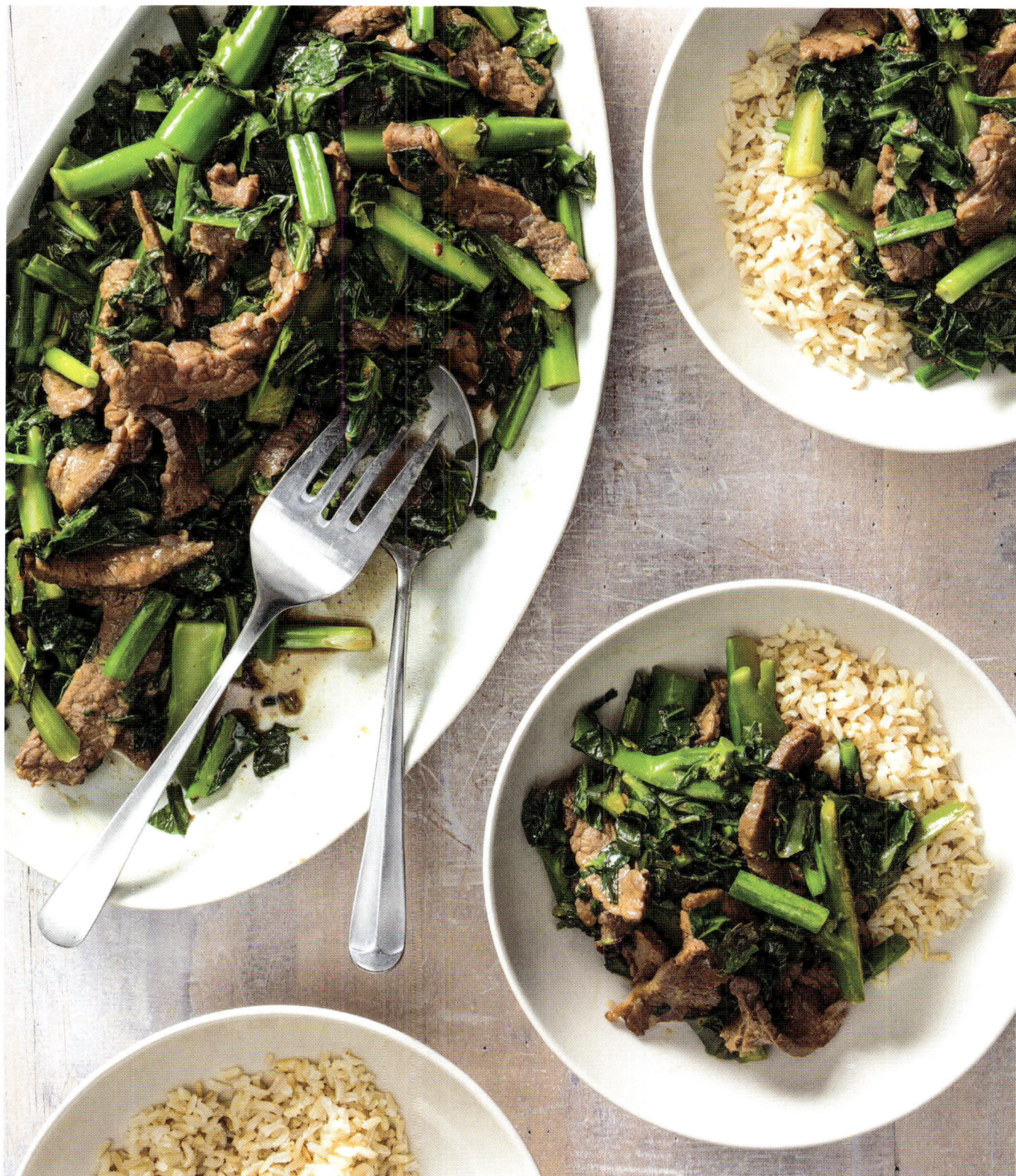

Stir-Fried Beef with Gai Lan and Oyster Sauce

3 Heat 2 teaspoons avocado oil in 12-inch nonstick skillet over medium-high heat until just smoking. Add half of beef mixture and increase heat to high. Cook, tossing beef slowly but constantly, until exuded juices have evaporated and meat begins to sizzle, 2 to 6 minutes; transfer to large bowl. Repeat with 2 teaspoons oil and remaining beef. Heat 2 teaspoons avocado oil in now-empty pan over high heat until just smoking. Add half of gai lan and cook, tossing slowly but constantly, until dry and beginning to brown, 2 to 3 minutes; transfer to bowl with beef. Repeat with 2 teaspoons avocado oil and remaining gai lan; transfer to bowl.

4 Add remaining 1 teaspoon avocado oil, ginger, and garlic to again-empty pan and cook over medium-high heat, mashing mixture into pan, until fragrant, about 15 seconds. Whisk soy sauce mixture to recombine and add to pan. Add beef–gai lan mixture and cook, tossing slowly but constantly, until sauce has thickened and beef and gai lan are well coated and heated through, about 1 minute. Stir in scallion greens and serve.

MAKE AHEAD • Prepped gai lan and steak can be refrigerated separately for up to 24 hours.

MAKE IT GLUTEN-FREE • Substitute gluten-free oyster sauce and low-sodium tamari for the oyster sauce and the low-sodium soy sauce.

Flank Steak with Farro and Mango Salsa

serves 4 • total time: 40 minutes **FAST**

why this recipe works • This easy steak supper combines hearty farro with a fruity, phytonutrient-loaded salad of fresh mango and red bell pepper that is far greater than the sum of its parts in the flavor department. Preparing the steak while the farro cooked was efficient. To make four equal-size steaks, we cut the steak in half lengthwise with the grain, then cut each piece in half crosswise against the grain. We prefer the flavor and texture of whole farro in this recipe. Do not use pearl, quick-cooking, or pre-steamed farro (check the ingredient list on the package to determine this) for the whole farro.

    2 cups whole farro
 1¼ teaspoons table salt, divided, plus salt for cooking farro
    1 (1-pound) flank steak, trimmed and cut into 4 equal steaks
 1½ teaspoons ground cumin
    ¾ teaspoon pepper, divided
    2 tablespoons avocado oil
    1 mango, peeled, pitted, and cut into ¼-inch pieces

    1 red bell pepper, stemmed, seeded, and cut into ¼-inch pieces
    ½ cup finely chopped red onion
    ½ cup chopped fresh cilantro
    2 tablespoons lime juice
    1 tablespoon extra-virgin olive oil

1 Bring 2 quarts water to boil in large saucepan. Add farro and 1 tablespoon salt. Return to boil, reduce heat to medium-low, and simmer until farro is tender with slight chew, 15 to 30 minutes. Drain well and set aside.

2 Meanwhile, pat steaks dry with paper towels and sprinkle with cumin, ½ teaspoon salt, and ¼ teaspoon pepper. Heat avocado oil in 12-inch nonstick skillet over medium-high heat until just smoking. Add steaks and cook until well browned and meat registers 120 to 125 degrees (for medium-rare) or 130 to 135 degrees (for medium), 5 to 7 minutes per side. Transfer to cutting board, tent with aluminum foil, and let rest for 5 minutes.

3 Combine mango, bell pepper, onion, cilantro, lime juice, olive oil, remaining ¾ teaspoon salt, and remaining ½ teaspoon pepper in large bowl. Measure out and reserve ½ cup salsa. Add farro to remaining salsa in bowl, tossing to combine. Slice steaks thin against grain on bias. Serve steaks with farro and reserved salsa.

MAKE AHEAD • Cooked farro can be refrigerated for up to 3 days. Prepped vegetables, mango, and steak can be refrigerated separately for up to 24 hours.

MAKE IT GLUTEN-FREE • Substitute oat berries for the farro.

Steak Fajitas

serves 6 • total time: 40 minutes **FAST**

why this recipe works • Fajitas are a sizzling spectacle, but we wanted a recipe that was more about flavor than theater and used only one baking sheet for easy weeknight clean-up. We chose flank steak, preferred by tasters for its beefy flavor, tenderness, and availability. We felt that a potent, dark-colored spice rub was needed to create both intense flavor and appealing color, and came up with a mix of chili powder and a bit of brown sugar plus salt and pepper that did the trick. After tossing strips of bell peppers, rings of red onion, and slices of garlic in oil, salt, and pepper, we spread them out on the baking sheet and slid it into the hot oven—on the lower-middle rack to ensure that the vegetables browned and didn't steam. This medley of vegetables packed lots of fiber into this recipe, resulting in a large meal—enough for 6 portions—from a single flank steak. We then pushed the vegetables to one side of the baking sheet and added the steak to the other side. In just 6 to 8 minutes, the meat was at our desired doneness: We found that the steak became less chewy and more ideal for slicing when cooked to medium instead of medium-rare. Finally, we tossed the tender vegetables with a spritz of lime juice to brighten the flavors and served them up with the meat and warm tortillas. Serve with your favorite tortilla toppings.

- 3 green, red, orange, and/or yellow bell peppers, stemmed, seeded, and cut into ½-inch-wide strips
- 1 large red onion, cut into ½-inch-thick rounds
- 3 garlic cloves, sliced thin
- 1 tablespoon extra-virgin olive oil
- 2 teaspoons table salt, divided
- 2 teaspoons pepper, divided
- 1½ tablespoons chili powder
- 1 teaspoon packed brown sugar
- 1 (1½-pound) flank steak, trimmed
- 1 tablespoon lime juice, plus lime wedges for serving
- 2 tablespoons chopped fresh cilantro
- 12 (6-inch) corn tortillas, warmed

1 Adjust oven rack to lower-middle position and heat oven to 475 degrees. Toss bell peppers, onion, garlic, oil, 1 teaspoon salt, and 1 teaspoon pepper together on rimmed baking sheet and spread into even layer. Roast until vegetables are lightly browned around edges, about 10 minutes.

2 Meanwhile, combine chili powder, sugar, remaining 1 teaspoon salt, and remaining 1 teaspoon pepper in bowl. Cut steak lengthwise with grain into 3 equal pieces. Pat steaks dry with paper towels, then sprinkle with spice mixture.

3 Remove sheet from oven. Using silicone spatula, push vegetables to 1 half of sheet. Place steaks on other half of sheet, leaving space between pieces. Roast until vegetables are spotty brown and meat registers 130 to 135 degrees (for medium), 6 to 8 minutes.

4 Remove sheet from oven, transfer steaks to cutting board, and let rest, uncovered, for 5 minutes. Transfer vegetables to serving platter and toss with lime juice.

5 Slice steaks thin against grain and transfer to platter with vegetables. Sprinkle with cilantro. Serve steak and vegetables with tortillas.

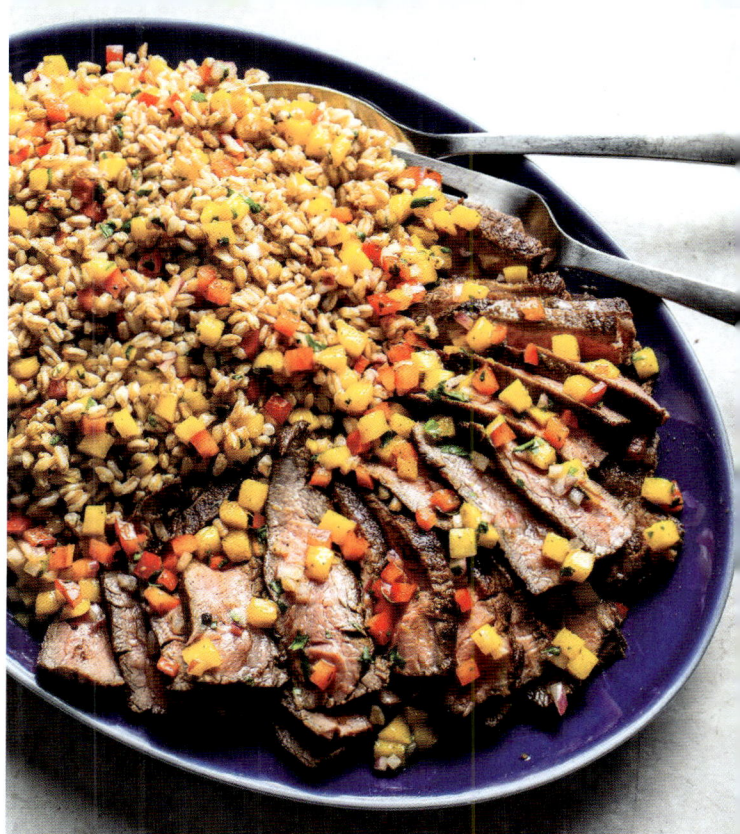

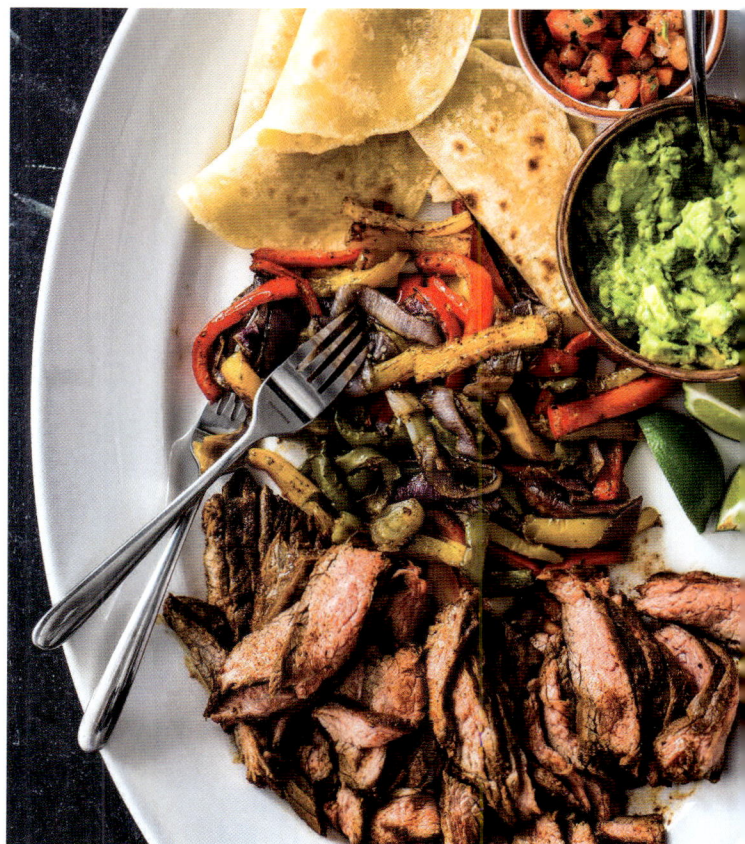

top | *Flank Steak with Farro and Mango Salsa*
bottom | *Steak Fajitas*

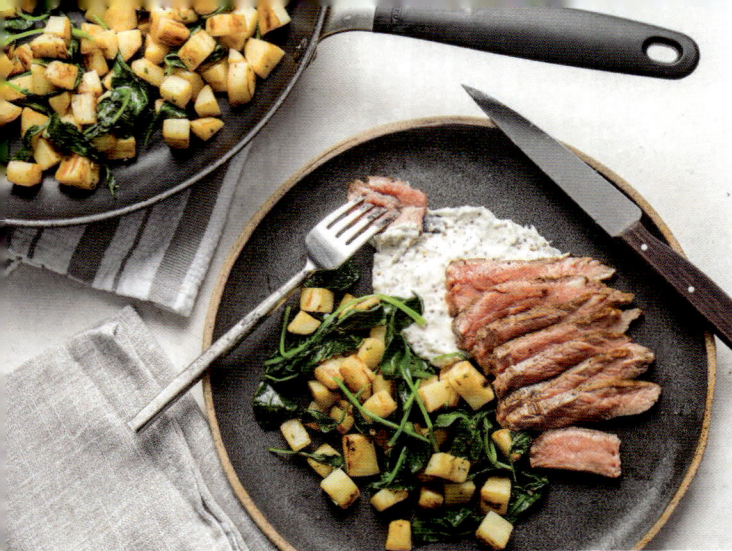

Flank Steak with Parsnips and Baby Kale

serves 4 · total time: 45 minutes **FAST**

why this recipe works • A thin cut of juicy steak with a side of crisped potatoes and a zesty horseradish sauce is a comforting bistro dish. While potatoes are high in fiber, we thought we could go higher: In this nutritious spin, we swapped in hearty parsnips, a vegetable with a remarkable amount of fiber. We were able to use one pan to cook our flank steak and parsnips, which made this a weeknight-friendly dish with minimal cleanup. Cooking the steak first allowed the savory steak juices to permeate the sweet parsnips (which we parcooked in the microwave to hasten the pan cooking). The parsnips' nutty flavor was enhanced in the skillet, and for extra seasoning and antioxidants we added fresh rosemary and garlic. Just before serving, we folded in a generous portion of kale, another excellent source of fiber. We kept the creamy, piquant sauce element—we loved how horseradish not only cuts the richness of the steak but offsets the sweetness of the parsnips—but gave it a probiotic spin with Greek yogurt.

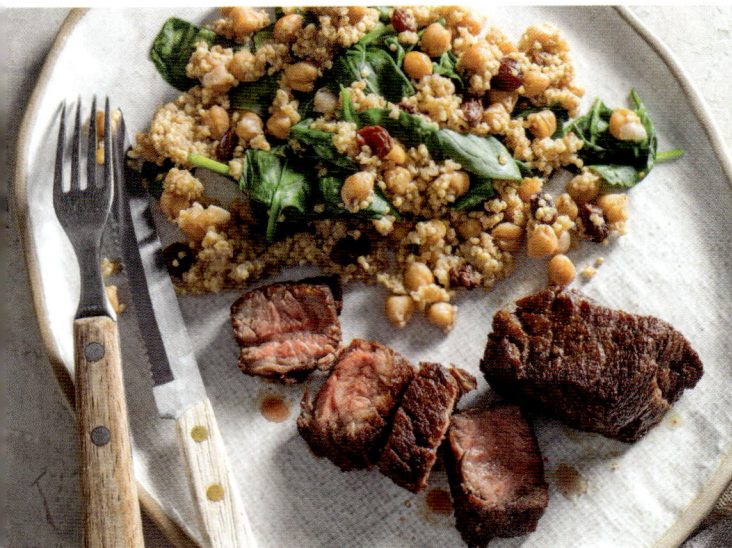

- ¼ cup plain Greek yogurt
- 1 tablespoon prepared horseradish, drained
- 1 tablespoon whole-grain mustard
- 1 teaspoon table salt, divided
- ¾ teaspoon pepper, divided
- 2 pounds parsnips, peeled and cut into ½-inch pieces
- 1 (1-pound) flank steak, trimmed and halved with grain
- 3 tablespoons avocado oil, divided
- 1 tablespoon minced fresh rosemary
- 2 garlic cloves, minced
- 3 ounces (3 cups) baby kale, chopped coarse

1 Whisk yogurt, horseradish, mustard, ¼ teaspoon salt, and ¼ teaspoon pepper together in small bowl; set aside for serving.

2 Microwave parsnips and 2 tablespoons water in large covered bowl, stirring occasionally, until parsnips are tender, 9 to 14 minutes. Drain parsnips and set aside.

3 Pat steaks dry with paper towels, then sprinkle with ¼ teaspoon salt and ¼ teaspoon pepper. Heat 1 tablespoon oil in 12-inch nonstick skillet over medium-high heat until just smoking. Add steaks and cook until well browned and meat registers 120 to 125 degrees (for medium-rare) or 130 to 135 degrees (for medium), 3 to 6 minutes per side. Transfer steaks to cutting board, tent with aluminum foil, and let rest while finishing parsnips.

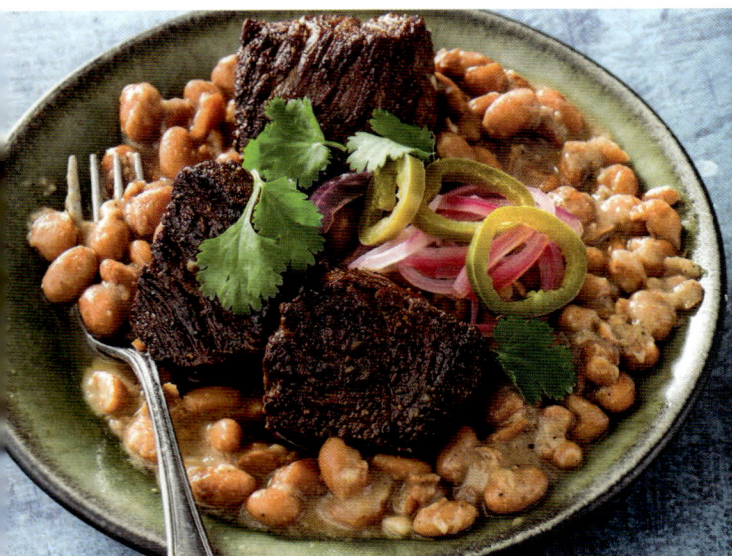

top	Flank Steak with Parsnips and Baby Kale
middle	Steak Tips with Spiced Millet and Spinach
bottom	Sirloin Steak Tips with Charro Beans

4 Heat 1 tablespoon oil in now-empty skillet over medium-high heat until shimmering. Add parsnips, remaining ½ teaspoon salt, and remaining ¼ teaspoon pepper and cook, stirring occasionally, until parsnips are lightly browned, 8 to 10 minutes.

5 Push parsnips to sides of skillet. Add rosemary, garlic, and remaining 1 tablespoon oil to center of skillet and cook until fragrant, 15 to 30 seconds. Stir rosemary mixture into parsnips. Stir kale into parsnips, 1 handful at a time, until wilted, about 2 minutes. Season with salt and pepper to taste. Slice steak thin against grain on bias and serve with parsnip mixture and horseradish sauce.

MAKE IT DAIRY-FREE • Substitute plant-based Greek yogurt for the dairy Greek yogurt.

Steak Tips with Spiced Millet and Spinach

serves 4 • total time: 30 minutes   **FAST**

why this recipe works • Inspired by the pairing of warm spices and dried fruit common in Morocco, we seasoned steak tips (a lean but deeply flavored cut) with a spice rub featuring cumin and cinnamon and then seared them in a skillet for flavorful browning. A side of tender millet, hearty chickpeas, and sunny-sweet golden raisins was a fitting accompaniment. Stirring baby spinach into the millet at the end of cooking allowed the leaves to wilt slightly before serving. Sirloin steak tips, also known as flap meat, can be sold as whole steaks, cubes, or strips; we prefer to purchase whole steaks and cut them ourselves. We found that, unlike other grains, millet can become gluey if allowed to steam off the heat, so be sure to serve immediately.

  1½ teaspoons ground cumin
    1 teaspoon ground cinnamon
  ¾ teaspoon table salt
  ¼ teaspoon pepper
    1 pound sirloin steak tips, trimmed and cut into 2-inch pieces
    1 tablespoon avocado oil
  1½ cups water
    1 (15-ounce) can no-salt-added chickpeas, rinsed
  ¾ cup millet, rinsed and dried thoroughly
  ¼ cup golden raisins
    5 ounces (5 cups) baby spinach, chopped

1 Combine cumin, cinnamon, salt, and pepper in bowl. Pat steak tips dry with paper towels and sprinkle with 1½ teaspoons spice mixture. Heat oil in 12-inch skillet over medium-high heat

until just smoking. Add steak and cook until browned on all sides and meat registers 120 to 125 degrees (for medium-rare) or 130 to 135 degrees (for medium), 6 to 10 minutes. Transfer steak tips to plate, tent with aluminum foil, and let rest for 5 minutes.

2 Meanwhile, combine water, chickpeas, millet, raisins, and remaining spice mixture in large saucepan and bring to boil over medium-high heat. Reduce heat to low, cover, and simmer until liquid is absorbed, 15 to 20 minutes. Fold in spinach, one handful at a time. Serve with steak tips.

Sirloin Steak Tips with Charro Beans

serves 4 • total time: 30 minutes   **FAST**

why this recipe works • This hearty weeknight meal delivers bold flavor and balanced nutrition in just half an hour. We started with sirloin steak tips, which provided a lean source of protein and iron. Taking inspiration from flavorful Mexican charro beans, we seasoned fiber-rich pinto beans with garlic and cumin, which added both plant-powered protein and antioxidants. Lightly mashing some of the beans created a creamy texture, and using no-salt-added beans and unsalted broth allowed for more control over sodium levels. A quick pickle of red onion and jalapeño, prepared in the microwave, contributed brightness and tang, enhancing the flavor profile. The result was a satisfying, nutrient-dense dish with just the right amount of kick. Sirloin steak tips, also known as flap meat, can be sold as whole steaks, cubes, or strips; we prefer to purchase whole steaks and cut them ourselves. For a spicier dish, include the seeds from the chile. Garnish with fresh cilantro leaves, if desired.

  ½ small red onion, sliced thin
  ¼ cup distilled white vinegar
    1 small jalapeño chile, stemmed, seeded, and sliced thin
    2 pounds sirloin steak tips, trimmed and cut into 2-inch pieces
    1 teaspoon table salt, divided
  2½ teaspoons ground cumin, divided
  1½ teaspoons pepper, divided
    2 tablespoons avocado oil
    3 garlic cloves, minced
    3 (15-ounce) cans no-salt-added pinto beans, rinsed
  1½ cups unsalted chicken or vegetable broth

1 Combine onion, vinegar, and jalapeño in small bowl. Cover and microwave until hot, about 2 minutes; set aside.

2   Pat steak tips dry with paper towels then sprinkle with ½ teaspoon salt, ½ teaspoon cumin, and 1 teaspoon pepper. Heat oil in 12-inch nonstick skillet over medium-high heat until just smoking. Add steak and cook until browned on all sides and meat registers 120 to 125 degrees (for medium-rare) or 130 to 135 degrees (for medium), 6 to 10 minutes. Transfer steak tips to plate, tent with aluminum foil, and let rest for 5 minutes.

3   Meanwhile, cook garlic and remaining 2 teaspoons cumin in now-empty skillet over medium heat until fragrant, about 30 seconds. Stir in beans, broth, remaining ½ teaspoon salt, and remaining ½ teaspoon pepper. Using potato masher, lightly mash beans until about one-quarter of beans are broken down. Bring to simmer and cook until thickened and liquid is fully incorporated into bean mixture, about 4 minutes. Serve steak with beans and pickled onion mixture.

MAKE AHEAD • Pickled onion mixture can be refrigerated for up to 3 days.

Coffee-Rubbed Steak with Sweet Potatoes and Apples

serves 4 • **total time: 1 hour**

why this recipe works • This autumnal sheet-pan meal of steak, sweet potatoes, and apples is just the easy, cozy meal you need when colder weather hits. The sweet potatoes, which we roasted alongside shallots for extra flavor and fiber, turned tender and caramelly in the oven. The sweetly floral apple slices that we added later to the pan with the steak echoed the sweetness of the potatoes. Rubbing boneless strip steaks with a bold blend of coffee, chili powder, and a touch of brown sugar created a crust full of flavor. Finally, tossing the vegetables and fruit with a quick parsley and vinegar dressing introduced bright, fresh notes—while adding a dose of antioxidants. The result was a well-balanced, anti-inflammatory meal that tasted equally comforting and nourishing. Look for shallots that weigh about 1 ounce each.

2   pounds sweet potatoes, unpeeled, cut lengthwise into 1-inch wedges

8   shallots, peeled and quartered lengthwise

¼   cup extra-virgin olive oil, divided

1   teaspoon table salt, divided

1   teaspoon pepper, divided

2   large apples, cored, halved, and sliced thin

2   teaspoons packed dark brown sugar

2   teaspoons finely ground coffee

2   teaspoons chili powder

2   (6- to 8-ounce) boneless strip steaks, 1 to 1½ inches thick, trimmed

¼   cup minced fresh parsley, plus extra for serving

2   tablespoons red wine vinegar

1   Adjust oven rack to lower-middle position and heat oven to 450 degrees. Toss potatoes and shallots with 4 teaspoons oil, ¼ teaspoon salt, and ½ teaspoon pepper in large bowl. Arrange potatoes skin side down on half of rimmed baking sheet and arrange shallots in single layer next to potatoes. Roast until vegetables are softened and lightly browned, 20 to 25 minutes.

2   Toss apples with 2 teaspoons oil and ¼ teaspoon salt in now-empty bowl. Combine sugar, coffee, chili powder, remaining ½ teaspoon salt, and remaining ½ teaspoon pepper in medium bowl. Pat steaks dry with paper towels and rub with spice mixture.

3   Place steak on empty side of sheet and arrange apple slices on top of shallots. Roast until potatoes, shallots, and apples are fully tender and meat registers 120 to 125 degrees (for medium-rare), 10 to 15 minutes. Transfer steak, bottom side up, to cutting board, tent loosely with aluminum foil, and let rest for 5 minutes.

4   Combine parsley, vinegar, and remaining 2 tablespoons oil in large bowl. Add potatoes, shallots, and apples and toss to combine. Season with salt and pepper to taste. Slice steak thin against grain and sprinkle with extra parsley. Serve steak with sweet potato mixture.

Braised Steaks with Root Vegetables

serves 4 • **total time: 2½ hours**

why this recipe works • Steak isn't always about the thick crust from a hard, fast sear. Tough blade steaks turn meltingly tender when simmered in liquid, producing an accompanying sauce full of beefy flavor. To achieve this effect, we purposely "overcooked" the meat—a 1½-hour braise allowed nearly all of the fat and connective tissue to dissolve, giving each bite a soft, silky texture. We started by searing the meat to get some browning—without pushing it into charred territory—then set it aside while we built a balanced braising liquid scented with garlic and thyme. We then returned the steaks to the pan, along with potatoes and carrots, to simmer for an hour in the oven, providing an easy one-pot meal. The root vegetables brought fiber and soaked up the savory, meaty juices. At the very end, we reduced the braising liquid to a savory sauce to spoon over the whole dish before serving. Make sure to buy steaks that are about the same size to ensure even cooking. You will need a 12-inch ovensafe skillet with a tight-fitting lid for this recipe.

- 4 (6- to 8-ounce) beef blade steaks, ¾ to 1 inch thick, trimmed
- ½ teaspoon table salt
- ⅛ teaspoon pepper
- 2 tablespoons avocado oil, divided
- 1 onion, halved and sliced thin
- 3 garlic cloves, minced
- 1 tablespoon minced fresh thyme or 1 teaspoon dried
- 1 tablespoon all-purpose flour
- 1½ cups unsalted beef broth
- 1 cup water
- ½ cup dry red wine
- 12 ounces red or yellow waxy potatoes, unpeeled, cut into 1-inch pieces
- 12 ounces carrots, celery root, and/or turnips, peeled and cut into 1-inch pieces
- 1 cup frozen peas
- 1 tablespoon minced fresh parsley

1 Adjust oven rack to lower-middle position and heat oven to 325 degrees. Pat steaks dry with paper towels and sprinkle with salt and pepper. Heat 1 tablespoon oil in 12-inch ovensafe skillet over medium-high heat until just smoking. Add steaks and cook until well browned, 3 to 5 minutes per side. Transfer steaks to plate.

2 Heat remaining 1 tablespoon oil in now-empty skillet over medium heat until shimmering. Add onion and cook until softened, about 5 minutes. Stir in garlic, thyme, and flour and cook until fragrant, about 1 minute. Stir in broth, water, and wine, scraping up any browned bits and smoothing out any lumps, and bring to simmer.

3 Add steaks to skillet, along with any accumulated juices. Nestle potatoes and carrots around steaks. Cover skillet, transfer to oven, and cook until steaks are tender and paring knife can be slipped in and out of meat with very little resistance, about 1½ hours.

4 Being careful of hot skillet handle, remove skillet from oven. Transfer steaks and vegetables to serving platter, tent with aluminum foil, and let rest while finishing sauce. Bring sauce to simmer over medium-high heat and cook until thickened and reduced to about ¾ cup, 10 to 15 minutes. Stir in peas and cook until warmed through, about 2 minutes. Season with salt and pepper to taste. Spoon sauce over steak and vegetables, sprinkle with parsley, and serve.

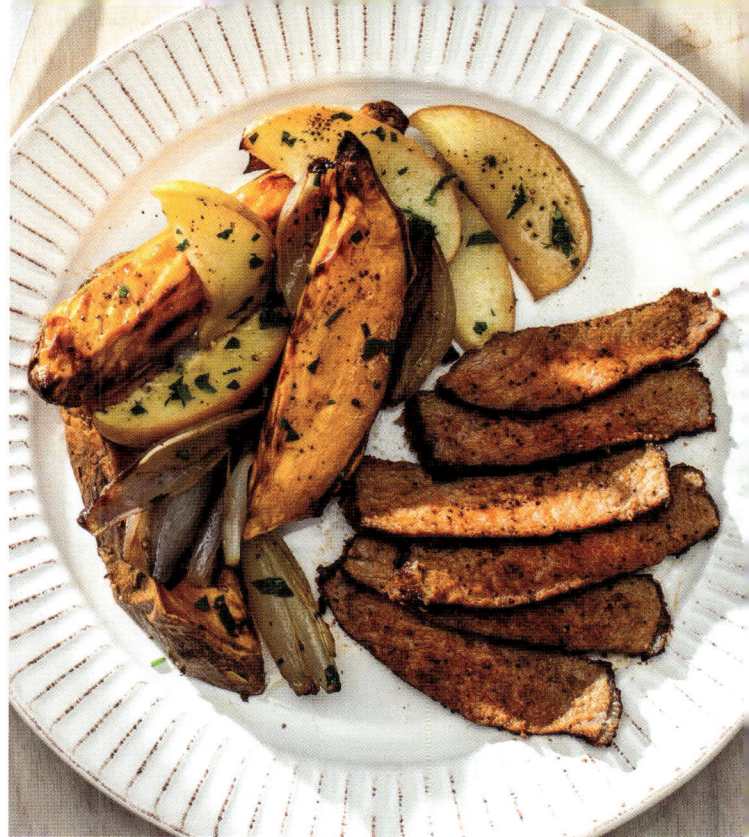

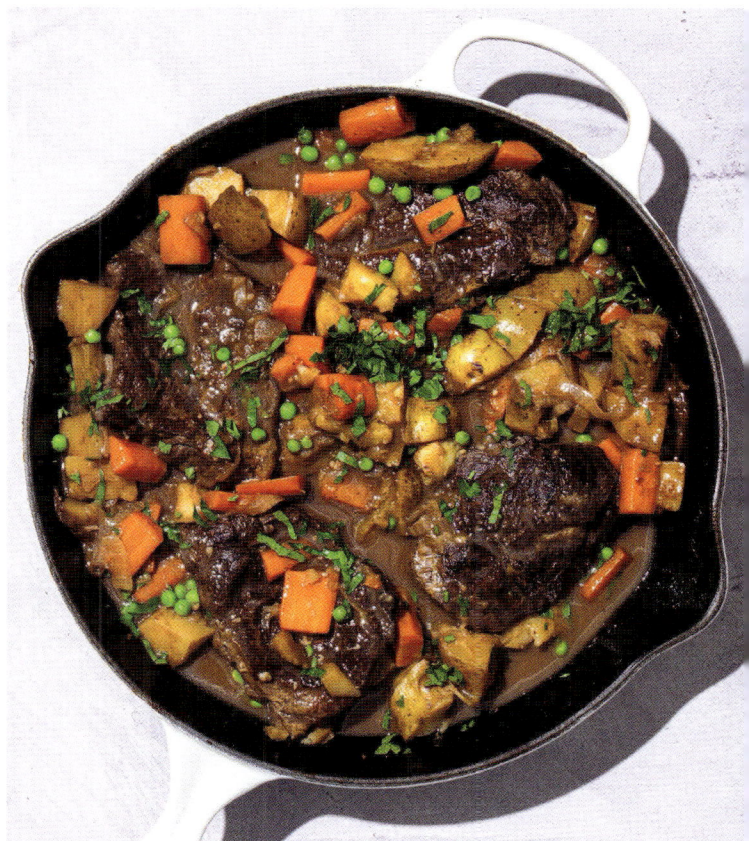

top | *Coffee-Rubbed Steak with Sweet Potatoes and Apples*
bottom | *Braised Steaks with Root Vegetables*

Spiced Meatballs, Carrots, and Radishes with Couscous and Dried Cherries

serves 4 to 6 • total time: 55 minutes `SUPERCHARGED`

why this recipe works • Perfumed with cumin and cinnamon, this weeknight-friendly dish pairs couscous and satisfyingly juicy meatballs with colorful and vitamin-rich carrots and radishes. Lightly browning the couscous in avocado oil before adding broth boosted the chewy pasta's toasty flavor. We further amped up the grains with dried tart cherries for even more antioxidants. We paired tart cherry juice—an antioxidant and anti-inflammatory hero—with broth to make a zingy cooking liquid for the vegetables. For the meatballs, we mixed ground beef with panko, yogurt, and an egg yolk to keep them moist. The fat they left behind after browning was perfect for cooking our vegetables and imbuing them with savory richness.

  2 tablespoons avocado oil, divided
  2 cups couscous
1¾ teaspoons ground cinnamon, divided
  1 teaspoon ground cumin, divided
3¼ cups unsalted chicken broth, divided
  ½ cup dried unsweetened tart cherries, chopped
1½ teaspoons table salt, divided
  1 cup plain yogurt, divided
  ⅓ cup panko bread crumbs
  ½ cup chopped fresh mint, divided
  1 large egg yolk
  2 garlic cloves, minced, divided
  ¼ teaspoon pepper
  1 pound 90 percent lean ground beef
  1 pound carrots, peeled and sliced ¼ inch thick on bias
 12 ounces radishes, halved if small, quartered if large
  1 cup unsweetened tart cherry juice
  2 teaspoons grated lemon zest plus 2 tablespoons juice, plus lemon wedges for serving

1 Heat 1 tablespoon oil in medium saucepan over medium-high heat until shimmering. Add couscous and cook, stirring frequently, until grains are just beginning to brown, 3 to 5 minutes. Add ½ teaspoon cinnamon and ¼ teaspoon cumin and cook until fragrant, about 30 seconds. Stir in 2¼ cups broth, cherries, and ½ teaspoon salt. Cover and let sit off heat until couscous is tender, about 7 minutes. Set aside.

2 Meanwhile, combine ⅓ cup yogurt, panko, 3 tablespoons mint, egg yolk, half of garlic, pepper, 1 teaspoon cinnamon, ½ teaspoon cumin, and ½ teaspoon salt in large bowl. Add beef

and mix with your hands until thoroughly combined. Form mixture into 20 tightly packed 1½-inch meatballs.

3 Heat remaining 1 tablespoon oil in 12-inch nonstick skillet over medium-high heat until just smoking. Add meatballs and cook until well browned all over and cooked through, 6 to 8 minutes; transfer to large plate and tent with aluminum foil.

4 To fat left in skillet, add carrots, radishes, remaining 1 cup broth, cherry juice, lemon zest, remaining garlic, remaining ¼ teaspoon cinnamon, remaining ¼ teaspoon cumin, and remaining ½ teaspoon salt. Bring to vigorous simmer and cook, stirring occasionally, until vegetables are just tender and liquid is reduced slightly, 8 to 10 minutes. Add meatballs to skillet and cook until warmed through, 1 to 2 minutes, stirring meatballs to coat in sauce.

5 Sprinkle couscous with lemon juice and 3 tablespoons mint and fluff with fork until well combined. Sprinkle meatballs and sauce with remaining 2 tablespoons mint. Serve with couscous, passing remaining ⅔ cup yogurt and lemon wedges separately.

Nutritional Knowledge   In this nutritionally well-rounded spiced meatball dish, tart cherry juice and dried cherries bring concentrated anthocyanins—potent antioxidants known to reduce joint pain and inflammation. Carrots and radishes provide beta-carotene and vitamin C to help combat oxidative stress. The ground beef has essential nutrients like iron and B_{12}. Seasonings like cinnamon, garlic, and mint support immune function.   —*Alicia*

Tamale Pie

serves 6 to 8 • total time: 1½ hours

why this recipe works • Tamale pie—lightly seasoned, tomatoey ground beef with a cornbread topping—borrows the flavor of traditional Mexican tamales. The addition of black beans made our pie heartier, not to mention higher in protein, while corn and tomatoes contributed additional flavor, texture, and nutrients. We first sautéed 90 percent lean ground beef, which contributed richness while allowing us to moderate the saturated fat content. Then we added onion and jalapeño to soften, followed by chili powder, oregano, and garlic to bloom and intensify their flavors. Next went in the beans, tomatoes, and corn and a final addition of

Monterey Jack cheese to enrich the filling and help thicken it. To finish our pie, we made a simple cornmeal batter to spread over the filling before baking. After 30 minutes in the oven, our rich, hearty pie had a crunchy, flavorful topping that was reminiscent of real tamale dough. To make the pie spicier, include the seeds from the chile.

- 3 tablespoons avocado oil, divided
- 1 pound 90 percent lean ground beef
- 1 onion, chopped fine
- 1 jalapeño chile, stemmed, seeded, and minced
- 1 teaspoon table salt, divided
- 2 tablespoons chili powder
- 1 tablespoon minced fresh oregano or 1 teaspoon dried
- 2 garlic cloves, minced
- 1 (15-ounce) can no-salt-added black beans, rinsed
- 1 (14.5-ounce) can no-salt-added diced tomatoes
- 1 cup fresh or frozen corn
- 2½ cups water
- ¾ cup coarse cornmeal
- 4 ounces Monterey Jack cheese, shredded (1 cup)

1 Adjust oven rack to lower-middle position and heat oven to 375 degrees. Heat 1 tablespoon oil in 12-inch skillet over medium-high heat until just smoking. Add beef and cook, breaking up meat with wooden spoon, until just beginning to brown, about 5 minutes.

2 Stir in onion, jalapeño, and ½ teaspoon salt and cook until softened, about 5 minutes. Stir in chili powder, oregano, and garlic and cook until fragrant, about 30 seconds. Stir in beans, tomatoes and their juice, and corn and simmer until most of liquid has evaporated, about 3 minutes. Off heat, season with salt and pepper to taste.

3 Bring water to boil in large saucepan. Add remaining ½ teaspoon salt and then slowly pour in cornmeal while whisking vigorously to prevent clumping. Reduce heat to medium and cook, whisking constantly, until cornmeal thickens, about 3 minutes. Stir in remaining 2 tablespoons oil.

4 Stir Monterey Jack into beef mixture, then scrape into deep-dish pie plate (or other 3-quart baking dish). Spread cornmeal mixture over top and seal against edge of dish. Cover with aluminum foil and bake until crust has set and filling is hot throughout, about 30 minutes. Let casserole cool for 10 minutes. Serve.

MAKE IT DAIRY-FREE • Substitute plant-based Monterey Jack cheese for the dairy Monterey Jack cheese.

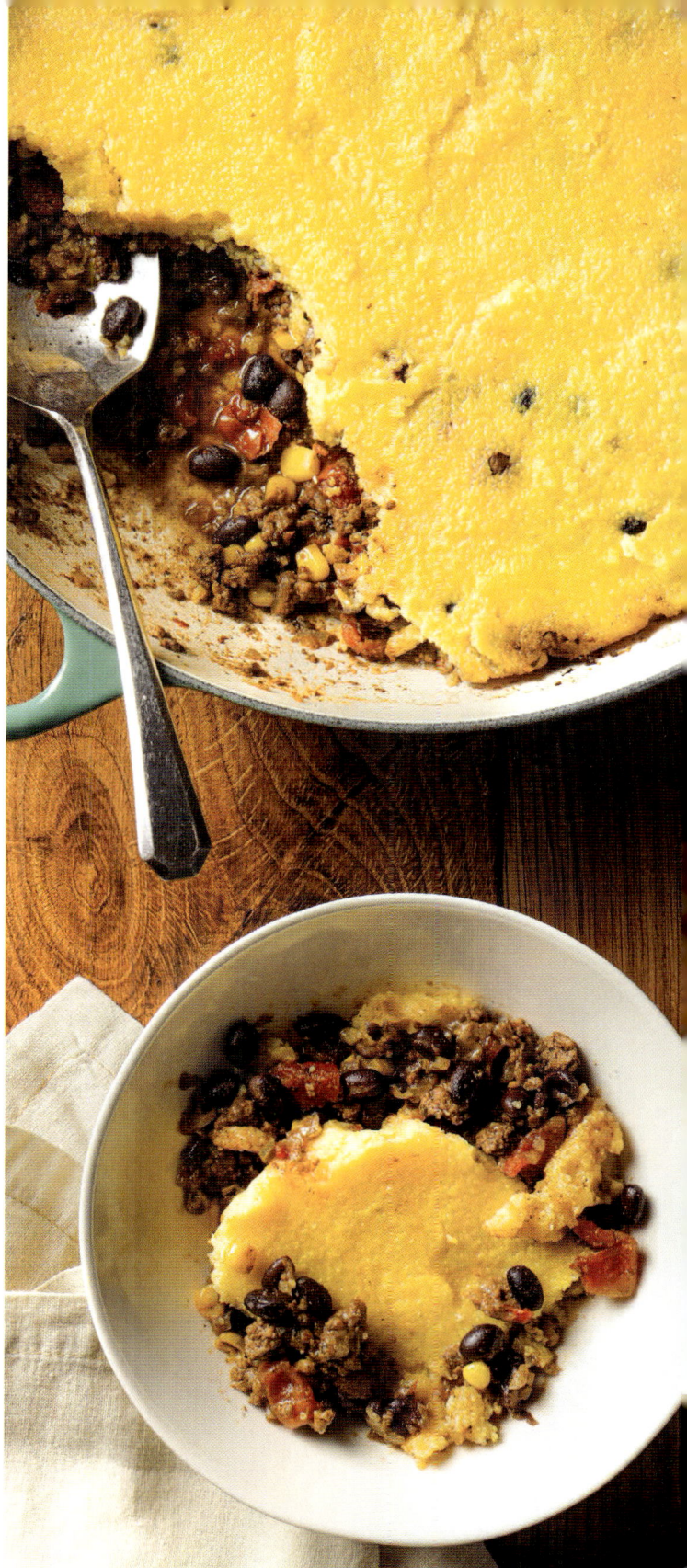

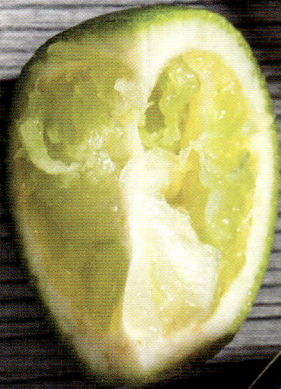

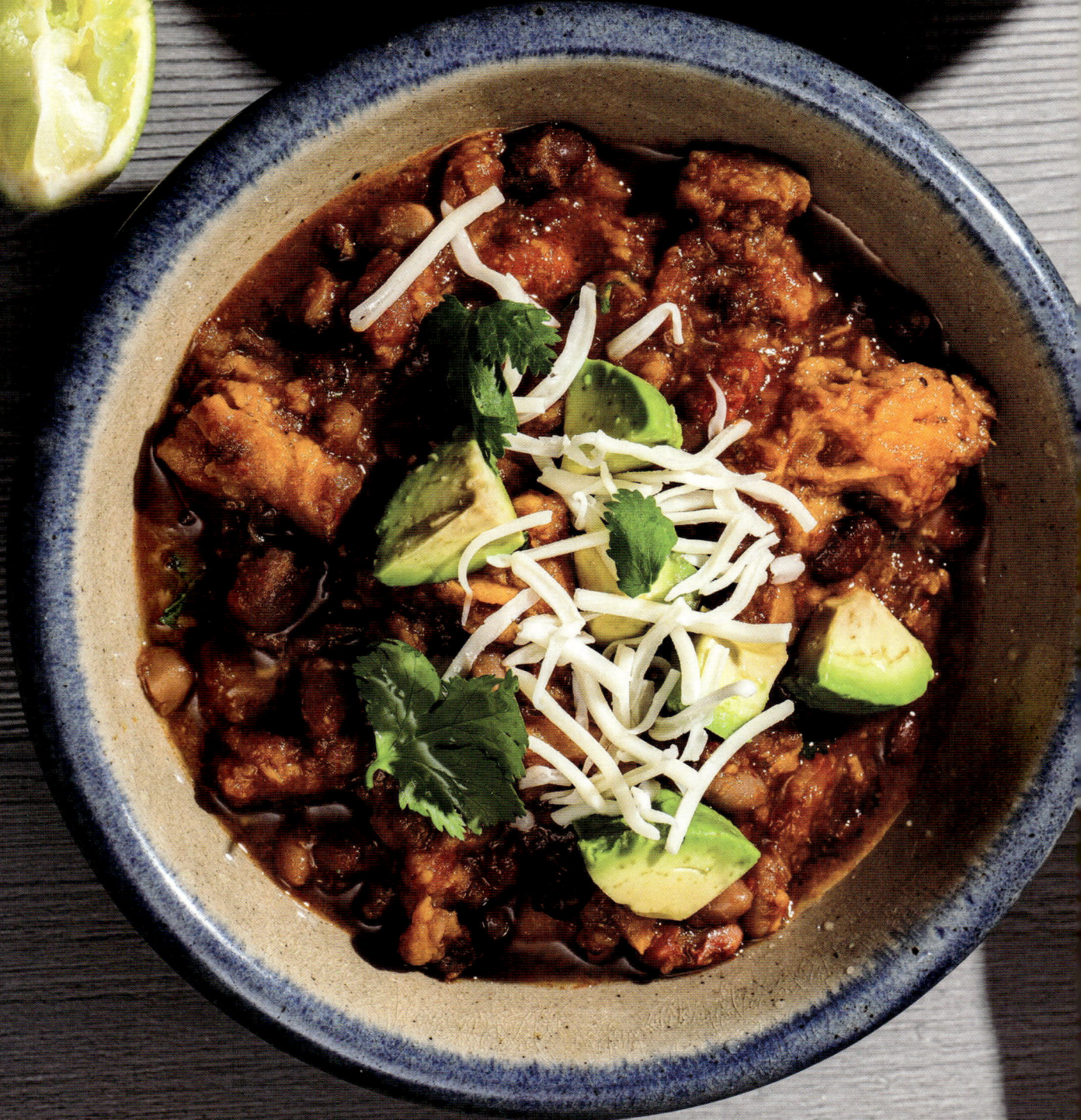

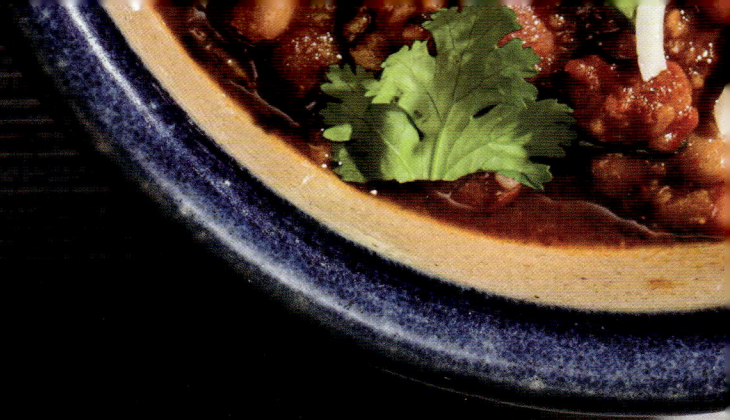

PRESSURE COOKER

■ FAST   ■ SUPERCHARGED

Pressure-Cooker Chicken Noodle Soup with Shells, Tomatoes, and Zucchini

serves 6 · total time: 1¼ hours

why this recipe works · Chicken noodle soup is a perfect candidate for the pressure cooker because the high-heat environment extracts tons of flavor from the meat, skin, and bones of a whole chicken. It's also a great candidate for bulking up with lots of anti-inflammatory vegetables. To prevent the meat from overcooking while ensuring a flavorful broth, it was crucial to get the timing right. Positioning the chicken with the breast side up exposed the dark meat thighs to more direct heat and shielded the delicate breast meat from overcooking. Once cooked, the tender meat was easy to shred and stir back in. We used the sauté function to simmer tomatoes and zucchini right in the broth toward the end of cooking so they could maintain their texture and flavor. Other small pasta shapes can be substituted for the shells.

- 1 tablespoon avocado oil
- 1 onion, chopped fine
- 1 tablespoon tomato paste
- 2 teaspoons minced fresh thyme or ½ teaspoon dried
- 8 cups water, divided
- 4 carrots, peeled, halved lengthwise, and cut into ½-inch pieces
- 2 celery ribs, halved lengthwise and cut into ½-inch pieces
- 2 tablespoons low-sodium soy sauce
- 1 teaspoon table salt
- 1 (4-pound) whole chicken, giblets discarded
- 1 (8-ounce) zucchini, quartered lengthwise and sliced ¼ inch thick
- 2 tomatoes, cored and chopped
- 4 ounces (1 cup) small pasta shells
- ¼ cup chopped fresh basil

1 Using highest sauté function, heat oil in electric pressure cooker until shimmering. Add onion and cook until softened, 3 to 5 minutes. Stir in tomato paste and thyme and cook until fragrant, about 30 seconds. Stir in 6 cups water, scraping up browned bits, then stir in carrots, celery, soy sauce, and salt. Place chicken breast side up in pot.

2 Lock lid into place and close pressure-release valve. Select high pressure-cook function and cook for 20 minutes. Turn off pressure cooker and quick-release pressure. Carefully remove lid, allowing steam to escape away from you. Transfer chicken to carving board, let cool slightly, then shred into bite-size pieces using 2 forks; discard skin and bones.

3 Meanwhile, stir zucchini, tomatoes, pasta, and remaining 2 cups water into soup and cook using highest sauté function until pasta is tender, about 8 minutes. Turn off pressure cooker. Return chicken and any accumulated juices to pot and let sit until heated through, about 2 minutes. Stir in basil and season with salt and pepper to taste. Serve.

MAKE IT GLUTEN-FREE · Substitute low-sodium tamari for the low-sodium soy sauce and gluten-free pasta for the pasta.

NOTES FROM THE TEST KITCHEN

Why Pressure Cookers Are Great for Anti-Inflammatory Cooking

Thanks to shorter cook times and less exposure to high heat, pressure cooking often preserves more nutrients than other cooking methods.

For lean or delicate proteins like chicken breasts and fish, a pressure cooker also minimizes the risk of overcooking and drying out. Cooking begins as pressure builds, so many recipes need only a few minutes (or less) at high pressure.

We especially like the hands-off nature of electric pressure cookers, which offer a "keep warm" function—an added bonus on busy days. With that in mind, we've written all the recipes in this chapter for an electric pressure cooker. However, the recipes can be easily modified to work on a stovetop model.

To use a stovetop pressure cooker:

Use medium heat when softening vegetables or aromatics, and medium-high for browning proteins.

Bring the cooker to high pressure over medium-high heat. As soon as the indicator signals that it has reached high pressure, reduce the heat to medium-low and begin counting the cook time stated in recipe, adjusting the heat as needed to maintain high pressure.

Remove the cooker from the heat before allowing pressure to quick release or naturally release.

Pressure-Cooker Chicken Harira

serves 6 · total time: 1 hour   **SUPERCHARGED**

why this recipe works · Moroccan harira is often eaten to break fast during Ramadan, as it is a filling and nutritious soup (made with lentils, tomatoes, fresh herbs, and often lamb). For our take, bone-in chicken breasts provided a lean protein source that was relatively low in saturated fat. After browning them on the sauté function, we bloomed an inflammation-fighting combination of ginger, cumin, paprika, and cinnamon for their nutrition and fragrance, then stirred in broth and lentils. After nestling the chicken into the mixture, we cooked the soup under pressure for 8 minutes. Tomatoes, stirred in at the end so they retained some structure, added bright flavor, while harissa gave us some heat. Brown or green lentils work well in this recipe; do not use lentilles du Puy (French green lentils). We like to use our homemade Harissa (page 106), but you can use store-bought if you prefer.

  2 (12-ounce) bone-in split chicken breasts, trimmed
  1 tablespoon avocado oil
  1 tablespoon all-purpose flour
  1 teaspoon grated fresh ginger
  1 teaspoon ground cumin
  ½ teaspoon paprika
  ¼ teaspoon ground cinnamon
     Pinch saffron threads, crumbled
 10 cups unsalted chicken broth
  1 cup dried brown or green lentils, picked over and rinsed
  4 plum tomatoes, cored and cut into ¾-inch pieces
  ⅓ cup minced fresh cilantro
  ¼ cup harissa, plus extra for serving

1   Pat chicken dry with paper towels. Using highest sauté function, heat oil in electric pressure cooker until just smoking. Place chicken skin side down in pot and cook until well browned on first side, about 5 minutes; transfer to plate. Turn off pressure cooker.

2   Add flour, ginger, cumin, paprika, cinnamon, and saffron to fat left in pot and cook, stirring frequently, until fragrant, about 30 seconds. Slowly whisk in broth, scraping up any browned bits and smoothing out any lumps. Stir in lentils, then nestle chicken skin side up into lentil mixture and add any accumulated juices.

3   Lock lid into place and close pressure-release valve. Select high pressure-cook function and cook for 8 minutes. Turn off pressure cooker and quick-release pressure. Carefully remove lid, allowing steam to escape away from you. Transfer chicken to cutting board, let cool slightly, then shred into bite-size pieces using 2 forks; discard skin and bones.

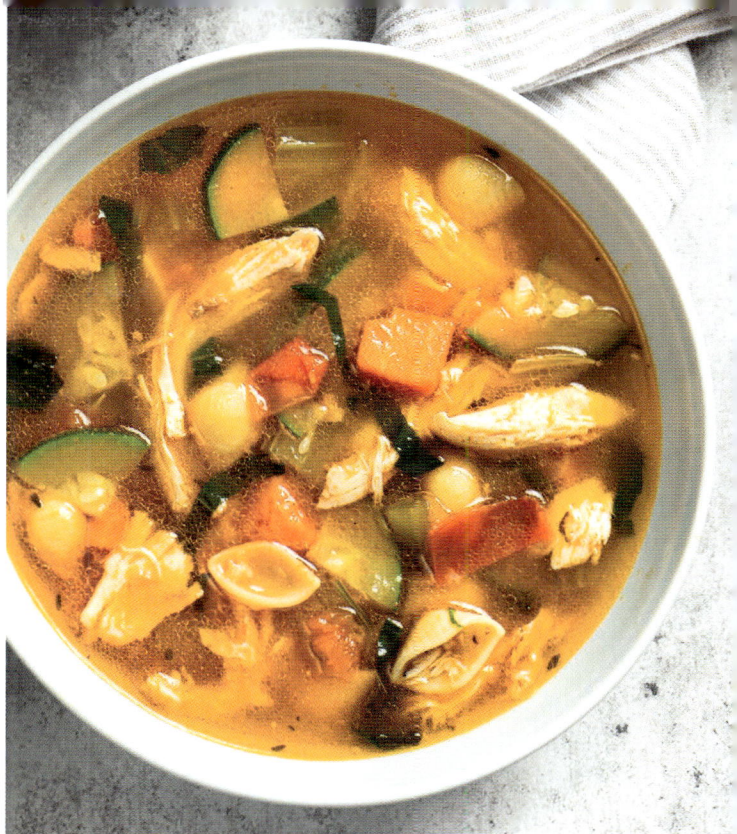

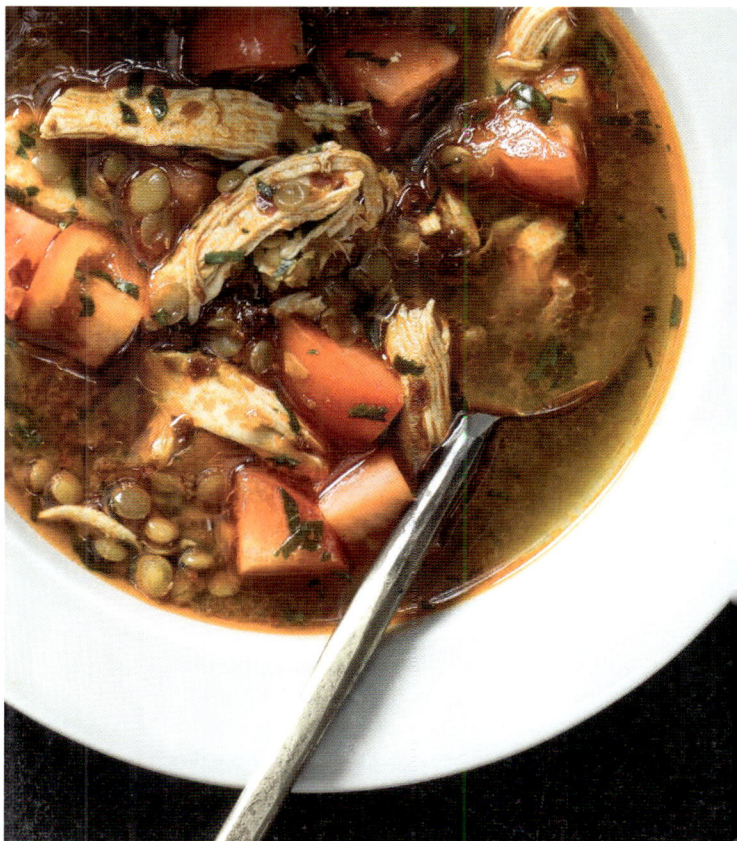

top | Pressure-Cooker Chicken Noodle Soup with Shells, Tomatoes, and Zucchini
bottom | Pressure-Cooker Chicken Harira

4   Meanwhile, continue to cook lentils using highest sauté function until just tender, about 5 minutes. Turn off pressure cooker. Stir in chicken and any juices and tomatoes, and let sit until heated through, about 2 minutes. Stir in cilantro and harissa and season with salt and pepper to taste. Serve, passing extra harissa separately.

❙ MAKE AHEAD • Soup can be refrigerated for up to 2 days.

Pressure-Cooker White Chicken Chili with Zucchini

serves 6 • total time: 1 hour, plus 8 hours brining

why this recipe works • What distinguishes a white chili from a red one is not its final hue, but rather the color of its ingredients—white poultry rather than beef or pork; white beans instead of red kidney beans; green chiles instead of red ones; and the absence of tomatoes. Using two kinds of chiles gave our white chili more complex flavor and more capsaicin: Jalapeños offered a vegetal taste, while poblanos brought earthiness. To thicken the chili, we pureed a portion of the fiber-rich white beans with some cilantro, then stirred this mixture back into the cooker to create a velvety texture that was vibrantly green and creamy (without any cream). Chicken thighs gave us a flavorful protein source and infused the chili with savory, meaty flavor. Simmering healthful zucchini in the stew after it cooked under pressure enabled the squash to retain some of its chewy texture. Serve with cubed avocado, lime wedges, and sour cream or Greek yogurt.

1½ tablespoons table salt for brining
8 ounces (1¼ cups) dried cannellini beans, picked over and rinsed
1 onion, chopped coarse
2 poblano chiles, stemmed, seeded, and chopped coarse
2 jalapeño chiles, stemmed, seeded, and chopped
1 tablespoon avocado oil
1¼ teaspoons table salt
4 garlic cloves, minced
1 tablespoon ground cumin
2 teaspoons ground coriander
2 cups unsalted chicken broth
1½ pounds boneless, skinless chicken thighs, trimmed
1½ cups fresh cilantro, trimmed and cut into 2-inch lengths, divided
2 zucchini (8 ounces each), quartered lengthwise and sliced ¼ inch thick

1   Dissolve 1½ tablespoons salt in 2 quarts cold water in large container. Add beans and soak at room temperature for at least 8 hours or up to 24 hours. Drain and rinse well.

2   Pulse onion, poblanos, and jalapeños in food processor until finely chopped, about 10 pulses, scraping down sides of bowl as needed. Transfer to bowl and set aside (do not wash food processor).

3   Using highest sauté function, heat oil in electric pressure cooker until shimmering. Add onion mixture and salt and cook until mixture is softened and lightly browned, 5 to 7 minutes. Stir in garlic, cumin, and coriander and cook until fragrant, about 30 seconds. Stir in beans and broth, scraping up any browned bits, then nestle chicken into bean mixture. Lock lid into place and close pressure-release valve. Select high pressure-cook function and cook for 9 minutes.

4   Turn off pressure cooker and quick-release pressure. Carefully remove lid, allowing steam to escape away from you. Transfer chicken to cutting board, let cool slightly, then shred into bite-size pieces using 2 forks.

5   Meanwhile, transfer 1 cup cooked bean mixture and 1 cup cilantro to food processor and process until smooth, about 1 minute. Stir zucchini into chili, partially cover, and cook, using highest sauté function, until just tender, about 4 minutes.

6   Stir in shredded chicken and any accumulated juices and processed bean mixture and cook until heated through, about 1 minute. Top individual portions with remaining cilantro and serve.

Pressure-Cooker Spiced Chicken Soup with Squash and Chickpeas

serves 6 • total time: 1¼ hours   **SUPERCHARGED**

why this recipe works • With a pressure cooker, cooking bone-in, skin-on chicken breasts until they are moist and tender is quick and easy—and produces a richly flavored, hands-off broth to boot. Here, this liquid becomes the ideal base for a chicken and vegetable soup packed with fiber and antioxidant-rich spices. Just 20 minutes under high pressure was enough to ensure the meat turned succulent and the star vegetable—fiberful butternut squash—was cooked to silky perfection. Inspired by hararat, a North African blend of spices such as cumin, coriander, and all-spice (also known as Libyan five-spice blend), we incorporated a

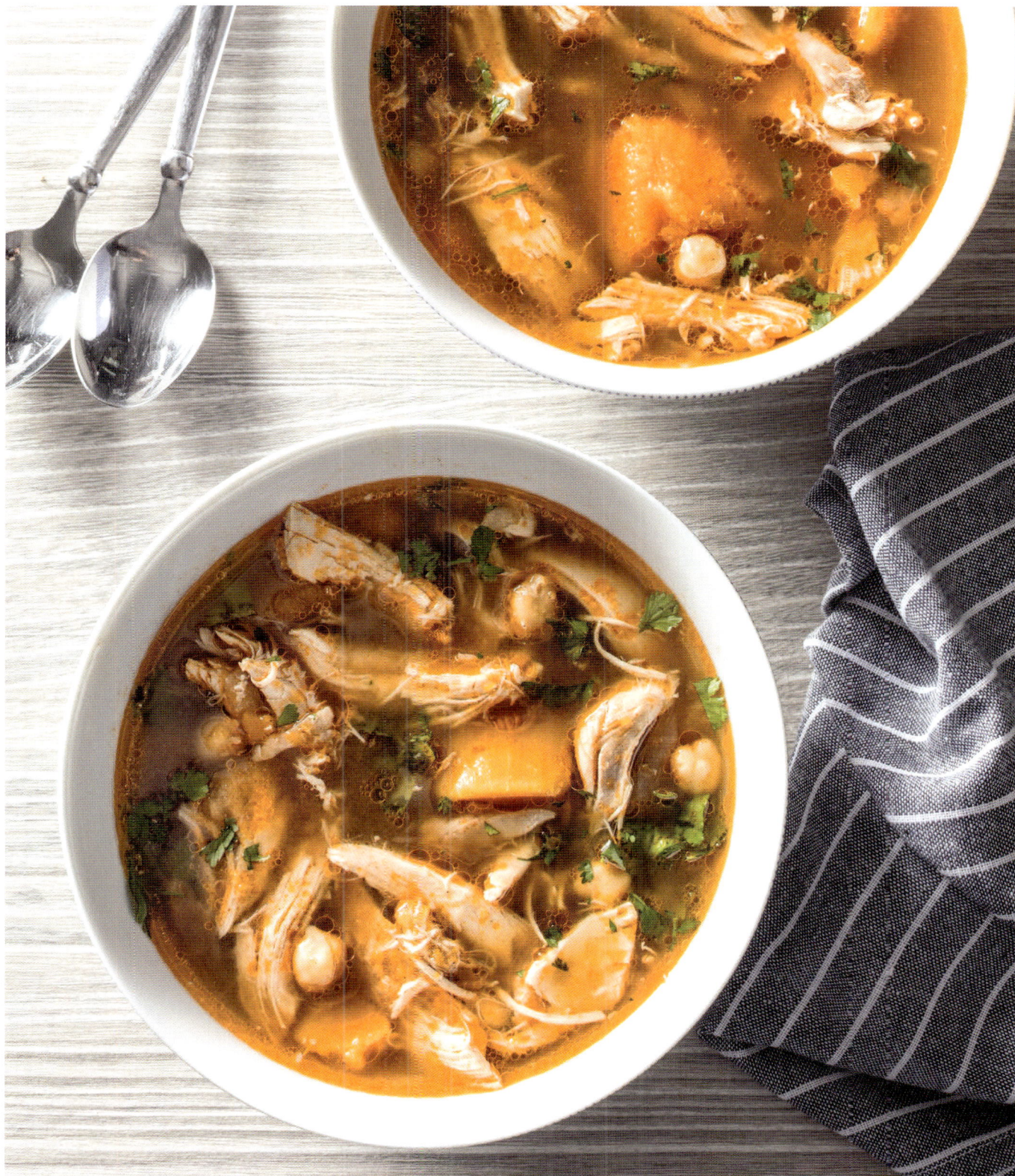

Pressure-Cooker Spiced Chicken Soup with Squash and Chickpeas

combination of warm spices that provided earthiness and subtle heat. After shredding the chicken and returning it to the pot, we stirred in canned chickpeas, a convenient source of plant-powered protein, until heated through. You can substitute 8 (5- to 7-ounce) bone-in chicken thighs for the breasts.

2 tablespoons extra-virgin olive oil
1 onion, chopped
1¾ teaspoons table salt
2 tablespoons no-salt-added tomato paste
4 garlic cloves, minced
1 tablespoon ground coriander
1½ teaspoons ground cumin
1 teaspoon ground cardamom
½ teaspoon ground allspice
¼ teaspoon cayenne pepper
7 cups water, divided
3 (12-ounce) bone-in split chicken breasts, trimmed
1½ pounds butternut squash, peeled, seeded, and cut into 1½-inch pieces (4 cups)
1 (15-ounce) can no-salt-added chickpeas, rinsed
½ cup chopped fresh cilantro

1 Using highest sauté function, heat oil in electric pressure cooker until shimmering. Add onion and salt and cook until onion is softened, about 5 minutes. Stir in tomato paste, garlic, coriander, cumin, cardamom, allspice, and cayenne and cook until fragrant, about 30 seconds. Stir in 5 cups water, scraping up any browned bits. Nestle chicken into pot, then arrange squash evenly around chicken.

2 Lock lid into place and close pressure release valve. Select high pressure-cook function and cook for 20 minutes. Turn off pressure cooker and quick-release pressure. Carefully remove lid, allowing steam to escape away from you.

3 Transfer chicken to cutting board, let cool slightly, then shred into bite-size pieces using 2 forks; discard skin and bones.

4 Using spoon, break squash into bite-size pieces. Stir shredded chicken along with any accumulated juices, chickpeas, and remaining 2 cups water into soup and let sit until heated through, about 2 minutes. Stir in cilantro and season with salt and pepper to taste. Serve.

❚ MAKE AHEAD • Soup can be refrigerated for up to 2 days.

Pressure-Cooker Smoky Turkey Meatball Soup with Kale and Manchego

serves 6 · total time: 1 hour

why this recipe works • For this sunset-hued meatball soup inspired by Spanish flavors, we started with a Spanish-style sofrito—a base of onion, bell pepper, and garlic—then added smoked paprika. After deglazing the pot with white wine, we added kale and chicken broth, then dropped in meatballs made with lean turkey (kept moist and tender thanks to a panade and a bit of Manchego, a sharp sheep's-milk cheese). The soup required a mere 3 minutes under pressure, after which we topped it off with a sprinkling of fresh parsley and a touch of extra Manchego. The meatballs stayed moist and juicy, and the kale turned tender. Be sure to use ground turkey, not ground turkey breast (also labeled 99 percent fat-free) in this recipe.

1 slice hearty white sandwich bread, torn into quarters
¼ cup milk
1 ounce Manchego cheese, grated (½ cup), plus extra for serving
5 tablespoons minced fresh parsley, divided
½ teaspoon table salt
1½ pounds ground turkey
3 tablespoons extra-virgin olive oil, divided
1 onion, chopped
1 red bell pepper, stemmed, seeded, and cut into ¾-inch pieces
4 garlic cloves, minced
1 tablespoon smoked paprika
½ cup dry white wine
8 cups unsalted chicken broth
12 ounces kale, stemmed and chopped

1 Using fork, mash bread and milk into paste in large bowl. Stir in Manchego, 3 tablespoons parsley, and salt until combined. Add turkey and knead mixture with hands until well combined. Pinch off and roll mixture into 1-tablespoon-size balls.

2 Using highest sauté function, heat 1 tablespoon oil in electric pressure cooker until shimmering. Add onion and bell pepper and cook until softened and lightly browned, 5 to 7 minutes. Stir in garlic and paprika and cook until fragrant, about 30 seconds. Stir in wine, scraping up any browned bits, and cook until nearly evaporated, about 1 minute. Stir in broth and kale, then gently submerge meatballs in broth mixture.

3 Lock lid into place and close pressure-release valve. Select high pressure-cook function and cook for 3 minutes. Turn off pressure cooker and quick-release pressure. Carefully remove lid, allowing steam to escape away from you.

4 Stir in remaining 2 tablespoons parsley and remaining 2 tablespoons oil. Season with salt and pepper to taste. Serve, passing extra Manchego separately.

> **MAKE IT GLUTEN-FREE** • Substitute gluten-free sandwich bread for the sandwich bread.

Pressure-Cooker Double Vegetable Beef Stew with Lemon Zest

serves 6 • **total time: 1½ hours**

why this recipe works • For a faster beef stew with inflammation-fighting prowess (thanks to double the amount of vegetables most recipes have), we turned to the pressure cooker to create a nourishing meal that kept its umami savor. After browning half of the boneless chuck-eye pieces (just enough for tasty fond without crowding the pot) and setting them aside, we sautéed healthful mushrooms and shallots and then added wine, broth, potatoes, and the beef (both browned and uncooked). Going under pressure for 25 minutes turned everything tender. Simmering a big helping of fiberful green beans and beta-carotene-rich carrots at the end of cooking kept their bite and flavor. A finishing sprinkle of lemon zest and parsley added bright flavor along with polyphenols. Boneless beef short ribs can be substituted for the chuck-eye roast. If using larger potatoes, cut them into 1½-inch pieces.

- 1½ pounds boneless beef chuck-eye roast, trimmed and cut into 1½-inch pieces
- 1¼ teaspoons table salt, divided
- 2 tablespoons avocado oil, divided
- 8 ounces cremini mushrooms, trimmed and halved if small or quartered if large
- 6 shallots, peeled and halved lengthwise
- ¼ cup all-purpose flour
- 1 tablespoon tomato paste
- 1 tablespoon minced fresh thyme or 1 teaspoon dried
- ¾ cup dry white wine
- 2 cups unsalted beef broth
- 1 pound small red or yellow potatoes, unpeeled, halved
- 12 ounces green beans, trimmed and cut into 1½-inch lengths on bias
- 3 carrots, peeled and sliced ¼ inch thick on bias
- 6 tablespoons chopped fresh parsley
- 1 tablespoon grated lemon zest

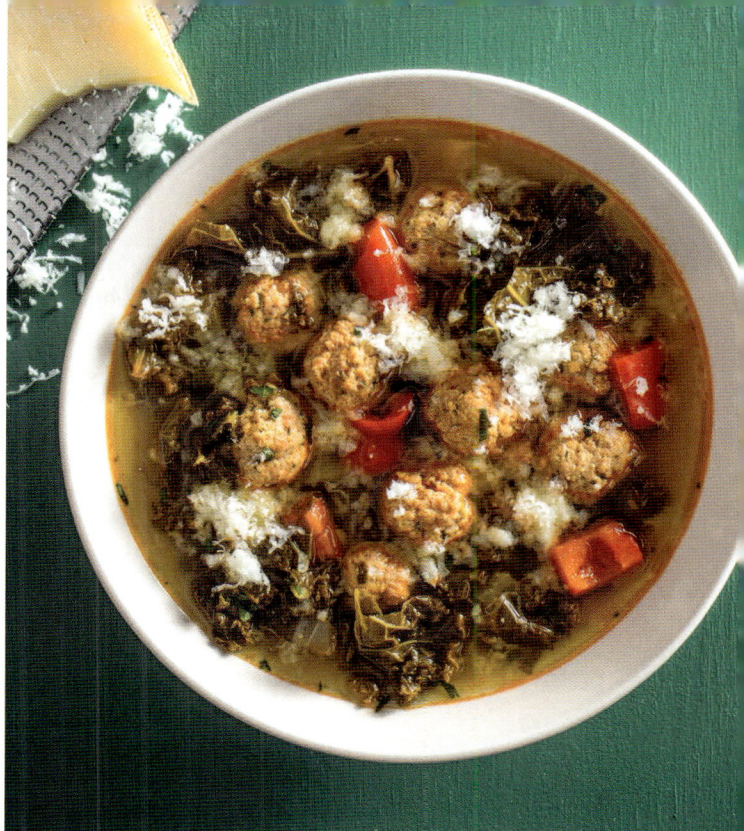

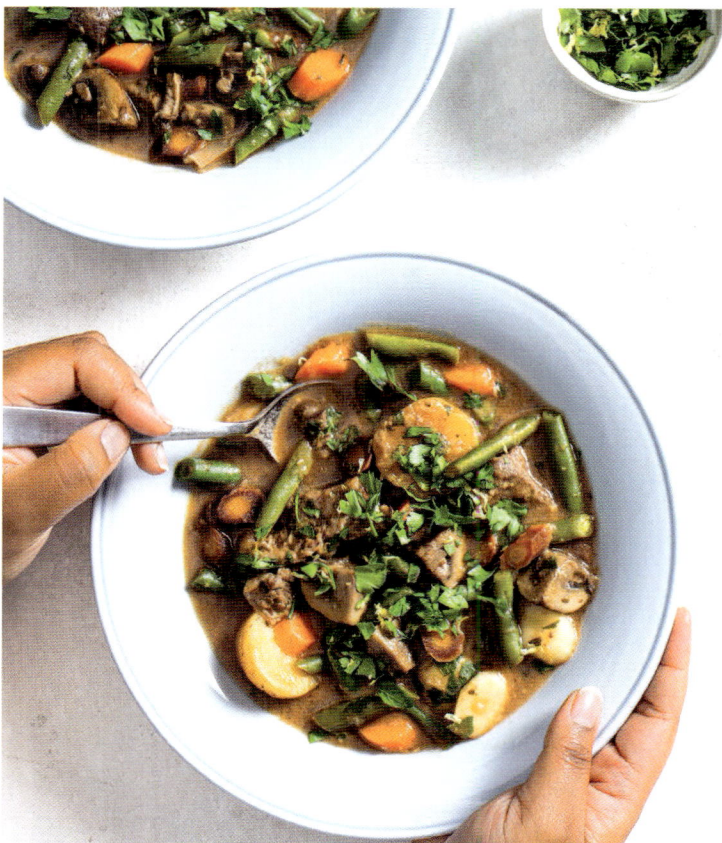

| top | Pressure-Cooker Smoky Turkey Meatball Soup with Kale and Manchego |
| bottom | Pressure-Cooker Double Vegetable Beef Stew with Lemon Zest |

1   Pat beef dry with paper towels and sprinkle with ½ teaspoon salt. Using highest sauté function, heat 1 tablespoon oil in electric pressure cooker until just smoking. Brown half of beef on all sides, 5 to 7 minutes; transfer to bowl. Set aside remaining uncooked beef.

2   Add mushrooms, shallots, and remaining 1 tablespoon oil to fat left in pot and cook, using lowest sauté function, until mushrooms are softened, about 3 minutes. Stir in flour, tomato paste, and thyme and cook until fragrant, about 30 seconds. Stir in wine, scraping up any browned bits, and cook until mixture forms thick paste, about 30 seconds. Whisk in broth, smoothing out any lumps. Stir in potatoes and remaining ¾ teaspoon salt, then stir in browned beef and any accumulated juices and remaining uncooked beef.

3   Lock lid into place and close pressure-release valve. Select high pressure-cook function and cook for 25 minutes. Turn off pressure cooker and quick-release pressure. Carefully remove lid, allowing steam to escape away from you.

4   Stir in green beans and carrots, partially cover, and cook, using lowest sauté function, until green beans and carrots are crisp-tender, 3 to 5 minutes. Combine parsley and lemon zest in bowl. Stir half of parsley mixture into stew and season with salt and pepper to taste. Sprinkle individual portions with remaining parsley mixture before serving.

❙   **MAKE AHEAD** • Stew can be refrigerated for up to 2 days.

Pressure-Cooker Pork Pozole Rojo

serves 6 • **total time: 1 hour, plus 8 hours soaking**

why this recipe works • A pressure cooker makes quick work of this Mexican soup of pork and hominy. For savory depth in less time, we skipped browning the pork and built a flavor-rich base of onion, ancho chile powder, and oregano. Country-style pork ribs are a fattier but deeply flavorful cut, so a judicious amount went a long way in flavoring this big-batch soup while moderating saturated fat. Dried hominy, which we soaked, released enough starches to give our pozole rojo plenty of body. You can substitute two (15-ounce) cans rinsed hominy for the soaked dried hominy. Boneless pork butt can be substituted for the ribs. Serve with shredded cabbage, thinly sliced radishes, diced avocado, cilantro, and lime wedges.

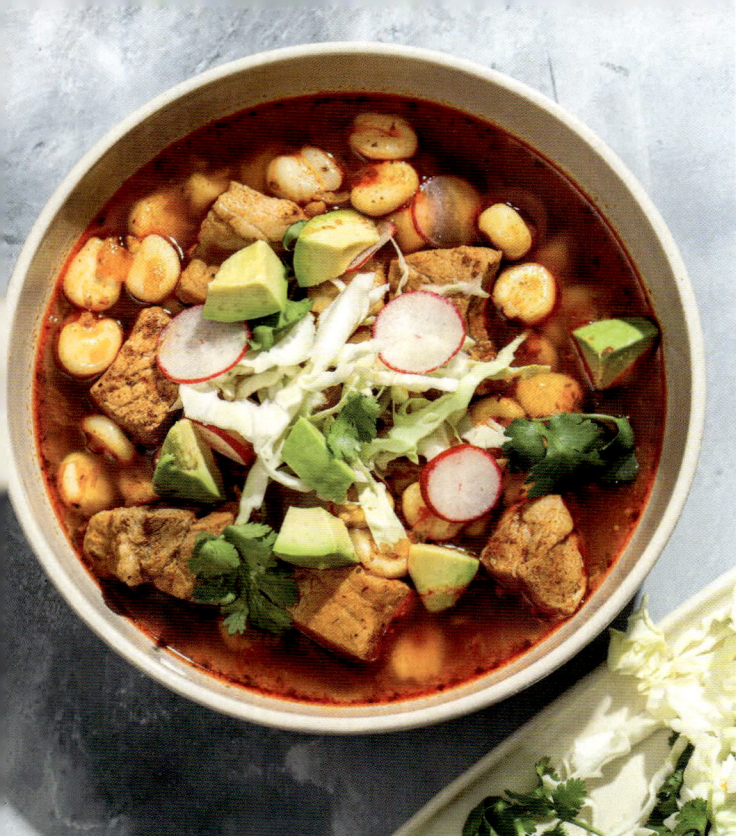

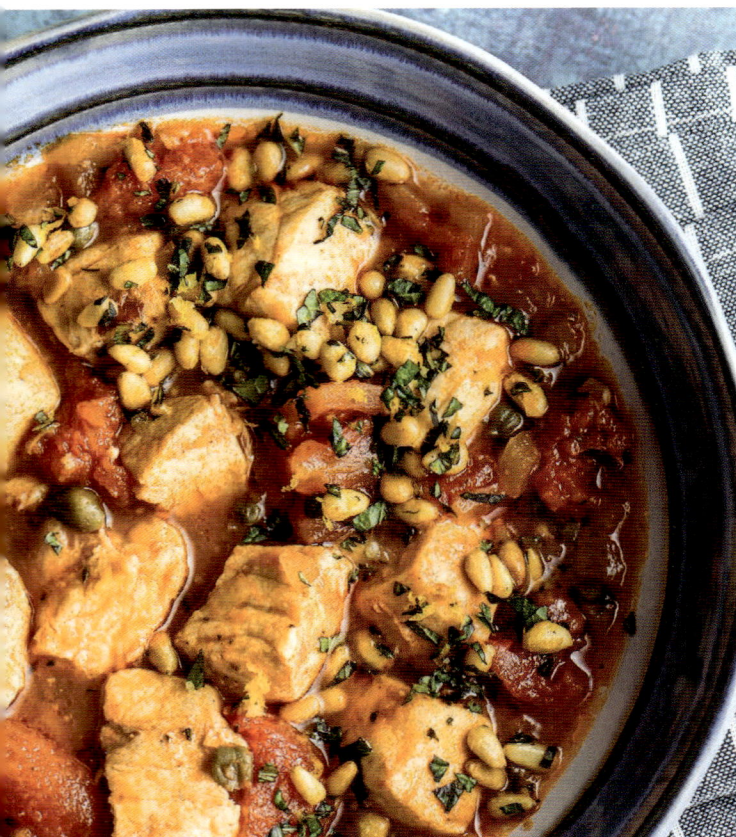

top | Pressure-Cooker Pork Pozole Rojo
bottom | Pressure-Cooker Swordfish Stew with Tomatoes, Capers, and Pine Nuts

8 ounces (1¼ cups) dried whole white or yellow hominy
1 tablespoon extra-virgin olive oil
1 onion, chopped fine
2 tablespoons ancho chile powder
5 garlic cloves, minced
1 teaspoon dried oregano
4 cups unsalted chicken broth
1½ pounds boneless country-style pork ribs, trimmed and cut into 1-inch pieces
1 teaspoon table salt
½ teaspoon pepper
2 bay leaves

1 Place hominy and 2 quarts cold water in large container. Let soak at room temperature for at least 8 hours or up to 24 hours. Drain and rinse well.

2 Using highest sauté function, heat oil in electric pressure cooker until shimmering. Add onion and cook until softened and lightly browned, 5 to 7 minutes. Add ancho chile powder, garlic, and oregano and cook, stirring frequently, until fragrant, about 30 seconds. Stir in broth, scraping up any browned bits. Stir in pork, hominy, salt, pepper, and bay leaves.

3 Lock lid into place and close pressure-release valve. Select high pressure-cook function and cook for 25 minutes. Turn off pressure cooker and quick-release pressure. Carefully remove lid, allowing steam to escape away from you.

4 Discard bay leaves. Using wide, shallow spoon, skim excess fat from surface of soup. Season with salt and pepper to taste, and serve.

❙ MAKE AHEAD • Soup can be refrigerated for up to 2 days.

Pressure-Cooker Swordfish Stew with Tomatoes, Capers, and Pine Nuts

serves 4 to 6 • **total time: 45 minutes**   **FAST**

why this recipe works • This Sicilian-inspired stew is the ultimate balance of sweet, sour, and salty notes. We chose swordfish for its meaty texture that could stand up to a symphony of bold flavors. For the base, we created an antioxidant-packed stock of onions, garlic, thyme, and red pepper flakes simmered in white wine,

canned tomatoes, and clam juice. We added raisins and capers for contrasting sweet and briny bursts. The swordfish only needed a minute under pressure to emerge tender and succulent. To top our stew, we combined orange zest, mint, and garlic, along with some pine nuts for crunch. Halibut, mahi-mahi, red snapper, and striped bass are good substitutes for the swordfish. If the swordfish has not reached at least 130 degrees after releasing the pressure, partially cover the pot and continue to cook using residual heat until it reaches 130 degrees. Serve with crusty bread.

2 tablespoons extra-virgin olive oil
2 onions, chopped fine
1 teaspoon minced fresh thyme or ¼ teaspoon dried
  Pinch red pepper flakes
4 garlic cloves, minced, divided
1 (8-ounce) bottle clam juice
¼ cup dry white wine
1 (28-ounce) can no-salt-added whole peeled tomatoes, drained with juice reserved, chopped coarse
¼ cup golden raisins
2 tablespoons capers, rinsed
½ teaspoon table salt
½ teaspoon pepper
1½ pounds skinless swordfish steaks, 1 to 1½ inches thick, cut into 1-inch pieces
¼ cup pine nuts, toasted
¼ cup minced fresh mint
1 teaspoon grated orange zest

1 Using highest sauté function, heat oil in electric pressure cooker until shimmering. Add onions and cook until softened and lightly browned, 3 to 5 minutes. Add thyme, pepper flakes, and three-quarters of garlic and cook, stirring frequently, until fragrant, about 30 seconds.

2 Stir in clam juice and wine, scraping up any browned bits, then stir in tomatoes and reserved juice, raisins, capers, salt, and pepper. Arrange swordfish pieces in even layer in pot and spoon some cooking liquid over top.

3 Lock lid into place and close pressure-release valve. Select high pressure-cook function and cook for 1 minute. Turn off pressure cooker and quick-release pressure. Carefully remove lid, allowing steam to escape away from you.

4 Combine pine nuts, mint, orange zest, and remaining garlic in bowl. Season stew with salt and pepper to taste. Sprinkle individual portions with pine nut mixture before serving.

Pressure-Cooker Chicken and Braised Radishes with Dukkah

serves 4 • total time: 1 hour

why this recipe works • A pressure cooker is perfect for braising radishes because the quick time under pressure turns them delicately sweet while maintaining their crunch. We browned some chicken breasts first, removed them from the pot, and then cooked garlic in the residual heat along with radishes and dukkah, an Egyptian spice blend, for sweetness and warmth, and lemon for brightness. We returned the chicken to the pot and cooked it all under pressure for just a few minutes so the flavors could meld. After releasing the pressure, we rested the chicken while we tossed the radishes with watercress for a fresh accent. A creamy sauce of nutty tahini, yogurt, and lemon juice was the perfect complement. If you can't find watercress, you can substitute baby arugula.

½ cup plain yogurt
¼ cup tahini
6 garlic cloves, minced, divided
4 teaspoons grated lemon zest, divided, plus 2 teaspoons juice
2 tablespoons minced fresh parsley
4 (6- to 8-ounce) boneless, skinless chicken breasts, trimmed
¾ teaspoon table salt, divided
¼ teaspoon pepper
4 teaspoons avocado oil, divided
1½ pounds radishes, trimmed and halved lengthwise
½ cup unsalted chicken broth
3 tablespoons dukkah, divided
2 ounces (2 cups) watercress

1 Combine yogurt, tahini, 1 teaspoon garlic, 1 teaspoon lemon zest, lemon juice, and parsley in small bowl and season with salt and pepper to taste; set aside for serving.

2 Cover chicken breasts with plastic wrap and pound thick ends gently with meat pounder until ¾ inch thick. Pat chicken dry with paper towels and sprinkle with ¼ teaspoon salt and pepper. Using highest sauté function, heat 1½ teaspoons oil in electric pressure cooker until just smoking. Add 2 pieces chicken smooth side down to pot and cook until well browned on first side, 3 to 5 minutes; transfer to plate. Repeat with 1½ teaspoons oil and remaining 2 pieces chicken; transfer to plate. Turn off pressure cooker.

3 Add remaining garlic and remaining 1 teaspoon oil to fat left in pot. Cook using residual heat, stirring frequently, until fragrant, about 30 seconds. Stir in radishes, broth, 1 tablespoon dukkah, remaining 1 tablespoon lemon zest, and remaining ½ teaspoon salt, scraping up any browned bits. Arrange chicken browned side

up in even layer on top of radishes and add any accumulated juices. Lock lid into place and close pressure-release valve. Select high pressure-cook function and cook for 4 minutes.

4 Turn off pressure cooker and quick-release pressure. Carefully remove lid, allowing steam to escape away from you. Transfer chicken to cutting board, tent with aluminum foil, and let rest while finishing radishes.

5 Drain radishes in colander and transfer to large bowl. Add watercress to bowl, 1 handful at a time, and toss with warm radishes until watercress is slightly wilted, about 1 minute. Slice chicken ½ inch thick. Divide yogurt mixture among 4 individual serving plates and spread into even layer. Arrange radish mixture and chicken on top and sprinkle with remaining 2 tablespoons dukkah. Serve.

MAKE IT DAIRY-FREE • Substitute plant-based yogurt for the dairy yogurt.

Pressure-Cooker Chicken and Black Rice Bowls with Peanut-Sesame Sauce

serves 4 • total time: 1 hour

why this recipe works • Black rice, rich in fiber and antioxidants, makes a perfectly chewy, hearty base for a nourishing and delicious chicken bowls with Thai-inspired flavors. To infuse the rice with a piquant, citrusy taste, we started by blooming fresh ginger and lemongrass. We enclosed the chicken thighs in a foil packet and cooked them with the rice. This ensured moist meat while keeping the chicken from soaking up the dark purple color of the rice. We rounded out the bowls with sweet snap peas, crisp-tender carrots, and crunchy bean sprouts. To finish, we drizzled the bowls with a savory peanut-sesame sauce. You can substitute long-grain brown rice for the black rice, if you prefer.

1½ pounds boneless, skinless chicken thighs, trimmed
1 tablespoon avocado oil
1 lemongrass stalk, trimmed to bottom 6 inches and minced
1 (2-inch) piece ginger, peeled and sliced thin
2 cups water
1½ cups black rice, rinsed
½ teaspoon table salt
4 ounces sugar snap peas, strings removed, sliced thin on bias
2 carrots, peeled and cut into 2-inch-long matchsticks
2 ounces (1 cup) bean sprouts
1 recipe Peanut-Sesame Sauce
½ cup fresh mint leaves, torn

1 Arrange chicken in even layer in center of 20 by 12-inch sheet of aluminum foil. Bring short sides of foil together and crimp edges to seal tightly. Crimp open edges of packet.

2 Using highest sauté function, cook oil, lemongrass, and ginger in electric pressure cooker until fragrant, about 30 seconds. Stir in water, rice, and salt, scraping up any browned bits. Place foil packet on top of rice mixture. Lock lid into place and close pressure-release valve. Select high pressure-cook function and cook for 18 minutes.

3 Turn off pressure cooker and quick-release pressure. Carefully remove lid, allowing steam to escape away from you. Transfer foil packet to plate, brushing any rice back into pot. Lay clean dish towel over pot, replace lid, and let sit for 5 minutes.

4 Meanwhile, carefully open foil packet and transfer chicken to cutting board; discard foil and any juices. Shred chicken into bite-size pieces using 2 forks. Fluff rice gently with fork. Transfer rice to individual serving bowls and top with chicken, snap peas, carrots, and bean sprouts. Drizzle with peanut-sesame sauce and sprinkle with mint. Serve.

| **MAKE AHEAD** • Cooked chicken and rice can be refrigerated for up to 3 days.

Peanut-Sesame Sauce

makes about ⅔ cup • total time: 10 minutes

    3   tablespoons smooth or chunky peanut butter
    3   tablespoons toasted sesame seeds
    2   tablespoons low-sodium soy sauce or
        low-sodium tamari
  1½   tablespoons unseasoned rice vinegar
  1½   tablespoons packed light brown sugar
  1½   teaspoons grated fresh ginger
    1   garlic clove, minced
    ¾   teaspoon sriracha

Process all ingredients in blender until mixture is smooth and has consistency of heavy cream, about 1 minute (adjust consistency with warm water, 1 tablespoon at a time, as needed). (Sauce can be refrigerated for up to 3 days.)

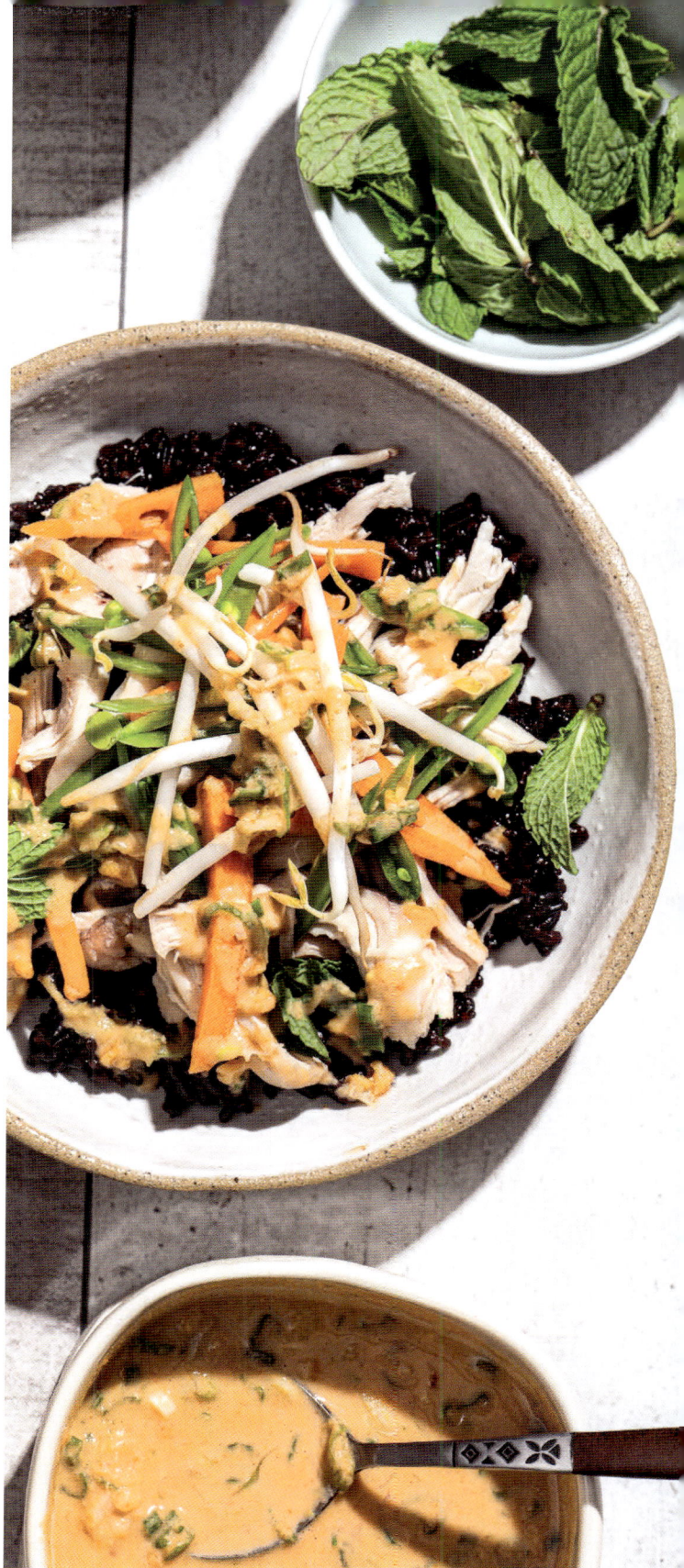

Pressure-Cooker Chicken and Black Rice Bowls with Peanut-Sesame Sauce

Pressure-Cooker Shredded Chicken Tacos with Mango Salsa

serves 4 • total time: 45 minutes **FAST**

why this recipe works • For truly flavor-packed chicken tacos from the pressure cooker, we chose boneless thighs, which are convenient and boast deeply savory flavor. For smokiness, we built a base of cumin, cinnamon, and chipotle in adobo—all of which boosted the complexity of the sauce. We added tomato sauce and nestled the chicken in the sauce, then relied on the moist heat of the pressure cooker to create saucy chicken that was meltingly tender in just 3 minutes. A potato masher allowed us to shred the chicken right in the pot, minimizing cleanup. Simmering the shredded chicken in the sauce before serving gave the sauce a chance to thicken and work its way into every crevice of the meat's abundant surface area. A sweet mango salsa was the perfect refreshing foil to the smoky, meaty filling and a sprinkle of salty cotija was the final touch to kick taco night up a notch.

Salsa
- 1   ripe but firm mango, peeled, pitted, and cut into ¼-inch pieces
- ¼   cup fresh cilantro leaves
- 1   jalapeño chile, stemmed, seeded, and minced
- 1   small shallot, minced
- 1   tablespoon lime juice

Filling
- 1   tablespoon avocado oil
- 4   garlic cloves, minced
- 1   teaspoon ground cumin
- ¼   teaspoon ground cinnamon
- 1   (8-ounce) can no-salt-added tomato sauce
- ½   cup unsalted chicken broth
- 2   tablespoons minced canned chipotle chile in adobo sauce plus 2 teaspoons adobo sauce
- ½   teaspoon table salt
- 1½ pounds boneless, skinless chicken thighs, trimmed and quartered

- 12 (6-inch) corn or flour tortillas, warmed
- 2   ounces cotija cheese, crumbled (½ cup)
     Lime wedges

1 **For the salsa** Combine all ingredients in bowl and season with salt and pepper to taste; set aside for serving.

2 **For the filling** Using highest sauté function, cook oil, garlic, cumin, and cinnamon in electric pressure cooker until fragrant, about 3 minutes. Stir in tomato sauce, broth, chipotle and adobo sauce, and salt, scraping up any browned bits. Stir in chicken. Lock lid into place and close pressure-release valve. Select high pressure-cook function and cook for 3 minutes.

3 Turn off pressure cooker and quick-release pressure. Carefully remove lid, allowing steam to escape away from you. Using potato masher, mash chicken until coarsely shredded. Using highest sauté function, cook chicken until sauce has thickened, 5 to 7 minutes. Season with salt and pepper to taste. Serve chicken with tortillas, passing salsa, cotija, and lime wedges separately.

MAKE AHEAD • Chicken filling can be refrigerated for up to 2 days.

MAKE IT DAIRY-FREE • Omit the cotija cheese.

Pressure-Cooker Chipotle Chicken and Black Beans with Pickled Cabbage

serves 4 • total time: 1 hour

why this recipe works • This recipe is an excellent showcase for the pressure cooker's versatility in streamlining almost every step of dinner, from searing to sautéing, blooming to braising. First, we seared bone-in chicken thighs to render the drippings, then bloomed chipotle, garlic, and oregano in the flavorful juices, which provided plenty of richness (without going overboard on saturated fat). The warming seasonings we chose weren't just bold in flavor; they also added anti-inflammatory compounds like capsaicin and allicin. Returning the chicken to the pot to cook in broth under pressure created a magnificent liquid. To sop up that deliciousness, we warmed canned black beans in the flavorful broth as the chicken rested. On the side, we made a vinegar and coriander brine to quick-pickle red cabbage into a shockingly pink accompaniment. The sweet and sour notes offered a fresh, crunchy counter to the succulent chicken and spiced beans. The result was a hearty meal full of savoriness and some heat. For a milder dish, omit the chipotle in step 6.

Pickled Cabbage
- ½   cup white wine vinegar
- 1   tablespoon sugar
- 1   teaspoon ground coriander
- 1½ cups shredded red cabbage

Chicken

- 4 (5- to 7-ounce) bone-in chicken thighs, trimmed
- 1 tablespoon avocado oil
- 1 onion, chopped
- 4 teaspoons minced canned chipotle chile in adobo sauce, divided
- 3 garlic cloves, minced
- 1 teaspoon minced fresh oregano or ½ teaspoon dried
- ¾ cup unsalted chicken broth
- 2 (15-ounce) cans no-salt-added black beans, rinsed
- 1 cup fresh cilantro, trimmed and cut into 2-inch lengths, divided

1 **For the pickled cabbage** Microwave vinegar, sugar, and coriander in medium bowl until steaming, 1 to 2 minutes; whisk to dissolve sugar. Add cabbage to hot brine and let sit, stirring occasionally, for 30 minutes. Drain cabbage and return to now-empty bowl; set aside for serving.

2 **For the chicken** Meanwhile, pat chicken dry with paper towels. Using highest sauté function, heat oil in electric pressure cooker until just smoking. Place chicken skin side down in pot and cook until well browned on first side, about 5 minutes; transfer to plate.

3 Add onion to fat left in pot and cook, using lowest sauté function, until softened, 3 to 5 minutes. Stir in 1 tablespoon chipotle, garlic, and oregano and cook until fragrant, about 30 seconds. Stir in broth, scraping up any browned bits.

4 Place chicken skin side up in pot, adding any accumulated juices, and spoon some cooking liquid over top. Lock lid into place and close pressure-release valve. Select high pressure-cook function and cook for 9 minutes.

5 Turn off pressure cooker and quick-release pressure. Carefully remove lid, allowing steam to escape away from you. Transfer chicken to clean plate and discard skin, if desired. Tent with aluminum foil and let rest while finishing beans.

6 Stir beans and remaining 1 teaspoon chipotle into braising liquid and cook, using highest sauté function, until beans are heated through, about 2 minutes. Turn off pressure cooker. Stir in ¾ cup cilantro and season with salt and pepper to taste. Serve chicken with beans and pickled cabbage and top with remaining cilantro.

MAKE AHEAD • Pickled cabbage, cooked chicken, and beans can be refrigerated for up to 3 days.

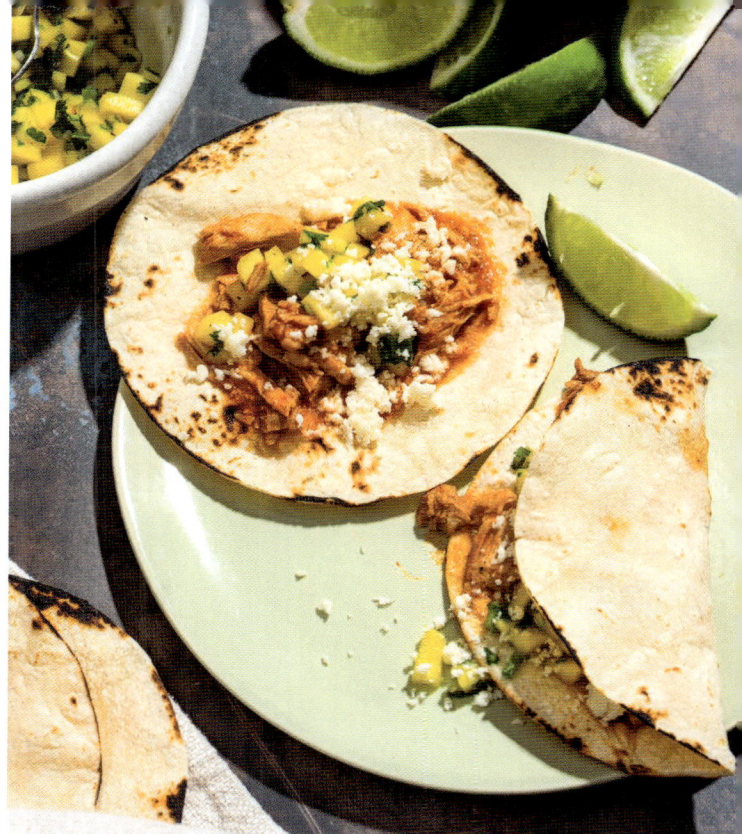

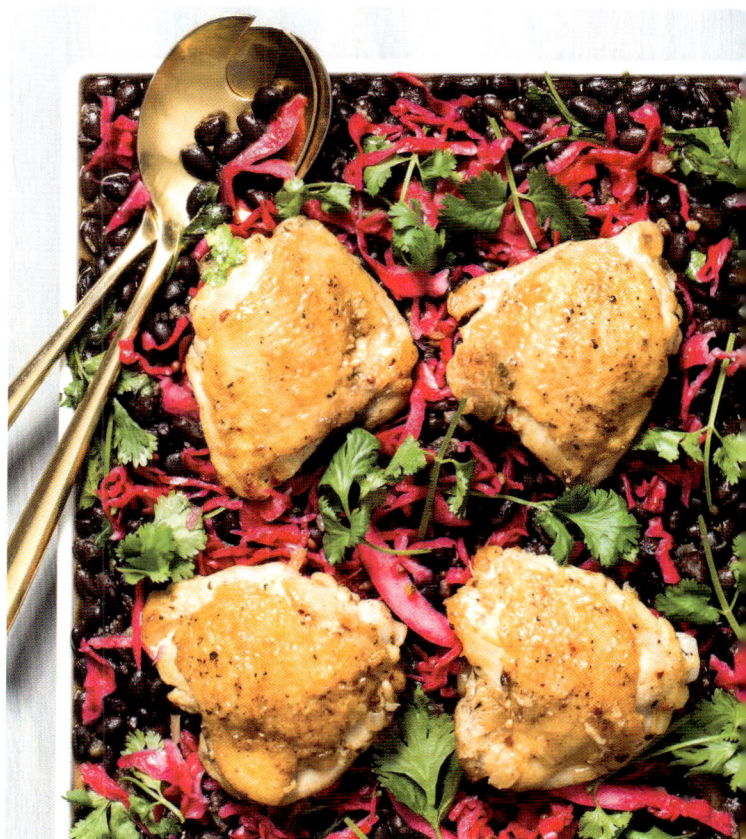

top | *Pressure-Cooker Shredded Chicken Tacos with Mango Salsa*
bottom | *Pressure-Cooker Chipotle Chicken and Black Beans with Pickled Cabbage*

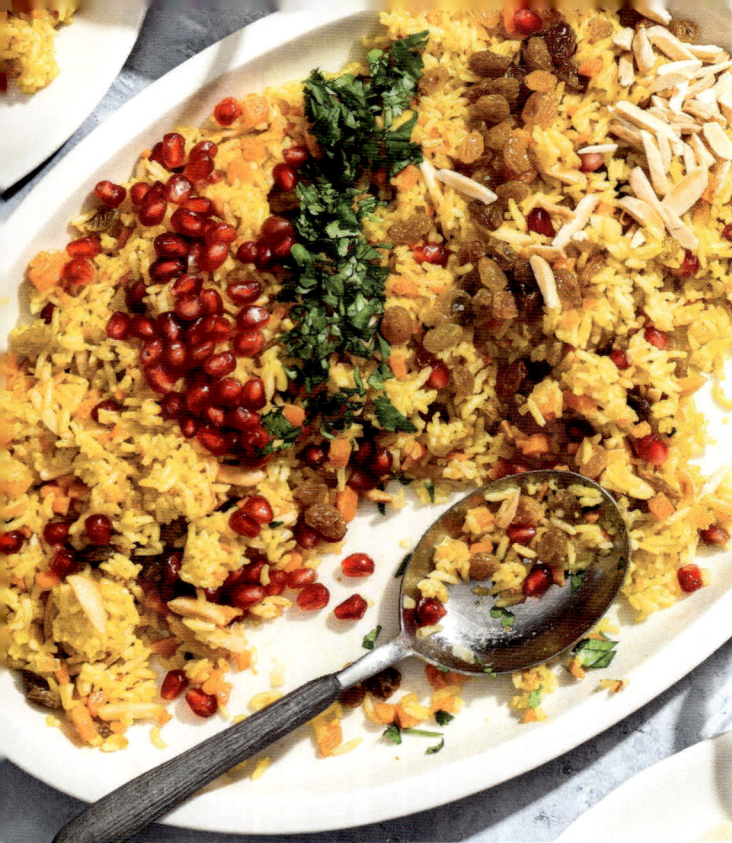

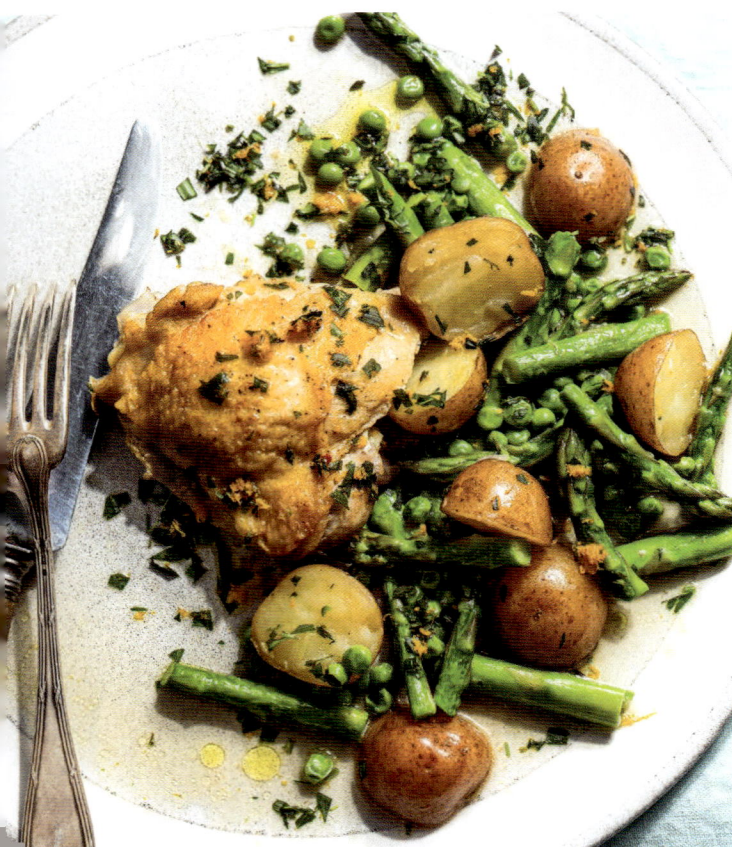

Pressure-Cooker Javaher Polo with Chicken

serves 4 · total time: 1 hour

why this recipe works · Javaher polo, a staple celebratory Persian dish of jeweled rice, is often served during wedding celebrations and special occasions. Consisting of basmati rice perfumed with saffron and cardamom, the dish gets its name from the colorful dried fruit and nuts that traditionally stud its appealingly golden surface in intricate designs. We love the dish's subtle balances between sweet and savory, nuts and fruit, and fresh and warm and were inspired to create a recipe for the pressure cooker. We first browned bone-in chicken breasts skin side down and then sautéed onion and carrot in the rendered fat. We then added rice, broth, and saffron, returned the chicken to the pot, and cooked under pressure until the rice was tender and the chicken cooked through. We finished the rice with golden raisins, toasted almonds, and pomegranate seeds for their diverse textures and anti-inflammatory compounds. For weeknight ease, we forewent any intricate design and instead folded a portion of the toppings into the cooked rice, saving some for a garnish that created a pleasing textural contrast. A drizzle of lemony yogurt sauce elevated the meal with bright creaminess and pleasant tang. You can use store-bought preserved lemons or make our Quick Preserved Lemon (page 209); you can also substitute 1 tablespoon lemon zest, though the flavor will be less complex. An equal amount of fresh lemon juice can be substituted for the preserved lemon brine. You can substitute long-grain white rice for the basmati.

½ cup plain yogurt

2 tablespoons rinsed and minced preserved lemon, plus 1 tablespoon brine

3 tablespoons chopped fresh cilantro, divided

1 teaspoon ground cardamom

1 teaspoon ground coriander

2 (12-ounce) bone-in split chicken breasts, trimmed and halved crosswise

¾ teaspoon table salt, divided

2 tablespoons avocado oil, divided

1 onion, chopped fine

2 carrots, peeled and chopped fine
  Pinch saffron threads, crumbled

2 cups unsalted chicken broth

1½ cups basmati rice, rinsed

¾ cup golden raisins, divided

½ cup slivered almonds, toasted, divided

½ cup pomegranate seeds, divided

1 Combine yogurt, preserved lemon brine, and 2 tablespoons cilantro in small bowl and season with salt and pepper to taste; set yogurt sauce aside for serving.

2 Combine cardamom and coriander in separate small bowl. Pat chicken dry with paper towels and sprinkle with 1 teaspoon spice mixture and ¼ teaspoon salt. Using highest sauté function, heat 1 tablespoon oil in electric pressure cooker until just smoking. Place chicken skin side down in pot and cook until well browned on first side, about 5 minutes; transfer to plate.

3 Add onion, carrots, remaining 1 tablespoon oil, and remaining ½ teaspoon salt to fat left in pot and cook, using highest sauté function, until vegetables are softened, 3 to 5 minutes. Stir in remaining 1 teaspoon spice mixture and saffron and cook until fragrant, about 30 seconds. Stir in broth and rice, scraping up any browned bits. Nestle chicken skin side up into rice mixture and add any accumulated juices. Lock lid into place and close pressure-release valve. Select high pressure-cook function and cook for 7 minutes.

4 Turn off pressure cooker and quick-release pressure. Carefully remove lid, allowing steam to escape away from you. Transfer chicken to cutting board and discard skin, if desired. Tent with aluminum foil and let rest while finishing rice.

5 Sprinkle minced preserved lemon, ½ cup raisins, ¼ cup almonds, and ¼ cup pomegranate seeds over rice in pot. Lay clean dish towel over pot, replace lid, and let sit for 5 minutes. Fluff rice gently with fork to combine, then transfer to serving platter. Sprinkle rice attractively with remaining 1 tablespoon cilantro, remaining ¼ cup raisins, remaining ¼ cup almonds, and remaining ¼ cup pomegranate seeds. Serve chicken with rice and yogurt sauce.

MAKE AHEAD • Cooked chicken and rice can be refrigerated for up to 3 days.

MAKE IT DAIRY-FREE • Substitute plant-based yogurt for the dairy yogurt.

Pressure-Cooker Chicken with Spring Vegetables

serves 4 • total time: 1 hour

why this recipe works • For this chicken recipe, we wanted to evoke the vibrant flavors of springtime. Red potatoes, asparagus, and peas offered a variety of textures and flavors to accompany meaty chicken thighs. These all cook at different rates, so we gave our chicken a head start by browning it before quickly sautéing garlic, shallot, and red pepper flakes. Then we added broth, red potatoes, and thyme and pressure-cooked the chicken atop the mixture. Red potatoes have a higher moisture content than other potatoes, so they held their shape well under pressure. We stirred asparagus and peas into the pot, and a garnish of tarragon and fresh orange zest woke up the dish and rounded everything out. If using larger potatoes, cut them into 1½-inch pieces. Look for asparagus spears that are about ½ inch thick at the base.

  4 (5- to 7-ounce) bone-in chicken thighs, trimmed
  ¾ teaspoon table salt, divided
  ¼ teaspoon pepper
  1 tablespoon avocado oil
  1 shallot, sliced thin
  2 garlic cloves, sliced thin
     Pinch red pepper flakes
  2 cups unsalted chicken broth
  1 pound small red potatoes, unpeeled, halved
  3 sprigs fresh thyme
  1 pound asparagus, trimmed and cut into 2-inch lengths
  2 cups frozen peas
  2 tablespoons chopped fresh tarragon
  2 teaspoons grated orange zest

1 Pat chicken dry with paper towels and sprinkle with ¼ teaspoon salt and pepper. Using highest sauté function, heat oil in electric pressure cooker until just smoking. Place chicken skin side down in pot and cook until well browned on first side, about 5 minutes; transfer to plate. Turn off pressure cooker.

2 Add shallot, garlic, and pepper flakes to fat left in pot and cook, using residual heat, until shallot is softened, about 1 minute. Stir in broth, potatoes, thyme sprigs, and remaining ½ teaspoon salt, scraping up any browned bits. Place chicken skin side up on top of potato mixture and add any accumulated juices. Lock lid into place and close pressure-release valve. Select high pressure-cook function and cook for 9 minutes.

3 Turn off pressure cooker and quick-release pressure. Carefully remove lid, allowing steam to escape away from you. Transfer chicken to serving platter and discard skin, if desired; tent with aluminum foil and let rest while finishing vegetables.

4 Discard thyme sprigs. Stir asparagus and peas into potato mixture, partially cover, and cook, using highest sauté function, until vegetables are crisp-tender, 3 to 5 minutes. Turn off pressure cooker.

5 Combine tarragon and orange zest in small bowl. Stir half of tarragon mixture into vegetables and season with salt and pepper to taste. Serve chicken with vegetables, sprinkling individual portions with remaining tarragon mixture.

Pressure-Cooker Chicken and Couscous with Prunes and Olives

serves 4 · total time: 1 hour

why this recipe works · This pressure-cooker chicken dish is inspired by the '80s sensation popularized by *The Silver Palate Cookbook*, chicken Marbella. Chicken Marbella includes a mixture of pungent ingredients like olives and capers, but they're all brought together by a sweet base of pureed prunes and brown sugar. To modernize the dish, we pressure-cook it to make it quick and eliminate pureeing the prunes (and the brown sugar), instead adding olives and capers after the chicken was cooked so they retain their brightness and individual textures. Cooking some prunes under pressure turned them jammy and brought out their natural sugars. We stirred the rest of the prunes into the dish, and their sweetness and texture shines against the vinegar and sherry. For an accurate measurement of boiling water, bring a full kettle of water to boil and then measure out the desired amount.

- 4 shallots, sliced thin, divided (¾ cup)
- 1½ teaspoons red wine vinegar, divided
- 4 teaspoons avocado oil, divided
- 4 (5- to 7-ounce) bone-in chicken thighs, trimmed
- ½ teaspoon table salt, divided
- 3 garlic cloves, minced
- 1 teaspoon dried oregano
- ¼ teaspoon red pepper flakes
- 1 cup unsalted chicken broth
- ¼ cup dry sherry
- ¾ cup chopped pitted prunes, divided
- 1 cup boiling water
- 1 cup couscous
- ⅓ cup pitted brine-cured green olives, halved
- 2 tablespoons capers, rinsed
- 1 cup fresh parsley leaves

1 Combine ¼ cup shallots, 1 teaspoon vinegar, and 1 teaspoon oil in small bowl; set aside. Pat chicken dry with paper towels and sprinkle with ¼ teaspoon salt. Using highest sauté function, heat remaining 1 tablespoon oil in electric pressure cooker until just smoking. Place chicken skin side down in pot and cook until well browned on first side, about 5 minutes; transfer to plate.

2 Add remaining shallots to fat left in pot and cook, using lowest sauté function, until shallots are softened, about 1 minute. Stir in garlic, oregano, and pepper flakes and cook until fragrant, about 30 seconds. Stir in broth, sherry, and ½ cup prunes, scraping up any browned bits. Place chicken skin side up in pot and add any accumulated juices. Lock lid into place and close pressure-release valve. Select high pressure-cook function and cook for 12 minutes.

3 Meanwhile, combine boiling water, couscous, and remaining ¼ teaspoon salt in large bowl. Cover and let sit for 10 minutes. Fluff couscous with fork and season with salt and pepper to taste; set aside.

4 Turn off pressure cooker and quick-release pressure. Carefully remove lid, allowing steam to escape away from you. Transfer chicken to serving platter and discard skin, if desired. Stir olives, capers, remaining ¼ cup prunes, and remaining ½ teaspoon vinegar into sauce in pot and season with salt and pepper to taste. Add parsley to shallot-vinegar mixture, toss to coat, and season with salt and pepper to taste. Serve chicken with couscous, sauce, and parsley salad.

Pressure-Cooker Shredded Beef Tacos with Jicama Slaw

serves 6 · total time: 1 hour

why this recipe works · Chuck roast turns meltingly tender and shreddable in a pressure cooker, becoming an ideal taco filling. Divided across six hearty servings, a judicious amount of the meat went a long way when paired with a flavorful jicama slaw. Cutting the roast into 1-inch pieces helped it cook faster and become even more tender. To make our well-spiced sauce, we combined a flavorful mixture of dried ancho chiles, tomato paste, garlic, cumin, and oregano; blooming these aromatics with oil in the pressure cooker brought out their full flavor. We then added our beef pieces and some beer to the pot and pressure-cooked everything for half an hour. To complement the warm spices of the beef, we created a cool, tangy jicama, radish, and carrot slaw, which we quickly brined while the beef cooked. Once the beef was pull-apart tender, we simply mashed it in the pot and simmered it briefly to the desired consistency. Boneless beef short ribs can be substituted for the chuck-eye roast. If jicama is unavailable, double the amount of radishes and carrot in the slaw.

Filling

- 3 tablespoons ancho chile powder
- 3 tablespoons no-salt-added tomato paste
- 2 tablespoons avocado oil
- 3 garlic cloves, minced
- 2 teaspoons ground cumin
- 2 teaspoons dried oregano
- ¼ teaspoon ground cloves
- ½ teaspoon table salt
- 1 cup full-bodied lager
- 1½ pounds boneless beef chuck-eye roast, trimmed and cut into 1-inch pieces

Jicama Slaw

- 1 cup distilled white vinegar
- 2 tablespoons sugar
- 6 radishes, trimmed and sliced thin
- 1 carrot, peeled and shredded
- 12 ounces jicama, peeled and cut into 2-inch-long matchsticks
- ¼ cup fresh cilantro leaves

- 12 (6-inch) corn tortillas, warmed

1   For the filling Combine ancho chile powder, tomato paste, oil, garlic, cumin, oregano, cloves, and salt in electric pressure cooker. Using highest sauté function, cook, stirring frequently, until fragrant, about 3 minutes. Whisk in beer, scraping up any browned bits and smoothing out any lumps. Stir in beef until evenly coated in spice mixture. Lock lid into place and close pressure-release valve. Select high pressure-cook function and cook for 30 minutes.

2   For the jicama slaw Meanwhile, microwave vinegar and sugar in medium bowl until steaming, 2 to 3 minutes; whisk to dissolve sugar. Add radishes and carrot to hot brine and let sit, stirring occasionally, for 30 minutes. Measure out and reserve 1 tablespoon brine, then drain vegetables and return to now-empty bowl. Add reserved brine and jicama and toss to combine; set aside.

3   Turn off pressure cooker and quick-release pressure. Carefully remove lid, allowing steam to escape away from you. Skim excess fat from top of filling using wide, shallow spoon. Using potato masher, smash beef until coarsely shredded. Using highest sauté function, cook filling until sauce has thickened, about 5 minutes. Season with salt and pepper to taste.

4   Stir cilantro into slaw. Serve beef with tortillas and slaw.

> **MAKE AHEAD** • Beef filling can be refrigerated for up to 3 days. Slaw can be refrigerated for up to 24 hours.

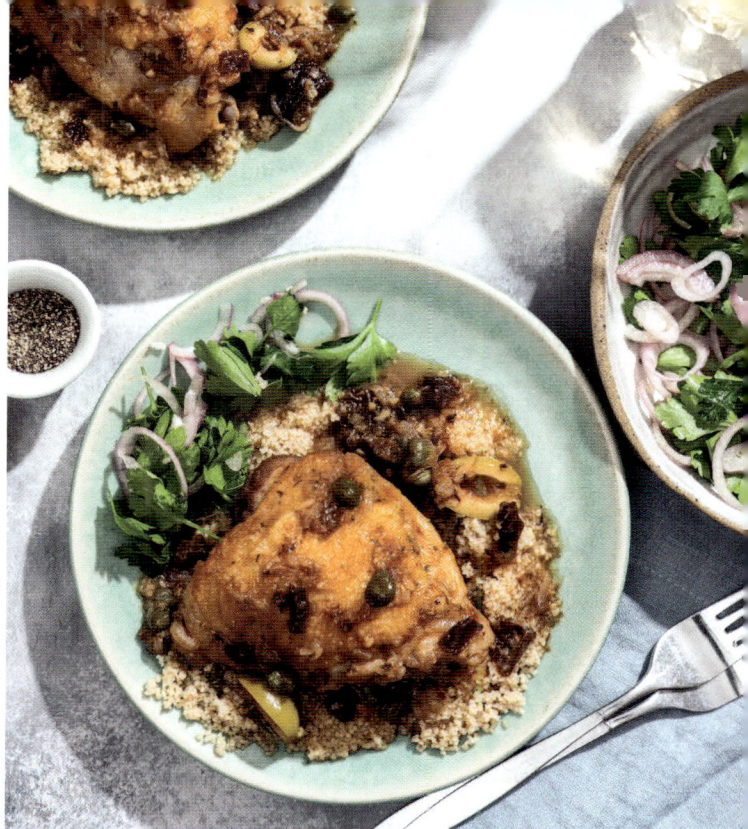

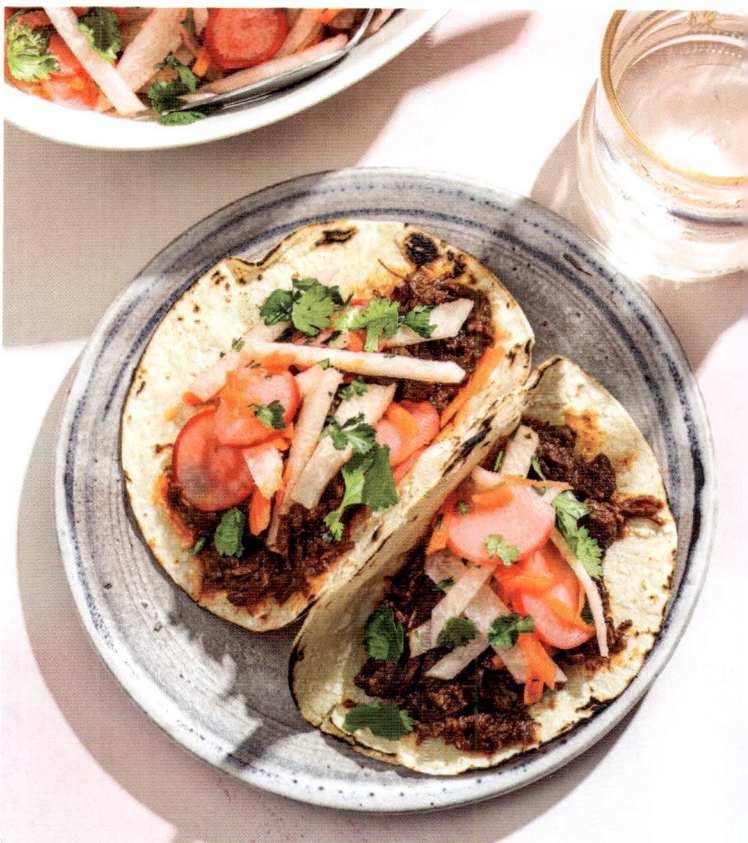

top	*Pressure-Cooker Chicken and Couscous with Prunes and Olives*
bottom	*Pressure-Cooker Shredded Beef Tacos with Jicama Slaw*

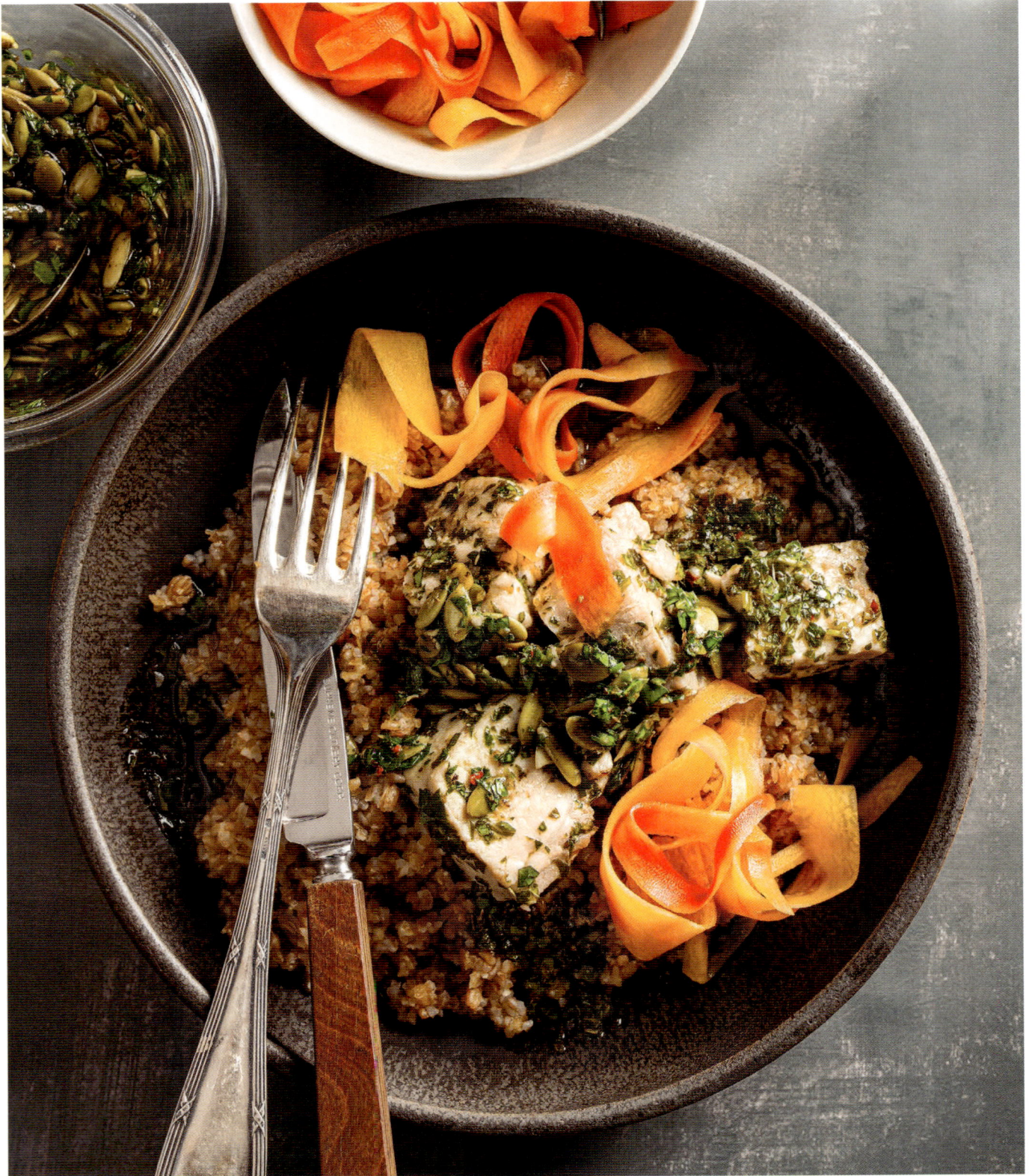

Pressure-Cooker Pork and Bulgur Bowls with Parsley-Pepita Sauce

Pressure-Cooker Pork and Bulgur Bowls with Parsley-Pepita Sauce

serves 4 · total time: 1½ hours

why this recipe works · Creating a grain bowl in a pressure cooker is an efficient method that uses one pot to cook many components successively. We concocted a flavorful braising liquid in the cooker for our pork ribs (a modest amount of this fattier cut went a long way in building intense flavor) that doubled as the bulgur cooking liquid. Next up was the bulgur, which was ideal for pressure cooking as it needed only 3 minutes to cook while the ribs rested. To serve, we arranged the pork over the grains and topped everything with quick-pickled carrots and a vibrant sauce seasoned with parsley, pepitas, and garlic. Boneless pork butt can be substituted for the ribs. Do not use cracked wheat; it has a longer cooking time and will not work in this recipe.

- 5 tablespoons extra-virgin olive oil, divided
- 3 garlic cloves, minced, divided
- 2 teaspoons dried oregano, divided
- ¼ cup dry white wine
- 1½ cups unsalted chicken broth, plus extra as needed
- 1 teaspoon table salt, divided
- 1 pound boneless country-style pork ribs, trimmed and cut into 1½-inch pieces
- ¾ cup minced fresh parsley
- ¼ cup roasted, unsalted pepitas
- ¼ teaspoon red pepper flakes
- 1½ cups medium-grind bulgur
- 1 recipe Quick-Pickled Vegetables with carrots (recipe follows)

1 Using highest sauté function, cook 1 tablespoon oil, two-thirds garlic, and 1 teaspoon oregano in electric pressure cooker, stirring frequently, until fragrant, about 3 minutes. Stir in wine, broth, and ½ teaspoon salt, scraping up any browned bits, then stir in pork. Lock lid into place and close pressure-release valve. Select high pressure-cook function and cook for 25 minutes.

2 Meanwhile, combine parsley, pepitas, pepper flakes, remaining ¼ cup oil, remaining garlic, and remaining 1 teaspoon oregano in bowl. Season with salt and pepper to taste. Set sauce aside for serving.

3 Turn off pressure cooker and quick-release pressure. Carefully remove lid, allowing steam to escape away from you. Using slotted spoon, transfer pork to serving platter, tent with aluminum foil, and let rest while cooking bulgur. Strain braising liquid through fine-mesh strainer into 4-cup liquid measuring cup; discard solids. Using wide, shallow spoon, skim excess fat from surface. Add extra broth as needed to equal 2½ cups.

4 Combine braising liquid, bulgur, and remaining ½ teaspoon salt in now-empty pot. Lock lid into place and close pressure-release valve. Select high pressure-cook function and cook for 3 minutes. Turn off pressure cooker and quick-release pressure. Carefully remove lid, allowing steam to escape away from you. Fluff bulgur gently with fork and divide among individual serving bowls. Arrange pork and pickled carrots over bulgur and top with parsley-pepita mixture. Serve.

Quick-Pickled Vegetables

makes about 2 cups · total time: 10 minutes, plus 45 minutes pickling

This recipe works well with a single variety or combination of vegetables such as onions, shallots, carrots, fennel, cabbage, and radishes. Trim and peel as needed. Halve and core fennel and cabbage before slicing. Shave carrots into ribbons for added contrast. Feel free to add up to 1 teaspoon of your favorite whole spices to the brine.

- 1 cup white or red wine vinegar
- ¼ cup sugar
- ⅛ teaspoon table salt
- 2 cups thinly sliced hearty vegetables

Microwave vinegar, sugar, and salt in medium bowl until steaming, 2 to 3 minutes; whisk to dissolve sugar and salt. Add vegetables to hot brine and press to submerge completely. Let sit for 45 minutes. Drain. (Drained pickled vegetables can be refrigerated for up to 1 week.)

Pressure-Cooker Haddock with Tomatoes, Escarole, and Crispy Garlic

serves 4 · total time: 45 minutes **FAST**

why this recipe works · Stovetop methods for steaming fish require careful monitoring to prevent overcooking. A pressure cooker—with its consistent moisture level and temperature—all but guarantees foolproof results. We chose flaky haddock and paired it with white wine, cherry tomatoes, thyme, and pepper flakes. The wine and tomatoes provided enough liquid to steam the fish and create an aromatic broth. A foil sling allowed the fish to flavor the broth while enabling us to easily transfer the cooked fish to a serving platter without it falling apart. To bulk up our

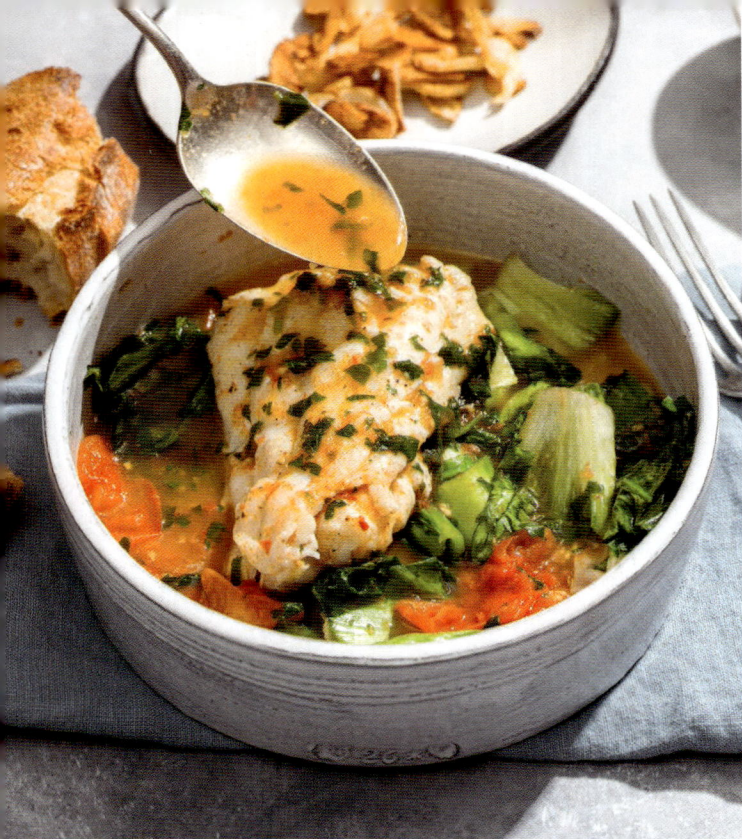

dish, we turned to fiber-rich escarole for a pleasantly bitter pairing with the fish. To amp up flavor, we cooked the escarole in an infused oil that we made by crisping thinly sliced garlic in the pot. You can substitute black sea bass, cod, hake, or pollock for the haddock. Tail-end fillets can be folded for proper thickness. If the haddock has not reached at least 135 degrees after releasing the pressure, partially cover the pot and continue to cook using residual heat until it reaches 135 degrees. Serve with crusty bread.

- 3 tablespoons extra-virgin olive oil, divided, plus extra for drizzling
- 4 garlic cloves, sliced thin
- 1 head escarole (1 pound), trimmed and cut into 1-inch pieces
- ¾ teaspoon table salt, divided
- 12 ounces cherry tomatoes, halved
- 1 cup dry white wine
- 2 sprigs fresh thyme
- ¼ teaspoon red pepper flakes
- 4 (6-ounce) skinless haddock fillets, 1 to 1½ inches thick
- ¼ teaspoon pepper
- 3 tablespoons chopped fresh parsley

1 Using highest sauté function, heat 2 tablespoons oil in electric pressure cooker until shimmering. Add garlic and cook, stirring often, until beginning to brown, 2 to 3 minutes. Turn off pressure cooker and continue to cook, using residual heat, until garlic is evenly golden brown and crisp, 2 to 3 minutes. Using slotted spoon, transfer garlic to paper towel–lined plate; set aside for serving.

2 Add escarole and ¼ teaspoon salt to oil left in pot and cook, using highest sauté function, until wilted, 2 to 4 minutes. Turn off pressure cooker. Transfer escarole to bowl and cover to keep warm.

3 Add tomatoes, wine, thyme sprigs, and pepper flakes to now-empty pot. Fold sheet of aluminum foil into 16 by 6-inch sling. Arrange haddock skinned side down in center of sling, brush with remaining 1 tablespoon oil, and sprinkle with pepper and remaining ½ teaspoon salt. Using sling, lower haddock into pot on top of tomato mixture; allow narrow edges of sling to rest along sides of pot.

4 Lock lid into place and close pressure-release valve. Select high pressure-cook function and cook for 4 minutes. Turn off pressure cooker and quick-release pressure. Carefully remove lid, allowing steam to escape away from you. Using sling, transfer haddock to large plate.

5 Discard thyme sprigs from tomato mixture. Stir in parsley and season with salt to taste. Serve haddock with escarole and tomato mixture, sprinkling individual portions with garlic and drizzling with extra oil.

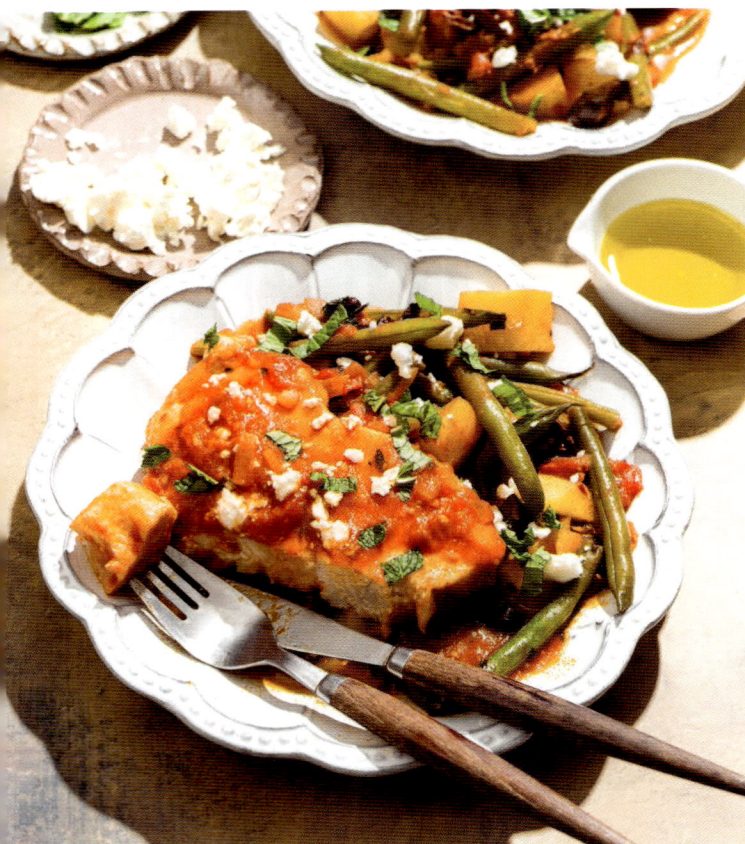

| top | *Pressure-Cooker Haddock with Tomatoes, Escarole, and Crispy Garlic* |
| bottom | *Pressure-Cooker Swordfish with Braised Green Beans, Tomatoes, and Feta* |

Pressure-Cooker Swordfish with Braised Green Beans, Tomatoes, and Feta

serves 4 · total time: 45 minutes   **FAST**

why this recipe works · This recipe transforms a few simple ingredients into a rich and satisfying dish full of flavor and inflammation-fighting power. We love swordfish because it packs in big, meaty flavor and texture and is high in minerals. Thanks to the pressure cooker's intense heat, canned whole peeled tomatoes and their juice became a concentrated broth. To keep the swordfish from overcooking, we placed it above the liquid and basted it with sauce just before going under pressure. Raw potatoes simmered in the liquid as well, giving off starches to help thicken the broth, while green beans melted to a tender texture. A smattering of olives and mint were added to the pot at the end of cooking so their flavor would remain fresh. A sprinkling of feta offered more pleasantly briny bites. A garnish of fresh mint added a clean finish. You can substitute halibut, mahi-mahi, red snapper, or striped bass for the swordfish. If the swordfish has not reached at least 130 degrees after releasing the pressure, partially cover the pot and continue to cook using residual heat until it reaches 130 degrees.

- 1 tablespoon extra-virgin olive oil, plus extra for drizzling
- 1 onion, chopped fine
- 3 garlic cloves, minced
- 1½ teaspoons chopped fresh oregano or ½ teaspoon dried
- ¼ teaspoon red pepper flakes
- 1 (28-ounce) can no-salt-added whole peeled tomatoes, drained with juice reserved, tomatoes halved
- 1 pound Yukon Gold potatoes, cut into ½-inch pieces
- 12 ounces green beans, trimmed
- ¼ teaspoon table salt, divided
- 4 (6-ounce) skinless swordfish steaks, 1 to 1½ inches thick
- 2 tablespoons chopped pitted kalamata olives
- 2 tablespoons chopped fresh mint, plus extra for serving
- 1 ounce feta cheese, crumbled (¼ cup)

1 Using highest sauté function, heat oil in electric pressure cooker until shimmering. Add onion and cook until softened and lightly browned, 3 to 5 minutes. Add garlic, oregano, and pepper flakes and cook, stirring frequently, until fragrant, about 30 seconds. Stir in tomatoes and their juice, scraping up any browned bits. Reserve ½ cup tomato mixture, then stir potatoes, green beans, and ⅛ teaspoon salt into pot.

2 Sprinkle swordfish with remaining ⅛ teaspoon salt. Nestle swordfish into pot and spoon reserved tomato mixture over tops. Lock lid into place and close pressure-release valve. Select high

pressure-cook function and cook for 1 minute. Turn off pressure cooker and quick-release pressure. Carefully remove lid, allowing steam to escape away from you.

3 Using spatula, transfer swordfish to large plate. Tent with aluminum foil and let rest while finishing vegetable mixture. Using highest sauté function, cook vegetable mixture until liquid has thickened slightly, 3 to 5 minutes. Stir in olives and mint and season with salt and pepper to taste. Serve swordfish with vegetable mixture, sprinkling individual portions with feta and extra mint and drizzling with extra oil.

MAKE IT DAIRY-FREE · Substitute plant-based feta for the feta cheese or omit.

Pressure-Cooker Braised Striped Bass with Zucchini and Tomatoes

serves 4 · total time: 1 hour

why this recipe works · This Greek-inspired one-pot meal is a celebration of summer vegetables and bright Mediterranean flavors. A light tomato stew forms a savory base that complements the clean flavor of striped bass. Once the bass was in the pot, we set the cooking time to 0 minutes, which allowed the fish to cook gently in the carryover heat. We stirred sautéed zucchini and briny olives into the sauce after cooking the fish for added bulk and a pop of flavor. The striped bass should register about 130 degrees after cooking; if it doesn't, partially cover the pot with the lid and continue to cook using the highest sauté function until the desired temperature is achieved.

- 2 tablespoons extra-virgin olive oil, divided, plus extra for drizzling
- 3 zucchini (8 ounces each), halved lengthwise and sliced ¼ inch thick
- 1 onion, chopped
- ¾ teaspoon table salt, divided
- 3 garlic cloves, minced
- 1 teaspoon minced fresh oregano or ¼ teaspoon dried
- ¼ teaspoon red pepper flakes
- 1 (28-ounce) can no-salt-added whole peeled tomatoes, drained with juice reserved, tomatoes halved
- 1½ pounds skinless striped bass, 1½ inches thick, cut into 2-inch pieces
- ¼ teaspoon pepper
- 2 tablespoons chopped pitted kalamata olives
- 2 tablespoons shredded fresh mint

1 Using highest sauté function, heat 1 tablespoon oil in electric pressure cooker until shimmering. Add zucchini and cook until tender, about 5 minutes; transfer to bowl and set aside.

2 Add remaining 1 tablespoon oil, onion, and ¼ teaspoon salt to now-empty pot and cook, using highest sauté function, until onion is softened, about 5 minutes. Stir in garlic, oregano, and pepper flakes and cook until fragrant, about 30 seconds. Stir in tomatoes and their juice.

3 Sprinkle bass with remaining ½ teaspoon salt and pepper. Nestle bass into tomato mixture and spoon some of cooking liquid on top of pieces. Lock lid into place and close pressure-release valve. Select high pressure-cook function and set cook time for 0 minutes. Once pressure cooker has reached pressure, immediately turn off pot and quick-release pressure. Carefully remove lid, allowing steam to escape away from you.

4 Transfer bass to plate, tent with aluminum foil, and let rest while finishing vegetables. Stir zucchini into pot and let sit until heated through, about 5 minutes. Stir in olives and season with salt and pepper to taste. Serve bass with vegetables, sprinkling individual portions with mint and drizzling with extra oil.

Pressure-Cooker Halibut with Couscous and Ras el Hanout

serves 4 • **total time: 45 minutes** FAST

why this recipe works • We love the delicate flavor of halibut, but because it is naturally low in fat, it can dry out quickly during cooking. Thanks to the pressure cooker, dry fish can be avoided. We rested the halibut on a bed of lemon slices in a foil sling in the pressure cooker, allowing us to remove the cooked halibut with ease after the lemon insulated the fish from direct heat and permeated it with citrusy flavor. The consistent internal environment of the pot produced moist fish in just 2 minutes. For a Moroccan-inspired side, we turned to couscous and ras el hanout. The warm spice blend, combined with garlic and lemon, infused the couscous with complex flavor. A cool, creamy yogurt-tahini sauce made a nice contrast to the nutty couscous, while a topping of toasted almonds made a crunchy garnish. You can substitute mahi-mahi, red snapper, striped bass, or swordfish for the halibut. If the fish has not reached at least 130 degrees after releasing the pressure, partially cover the pot and continue to cook using residual heat until it reaches 130 degrees.

½ cup plain yogurt
2 tablespoons tahini
4 garlic cloves, minced, divided
2 lemons, plus 2 teaspoons grated lemon zest, divided, plus 1 tablespoon lemon juice
3 tablespoons extra-virgin olive oil
2 teaspoons ras el hanout
1 cup couscous
1 cup jarred roasted red peppers, rinsed, patted dry, and sliced ¼ inch thick
¾ teaspoon table salt, divided
3 tablespoons chopped fresh mint, divided
4 (6-ounce) skinless halibut fillets, 1 to 1½ inches thick
¼ teaspoon pepper
¼ cup sliced almonds, toasted

1 Whisk yogurt, tahini, one-quarter of garlic, and 1 teaspoon lemon zest together in small bowl and season with salt and pepper to taste; set aside for serving. Microwave oil, ras el hanout, remaining garlic, and remaining 1 teaspoon lemon zest in large bowl until fragrant, about 30 seconds, stirring halfway through microwaving.

2 Stir 1 cup boiling water, couscous, red peppers, and ½ teaspoon salt into spice mixture; cover and let sit for 10 minutes. Drizzle lemon juice over couscous and sprinkle with 2 tablespoons mint. Fluff couscous with fork and season with salt and pepper to taste; set aside for serving.

3 Meanwhile, add ½ cup water to electric pressure cooker. Fold sheet of aluminum foil into 16 by 6-inch sling. Slice lemons ¼ inch thick and shingle widthwise in 3 rows across center of sling. Arrange halibut skinned side down on top of lemon slices and sprinkle with pepper and remaining ¼ teaspoon salt.

4 Using sling, lower halibut into pot on top of water; allow narrow edges of sling to rest along sides of pot. Lock lid into place and close pressure-release valve. Select high pressure-cook function and cook for 2 minutes.

5 Turn off pressure cooker and quick-release pressure. Carefully remove lid, allowing steam to escape away from you. Using sling, transfer halibut to large plate. Gently lift and tilt fillets with spatula to remove lemon slices. Serve halibut with couscous, drizzling individual portions with yogurt-tahini sauce and sprinkling with almonds and remaining 1 tablespoon mint.

MAKE IT DAIRY-FREE • Substitute plant-based yogurt for the dairy yogurt.

Pressure-Cooker Southwestern Shrimp and Oat Berry Bowls

serves 4 · total time: 1 hour SUPERCHARGED

why this recipe works · Oat berries (also known as groats) are a favorite healthy base for bowls because of their high nutritional content, hearty chew, and pleasant nuttiness. Rich in fiber, they help support gut health, which makes them a win for anti-inflammation. On the stove, they can take at least 45 minutes to cook, but the high-pressure function on the pressure cooker cuts that time in half. Inspired by the Southwestern flavors of fast-casual burrito bowls, we set out to create a nutrient-dense at-home bowl. We seasoned the oat berries by browning poblano peppers with garlic, chili powder, and coriander—which added antioxidant benefits—then tossed the mixture with the grains. After cooking the oat berries, we seared shrimp in the pot to double down on the flavors left behind. Finally, we added an abundance of toppings: corn salsa for zesty sweetness, avocado for rich creaminess, a chipotle-yogurt sauce for cool heat, and salty tortilla chips to add fun crunch. Extra-large shrimp (21 to 25 per pound) also work in this recipe.

1½ cups oat berries, rinsed
3 tablespoons avocado oil, divided
½ teaspoon table salt, divided, plus salt for cooking oat berries
1 cup frozen corn, thawed
¼ cup finely chopped red onion
1 tablespoon grated lime zest plus 1 tablespoon juice
½ cup fresh cilantro leaves
2 poblano chiles, stemmed, seeded, and sliced thin
4 garlic cloves, minced
¾ teaspoon chili powder
¾ teaspoon ground coriander
1 pound large shrimp (26 to 30 per pound), peeled, deveined, and tails removed
1 avocado, halved, pitted, and cut into ½-inch pieces
1½ ounces corn tortilla chips, broken into 1-inch pieces (½ cup)
½ recipe Chipotle-Yogurt Sauce (page 320)

1 Combine 6 cups water, oat berries, 1 tablespoon oil, and 1½ teaspoons salt in electric pressure cooker. Lock lid into place and close pressure-release valve. Select high pressure-cook function and cook for 20 minutes.

2 Turn off pressure cooker and let pressure release naturally for 15 minutes. Quick-release any remaining pressure, then carefully remove lid, allowing steam to escape away from you. Drain oat berries, transfer to large bowl, and cover to keep warm. Wipe pot clean with paper towels.

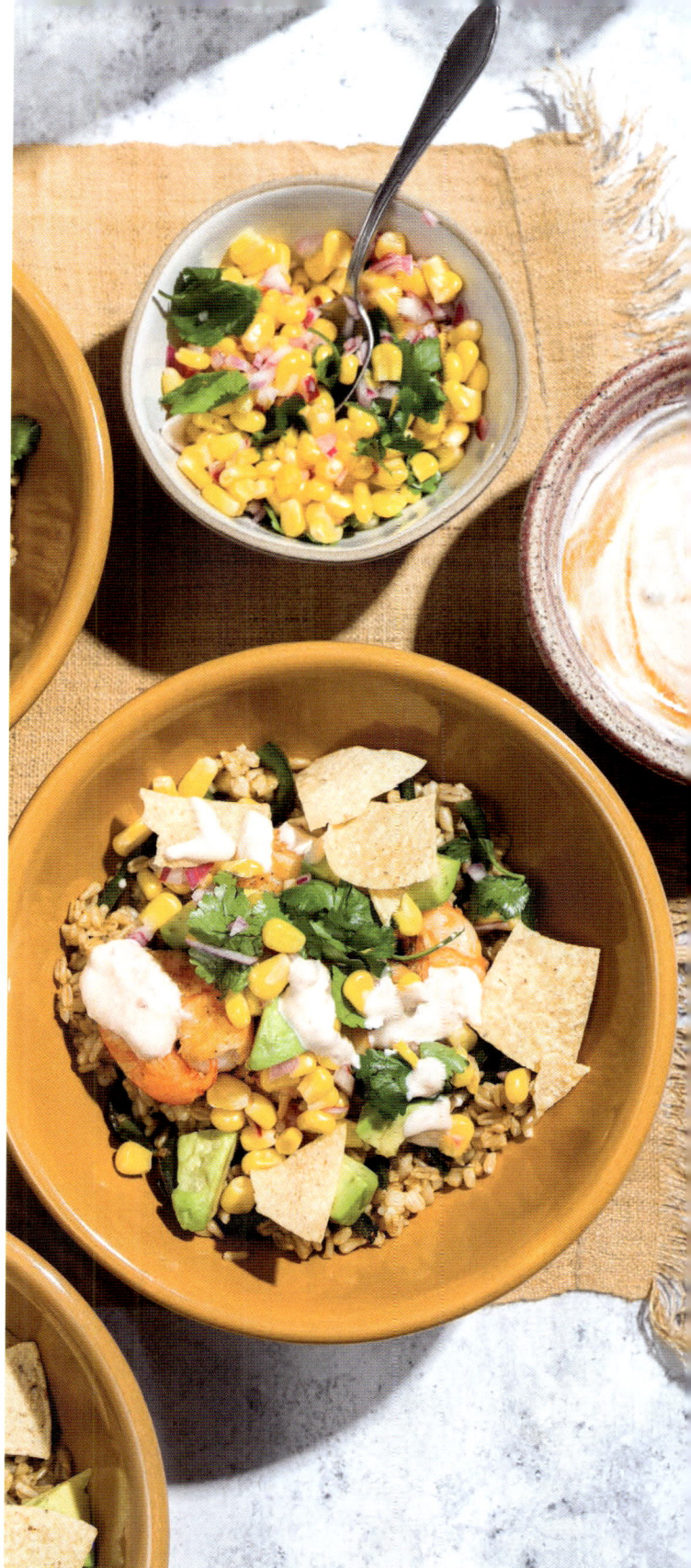

Pressure-Cooker Southwestern Shrimp and Oat Berry Bowls

3 Meanwhile, stir corn, onion, lime juice, cilantro, and ¼ teaspoon salt together in small bowl; set salsa aside for serving.

4 Using highest sauté function, heat 1 tablespoon oil in now-empty pot until shimmering. Add poblanos and cook until softened and lightly browned, 3 to 5 minutes. Add lime zest, garlic, chili powder, coriander, and remaining ¼ teaspoon salt and cook, stirring frequently, until fragrant, about 30 seconds. Transfer poblano mixture to bowl with oat berries, toss to combine, and season with salt and pepper to taste; set aside.

5 Using highest sauté function, heat remaining 1 tablespoon oil in again-empty pot until just smoking. Add shrimp and cook, tossing constantly, until all but very center is opaque, about 3 minutes.

6 Divide oat berries among individual serving bowls. Top with shrimp, avocado, tortilla chips, and corn salsa. Serve, passing yogurt sauce separately.

> **Nutritional Knowledge** These vibrant shrimp bowls are loaded with anti-inflammatory goodness—starting with oat berries. Packed with beta-glucan, a soluble fiber known to reduce inflammation and support heart and gut health, oat berries provide a hearty base with a pleasantly chewy bite. Poblano chiles, garlic, and coriander offer anti-oxidant and immune-boosting benefits, while creamy avocado contributes monounsaturated fats that help absorb fat-soluble phytonutrients. —*Alicia*

Chipotle-Yogurt Sauce

makes about 1 cup • total time: 5 minutes, plus 30 minutes resting

- 1 cup plain dairy yogurt or plant-based yogurt
- 1 tablespoon minced canned chipotle chile in adobo sauce
- 1 teaspoon grated lime zest plus 2 tablespoons juice
- 1 garlic clove, minced

Whisk all ingredients together in bowl. Cover and refrigerate until flavors meld, at least 30 minutes. Season with salt and pepper to taste. (Sauce can be refrigerated for up to 4 days.)

Pressure-Cooker Shrimp and White Beans with Butternut Squash and Sage

serves 4 • total time: 45 minutes `FAST`

why this recipe works • Turning chunks of dense vegetables into tender bites is one of the things a pressure cooker does best. We combined antioxidant-packed butternut squash with fiber-laden cannellini beans for a comforting and nutrient-rich meal. Sage pairs well with beans, squash, and shrimp separately, but it's magic with all three together. As well as adding minced sage to the base, we also used the sauté function to produce fried sage leaves for a crispy garnish. Our favored method for cooking shrimp in the pressure cooker is stirring them in raw at the end of cooking and letting the residual heat cook them through. The gentle heat virtually eliminates the chance of overcooking this delicate protein. Extra-large shrimp (21 to 25 per pound) also work in this recipe.

- 2 tablespoons extra-virgin olive oil, plus extra for drizzling
- 12 fresh sage leaves, plus 1 tablespoon minced fresh sage
- 1 onion, chopped fine
- 4 garlic cloves, minced
- ½ cup dry white wine
- 2 (15-ounce) cans no-salt-added cannellini beans, drained with ½ cup canning liquid reserved, rinsed
- 1½ pounds butternut squash, peeled, seeded, and cut into 1-inch pieces (4 cups)
- ½ teaspoon table salt
- 1 pound large shrimp (26 to 30 per pound), peeled, deveined, and tails removed
- 1 teaspoon grated lemon zest plus 2 teaspoons juice, plus lemon wedges for serving
- 2 tablespoons toasted sliced almonds

1 Using highest sauté function, cook oil and sage leaves in electric pressure cooker until dark green and crisp, 3 to 5 minutes, flipping leaves halfway through cooking. Using slotted spoon, transfer sage leaves to paper towel–lined plate.

2 Add onion to oil left in pot and cook until softened and lightly browned, 3 to 5 minutes. Add minced sage and garlic and cook, stirring frequently, until fragrant, about 30 seconds. Stir in wine, scraping up any browned bits, and cook until mostly evaporated, about 1 minute. Stir in beans and reserved liquid, squash, and salt.

3 Lock lid into place and close pressure-release valve. Select high pressure-cook function and cook for 3 minutes. Turn off pressure cooker and quick-release pressure. Carefully remove lid, allowing steam to escape away from you.

4 Stir shrimp gently into squash mixture, cover, and let sit until shrimp are opaque throughout, 5 to 8 minutes. Stir in lemon zest and juice and season with salt and pepper to taste. Sprinkle individual portions with almonds and sage leaves and drizzle with extra oil. Serve with lemon wedges.

Pressure-Cooker Bulgur with Chickpeas, Spinach, and Za'atar

serves 4 · total time: 45 minutes **FAST**

why this recipe works · Hearty bulgur, creamy and nutty chickpeas, and fresh spinach come together to spectacular effect in this recipe. To give it a flavor boost, we added the aromatic eastern Mediterranean spice blend za'atar for its fragrant wild herbs, toasted sesame seeds, and tangy sumac. Fluffing the bulgur right after cooking and then letting it sit was crucial to achieving perfectly cooked grains that weren't soggy: Agitating the grains and putting a towel under the lid allows the towel to absorb the grains' excess moisture. We used the residual heat from the bulgur to wilt baby spinach gently without turning it mushy. When shopping, don't confuse bulgur with cracked wheat, which has a much longer cooking time and will not work in this recipe. We like to use our homemade Za'atar (page 186), but you can use store-bought if you prefer.

- 3 tablespoons extra-virgin olive oil, divided
- 1 onion, chopped fine
- ½ teaspoon table salt
- 3 garlic cloves, minced
- 2 tablespoons za'atar, divided
- 1 cup medium-grind bulgur, rinsed
- 1 (15-ounce) can chickpeas, rinsed
- 1½ cups water
- 5 ounces (5 cups) baby spinach, chopped
- 1 tablespoon lemon juice, plus lemon wedges for serving

1 Using highest sauté function, heat 2 tablespoons oil in electric pressure cooker until shimmering. Add onion and salt and cook until onion is softened, about 5 minutes. Stir in garlic and 1 tablespoon za'atar and cook until fragrant, about 30 seconds. Stir in bulgur, chickpeas, and water.

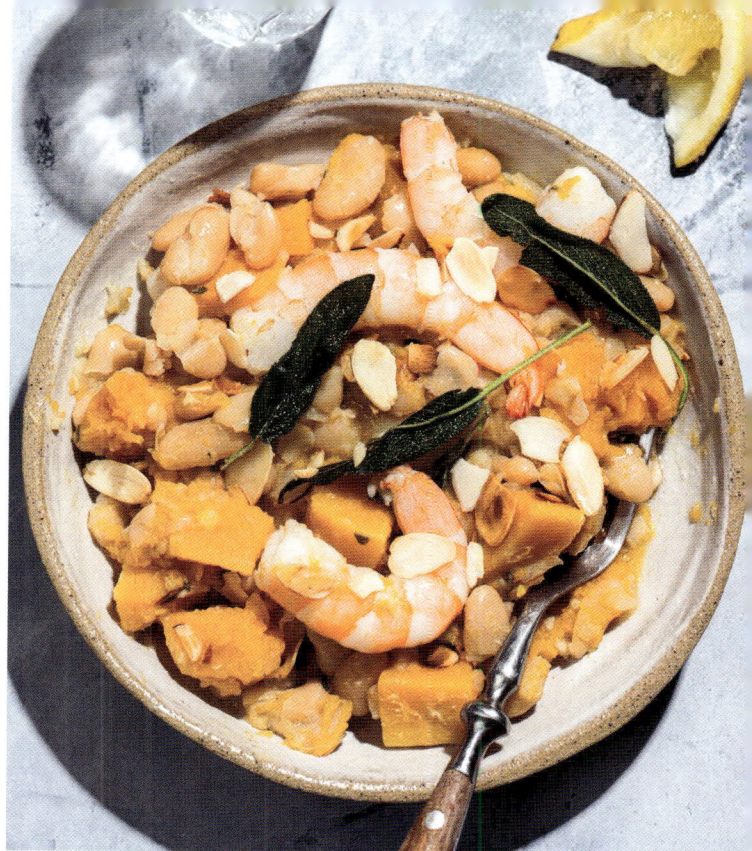

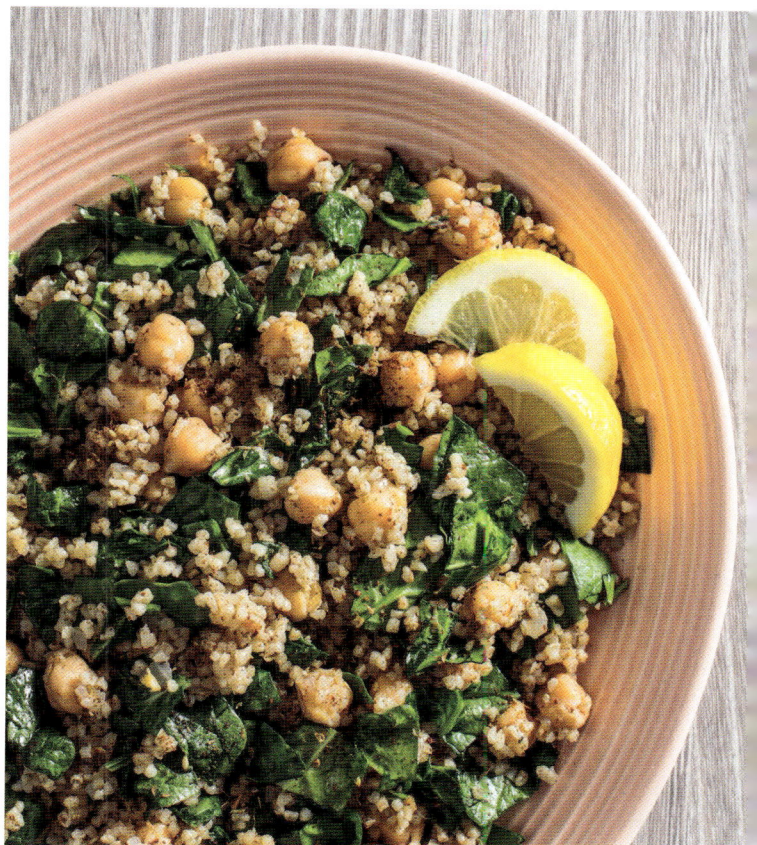

top | Pressure-Cooker Shrimp and White Beans with Butternut Squash and Sage
bottom | Pressure-Cooker Bulgur with Chickpeas, Spinach, and Za'atar

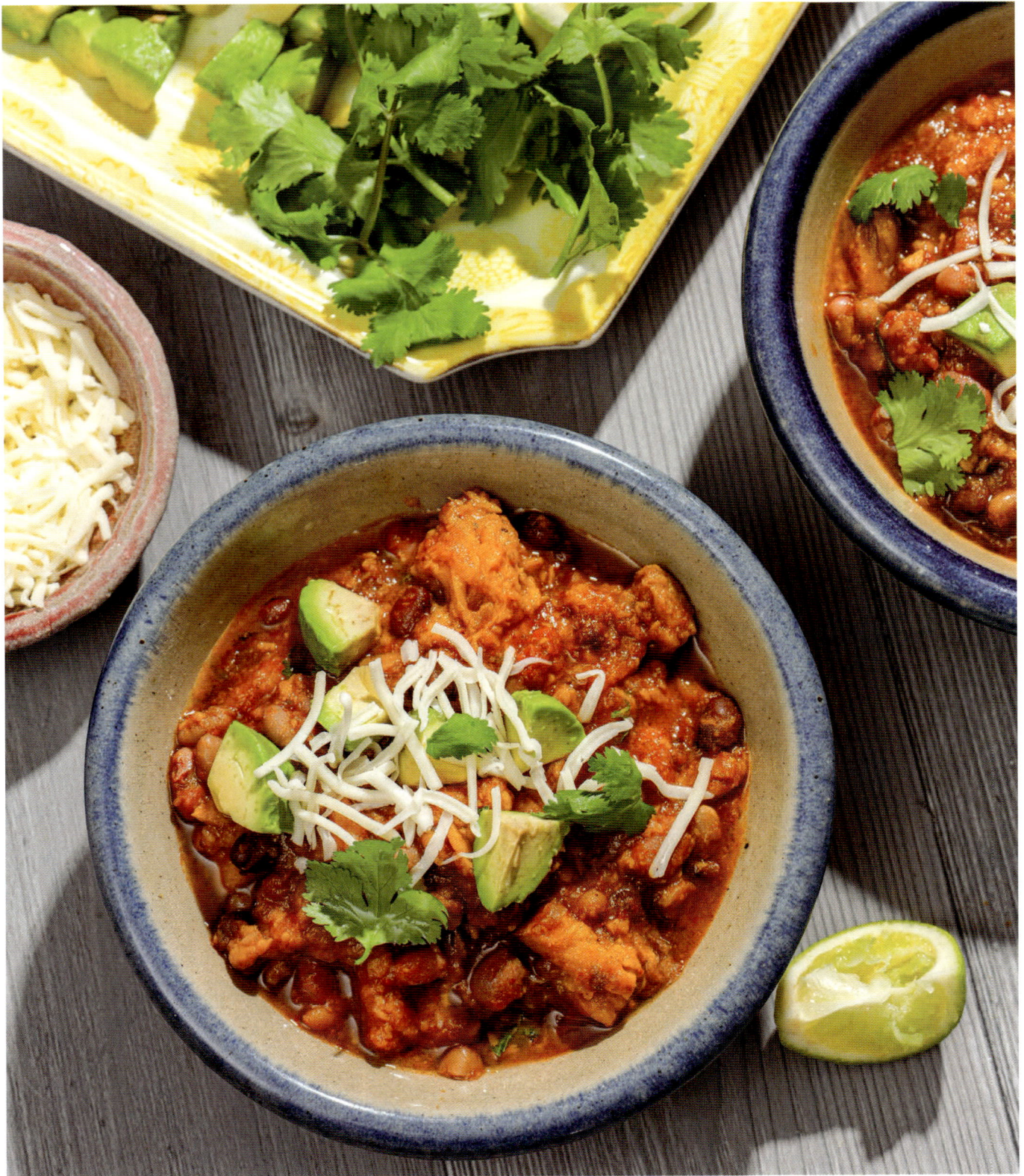

Pressure-Cooker Bean and Sweet Potato Chili

2   Lock lid into place and close pressure-release valve. Select high pressure-cook function and cook for 1 minute. Turn off pressure cooker and quick-release pressure. Carefully remove lid, allowing steam to escape away from you.

3   Gently fluff bulgur with fork. Lay clean dish towel over pot, replace lid, and let sit for 5 minutes. Add spinach, lemon juice, remaining 1 tablespoon za'atar, and remaining 1 tablespoon oil and gently toss to combine. Season with salt and pepper to taste. Serve with lemon wedges.

Pressure-Cooker Bean and Sweet Potato Chili

serves 6 to 8 • **total time: 1¼ hours, plus 8 hours brining**

why this recipe works • For familiar chili flavors with an anti-inflammatory spin, we paired beans with hearty chunks of nutritious sweet potato. To bring classically spiced flavor to our vegetarian chili, we bloomed ancho chile powder, coriander, cumin, oregano, and garlic powder in the pot with chopped onion—creating a flavorful and antioxidant-rich foundation. Adding a can of crushed tomatoes with the beans and sweet potatoes made an ideal base because the tomatoes broke down into a stewy consistency while maintaining some individual tomato pieces. We like a combination of beans, but a single variety will also work. Serve with diced avocado, yogurt, and/or shredded Monterey Jack or cheddar cheese, if desired.

1½   tablespoons table salt for brining
1   pound (2½ cups) dried black, navy, pinto, and/or small red beans, rinsed
2   tablespoons ancho chile powder
1   tablespoon ground coriander
2   teaspoons ground cumin
2   teaspoons dried oregano
1   teaspoon garlic powder
1½   teaspoons table salt
¼   cup extra-virgin olive oil
1   onion, chopped fine
1   (28-ounce) can no-salt-added crushed tomatoes
2   pounds sweet potatoes, peeled and cut into 1-inch pieces
¼   teaspoon baking soda
½   cup chopped fresh cilantro, divided
   Lime wedges

1   Dissolve 1½ tablespoons salt in 2 quarts cold water in large container. Add beans and soak at room temperature for at least 8 hours or up to 24 hours. Drain and rinse well.

2   Combine chile powder, coriander, cumin, oregano, garlic powder, and salt in bowl. Using highest sauté function, heat oil in electric pressure cooker until shimmering. Add onion and cook until softened, 3 to 5 minutes. Add spice mixture and cook, stirring frequently, until fragrant, about 30 seconds. Stir in tomatoes and 3 cups water, scraping up any browned bits, then stir in beans, potatoes, and baking soda.

3   Lock lid into place and close pressure-release valve. Select high pressure-cook function and cook for 30 minutes. Turn off pressure cooker and quick-release pressure. Carefully remove lid, allowing steam to escape away from you.

4   Adjust consistency with hot water as needed. Stir in ¼ cup cilantro and season with salt and pepper to taste. Sprinkle individual portions with remaining ¼ cup cilantro and serve with lime wedges.

❙   MAKE AHEAD • Chili can be refrigerated for up to 3 days.

Pressure-Cooker Farro Salad with Asparagus, Snap Peas, and Tomatoes

serves 4 to 6 • **total time: 1 hour**

why this recipe works • Since a pressure cooker is a convenient way to cook your favorite fiber-rich whole grains, we wanted to highlight this with a hearty farro salad. Our experience with cooking rice and grains in the pressure cooker taught us the importance of using enough water for even cooking and adding a little oil to reduce starchy foam. The farro cooked so quickly under pressure that we found it was best to cook for just 1 minute, then turn off the cooker and let the cooking take place while the pot depressurized for 15 minutes. To make sure this salad packed in anti-inflammatory goodness, we briefly blanched bite-size pieces of nutrient-packed asparagus and snap peas in the hot cooking liquid before draining the farro. This brought out their vibrant color and crisp-tender bite. A lemon-herb dressing served as a complement to the earthy farro, while cherry tomatoes and feta cheese offered a full-flavored finish. Do not use quick-cooking or presteamed farro in this recipe.

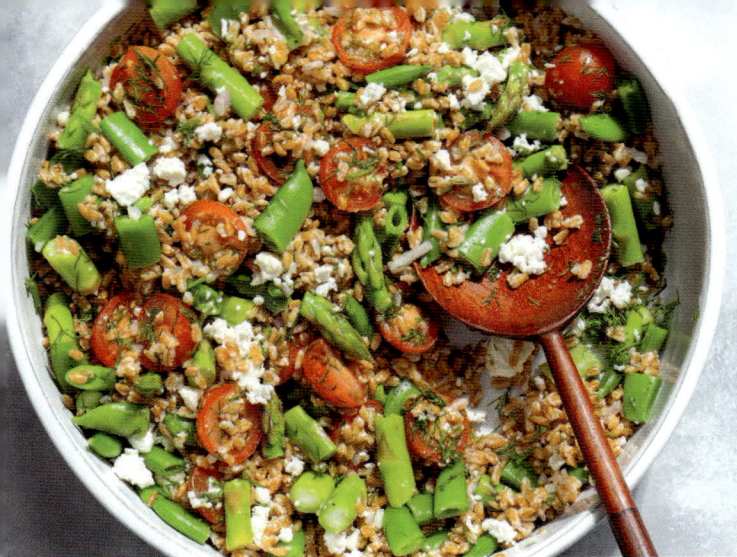

1½ cups whole farro

¼ cup extra-virgin olive oil, divided

½ teaspoon salt, plus salt for cooking farro

6 ounces asparagus, trimmed and cut into 1-inch lengths

6 ounces sugar snap peas, strings removed and cut into 1-inch lengths

2 tablespoons lemon juice

2 tablespoons minced shallot

1 teaspoon Dijon mustard

¼ teaspoon pepper

6 ounces cherry tomatoes, halved

3 tablespoons chopped fresh dill, basil, and/or parsley

2 ounces feta cheese, crumbled (½ cup), divided

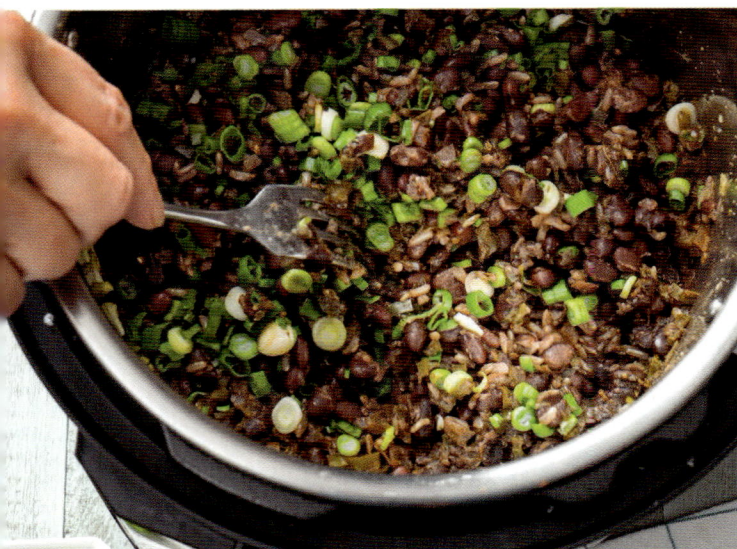

1 Combine 6 cups water, farro, 1 tablespoon oil, and 1½ teaspoons salt in electric pressure cooker. Lock lid into place and close pressure-release valve. Select high pressure-cook function and set cook time for 1 minute. Once pressure cooker has reached pressure, immediately turn off pot and let pressure release naturally for 15 minutes. Quick-release any remaining pressure, then carefully remove lid, allowing steam to escape away from you.

2 Stir asparagus and snap peas into pot and let sit until crisp-tender, about 3 minutes. Drain farro and vegetables, rinse with cold water, and drain again.

3 Whisk remaining 3 tablespoons oil, salt, lemon juice, shallot, mustard, and pepper together in large bowl. Add farro and vegetables, tomatoes, dill, and ¼ cup feta and toss gently to combine. Season with salt and pepper to taste. Transfer to serving platter and sprinkle with remaining ¼ cup feta. Serve.

MAKE AHEAD • Farro and vegetables, prepared through step 2, can be refrigerated for up to 3 days.

MAKE IT DAIRY-FREE • Substitute plant-based feta for the dairy feta.

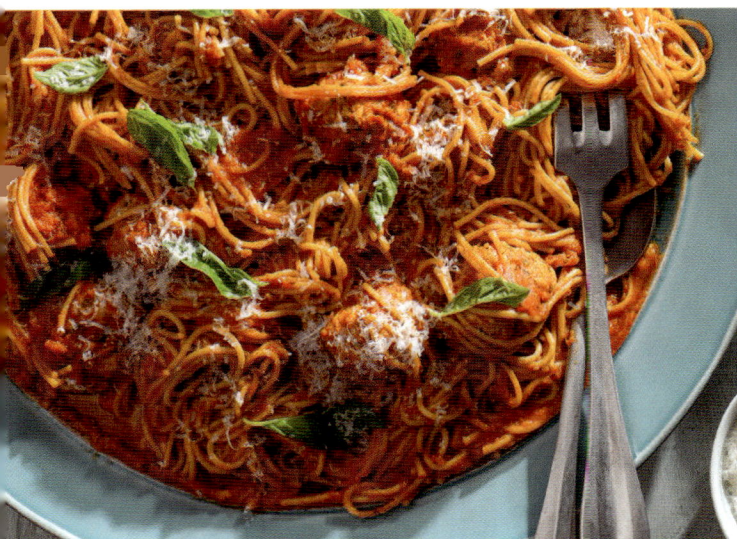

top	Pressure-Cooker Farro Salad with Asparagus, Snap Peas, and Tomatoes
middle	Pressure-Cooker Black Beans and Brown Rice
bottom	Pressure-Cooker Spaghetti and Turkey Meatballs

Pressure-Cooker Black Beans and Brown Rice

serves 4 to 6 • total time: 1 hour, plus 8 hours brining

why this recipe works • Beans and rice is classic one-pot comfort food the world over. But stovetop recipes can sometimes lead to blown-out rice or undercooked beans. Luckily, a pressure cooker can be calibrated with just the right amount of liquid and time to consistently produce fluffy rice and tender beans. We chose brown rice for its high fiber content and hearty texture. The beans are the stars of this meal, so we chose dried over canned for their superior taste and texture. For a savory base, we started by sautéing bell peppers, onions, and jalapeños with garlic, oregano, cumin, and tomato paste. We then added broth and the rice and beans and pressure-cooked it all for 22 minutes. As the beans cooked, they imparted flavor and color into the rice while maintaining structural integrity. The result was a warm, perfect pot of rice and beans. We finished this simple, flavor-packed dish with scallions and a splash of red wine vinegar. Do not substitute white rice here.

1½ tablespoons table salt for brining
8 ounces (1¼ cups) dried black beans, picked over and rinsed
1 tablespoon avocado oil
2 green bell peppers, stemmed, seeded, and chopped fine
1 onion, chopped fine
2 jalapeño chiles, stemmed, seeded, and minced
6 garlic cloves, minced
1 tablespoon no-salt-added tomato paste
2 teaspoons dried oregano
2 teaspoons ground cumin
1¼ teaspoons table salt
2¾ cups unsalted vegetable broth
1½ cups long-grain brown rice, rinsed
4 scallions, sliced thin
2 tablespoons red wine vinegar
Lime wedges

1 Dissolve 1½ tablespoons salt in 2 quarts cold water in large container. Add beans and soak at room temperature for at least 8 hours or up to 24 hours. Drain and rinse well.

2 Using highest sauté function, heat oil in electric pressure cooker until shimmering. Add bell peppers, onion, and jalapeños and cook until vegetables are softened and lightly browned, 5 to 7 minutes. Add garlic, tomato paste, oregano, cumin, and salt and cook, stirring frequently, until fragrant, about 30 seconds. Stir in broth, scraping up any browned bits, then stir in beans and rice.

3 Lock lid into place and close pressure-release valve. Select high pressure-cook function and cook for 22 minutes. Turn off pressure cooker and quick-release pressure. Carefully remove lid, allowing steam to escape away from you.

4 Lay clean dish towel over pot, replace lid, and let sit for 5 minutes. Sprinkle scallions and vinegar over rice and beans and fluff gently with fork to combine. Season with salt and pepper to taste. Serve with lime wedges.

Pressure-Cooker Spaghetti and Turkey Meatballs

serves 4 to 6 • total time: 1 hour

why this recipe works • Spaghetti and meatballs is a comforting favorite that can also deliver anti-inflammatory benefits when cooked right. With some help from the pressure cooker, we were able to deliver a mess-free, inflammation-fighting version that still satisfied. For our meatballs, instead of beef or pork, we used lighter ground turkey—mixed with Parmesan, fresh basil, and an egg for moisture—to moderate the saturated fat content. To infuse our dish with familiar flavors, we began by blooming oregano, tomato paste, and garlic using the high sauté function. One can of crushed tomatoes, plus broth and water, provided the right amount of liquid to cook our whole-wheat pasta and meatballs under pressure. Breaking the pasta into 6-inch lengths helped ensure all noodles were fully submerged for even cooking. Be sure to use ground turkey, not ground turkey breast (also labeled 99 percent fat-free). You can substitute traditional spaghetti for the whole-wheat. Do not substitute other pasta shapes.

1 pound 100 percent whole-wheat spaghetti
1 ounce Parmesan cheese, grated (½ cup), plus extra for serving
¼ cup panko bread crumbs
3 tablespoons plus ¼ cup chopped fresh basil, divided
1 large egg
6 garlic cloves, minced, divided
¾ teaspoon table salt, divided
1 pound ground turkey
2 tablespoons extra-virgin olive oil
2 tablespoons minced fresh oregano or 2 teaspoons dried
1 tablespoon no-salt-added tomato paste
1 (28-ounce) can no-salt-added crushed tomatoes
2 cups unsalted chicken or vegetable broth
2 cups water

1   Loosely wrap half of pasta in dish towel, then press bundle against corner of counter to break noodles into 6-inch lengths; repeat with remaining pasta. Set aside.

2   Combine Parmesan, panko, 3 tablespoons basil, egg, half of garlic, and ¼ teaspoon salt in large bowl. Add turkey and knead with hands until thoroughly combined. Pinch off and roll mixture into twelve 1½-inch meatballs.

3   Using highest sauté function, heat oil in electric pressure cooker until shimmering. Add oregano, tomato paste, and remaining garlic and cook, stirring frequently, until fragrant, about 30 seconds. Stir in tomatoes, broth, water, and remaining ½ teaspoon salt, scraping up any browned bits. Nestle meatballs into sauce, then arrange pasta in even layer on top of meatballs.

4   Lock lid into place and close pressure-release valve. Select high pressure-cook function and cook for 6 minutes. Turn off pressure cooker and quick-release pressure. Carefully remove lid, allowing steam to escape away from you.

5   Gently stir spaghetti, meatballs, and sauce to combine. Partially cover pot and let sit until spaghetti is tender and sauce is thickened, 5 to 8 minutes. Stir in remaining ¼ cup basil and season with salt and pepper to taste. Serve, passing extra Parmesan separately.

MAKE IT DAIRY-FREE • Substitute plant-based Parmesan for the Parmesan cheese.

Pressure-Cooker Parmesan Penne with Chicken and Asparagus

serves 4 to 6 • total time: 45 minutes   **FAST**

why this recipe works • You might think that cooking pasta under pressure means it's impossible to check for doneness partway through cooking, so what you might gain in speed you lose in accuracy. However, through our testing, we discovered a trick: We slightly undercook the pasta under pressure; then, using a combination of the sauté function and residual heat (depending on the recipe), we could simmer or rest the contents of the pot until the pasta and any add-ins are completely cooked. Using this approach, we created a crowd-pleasing dish of whole-wheat penne pasta tossed in a garlicky Parmesan sauce with chicken breasts, asparagus, tomatoes, and fresh basil. We started by creating a potent base of lightly toasted garlic, pepper flakes, and a splash of white wine. After testing our way through the ideal cook times for the pasta and the chicken, we found that we could cook both together, which allowed the pasta to simmer in the flavorful chicken liquid. After turning off the pot and releasing pressure, we removed and shredded the chicken; meanwhile, we stirred asparagus and tomatoes into the pasta and used the high sauté function to soften the vegetables while thickening the pasta sauce. To finish the dish, we returned the shredded chicken to the pot and added Parmesan and fresh basil. For a spicier dish, use the higher amount of pepper flakes.

10	garlic cloves, minced
2	tablespoons extra-virgin olive oil
⅛–¼	teaspoon red pepper flakes
½	cup dry white wine
4	cups unsalted chicken broth
1	cup water
1	pound whole-wheat penne
¾	teaspoon table salt
2	(6- to 8-ounce) boneless, skinless chicken breasts, trimmed and halved lengthwise
1	pound asparagus, trimmed and sliced ¼ inch thick on bias
10	ounces cherry tomatoes, halved
2	ounces Parmesan cheese, grated (1 cup), plus extra for serving
¼	cup chopped fresh basil, plus extra for serving

1   Using highest sauté function, cook garlic, oil, and pepper flakes in electric pressure cooker until fragrant, about 3 minutes. Stir in wine, scraping up any browned bits, and cook until mostly evaporated, about 1 minute. Stir in broth, water, pasta, and salt, then nestle chicken into pasta mixture.

2   Lock lid into place and close pressure-release valve. Select high pressure-cook function and cook for 4 minutes. Turn off pressure cooker and quick-release pressure. Carefully remove lid, allowing steam to escape away from you. Transfer chicken to cutting board, let cool slightly, then shred into bite-size pieces using 2 forks.

3   Meanwhile, stir asparagus and tomatoes into pasta. Cook, using highest sauté function, until pasta and asparagus are tender and sauce is thickened, 5 to 8 minutes. Stir in shredded chicken and any accumulated juices, Parmesan, and basil. Season with salt and pepper to taste. Serve, passing extra Parmesan and basil separately.

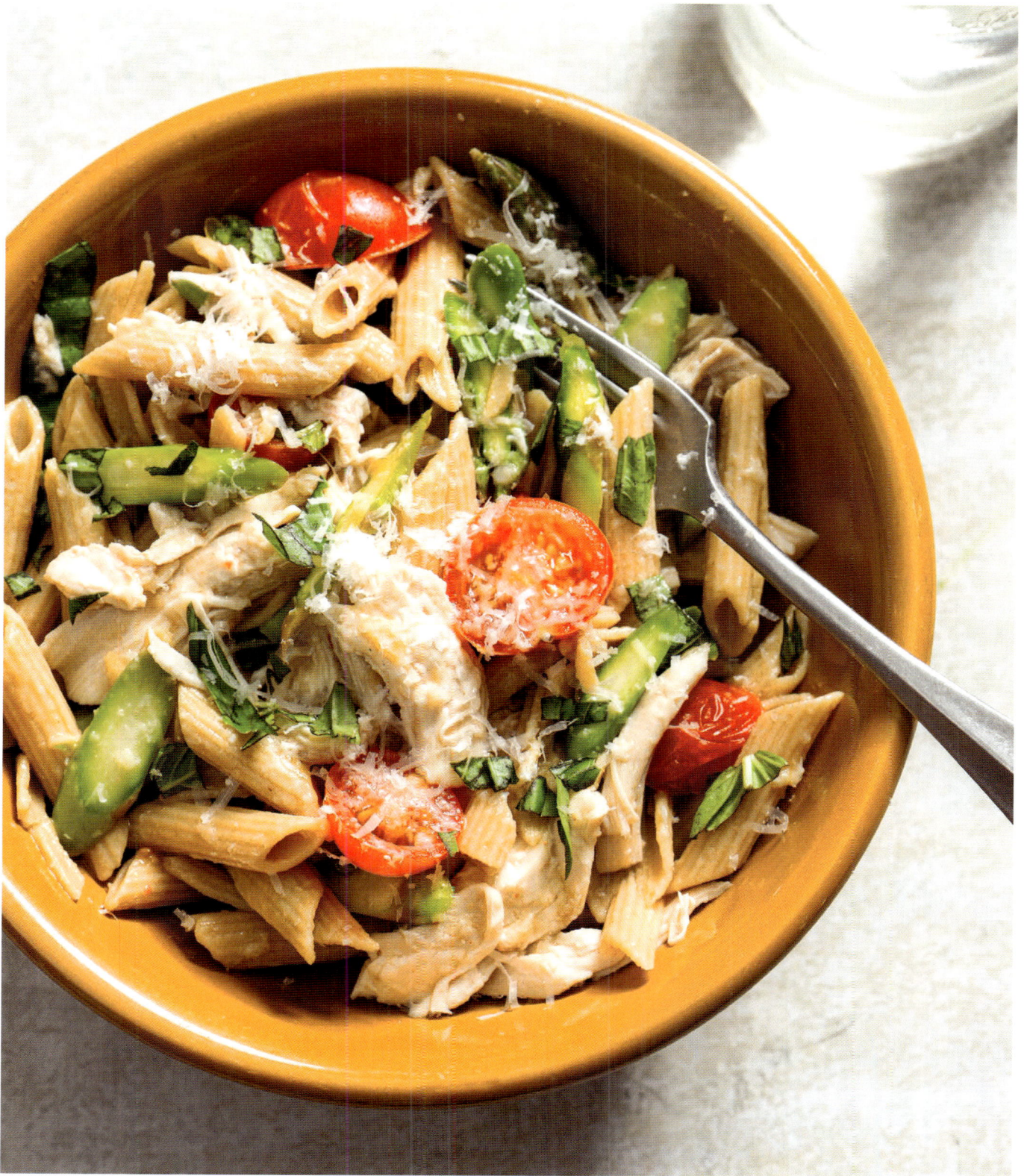

Pressure-Cooker Parmesan Penne with Chicken and Asparagus

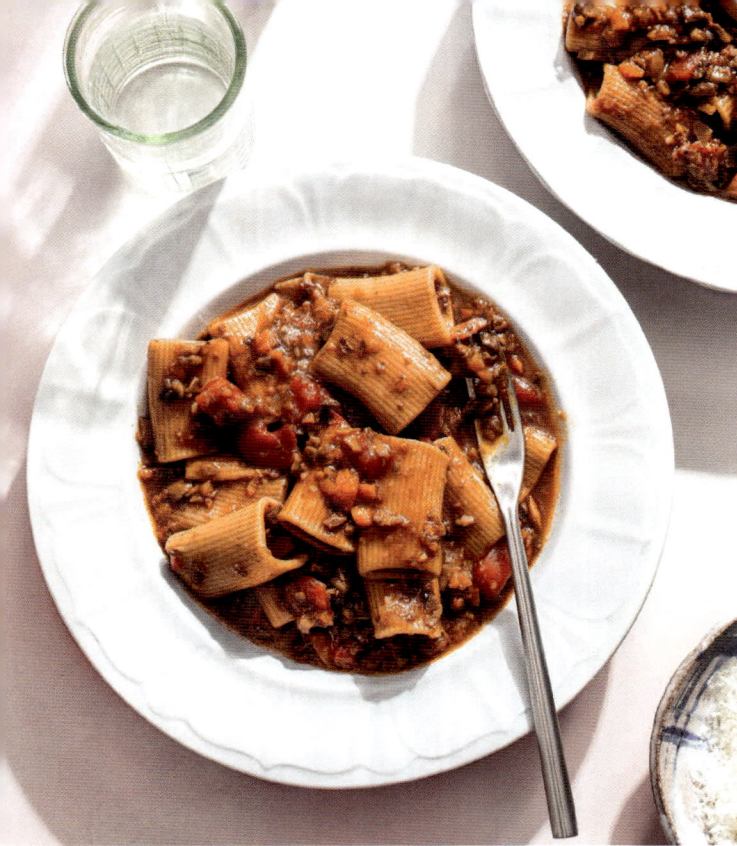

Pressure-Cooker Rigatoni with Mushroom Ragu

serves 4 to 6 • total time: 1 hour

why this recipe works • We wanted to develop a classic Italian-style pasta sauce that would have long-cooked flavor and hearty texture—but swapping antioxidant-rich mushrooms in for the meat. Dried porcini delivered depth of flavor, while a whopping 1½ pounds of fresh cremini gave our sauce a hearty and meaty bite. To round out the sauce's umami qualities, we added a splash of soy sauce and some tomato paste, while a bit of red wine and diced tomatoes added the right amount of fruity acidity and body. To make prep easy, we used the food processor to chop the cremini, onion, and carrot. The key to success was pairing the rich sauce with the right pasta: Rigatoni proved to be a great match, with its sturdy body (to stand up to the heavy sauce) and its ridges (to hold onto the sauce's bits of vegetables). After cooking everything under pressure, we let the pasta and sauce rest until the sauce was perfectly thickened. A sprinkle of grated Parmesan cheese was a simple, classic finish. You can substitute traditional rigatoni for the whole-wheat; however, do not substitute other pasta shapes. If using traditional pasta, decrease the water to ¾ cup.

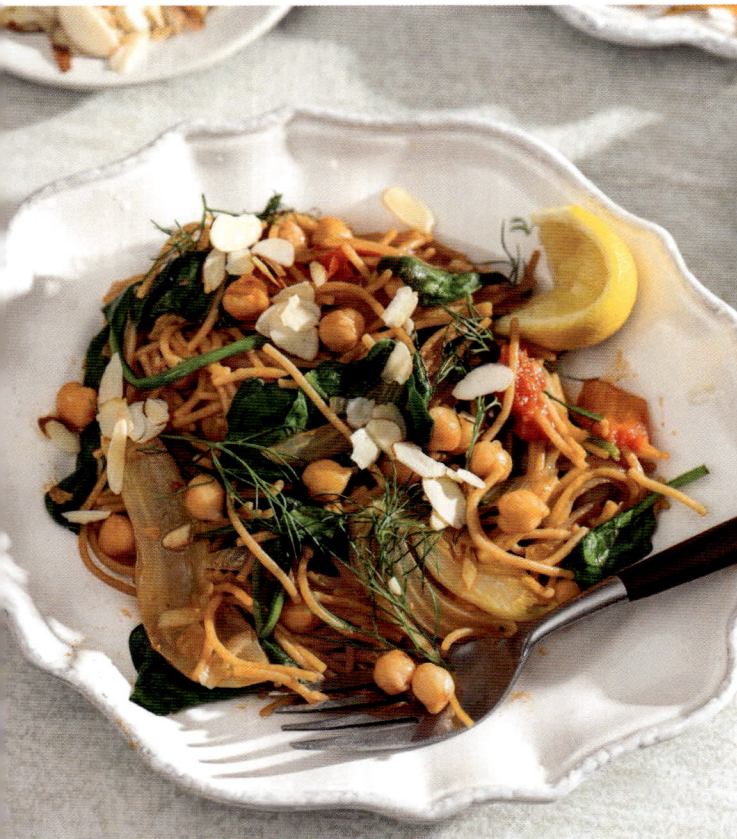

1½ pounds cremini mushrooms, trimmed and quartered
1 carrot, peeled and chopped
1 small onion, chopped
3 tablespoons extra-virgin olive oil
½ ounce dried porcini mushrooms, rinsed and minced
3 garlic cloves, minced
2 tablespoons no-salt-added tomato paste
¾ cup dry red wine
1 (28-ounce) can diced tomatoes
1 pound 100 percent whole-wheat rigatoni
2 cups unsalted vegetable or chicken broth
1½ cups water
1 tablespoon low-sodium soy sauce
   Grated Parmesan cheese

1 Working in batches, pulse cremini mushrooms in food processor until pieces are no larger than ½ inch, 5 to 7 pulses; transfer to large bowl. Pulse carrot and onion in now-empty processor until finely chopped, 5 to 7 pulses; transfer to bowl with mushrooms.

2 Using highest sauté function, heat oil in electric pressure cooker until shimmering. Add processed vegetables and porcini mushrooms, partially cover pot, and cook, stirring occasionally, until vegetables release their liquid, about 5 minutes. Uncover and continue to cook until liquid has evaporated and vegetables begin to brown, 8 to 10 minutes.

3 Add garlic and tomato paste and cook, stirring frequently, until fragrant, about 30 seconds. Stir in wine, scraping up any browned bits, and cook until mostly evaporated, about 1 minute. Stir in tomatoes and their juice, pasta, broth, water, and soy sauce.

4 Lock lid into place and close pressure-release valve. Select high pressure-cook function and cook for 5 minutes. Turn off pressure cooker and quick-release pressure. Carefully remove lid, allowing steam to escape away from you.

5 Stir pasta and sauce to combine. Partially cover pot and let sit until pasta is tender and sauce is thickened, 5 to 8 minutes. Season with salt and pepper to taste. Serve, passing Parmesan separately.

❙ **MAKE IT DAIRY-FREE** • Omit the Parmesan cheese.

Pressure-Cooker Fideos with Chickpeas, Fennel, and Spinach

serves 4 • total time: 45 minutes   `FAST`

why this recipe works • Fideos, traditional to Spanish cooking, is a richly flavored dish in which thin noodles are toasted until nut-brown, then cooked in a garlicky, tomatoey sauce, sometimes with seafood. Recipes often involve a homemade stock, a sofrito base of slowly reduced fresh tomatoes with seasonings, and time in the oven. The complex flavors are undeniably exciting, but the preparation can be time-consuming. We streamlined the sofrito base by finely chopping onion (so it softened and browned quickly with the sauté function), thinly slicing fennel, and using canned tomatoes instead of fresh. Garlic, smoked paprika, and wine added even more depth to the broth. Canned chickpeas were a convenient way to up the protein and fiber. We chose whole-wheat spaghetti because it retained its bite under pressure, not to mention gave us a nice dose of fiber. After cooking everything under pressure, we stirred spinach into the pasta to wilt while the

sauce thickened. A final garnish of fennel fronds and sliced almonds provided welcome textural contrast. You can substitute traditional spaghetti for the whole-wheat spaghetti; however, do not substitute other pasta shapes. If your fennel bulb does not come with fronds, substitute 1 tablespoon chopped fresh dill or parsley for the fronds.

> 8 ounces 100 percent whole-wheat spaghetti
> 2 tablespoons extra-virgin olive oil
> 1 onion, chopped fine
> 1 fennel bulb, 1 tablespoon fronds minced, stalks discarded, bulb halved, cored, and sliced thin
> 3 garlic cloves, minced
> 1½ teaspoons smoked paprika
> 1½ cups unsalted vegetable or chicken broth
> 1 (15-ounce) can chickpeas, rinsed
> 1 (14.5-ounce) can diced tomatoes
> ¼ cup dry white wine
> ¼ teaspoon table salt
> ¼ teaspoon pepper
> 4 ounces (4 cups) baby spinach
> ¼ cup sliced almonds, toasted
>   Lemon wedges

1 Loosely wrap pasta in dish towel, then press bundle against corner of counter to break noodles into 1- to 2-inch lengths.

2 Using highest sauté function, heat oil in electric pressure cooker until shimmering. Add onion and sliced fennel and cook until softened, about 5 minutes. Add pasta and cook, stirring frequently, until lightly toasted, about 2 minutes.

3 Add garlic and paprika and cook, stirring frequently, until fragrant, about 30 seconds. Stir in broth, chickpeas, tomatoes and their juice, wine, salt, and pepper.

4 Lock lid into place and close pressure-release valve. Select high pressure-cook function and cook for 1 minute. Turn off pressure cooker and quick-release pressure. Carefully remove lid, allowing steam to escape away from you.

5 Stir spinach into pasta. Partially cover pot and let sit until pasta is tender and sauce is thickened, 5 to 8 minutes. Season with salt and pepper to taste. Sprinkle with fennel fronds and almonds and serve with lemon wedges.

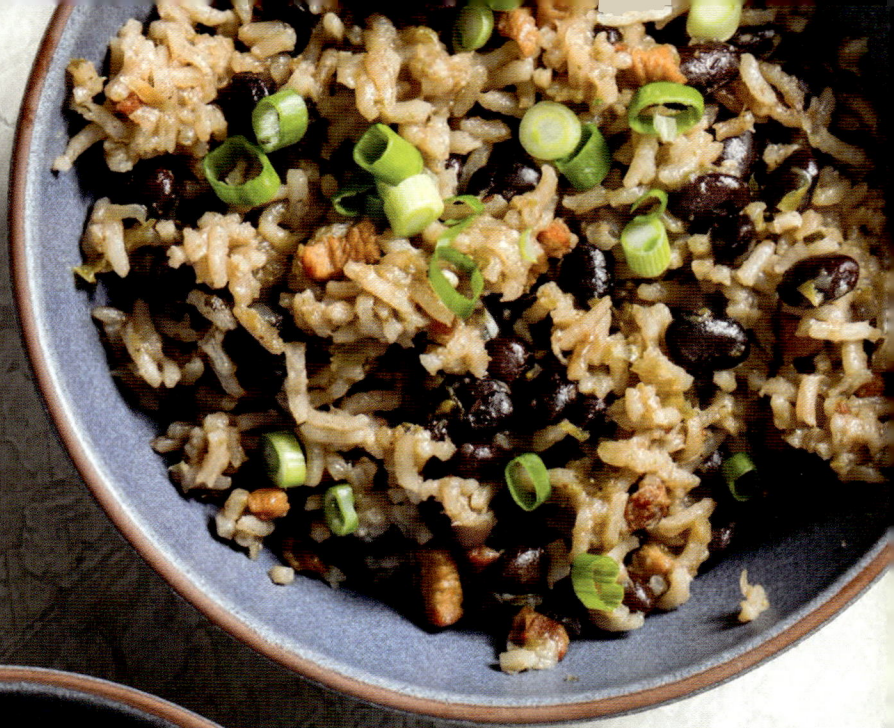

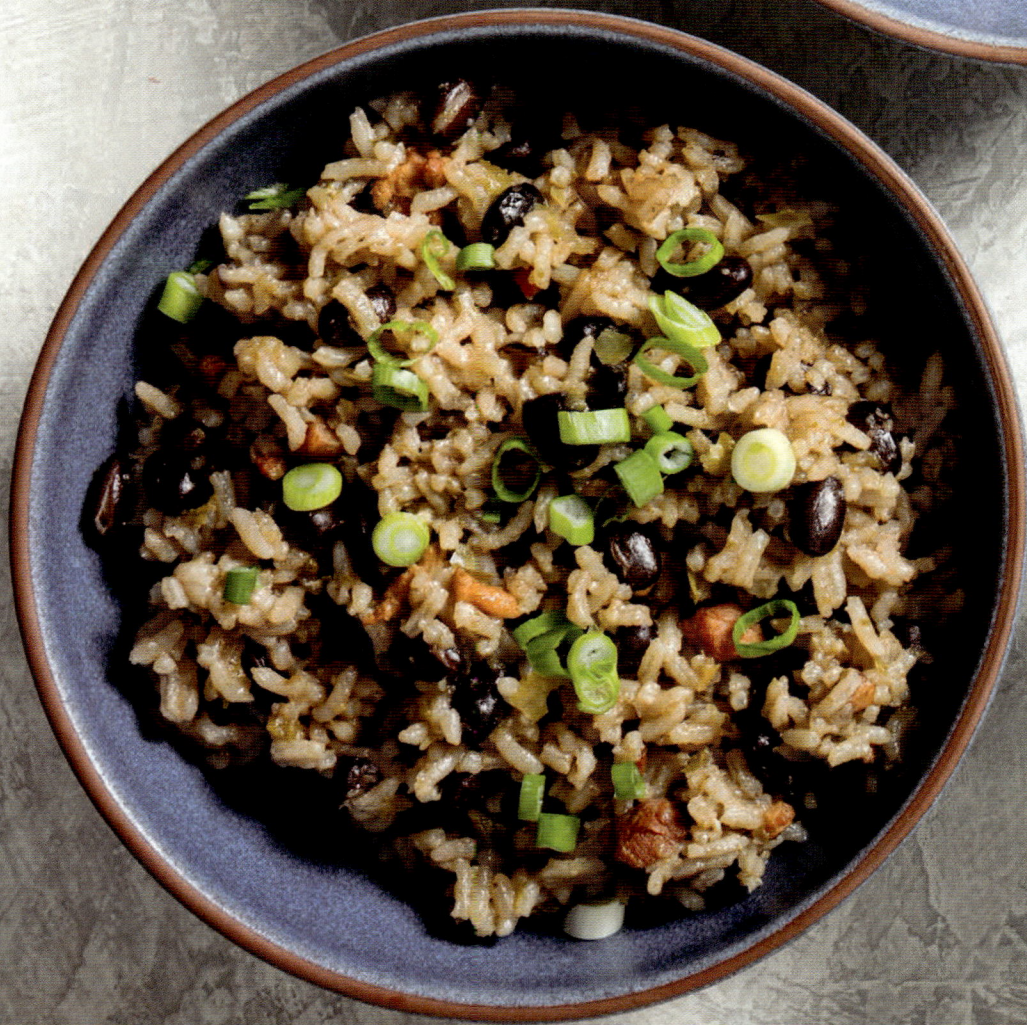

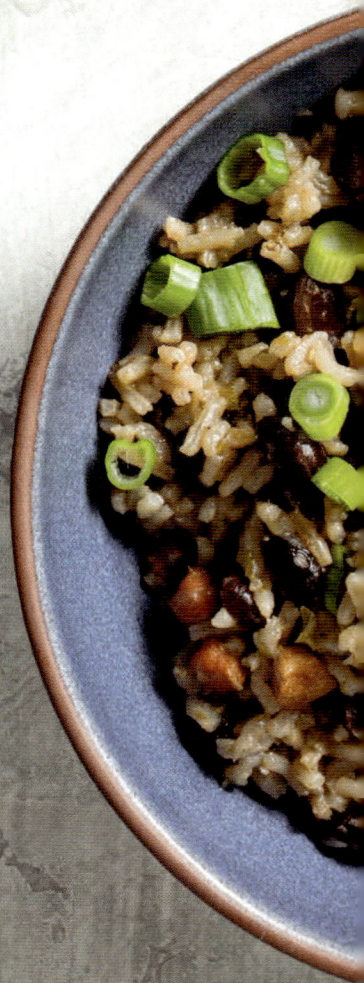

BEAN, GRAIN & VEGETABLE SIDES

■ FAST   ■ SUPERCHARGED

bean & grain basics

Grain Cooking Methods

Grains can be cooked a variety of ways. We especially like simmering, boiling, and microwaving. Boiling is usually the best choice for longer-cooking grains such as farro and wheat berries, while simmering and microwaving tend to be good choices for shorter-cooking grains such as quinoa.

Boiling (the pasta method)

This approach involves boiling the grains in a large amount of water that is later drained off. Bring 2 or 4 quarts water (depending on the grain) to a boil in a large saucepan. Stir in the grains and ½ teaspoon salt. Return to a boil, then reduce to a simmer and cook until the grains are tender, following the times in the cooking chart (page 333). Drain.

Simmering (the pilaf method)

This technique calls for simmering a measured amount of grains in a specific amount of water in a covered pot until the water is absorbed. Rinse and dry the grains on a towel. Heat 1 tablespoon oil in a medium saucepan (preferably nonstick) over medium-high heat until shimmering. Stir in the grains and toast until lightly golden and fragrant, 2 to 3 minutes. Stir in the water and ¼ teaspoon salt. Bring the mixture to a simmer, then reduce the heat to low, cover, and continue to simmer until the grains are tender and have absorbed all of the liquid, following the times in the cooking chart (page 333). Off the heat, let the grains stand for 10 minutes, then fluff with a fork.

Microwaving

Rinse the grains. Combine the grains, 1 or 2 cups water, and ¼ teaspoon salt in a bowl. Cover and cook following the times and temperatures in the cooking chart (page 333) until the grains are tender and have absorbed all of the liquid. Carefully remove the bowl from the microwave and let sit covered for 5 minutes, then fluff with a fork.

Quinoa Pilaf with Herbs and Lemon

serves 4 to 6 • total time: 1 hour

- 1½ cups prewashed white quinoa
- 2 tablespoons extra-virgin olive oil
- 1 small onion, chopped fine
- ¾ teaspoon table salt
- 1¾ cups water
- 3 tablespoons chopped fresh parsley, cilantro, chives, and/or tarragon
- 1 tablespoon lemon juice

1 Toast quinoa in medium saucepan over medium-high heat, stirring frequently, until quinoa is very fragrant and makes continuous popping sound, 5 to 7 minutes. Transfer quinoa to bowl and set aside.

2 Heat oil in now-empty saucepan over medium-low heat until shimmering. Add onion and salt and cook until softened and lightly browned, 5 to 7 minutes.

3 Increase heat to medium-high, stir in water and quinoa, and bring to simmer. Cover, reduce heat to low, and simmer until grains are just tender and liquid has been fully absorbed, 18 to 20 minutes, stirring once halfway through cooking. Remove saucepan from heat and let sit, covered, for 10 minutes. Fluff quinoa with fork, stir in herbs and lemon juice, and season with salt and pepper to taste. Serve.

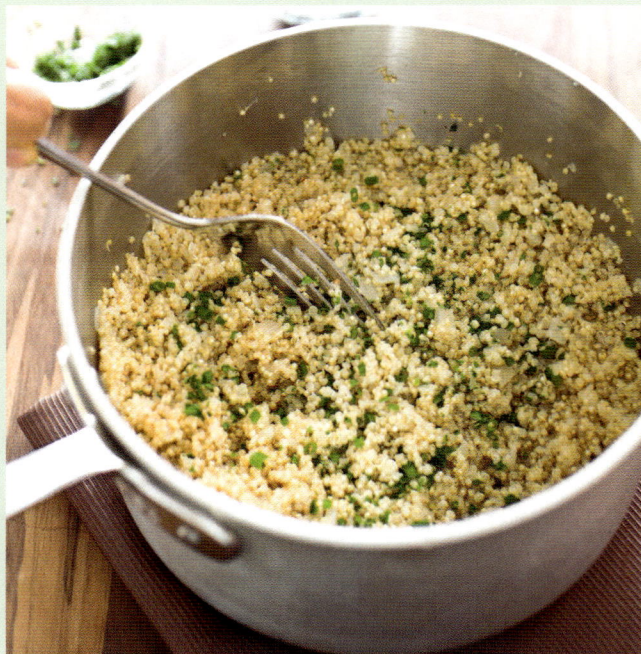

Quinoa Pilaf with Herbs and Lemon

Grain Cooking Chart

For the grains below, 1 cup dry grains = 2½ cups cooked; 1½ cups dry grains = 4 cups cooked.

Recipes can be scaled up by increasing the amounts proportionally. Cooking times do not change.

TYPE OF GRAIN	COOKING METHOD	AMOUNT OF GRAIN	AMOUNT OF WATER	COOKING TIME
Pearl Barley	Boiled	1½ cups	4 quarts	20 to 40 minutes
	Pilaf-Style	X	X	X
	Microwave	X	X	X
Bulgur (medium- to coarse-grind)	Boiled	1 cup	4 quarts	15 to 20 minutes
	Pilaf-Style*	1 cup	1 cup	16 to 18 minutes
	Microwave	1 cup	1 cup	5 to 10 minutes
Bulgur (fine-grind)	Boiled	X	X	X
	Pilaf-Style	X	X	X
	Microwave	1 cup	2 cups	4 minutes
Buckwheat	Boiled	1 cup	2 quarts	10 to 12 minutes
	Pilaf-Style	1 cup	1½ cups	12 minutes
	Microwave	X	X	X
Farro	Boiled	1 cup	4 quarts	15 to 20 minutes
	Pilaf-Style	X	X	X
	Microwave	X	X	X
Fonio	Boiled	X	X	X
	Pilaf-Style	X	X	X
	Microwave	1 cup	2 cups	5 minutes
Freekeh	Boiled	1½ cups	4 quarts	30 to 45 minutes
	Pilaf-Style	X	X	X
	Microwave	X	X	X
Kamut	Boiled	1 cup	2 quarts	55 minutes to 1¼ hours
	Pilaf-Style	X	X	X
	Microwave	X	X	X
Millet	Boiled	X	X	X
	Pilaf-Style**	1 cup	2 cups	15 to 20 minutes
	Microwave	X	X	X
Oat Berries	Boiled	1 cup	4 quarts	30 to 40 minutes
	Pilaf-Style	1 cup	1½ cups	30 to 40 minutes
	Microwave	X	X	X
Quinoa (any color)	Boiled	X	X	X
	Pilaf-Style	1 cup	1 cup + 3 tablespoons	18 to 20 minutes
	Microwave	1 cup	2 cups	5 minutes on medium, then 5 minutes on high
Spelt	Boiled	1 cup	2 quarts	50 minutes to 1 hour 5 minutes
	Pilaf-Style	X	X	X
	Microwave	X	X	X
Wheat Berries	Boiled	1 cup	4 quarts	1 hour
	Pilaf-Style	X	X	X
	Microwave	X	X	X

* For pilaf, do not rinse, and skip the toasting step, adding the grain to the pot with the liquid.

** For pilaf, increase the toasting time until the grains begin to pop, about 12 minutes.

X = Not recommended

Basic Beans

makes about 7 cups · total time: 1¼ hours, plus 8 hours brining

1½ tablespoons table salt for brining
 1 pound (2½ cups) dried beans, picked over and rinsed
1½ teaspoons table salt

1 Dissolve 1½ tablespoons salt in 2 quarts cold water in large container. Add beans and soak at room temperature for at least 8 hours or up to 24 hours. Drain and rinse well.

2 Bring soaked beans and 7 cups water to simmer in Dutch oven over medium heat. Reduce heat to medium-low and simmer, uncovered, until beans are tender, about 40 minutes. Off heat, stir in salt and let sit for 15 minutes. Drain and serve.

MAKE AHEAD · Brined and drained beans can be refrigerated for up to 4 days or frozen up to 1 month. Pat dry with paper towels and transfer to a zipper-lock bag for freezing.

NOTES FROM THE TEST KITCHEN

Quick-Brining Beans

If you are pressed for time, a quick brine (water plus salt) for an hour is better than nothing, but the test kitchen strongly recommends overnight brining. Longer brining results in superior texture and the creamiest beans. Quick brined dried beans will be less creamy and may take longer to cook

To quick-brine beans Combine dried beans with 1½ tablespoons salt in 2 quarts cold water in a large Dutch oven and bring to a boil. Remove from the heat, cover, and let sit for 1 hour. Drain and rinse well under cold water before continuing with the recipe.

Baked Brown Rice

serves 4 to 6 · total time: 1¾ hours

 1 tablespoon extra-virgin olive oil
 1 small onion, chopped fine
 ¼ teaspoon table salt
2¼ cups water
 1 cup unsalted vegetable or chicken broth
1½ cups long-grain brown rice, rinsed

1 Adjust oven rack to middle position and heat oven to 375 degrees. Heat oil in Dutch oven over medium heat until shimmering. Add onion and salt and cook until softened and lightly browned, 5 to 7 minutes.

2 Add water and broth, cover, and bring to boil. Off heat, stir in rice. Cover, transfer pot to oven, and bake rice until tender and liquid has been fully absorbed, 60 to 75 minutes.

3 Remove pot from oven. Fluff rice with fork, scraping up any rice that has stuck to bottom. Place folded clean dish towel over pot, then replace lid and let sit for 10 minutes. Serve.

Rice and Bean Pilaf

serves 4 · total time: 45 minutes **FAST**

 1 tablespoon extra-virgin olive oil
 1 small shallot, minced
 ¾ cup long-grain white rice, rinsed
 1 cup water
 ¼ teaspoon table salt
 1 (15-ounce) can no-salt-added chickpeas, rinsed

1 Heat oil in small saucepan over medium heat until shimmering. Add shallot and cook until softened, about 2 minutes. Stir in rice and cook until edges of grains begin to turn translucent, about 2 minutes. Stir in water and salt and bring to boil. Add chickpeas (do not stir into rice), reduce heat to low, cover, and simmer until all liquid is absorbed, 12 to 15 minutes.

2 Remove saucepan from heat. Remove lid, place folded clean dish towel over saucepan, then replace lid. Let rice and beans sit for 10 minutes. Gently fluff rice and beans with fork. Serve.

Southwestern Black Bean Salad

serves 4 · total time: 25 minutes **FAST**

why this recipe works · For a light, summery bean salad, we combined fiber-rich black beans with fresh corn, bright tomato, and creamy avocado. Toasting the corn in a skillet until golden brown brought out its natural sweetness. Chipotle chile in adobo sauce, cilantro, and lime juice created a Southwestern flavor profile—plus lots of phytonutrients—for this easy-to-prepare salad. Fresh corn is important for the flavor of the salad, so we don't recommend substituting frozen or canned corn in this recipe.

- 2 scallions, sliced thin
- 3 tablespoons lime juice (2 limes)
- 2 tablespoons extra-virgin olive oil, divided
- 1½ teaspoons minced canned chipotle chile in adobo sauce
- ¼ teaspoon plus ⅛ teaspoon table salt, divided
- ¼ teaspoon pepper
- 2 ears corn, kernels cut from cobs
- 1 (15-ounce) can no-salt-added black beans, rinsed
- 1 tomato, cored and chopped
- 1 avocado, halved, pitted, and cut into ½-inch pieces
- 3 tablespoons minced fresh cilantro

1 Whisk scallions, lime juice, 1 tablespoon oil, chipotle, ¼ teaspoon salt, and pepper together in large bowl.

2 Heat remaining 1 tablespoon oil in 10-inch skillet over medium-high heat until just smoking. Add corn and remaining ⅛ teaspoon salt and cook, stirring occasionally, until golden brown, 6 to 8 minutes. Transfer corn, beans, and tomato to bowl with dressing and toss gently to coat. Gently fold in avocado and cilantro. Season with pepper to taste, and serve.

Cuban-Style Black Beans and Rice

serves 6 to 8 · total time: 1¾ hours, plus 8 hours brining

why this recipe works · Beans and rice is a familiar combination the world over, with good reason: It's healthful, inexpensive, and full of fiber and nutrients. Cuban black beans and rice is unique in that the rice is cooked in the inky, concentrated liquid left over from cooking the beans. For our take inspired by this technique, we brined the beans overnight before cooking. We reserved half of our sofrito ingredients (a combination of garlic, bell pepper, and onion) and added them to the cooking liquid to infuse the beans with aromatic flavor. Lightly browning the remaining sofrito vegetables along with spices and tomato paste added complex

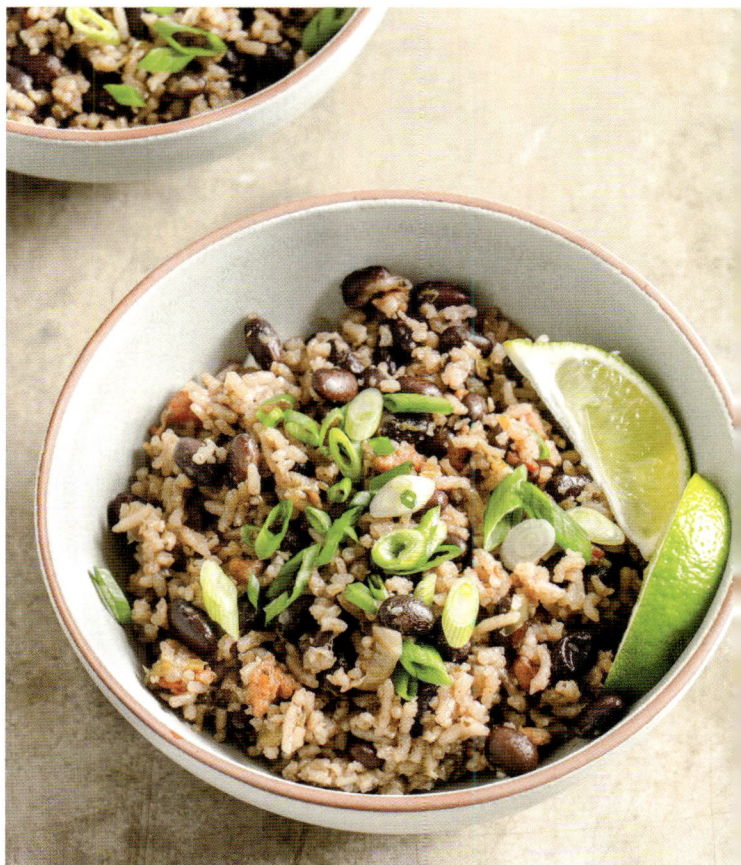

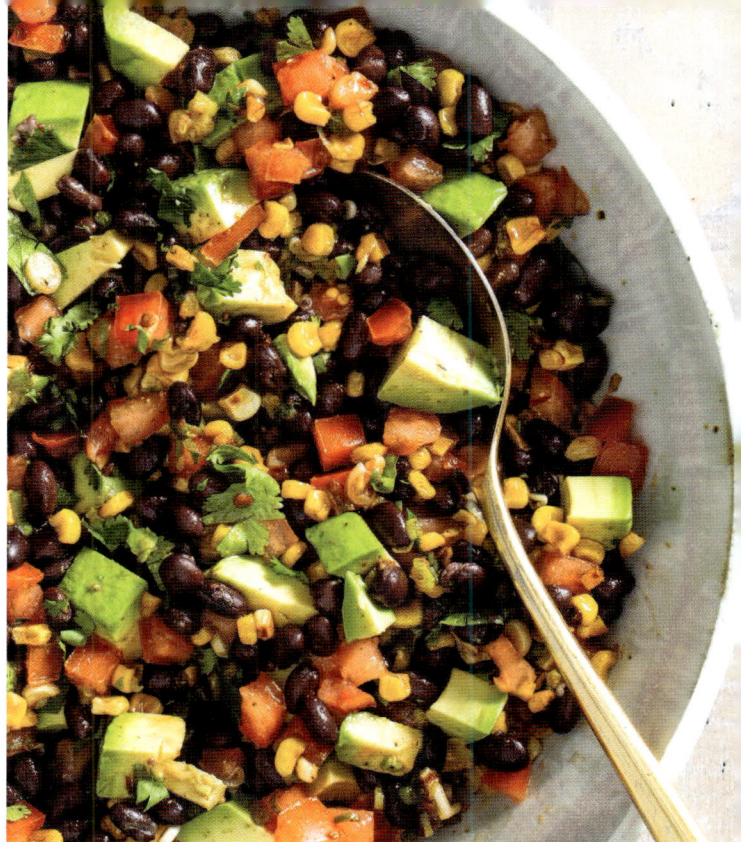

top | Southwestern Black Bean Salad
bottom | Cuban-Style Black Beans and Rice

flavor to this simple dish. Once the beans were soft, we combined them with the sofrito and rice to finish cooking. Baking the rice and beans eliminated the crusty bottom that can form when the dish is cooked on the stovetop.

1½ tablespoons table salt for brining
1 cup dried black beans, picked over and rinsed
2 large green bell peppers, halved, stemmed, and seeded, divided
1 large onion, halved crosswise and peeled, root end left intact, divided
1 garlic head, 5 cloves minced, rest of head halved crosswise with skin left intact, divided
2 bay leaves
1½ teaspoons table salt, plus salt for cooking beans
2 tablespoons extra-virgin olive oil
4 teaspoons ground cumin
1 tablespoon minced fresh oregano or 1 teaspoon dried
1 tablespoon no-salt-added tomato paste
1½ cups long-grain white rice
2 tablespoons red wine vinegar
2 scallions, sliced thin
Lime wedges

1 Dissolve 1½ tablespoons salt in 2 quarts cold water in large bowl or container. Add beans and soak at room temperature for at least 8 hours or up to 24 hours. Drain and rinse well. (If you're pressed for time, see page 334 for information on quick-brining your beans.)

2 Combine beans, 4 cups water, 1 bell pepper half, 1 onion half (with root end), halved garlic head, bay leaves, and 1 teaspoon salt in Dutch oven. Bring to simmer over medium-high heat, cover, and reduce heat to low. Cook until beans are just soft, 30 to 40 minutes.

3 Discard bell pepper, onion, garlic, and bay leaves. Drain beans in colander set over large bowl, reserving 2½ cups bean cooking liquid. (If you don't have enough cooking liquid, add water as needed to measure 2½ cups.) Do not wash pot.

4 Adjust oven rack to middle position and heat oven to 350 degrees. Cut remaining bell peppers and onion into 2-inch pieces and pulse in food processor until chopped into rough ¼-inch pieces, about 8 pulses, scraping down bowl as needed.

5 Add oil to now-empty pot and heat over medium heat until shimmering. Add processed bell peppers and onion, cumin, oregano, and tomato paste and cook, stirring often, until vegetables are softened and beginning to brown, 10 to 15 minutes. Stir in minced garlic and cook until fragrant, about 1 minute. Stir in rice and cook for 30 seconds.

6 Stir in beans, reserved bean cooking liquid, vinegar, and remaining 1½ teaspoons salt. Increase heat to medium-high and bring to simmer. Cover, transfer to oven, and cook until liquid is absorbed and rice is tender, about 30 minutes. Fluff rice with fork and let rest, uncovered, for 5 minutes. Serve with scallions and lime wedges.

MAKE AHEAD • Brined and drained beans can be refrigerated for up to 4 days or frozen up to 1 month. Pat dry with paper towels and transfer to a zipper-lock bag for freezing.

Succotash Salad with Butter Beans and Basil

serves 4 to 6 • total time: 25 minutes, plus 30 minutes resting

why this recipe works • When seasonal summer produce is at its best, it should be allowed to shine, as it does here in this fresh, bright succotash. Here, we combined sweet corn (browned to add a hint of caramelized complexity) with mild, creamy butter beans; zucchini; and cherry tomatoes and then doused the mixture in an ultrarefreshing white wine vinaigrette. To keep the dish in anti-inflammatory territory, we skipped cream or butter, allowing the fresh flavors to take center stage. We stirred in fresh basil, which brought a licorice-like note, and scallions, which contributed a light savoriness and a pop of green. Fresh corn is important for the flavor of the salad—we don't recommend substituting frozen or canned corn here.

⅓ cup extra-virgin olive oil, divided
¼ cup white wine vinegar
2 teaspoons table salt, divided
1 teaspoon pepper
1 (15-ounce) can no-salt-added butter beans, rinsed
8 ounces cherry tomatoes, halved
1 zucchini, cut into ½-inch pieces
4 scallions, sliced thin
4 ears corn, kernels cut from cobs (3 cups)
1 garlic clove, minced
2 tablespoons chopped fresh basil

1 Whisk ¼ cup oil, vinegar, 1½ teaspoons salt, and pepper together in large bowl. Add butter beans, tomatoes, zucchini, and scallions and toss to combine.

2   Heat remaining oil in 12-inch nonstick skillet over medium-high heat until shimmering. Add corn and remaining ½ teaspoon salt and cook, stirring occasionally, until softened and just beginning to brown, 5 to 7 minutes. Add garlic and cook until fragrant, about 30 seconds.

3   Transfer corn mixture to bowl with butter bean mixture and toss to combine. Let sit for at least 30 minutes to allow flavors to meld. Stir in basil and season with salt and pepper to taste. Serve.

Black-Eyed Pea Salad with Peaches and Pecans

serves 4 to 6 • total time: 15 minutes   **FAST**   **SUPERCHARGED**

why this recipe works • With their delicate skins and creamy interiors, black-eyed peas are a hearty, fiberful addition to salads and are especially popular in the South, so we looked to Southern cuisine for inspiration to create this ultrasimple dish. We used canned black-eyed peas, which are convenient and have great flavor and texture. Peaches added sweet juiciness and fiber, while pecans lent crunch and healthy fats. For a little spice, we chopped a jalapeño, removing its seeds to mellow its fruity heat. We felt greens were necessary but wanted something other than humdrum romaine. We turned to frisée, a delicate but slightly bitter-tasting lettuce with more anti-inflammatory compounds. Finely chopped red onion added a nice bite, and basil added freshness. The tartness of our lime vinaigrette nicely counterbalanced the peaches. If you can't find good ripe peaches, you can substitute 1 orange, peeled and chopped into ½-inch pieces.

  1   teaspoon grated lime zest plus 2½ tablespoons juice (2 limes)
  1   small garlic clove, minced
  ¾   teaspoon table salt
  2   tablespoons extra-virgin olive oil
  2   (15-ounce) cans no-salt-added black-eyed peas, rinsed
  2   peaches, halved, pitted, and chopped coarse
  3   ounces frisée, trimmed and chopped into 2-inch pieces
  ¼   cup finely chopped red onion
  ¼   cup pecans, toasted and chopped
  ¼   cup fresh basil leaves, torn into ½-inch pieces
  1   jalapeño chile, stemmed, seeded, and chopped fine

Whisk lime zest and juice, garlic, and salt together in large bowl. Slowly whisk in oil until incorporated. Add beans, peaches, frisée, onion, pecans, basil, and jalapeño and toss to combine. Season with salt and pepper to taste, and serve.

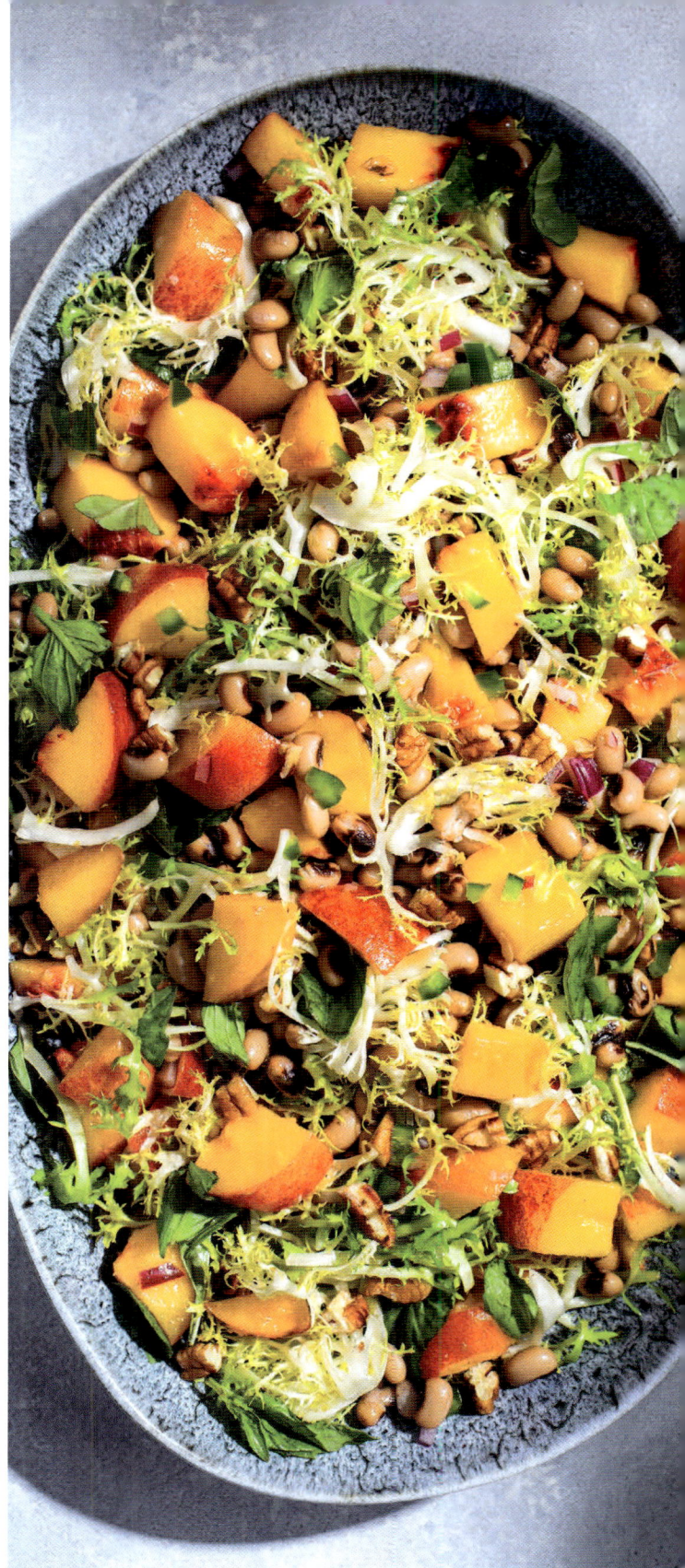

Black-Eyed Pea Salad with Peaches and Pecans

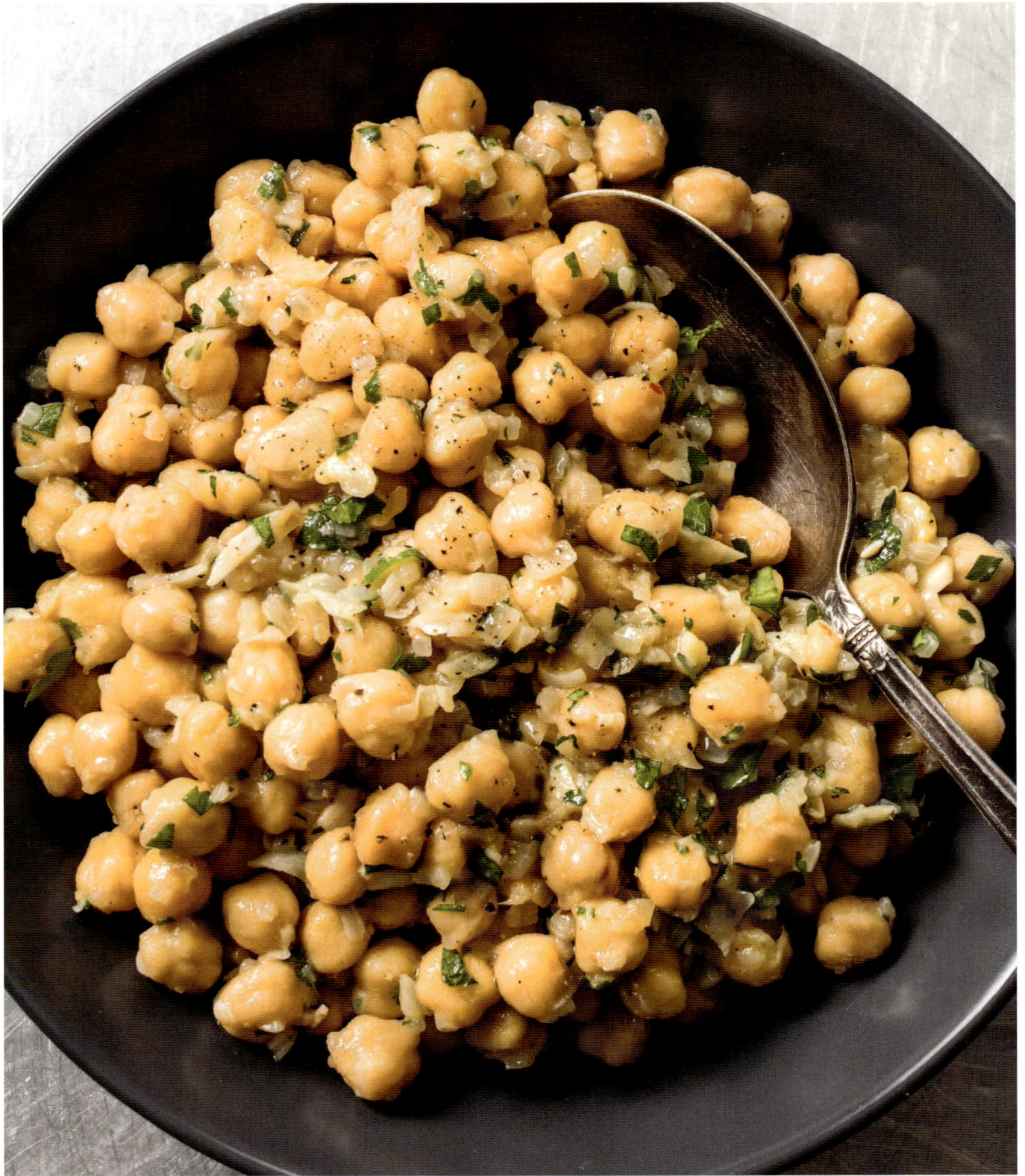

Chickpeas with Garlic and Parsley

Stewed Chickpeas and Spinach with Dill and Lemon

serves 4 to 6 • total time: 20 minutes **FAST**

why this recipe works • For this protein-rich Greek-inspired side, we wanted chickpeas tossed with a tangle of wilted spinach in a vibrant lemon-and-dill-flavored broth. We heated garlic and pepper flakes in olive oil to infuse the oil with spicy flavor. Canned chickpeas kept this weeknight-friendly. Instead of curly-leaf spinach, which required stemming and chopping, we opted for prep-free baby spinach. A little broth provided a savory backbone that tied the dish together. To give the broth body, we added the starchy liquid from a can of chickpeas along with the beans. Lemon juice and a handful of fresh dill added bright freshness.

- 2 tablespoons extra-virgin olive oil, plus extra for drizzling
- 3 garlic cloves, sliced thin
- ¼ teaspoon red pepper flakes
- 2 (15-ounce) cans no-salt-added chickpeas (1 can drained and rinsed, 1 can left undrained)
- 10 ounces (10 cups) baby spinach
- ½ cup unsalted vegetable or chicken broth
- ¼ teaspoon table salt
- ¼ cup chopped fresh dill
- 1 tablespoon lemon juice

Cook oil, garlic, and pepper flakes in Dutch oven over medium heat until garlic is golden brown, 3 to 5 minutes. Stir in 1 can drained chickpeas, 1 can chickpeas and their liquid, spinach, broth, and salt. Increase heat to medium-high and cook, stirring occasionally, until spinach is wilted and liquid is slightly thickened, about 5 minutes. Off heat, stir in dill and lemon juice. Season with salt and pepper to taste. Drizzle with extra oil and serve.

Chickpeas with Garlic and Parsley

serves 4 to 6 • total time: 30 minutes **FAST**

why this recipe works • Chickpeas are an ultraversatile ingredient that tastes terrific even when simply sautéed with a few flavorful ingredients. To build an aromatic base, we turned to garlic and red pepper flakes. Instead of mincing the garlic, we cut it into thin slices and sautéed them in extra-virgin olive oil for caramelized, more complex flavor that shone through in the finished dish. We softened an onion along with this aromatic base and then added the chickpeas along with a cup of broth, which imparted a savory richness to the dish without overpowering it. Parsley made for a perfectly herbaceous finish.

- ¼ cup extra-virgin olive oil, divided
- 4 garlic cloves, sliced thin
- ⅛ teaspoon red pepper flakes
- 1 onion, chopped fine
- ¼ teaspoon table salt
- 2 (15-ounce) cans no-salt-added chickpeas, rinsed
- 1 cup unsalted vegetable or chicken broth
- 2 tablespoons minced fresh parsley
- 2 teaspoons lemon juice

1 Cook 3 tablespoons oil, garlic, and pepper flakes in 12-inch skillet over medium heat, stirring frequently, until garlic turns golden but not brown, about 3 minutes. Stir in onion and salt and cook until softened and lightly browned, 5 to 7 minutes. Stir in chickpeas and broth and bring to simmer. Reduce heat to medium-low, cover, and cook until chickpeas are heated through and flavors meld, about 7 minutes.

2 Uncover, increase heat to high, and continue to cook until nearly all liquid has evaporated, about 3 minutes. Off heat, stir in parsley and lemon juice. Season with salt and pepper to taste and drizzle with remaining 1 tablespoon oil. Serve.

Edamame Salad with Arugula and Radishes

serves 6 • total time: 20 minutes **FAST** **SUPERCHARGED**

why this recipe works • We love snacking on edamame steamed in their shells, but to turn these immature soybeans into a more substantial salad, we took advantage of frozen, shelled edamame—a great source of plant-based protein and anti-inflammatory compounds—and tossed them with a vibrant mix of arugula, basil, and mint. The herbaceous basil and mint complemented the peppery arugula, and the edamame's neutral flavor and satisfying pop of texture paired well with the fragrant greens. Though fresh herbs are often used in minimal amounts for seasoning, we wanted to treat them like salad greens so used a handful of each, ensuring tons of flavor and a medley of extra vitamins and minerals. Thinly sliced shallot added mild onion flavor, and just a couple of radishes added crunch and color. For the vinaigrette, we chose to use rice vinegar for its mild acidity, which would complement and not overpower the edamame; we added a little honey for sweetness and to help emulsify the dressing. One small garlic clove added flavor without taking over the dish. The finishing touch was a sprinkling of roasted sunflower seeds, which contributed nuttiness and depth to our bright salad.

2 tablespoons unseasoned rice vinegar
1 tablespoon honey
1 small garlic clove, minced
¾ teaspoon table salt
3 tablespoons extra-virgin olive oil
20 ounces frozen shelled edamame beans, thawed and patted dry
2 ounces (2 cups) baby arugula
½ cup shredded fresh basil
½ cup chopped fresh mint
2 radishes, trimmed, halved, and sliced thin
1 shallot, halved and sliced thin
¼ cup roasted sunflower seeds

1 Whisk vinegar, honey, garlic, and salt together in large bowl. Whisking constantly, drizzle in oil until combined.

2 Add edamame, arugula, basil, mint, radishes, and shallot to bowl and toss to combine. Sprinkle with sunflower seeds and season with salt and pepper to taste. Serve.

Sautéed Fava Beans, Asparagus, and Leek

serves 6 • total time: 45 minutes **FAST**

why this recipe works • We love the mildly earthy flavor and toothsome texture of fava beans. Quickly sautéing these buttery beans with asparagus, leek, and fresh herbs made for an ultra-springy side dish. We shelled and blanched the favas and then added them at the end of cooking to preserve their vibrant color and creamy bite. This recipe works best with fresh fava beans; look for them at farmers' markets or supermarkets and choose bright-green, unblemished pods. You can use 12 ounces (2½ cups) frozen shelled fava beans, thawed, in place of the fresh favas; skip step 1. Do not use dried beans.

2½ pounds fava beans, shelled (2½ cups)
2 tablespoons extra-virgin olive oil
1 leek, white and light green parts only, sliced thin, and washed thoroughly (1½ cups)
1 pound asparagus, trimmed and cut on bias into 1-inch lengths
½ teaspoon table salt
⅛ teaspoon pepper
1 teaspoon grated lemon zest, plus lemon wedges for serving
1 tablespoon chopped fresh parsley, mint, tarragon, or cilantro

1 Bring 1 quart water to boil in medium saucepan. Fill large bowl halfway with ice and water. Nestle fine-mesh strainer into ice bath. Add beans to boiling water and cook for 4 minutes. Using spider skimmer or slotted spoon, transfer beans to strainer set in ice water and let cool, about 2 minutes. Transfer fava beans to double layer of paper towels and dry well. Using paring knife, make small cut along edge of each bean through waxy sheath, then gently squeeze sheath to release bean; discard sheath.

2 Heat oil in 12-inch nonstick skillet over medium heat until shimmering. Add leek and cook, stirring frequently until softened, about 4 minutes. Add asparagus, salt, and pepper and stir well. Continue to cook, stirring occasionally, until asparagus is crisp-tender, 3 to 6 minutes. Stir in beans and cook just until beans are warmed through, about 2 minutes. Remove from heat and stir in lemon zest. Season with salt to taste, and transfer to serving bowl. Sprinkle with parsley and serve with lemon wedges.

Lentil Salad with Olives, Mint, and Feta

serves 4 • total time: 1 hour, plus 1 hour brining

why this recipe works • For this Greek-inspired lentil salad, we first needed lentils that would stay intact during cooking. Lentilles du Puy were perfect, since they are small, firm, and hold their shape better than standard green or brown lentils. A salt soak softened their skins, leading to fewer blowouts. Cooking the lentils in the oven heated them gently, and we boosted their flavor by adding crushed garlic and a bay leaf. A simple tart vinaigrette further enlivened the lentils. We chose several bold mix-ins to bring our salad to life: mint, shallot, and kalamata olives. Lentilles du Puy, also called French green lentils, are our first choice for this recipe, but brown, black, or regular green lentils will also work here (note that cooking times will vary depending on the type used). Salt-soaking helps keep the lentils intact, but if you don't have time, you can skip that step and they will still taste good. You will need a medium ovensafe saucepan for this recipe.

1 teaspoon table salt for brining
1 cup dried lentilles du Puy, picked over and rinsed
5 garlic cloves, lightly crushed and peeled
1 bay leaf
   Table salt for cooking lentils
5 tablespoons extra-virgin olive oil
3 tablespoons white wine vinegar
½ cup pitted kalamata olives, chopped coarse
½ cup chopped fresh mint
1 large shallot, minced
1 ounce feta cheese, crumbled (¼ cup)

1 Dissolve 1 teaspoon salt in 1 quart water in bowl. Add lentils and brine at room temperature for at least 1 hour or up to 24 hours. Drain and rinse well.

2 Adjust oven rack to middle position and heat oven to 325 degrees. Combine lentils, 4 cups water, garlic, bay leaf, and ½ teaspoon salt in medium saucepan. Cover, transfer to oven, and bake until lentils are tender, 40 minutes to 1 hour.

3 Drain lentils well, discarding garlic and bay leaf. In large bowl, whisk oil and vinegar together. Add lentils, olives, mint, and shallot and toss to combine. Season with salt and pepper to taste. Transfer to serving dish and sprinkle with feta. Serve warm or at room temperature.

MAKE AHEAD · Brined and drained lentils can be refrigerated for up to 4 days or frozen up to 1 month. Pat dry with paper towels and transfer to a zipper-lock bag for freezing.

MAKE IT DAIRY-FREE · Substitute plant-based feta cheese for the feta cheese or omit.

VARIATIONS

Lentil Salad with Hazelnuts and Goat Cheese

Substitute 3 tablespoons red wine vinegar for white wine vinegar and add 2 teaspoons Dijon mustard to dressing. Omit olives and substitute ¼ cup chopped fresh parsley for mint. Substitute ¼ cup crumbled goat cheese for feta and sprinkle salad with ¼ cup coarsely chopped toasted hazelnuts before serving.

Lentil Salad with Carrots and Cilantro

Omit shallot and feta. Toss 2 carrots, peeled and cut into 2-inch-long matchsticks, with 1 teaspoon ground cumin, ½ teaspoon ground cinnamon, and ⅛ teaspoon cayenne pepper in bowl; cover and microwave until carrots are tender but still crisp, 2 to 4 minutes. Substitute 3 tablespoons lemon juice for white wine vinegar, carrots for olives, and ¼ cup chopped fresh cilantro for mint.

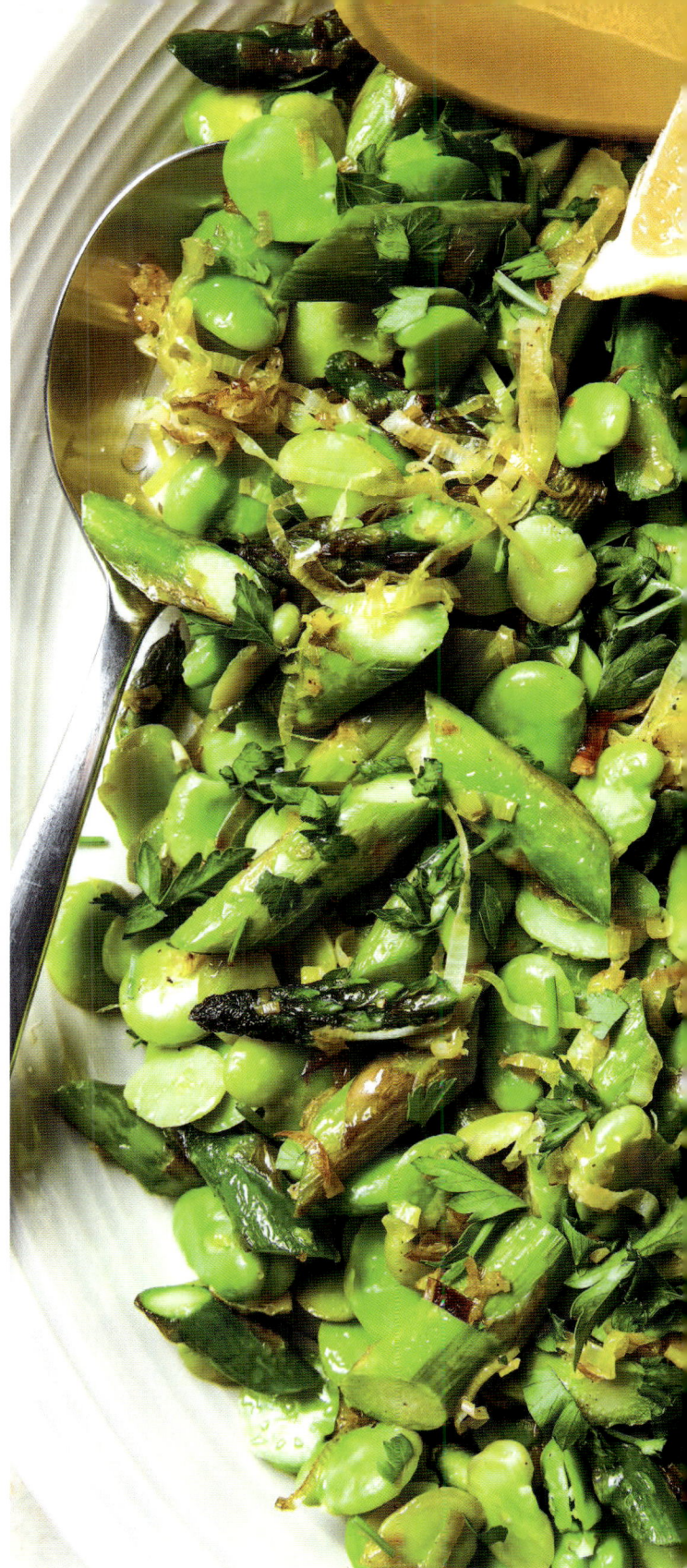

Sautéed Fava Beans, Asparagus, and Leek

Lentilles du Puy with Spinach and Crème Fraîche

serves 4 to 6 · total time: 1 hour

why this recipe works · This nutrient-dense lentil side dish is made with lentilles du Puy, which are French green lentils. To flavor the lentils, we started with a mirepoix of aromatic onion, carrot, and celery. We cooked the vegetables in olive oil before adding the lentils and cooking them with broth for depth of flavor. The lentils held their shape but still resulted in a pleasingly creamy texture. We folded in spinach for a bit of greenery and Dijon for a mustard kick. A dollop of crème fraîche made for a luxurious finish. By the end of step 1, the lentils should have absorbed most, but not all, of the broth. If the bottom of the saucepan looks dry and the lentils are still somewhat firm, add hot water and continue to cook until the lentils are tender. If you can't find crème fraîche, you can substitute sour cream. You can use other French green lentils in place of the lentilles du Puy. Do not substitute other types of green lentils or black, brown, or red lentils; the cooking times of the other lentil varieties can vary greatly.

  1 tablespoon extra-virgin olive oil
  ½ cup finely chopped onion
  ¼ cup finely chopped carrot
  ¼ cup finely chopped celery
  ½ teaspoon table salt
  2 cups unsalted vegetable or chicken broth
  1 cup dried lentilles du Puy, picked over and rinsed
  2 ounces (2 cups) baby spinach
  2 tablespoons Dijon mustard
  ¼ cup crème fraiche

1 Heat oil in large saucepan over medium heat until shimmering. Add onion, carrot, celery, and salt and cook until vegetables are tender, about 5 minutes. Stir in broth and lentils and bring to simmer. Reduce heat to medium-low; cover; and cook, stirring occasionally, until lentils are tender but still hold their shape, about 30 minutes. (Add hot water, ¼ cup at a time, if saucepan becomes dry before lentils are cooked through.)

2 Gently fold in spinach and mustard. Let sit off heat for 5 minutes. Transfer to serving bowl and dollop with crème fraîche. Serve.

MAKE IT DAIRY-FREE · Substitute plant-based yogurt or plant-based sour cream for the crème fraiche or omit.

Turkish Pinto Bean Salad with Tomatoes, Eggs, and Parsley

serves 4 to 6 · total time: 45 minutes   `FAST`

why this recipe works · Fasulye piyazi is a traditional Turkish bean salad that is often made with small white beans and usually features tomatoes, parsley, hard-cooked eggs, and more. For our version we opted for pinto beans instead, which offered a nuttier, more robust flavor. To further enhance the flavor profile, we infused the beans with aromatics by warming them briefly in a toasted garlic broth. The traditional dressing of olive oil and lemon juice proved underwhelming when paired with the stronger-flavored pinto beans, so we decided to incorporate another eastern Mediterranean staple ingredient: tahini. A generous amount of Aleppo pepper complemented the tart acidity of the dressing. We also added cherry tomatoes, onion, and parsley, which gave our salad bright, fresh flavor and a wider panel of nutrients. A sprinkle of sesame seeds offered healthy fats and highlighted the tahini nicely. Last, the traditional addition of hard-cooked eggs provided extra protein. If you can't find Aleppo pepper, you can substitute ¾ teaspoon of paprika and ¾ teaspoon of finely chopped red pepper flakes.

  ¼ cup extra-virgin olive oil, divided
  3 garlic cloves, lightly crushed and peeled
  2 (15-ounce) cans no-salt-added pinto beans, rinsed
  ¼ teaspoon table salt, plus salt for cooking beans
  ¼ cup tahini
  3 tablespoons lemon juice
  1 tablespoon ground dried Aleppo pepper, plus
     extra for serving
  8 ounces cherry tomatoes, halved
  ¼ red onion, sliced thin
  ½ cup fresh parsley leaves
  2 Easy-Peel Hard-Cooked Eggs (page 31), quartered
  1 tablespoon toasted sesame seeds

1 Cook 1 tablespoon oil and garlic in medium saucepan over medium heat, stirring often, until garlic turns golden but not brown, about 3 minutes. Add beans, 2 cups water, and 1 teaspoon salt and bring to simmer. Remove from heat, cover, and let sit for 15 minutes.

2 Drain beans and discard garlic. Whisk remaining 3 tablespoons oil, tahini, lemon juice, Aleppo pepper, 1 tablespoon water, and salt together in large bowl. Add beans, tomatoes, onion, and parsley and toss gently to combine. Season with salt and pepper to taste. Transfer to serving platter and arrange eggs on top. Sprinkle with sesame seeds and extra Aleppo pepper and serve.

Cannellini Beans with Roasted Red Peppers and Kale

serves 4 to 6 • total time: 45 minutes **FAST**

why this recipe works • This bean recipe gets a shot of freshness and ultranutritious heartiness with the addition kale for an anti-oxidant-packed, fiberful side dish. Convenient jarred roasted red peppers add sweetness plus vitamins. To make a full-flavored side, we first sautéed garlic and onion with hot red pepper flakes; the subtle spiciness balanced the sweetness of the beans and roasted peppers. Slicing the kale into thin ribbons and wilting it helped it meld with the other ingredients. Simmering the kale and beans in equal parts water and white wine added light body and brightness. Swiss chard can be substituted for the kale.

- ¼   cup extra-virgin olive oil, plus extra for serving
- 4   garlic cloves, minced
- ¼   teaspoon red pepper flakes
- 1   small red onion, halved and sliced thin
- ¼   teaspoon table salt
- 1   cup jarred roasted red peppers, sliced thin lengthwise
- 1   pound kale, stemmed and sliced thin crosswise
- 2   (15-ounce) cans no-salt-added cannellini beans, rinsed
- ½   cup dry white wine
- ½   cup water
- 1   ounce Parmesan cheese, grated (½ cup)
    Lemon wedges

1   Cook oil, garlic, and pepper flakes in 12-inch skillet over medium-high heat until garlic turns golden brown, about 2 minutes. Stir in onion and salt, reduce heat to medium, and cook until onion is softened, about 5 minutes. Stir in red peppers and cook until softened and glossy, about 3 minutes.

2   Stir in kale, 1 handful at a time, and cook until wilted, about 3 minutes. Stir in beans, wine, and water and bring to simmer. Reduce heat to medium-low, cover, and cook until flavors meld and kale is tender, 15 to 20 minutes. Season with salt and pepper to taste. Serve with Parmesan, lemon wedges, and extra oil.

MAKE IT DAIRY-FREE • Substitute plant-based Parmesan cheese for the dairy Parmesan cheese or omit.

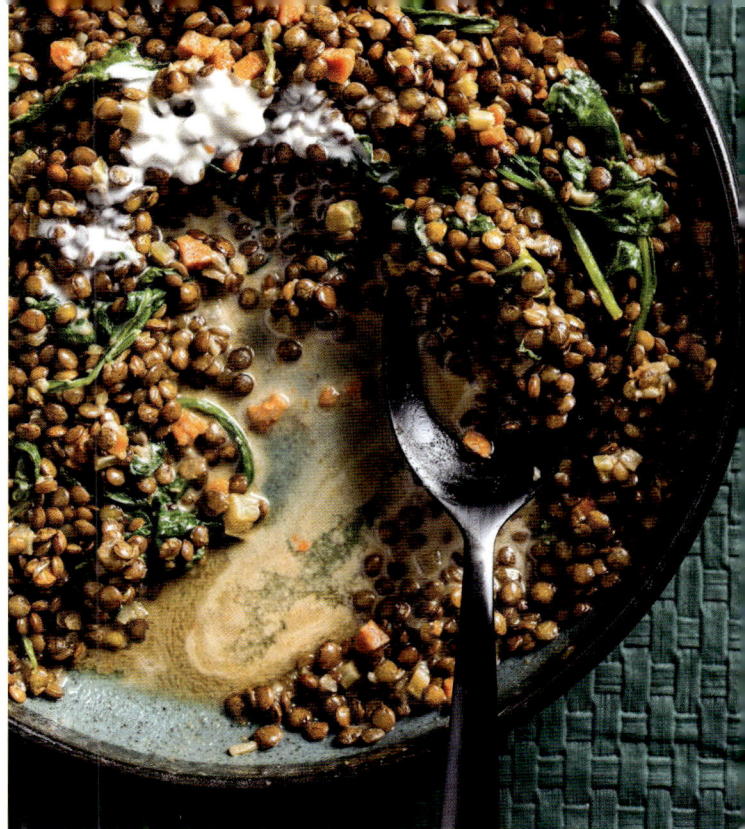

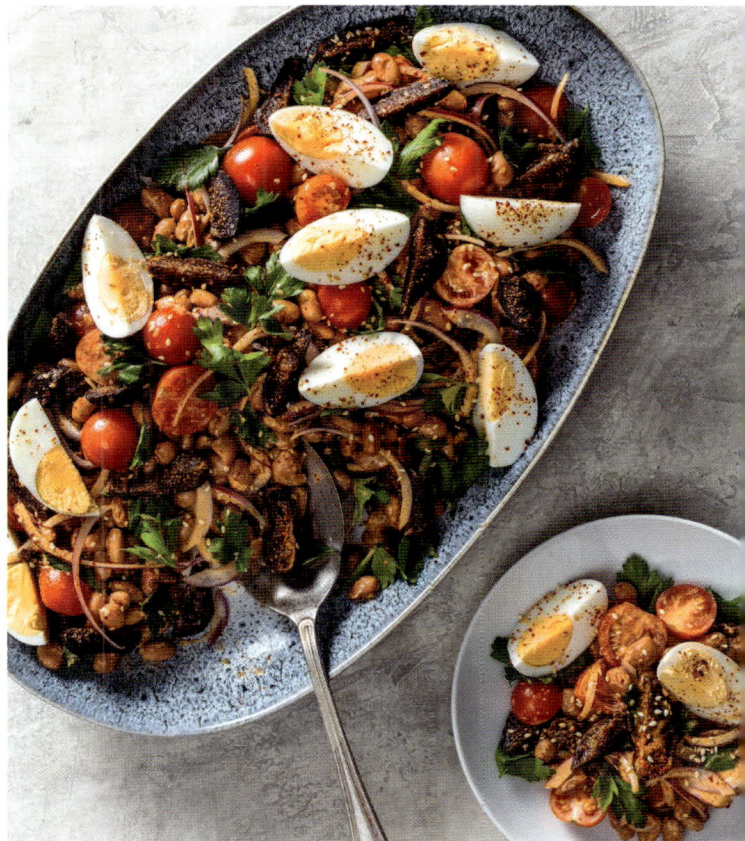

top | *Lentilles du Puy with Spinach and Crème Fraîche*
bottom | *Turkish Pinto Bean Salad with Tomatoes, Eggs, and Parsley*

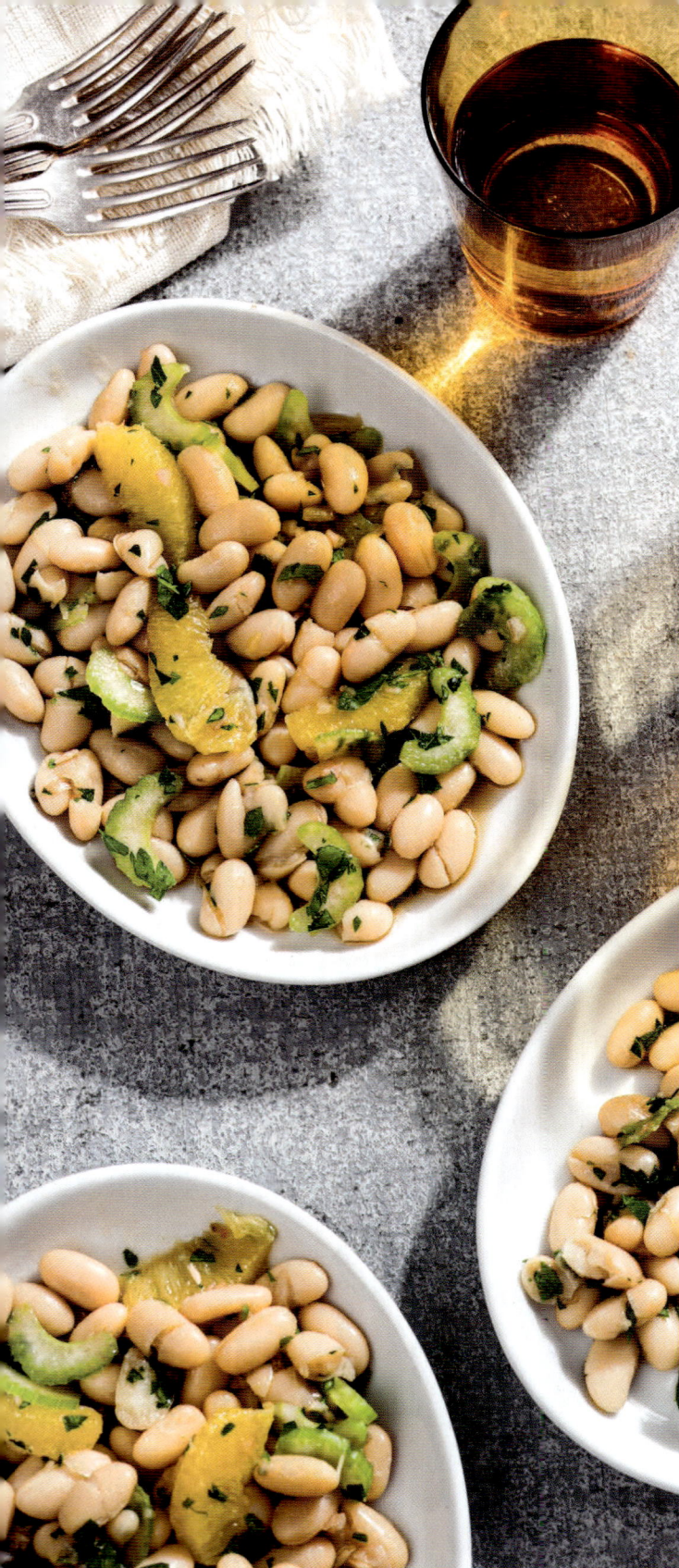

Sicilian White Beans and Escarole

serves 4 • total time: 45 minutes   **FAST**

Why This Recipe Works • White beans and escarole are a classic pairing in Sicilian cooking; the creamy beans are the perfect counterpoint to the tender, mildly bitter escarole, a vitamin-rich member of the chicory family. We first sautéed onions with garlic and red pepper flakes to build a flavor base. We then added the escarole and beans along with broth and water and cooked the greens just until the leaves wilted before cranking up the heat so that the liquid would quickly evaporate. This short stint on high heat prevented the beans from breaking down. Off heat, we stirred in lemon juice for a bright finish and drizzled on some extra olive oil for richness. Chicory can be substituted for the escarole, though its flavor will be stronger.

- 1 tablespoon extra-virgin olive oil, plus extra for serving
- 2 onions, chopped fine
- ½ teaspoon table salt
- 4 garlic cloves, minced
- ⅛ teaspoon red pepper flakes
- 1 head escarole (1 pound), trimmed and sliced 1 inch thick
- 1 (15-ounce) can no-salt-added cannellini beans, rinsed
- 1 cup unsalted vegetable or chicken broth
- 1 cup water
- 2 teaspoons lemon juice

1   Heat oil in Dutch oven over medium heat until shimmering. Add onions and salt and cook until softened and lightly browned, 5 to 7 minutes. Stir in garlic and pepper flakes and cook until fragrant, about 30 seconds.

2   Stir in escarole, beans, broth, and water and bring to simmer. Cook, stirring occasionally, until escarole is wilted, about 5 minutes. Increase heat to high and cook until liquid is nearly evaporated, 10 to 15 minutes. Stir in lemon juice and season with salt and pepper to taste. Drizzle with extra oil and serve.

White Bean Salad with Oranges and Celery

serves 6 • total time: 20 minutes, plus 40 minutes resting

why this recipe works • We took ordinary canned beans and turned them into the rightful stars of this flavorful, satisfying salad. The key was steeping the beans in a garlicky broth first. This afforded us time to tame the bite of a raw shallot by soaking it in vinegar. Once the beans were steeped and the shallot soaked, this salad came together in a minute. Canned beans are a convenient shortcut, but the complex flavors of this side salad could fool eaters into thinking you spent a lot of time in the kitchen. This recipe will also work with other types of canned beans. It's important to let the salad sit for 20 minutes before serving so that the beans absorb the flavors of the other ingredients.

⅓ cup extra-virgin olive oil, divided
4 garlic cloves, smashed and peeled
  Table salt for cooking beans
3 (15-ounce) cans no-salt-added cannellini or small white beans, rinsed
¼ cup sherry vinegar
1 shallot, minced
2 oranges
¾ cup thinly sliced celery
½ cup chopped fresh parsley or cilantro

1 Heat 1 tablespoon oil and garlic in medium saucepan over medium-high heat until just beginning to brown, about 2 minutes. Add 2 cups water and 1 teaspoon salt and bring to simmer. Off heat, add beans, cover, and let sit for 20 minutes. Combine vinegar and shallot in large bowl and let sit for 20 minutes.

2 Cut away peel and pith from oranges. Holding fruit over bowl, use paring knife to slice between membranes to release segments. Drain beans and discard garlic. Add beans, oranges, celery, parsley, and remaining oil to shallot mixture and toss until thoroughly combined. Season with salt and pepper to taste. Let sit until flavors meld, about 20 minutes. Serve.

Wild Rice Pilaf with Pecans and Cranberries

serves 6 to 8 · total time: 1 hour

why this recipe works · Properly cooked wild rice is tender yet chewy and pleasingly rustic—never crunchy or gluey. Simmering the wild rice in a flavorful liquid and then draining off the excess is the surest way to produce fluffy, evenly cooked wild rice every time. To enhance the rice's earthy nuttiness, we cooked it in a combination of broth and water. We also added some white rice to our pilaf to mellow the wild rice's assertive flavor, and we finished our dish with nuts and dried fruit. Do not use quick-cooking or presteamed wild rice in this recipe.

2½ cups water, divided
1¾ cups unsalted vegetable or chicken broth
2 bay leaves
8 sprigs fresh thyme, divided into 2 bundles, each tied together with kitchen twine
1 cup wild rice, rinsed
2 tablespoons extra-virgin olive oil
1 onion, chopped fine
1 large carrot, peeled and chopped fine
1 teaspoon table salt
1½ cups long-grain white rice, rinsed
¾ cup dried cranberries
¾ cup pecans, toasted and chopped coarse
2 tablespoons minced fresh parsley

1 Bring ¼ cup water, broth, bay leaves, and 1 bundle thyme to boil in medium saucepan over medium-high heat. Add wild rice and reduce heat to low. Cover and simmer gently until rice is plump and tender and most of liquid has been absorbed, 35 to 45 minutes. Drain rice and discard bay leaves and thyme. Transfer rice to large bowl, cover, and set aside.

2 Meanwhile, heat oil in large saucepan over medium-high heat until shimmering. Add onion, carrot, and salt and cook until vegetables are softened, about 5 minutes. Add white rice and cook, stirring constantly, until grains become chalky and opaque, 1 to 3 minutes.

3 Stir in remaining 2¼ cups water and remaining thyme bundle and bring to boil. Reduce heat to low, cover, and simmer gently until rice is tender and water has been fully absorbed, 16 to 18 minutes. Off heat, lay clean dish towel underneath lid and let sit, covered, for 10 minutes. Discard thyme and fluff rice with fork.

4 Add white rice, cranberries, pecans, and parsley to bowl with wild rice and toss to combine. Season with salt and pepper to taste. Serve.

VARIATION

Wild Rice Pilaf with Scallions, Cilantro, and Almonds
Omit dried cranberries. Substitute toasted sliced almonds for pecans and cilantro for parsley. Add 2 thinly sliced scallions and 1 teaspoon lime juice to pilaf before serving.

Barley Salad with Celery and Miso Dressing

serves 6 to 8 · **total time: 1¼ hours**

why this recipe works · Barley is a nutty but neutral grain, so it pairs well with most seasonings and also delivers satisfying chew and heartiness. In this simple salad, we combined barley with soy sauce, miso, toasted sesame oil, and rice vinegar. For grains that were distinct and boasted a tender chew, we cooked barley like pasta—boiled in a large volume of salted water and then drained—to rid the grains of much of their sticky starch, which would otherwise cause them to clump. Once the barley was cooked, we let it cool briefly on a rimmed baking sheet to help it dry thoroughly and then tossed it with a bright dressing, crunchy celery and carrots, and aromatics and herbs. The result was a colorful, textured, and refreshing salad. Do not use hulled, hull-less, quick-cooking, or presteamed barley in this recipe.

- 1½ cups pearl barley
- Table salt for cooking barley
- 3 tablespoons unseasoned rice vinegar
- 1 tablespoon white miso
- 1 tablespoon low-sodium soy sauce
- 1 tablespoon toasted sesame oil
- 1 tablespoon avocado oil
- 2 teaspoons grated fresh ginger
- 1 garlic clove, minced
- ¼ teaspoon red pepper flakes
- 2 celery ribs, sliced thin on bias
- 2 carrots, peeled and shredded
- ½ cup minced fresh cilantro

1 Bring 4 quarts water to boil in large pot. Add barley and 1 tablespoon salt and boil gently until grains are tender with slight chew, 25 to 45 minutes. Drain barley, spread on rimmed baking sheet, and let cool until no longer steaming, 5 to 7 minutes.

2 Whisk vinegar, miso, soy sauce, sesame oil, avocado oil, ginger, garlic, and pepper flakes together in large bowl. Add barley and toss to coat. Add celery, carrots, and cilantro and toss to combine. Season with salt and pepper to taste. Serve.

MAKE AHEAD · Cooked barley can be refrigerated for up to 2 days.

Barley Salad with Pomegranate, Pistachios, and Feta

serves 6 to 8 · **total time: 1 hour**

why this recipe works · This vibrantly spiced pearl barley salad is as aesthetically stunning as it is flavorful. Inspired by the flavors of Egypt, where barley is a staple, we incorporated toasty pistachios and bright cilantro and balanced their flavors with warm, earthy spices and sweet golden raisins. Salty feta cheese, pungent scallions, and pomegranate seeds adorned the dish for a colorful composed salad with dynamic flavors and textures. For the dressing, we used pomegranate molasses—another prominent ingredient in Egyptian cuisine—combined with olive oil, lemon, cumin, and cinnamon. Do not use hulled, hull-less, quick-cooking, or presteamed barley in this recipe.

- 1½ cups pearl barley
- ½ teaspoon table salt, plus salt for cooking barley
- 3 tablespoons extra-virgin olive oil, plus extra for serving
- 2 tablespoons pomegranate molasses
- 1 teaspoon lemon juice
- ½ teaspoon ground cinnamon
- ¼ teaspoon ground cumin
- ½ cup chopped fresh cilantro
- ⅓ cup golden raisins
- ¼ cup shelled pistachios, toasted and chopped
- 3 ounces feta cheese, cut into ½-inch cubes (¾ cup)
- 6 scallions, green parts only, sliced thin
- ½ cup pomegranate seeds

1 Bring 4 quarts water to boil in large pot. Add barley and 1 tablespoon salt and boil gently until grains are tender with slight chew, 25 to 45 minutes. Drain barley, spread on rimmed baking sheet, and let cool for at least 10 minutes.

2 Whisk oil, pomegranate molasses, lemon juice, cinnamon, cumin, and salt together in large bowl.

3 Add barley, cilantro, raisins, and pistachios and toss gently to combine. Season with salt and pepper to taste. Spread barley salad evenly on serving platter and arrange feta, scallions, and pomegranate seeds in separate diagonal rows on top. Drizzle with extra oil and serve.

MAKE AHEAD · Cooked barley can be refrigerated for up to 2 days.

MAKE IT DAIRY-FREE · Substitute plant-based feta cheese for the dairy feta cheese or omit.

Buckwheat Tabbouleh

serves 4 · total time: 35 minutes, plus 45 minutes resting

why this recipe works · Classic Mediterranean tabbouleh—featuring bulgur, parsley, mint, and chopped tomatoes tossed in a bright lemon vinaigrette—has a refreshing flavor profile that makes it a light yet nutrient-dense side. To give this classic our own spin, we swapped the bulgur for another grain: mild, appealingly earthy buckwheat groats. Because buckwheat contains a fair amount of starch, we cooked it pasta-style in plenty of water; the water washed away the excess starch, producing separate, evenly cooked kernels. For the herbs, we added plenty of fresh, peppery parsley; 1½ cups was just enough of a presence to balance well with ½ cup of fresh mint. To ensure undiluted, bright flavor in the final tabbouleh, we salted the tomatoes to rid them of excess moisture before tossing them into the salad.

- ¾   cup buckwheat groats, rinsed
- ½   teaspoon table salt, divided, plus salt for cooking buckwheat
- 3   tomatoes, cored and cut into ½-inch pieces
- 2   tablespoons lemon juice
    Pinch cayenne pepper
- ¼   cup extra-virgin olive oil
- 1½   cups minced fresh parsley
- ½   cup minced fresh mint
- 2   scallions, sliced thin

1   Bring 2 quarts water to boil in large saucepan. Stir in buckwheat and 2 teaspoons salt. Return to boil, then reduce to simmer and cook until tender, 10 to 12 minutes. Drain well. Spread buckwheat on rimmed baking sheet and let cool for at least 10 minutes.

2   Meanwhile, toss tomatoes with ¼ teaspoon salt in bowl. Transfer to fine-mesh strainer, set strainer in bowl, and let sit for 30 minutes, tossing occasionally.

3   Whisk lemon juice, cayenne, and remaining ¼ teaspoon salt together in large bowl. Whisking constantly, drizzle in oil.

4   Add drained tomatoes, cooled buckwheat, parsley, mint, and scallions and toss gently to combine. Cover and let sit at room temperature until flavors meld, at least 30 minutes or up to 2 hours. Toss to recombine and season with salt and pepper to taste. Serve.

MAKE AHEAD · Cooked buckwheat can be refrigerated for up to 2 days.

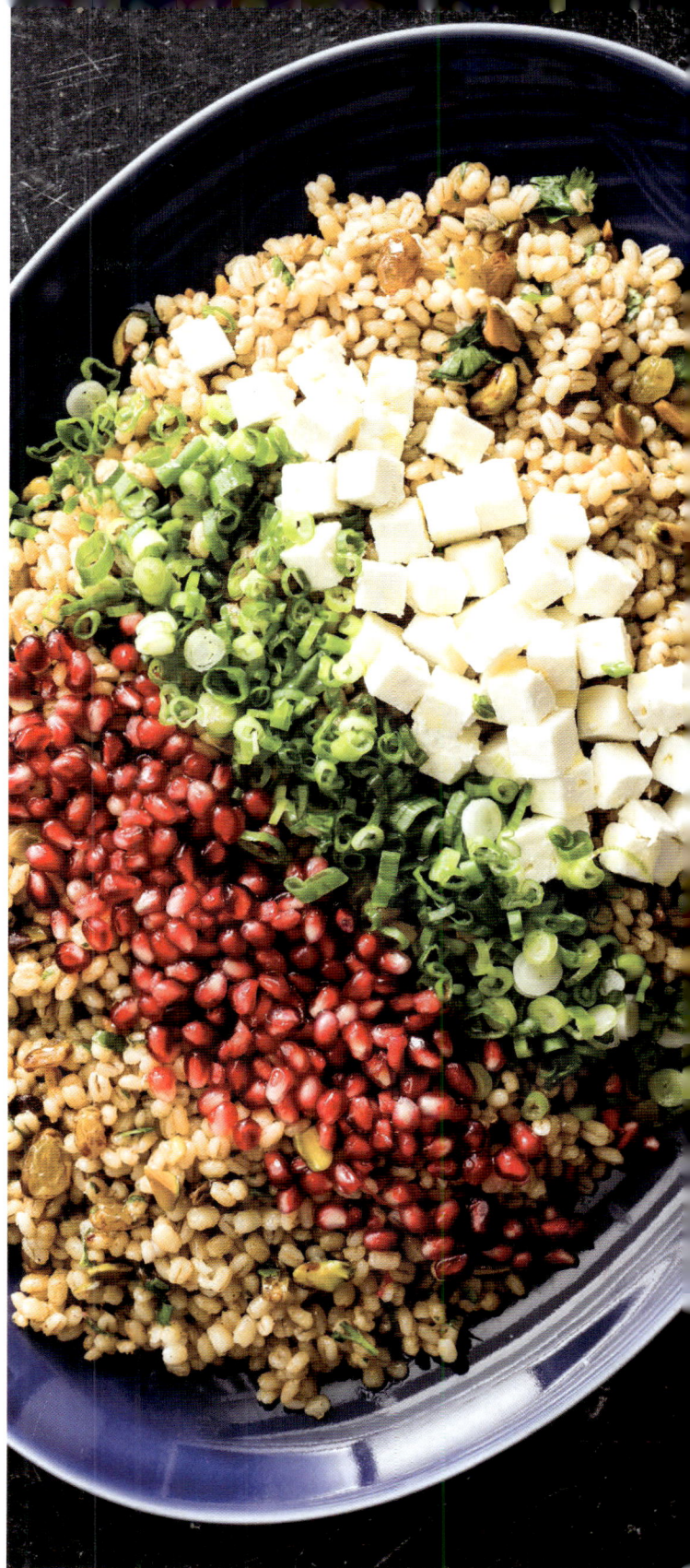

Barley Salad with Pomegranate, Pistachios, and Feta

Bulgur with Chickpeas, Spinach, and Za'atar

serves 4 to 6 · **total time: 50 minutes**

why this recipe works · This robust and very simple side dish combines creamy, nutty chickpeas and hearty bulgur with the clean, vegetal punch of fresh spinach. The aromatic Eastern Mediterranean spice blend za'atar, with its fragrant wild herbs, toasted sesame seeds, and tangy sumac, elevated the flavors with little effort. We found that incorporating the za'atar at two points in the cooking process brought out its complexity. First, to release its deep earthiness, we bloomed half of the za'atar in an aromatic base of onion and garlic before adding the bulgur, chickpeas, and cooking liquid. We added the remainder of the za'atar, along with the fresh baby spinach, off the heat; the residual heat in the bulgur was enough to perfectly soften the spinach and to highlight the za'atar's more delicate aromas. When shopping, don't confuse bulgur with cracked wheat, which has a much longercooking time and will not work in this recipe. We like to use our homemade Za'atar (page 186) in this recipe, but you can use store-bought if you prefer.

- 3 tablespoons extra-virgin olive oil, divided
- 1 onion, chopped fine
- ½ teaspoon table salt
- 3 garlic cloves, minced
- 2 tablespoons za'atar, divided
- 1 cup medium-grind bulgur, rinsed
- 1 (15-ounce) can no-salt-added chickpeas, rinsed
- ¾ cup unsalted vegetable or chicken broth
- ¾ cup water
- 3 ounces (3 cups) baby spinach, chopped
- 1 tablespoon lemon juice

1 Heat 2 tablespoons oil in large saucepan over medium heat until shimmering. Add onion and salt and cook until softened, about 5 minutes. Stir in garlic and 1 tablespoon za'atar and cook until fragrant, about 30 seconds.

2 Stir in bulgur, chickpeas, broth, and water and bring to simmer. Reduce heat to low, cover, and simmer gently until bulgur is tender, 16 to 18 minutes.

3 Remove saucepan from heat. Remove lid, place folded clean dish towel over saucepan, then replace lid. Let bulgur sit for 10 minutes. Add spinach, lemon juice, remaining 1 tablespoon oil, and remaining 1 tablespoon za'atar and fluff gently with fork to combine. Season with salt and pepper to taste. Serve.

Farro Salad with Asparagus, Snap Peas, and Tomatoes

serves 4 to 6 · **total time: 30 minutes, plus 30 minutes cooling**

why this recipe works · This nutrient-packed salad looks as good as it tastes, with vibrant green and red produce plus golden grains. Using the pasta method to cook the farro ensured that the grains cooked evenly. We briefly boiled bite-size pieces of asparagus and snap peas to enhance their color and retain their crisp-tenderness. Cherry tomatoes and herby dill offered notes of freshness. Do not use pearl, quick-cooking, or presteamed farro (check the ingredient list on the package to determine this) in place of the whole farro. You can use any whole grain in place of the farro; note that cooking times may change (see the chart on page 333).

- 6 ounces asparagus, trimmed and cut into 1-inch lengths
- 6 ounces sugar snap peas, strings removed, cut into 1-inch lengths
- ¼ teaspoon table salt, plus salt for cooking vegetables and farro
- 1½ cups whole farro
- 3 tablespoons extra-virgin olive oil
- 2 tablespoons lemon juice
- 2 tablespoons minced shallot
- 1 teaspoon Dijon mustard
- ¼ teaspoon pepper
- 6 ounces cherry tomatoes, halved
- 3 tablespoons chopped fresh dill
- 2 ounces feta cheese, crumbled (½ cup), divided (optional)

1 Bring 4 quarts water to boil in large pot. Add asparagus, snap peas, and 1 tablespoon salt and cook until crisp-tender, about 3 minutes. Using slotted spoon, transfer vegetables to large plate and let cool completely, about 15 minutes.

2 Add farro to water, return to boil, and cook until grains are tender with slight chew, 15 to 30 minutes. Drain farro, spread on rimmed baking sheet, and let cool for at least 10 minutes.

3 Whisk oil, lemon juice, shallot, mustard, pepper, and salt together in large bowl. Add asparagus and snap peas; farro; tomatoes; dill; and ¼ cup feta, if using, and toss gently to combine. Season with salt and pepper to taste. Transfer to serving platter; sprinkle with remaining ¼ cup feta, if using; and serve.

MAKE AHEAD · Cooked farro can be refrigerated for up to 2 days.

MAKE IT DAIRY-FREE · Substitute plant-based feta cheese for the dairy feta cheese, if using.

Warm Farro with Mushrooms and Thyme

serves 4 to 6 · total time: 40 minutes **FAST**

why this recipe works · In this warm grain side, mushrooms sautéed with shallot and thyme lend farro plenty of meatiness. Using sherry to deglaze the pan after the mushrooms browned added complexity to the dish. Finishing with sherry vinegar and a few of tablespoons of fresh parsley gave a brightness and freshness that balanced the hearty, savory flavors. White mushrooms can be substituted for the cremini. Do not use pearl, quick-cooking, or presteamed farro (check the ingredient list on the package to determine this) in place of the whole farro. You can use any whole grain in place of the farro; note that cooking times may change (see the chart on page 333).

- 1½ cups whole farro
- ¼ teaspoon table salt, plus salt for cooking farro
- 3 tablespoons extra-virgin olive oil, divided
- 12 ounces cremini mushrooms, trimmed and chopped coarse
- 1 shallot, minced
- 1½ teaspoons minced fresh thyme or ½ teaspoon dried
- 3 tablespoons dry sherry
- 3 tablespoons minced fresh parsley
- 1½ teaspoons sherry vinegar, plus extra for serving

1 Bring 4 quarts water to boil in Dutch oven. Add farro and 1 tablespoon salt, return to boil, and cook until grains are tender with slight chew, 15 to 30 minutes. Drain farro, return to now-empty pot, and cover to keep warm.

2 Heat 2 tablespoons oil in 12-inch skillet over medium heat until shimmering. Add mushrooms, shallot, thyme, and salt and cook, stirring occasionally, until moisture has evaporated and vegetables start to brown, 8 to 10 minutes. Stir in sherry and cook, scraping up any browned bits, until skillet is almost dry.

3 Add remaining 1 tablespoon oil and farro and cook, stirring frequently, until heated through, about 2 minutes. Off heat, stir in parsley and vinegar. Season with salt, pepper, and extra vinegar to taste, and serve.

MAKE AHEAD · Cooked farro can be refrigerated for up to 2 days.

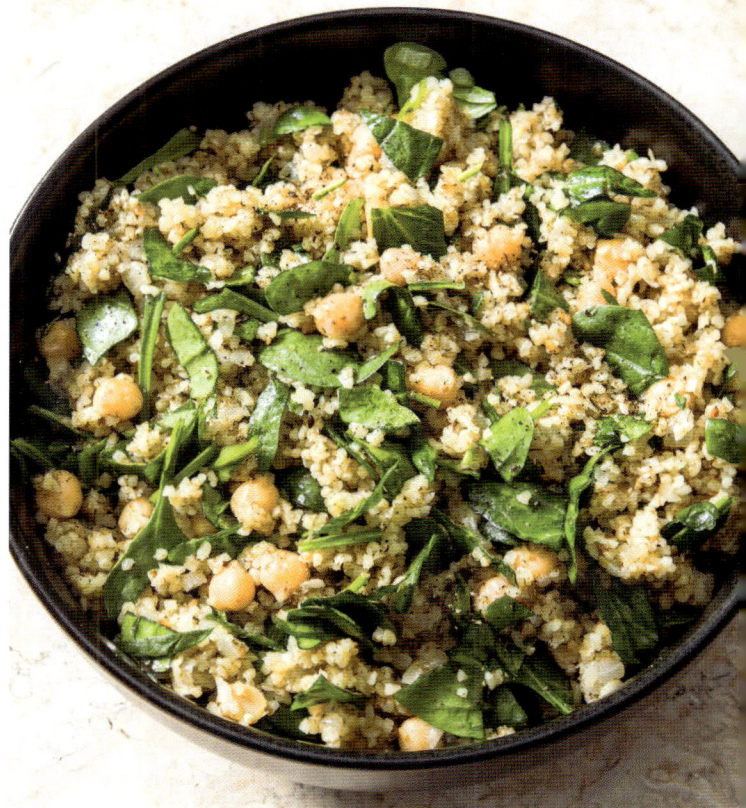

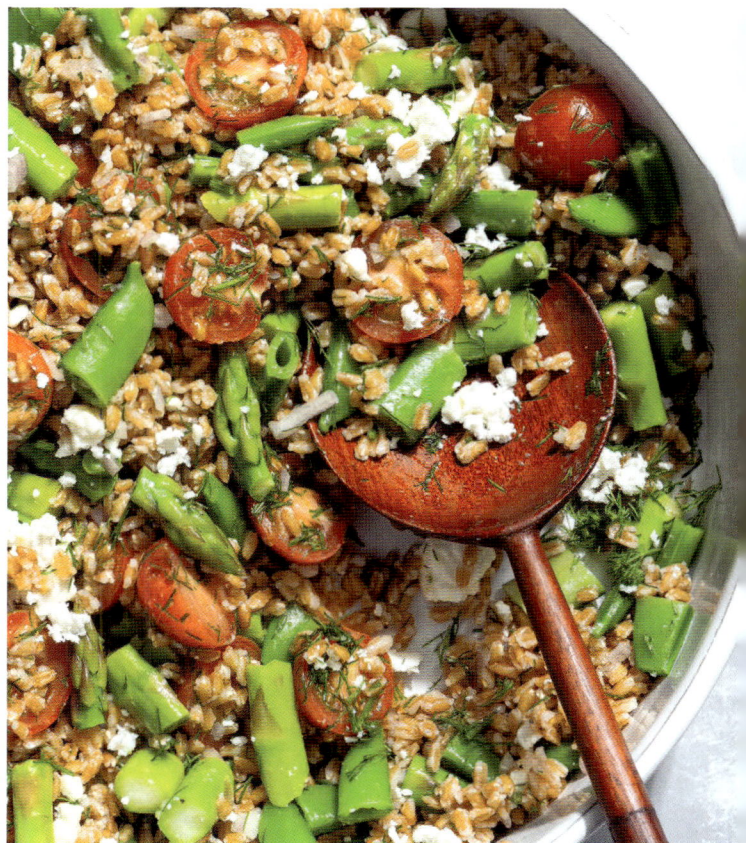

top | *Bulgur with Chickpeas, Spinach, and Za'atar*
bottom | *Farro Salad with Asparagus, Snap Peas, and Tomatoes*

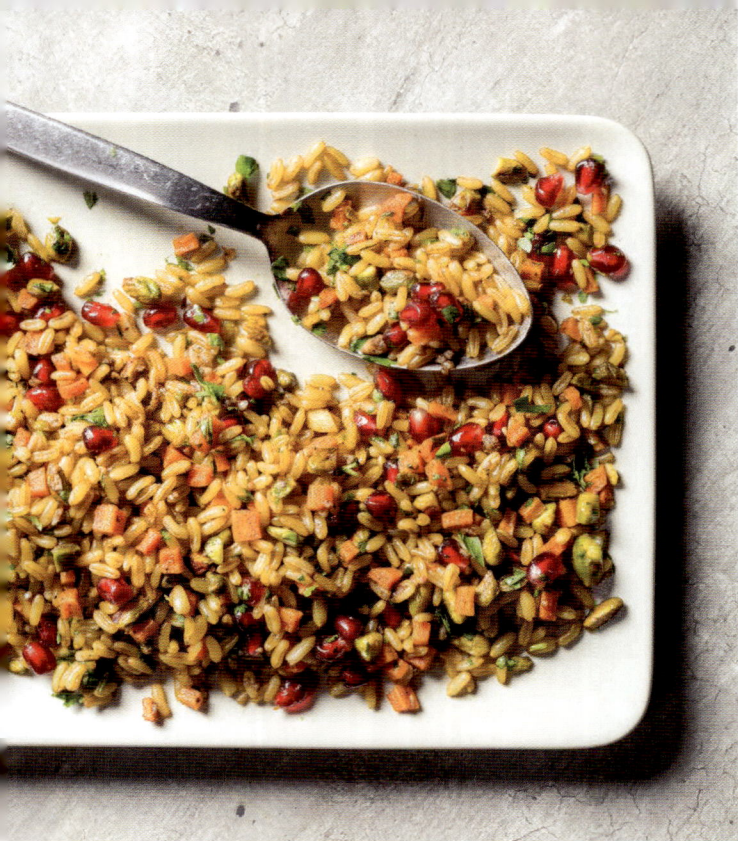

Warm Kamut with Carrots and Pomegranate

serves 4 to 6 • total time: 1½ hours   SUPERCHARGED

why this recipe works • The nutty flavor and firm texture of the ancient grain Kamut help it stand out even when paired with other assertive ingredients, making it a great candidate for the grain salad treatment. We combined Kamut with carrots, pistachios, cilantro, and pomegranate seeds for a side dish that turned out to be a riot of color, texture, and anti-inflammatory compounds. Garam masala and garlic added their pungent flavors and antioxidants to the mix. To shorten the Kamut cooking time to 35 to 50 minutes, soak it in water overnight. Kamut is also sold as Khorasan wheat. You can use any whole grain in place of the Kamut; note that cooking times may change (see the chart on page 333).

- 1   cup Kamut, rinsed and drained
- ¼   teaspoon table salt, plus salt for cooking Kamut
- 2   tablespoons extra-virgin olive oil
- 2   carrots, peeled and cut into ¼-inch pieces
- 2   garlic cloves, minced
- ¾   teaspoon garam masala
- ¼   cup shelled pistachios, lightly toasted and chopped coarse, divided
- 3   tablespoons chopped fresh cilantro, divided
- 1   teaspoon lemon juice
- ¼   cup pomegranate seeds

1   Bring 2 quarts water to boil in large saucepan. Stir in Kamut and 2 teaspoons salt. Return to boil, then reduce to simmer and cook until tender, 55 minutes to 1 hour 15 minutes. Drain well. Spread Kamut on rimmed baking sheet and let cool for at least 10 minutes.

2   Heat oil in 12-inch skillet over medium heat until shimmering. Add carrots and salt and cook, stirring frequently, until carrots are softened and lightly browned, 4 to 6 minutes. Add garlic and garam masala and cook, stirring constantly, until fragrant, about 1 minute. Add Kamut and cook until warmed through, 2 to 5 minutes. Off heat, stir in 2 tablespoons pistachios, 2 tablespoons cilantro, and lemon juice. Season with salt and pepper to taste. Transfer to serving bowl and sprinkle with pomegranate seeds, remaining 2 tablespoons pistachios, and remaining 1 tablespoon cilantro. Serve.

MAKE AHEAD • Cooked Kamut can be refrigerated for up to 2 days.

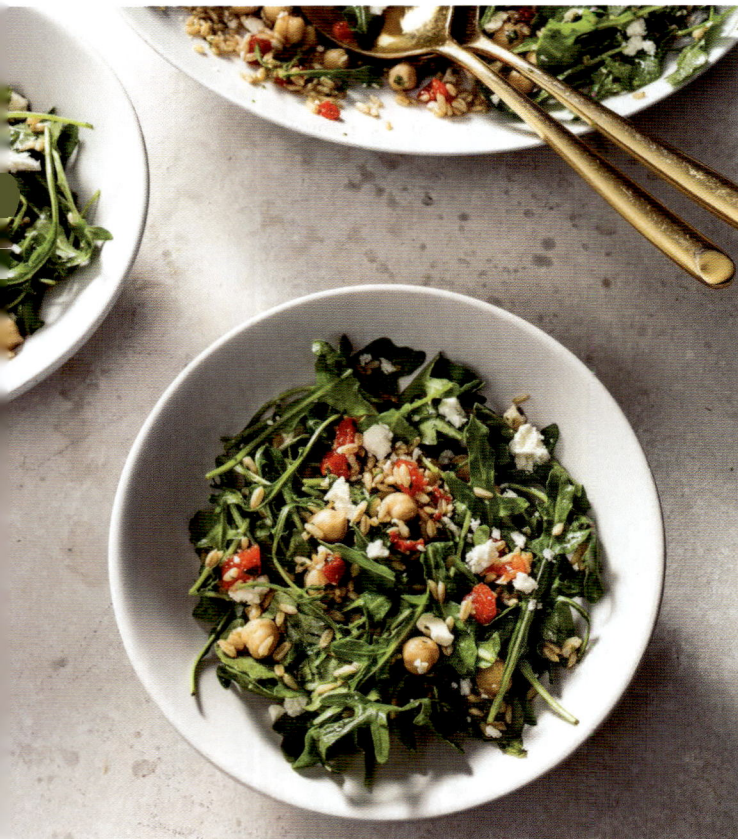

top	*Warm Kamut with Carrots and Pomegranate*
bottom	*Oat Berry, Chickpea, and Arugula Salad*

Oat Berry, Chickpea, and Arugula Salad

serves 4 to 6 • total time: 1¼ hours **SUPERCHARGED**

why this recipe works • Oats are not just for breakfast. Chewy, nutty oat berries (whole oats that have been hulled) make a wonderful base for a substantial grain salad. To ensure that the oat berries retained the perfect chewy texture when served cold, we cooked them in a large amount of water, pasta-style, and then drained and rinsed them under cold water to stop the cooking so that the grains didn't end up mushy. Assertive, peppery arugula paired well with the oat berries. We also added chickpeas for more heft plus a dose of plant protein. Roasted red peppers brought sweetness and some more vitamins, while feta added creaminess and salty bite. A simple lemon-cilantro dressing spiked with cumin, paprika, and cayenne provided bright heat. You can use any whole grain in place of the oat berries; note that cooking times may change (see the chart on page 333).

- 1 cup oat berry groats, rinsed
- ¼ teaspoon table salt, plus salt for cooking oat berries
- 2 tablespoons lemon juice
- 2 tablespoons minced fresh cilantro
- 1 teaspoon honey
- 1 garlic clove, minced
- ¼ teaspoon ground cumin
- ⅛ teaspoon paprika
  Pinch cayenne pepper
- 3 tablespoons extra-virgin olive oil
- 1 (15-ounce) can no-salt-added chickpeas, rinsed
- 6 ounces (6 cups) baby arugula
- ½ cup jarred roasted red peppers, patted dry and chopped
- 2 ounces feta cheese, crumbled (½ cup)

1 Bring 2 quarts water to boil in large saucepan. Add oat berries and ½ teaspoon salt and cook, partially covered, until grains are tender but still chewy, 45 to 50 minutes. Drain oat berries and rinse under cold running water until cool. Drain well.

2 Whisk lemon juice, cilantro, honey, garlic, cumin, paprika, cayenne, and salt together in large bowl. Whisking constantly, slowly drizzle in oil until emulsified, then stir in drained oat berries, chickpeas, arugula, red peppers, and feta. Season with salt and pepper to taste. Serve.

> **MAKE AHEAD** • Cooked oat berries can be refrigerated for up to 2 days.

> **MAKE IT DAIRY-FREE** • Substitute plant-based feta cheese for the dairy feta cheese or omit.

Butternut Squash Polenta

serves 8 • total time: 1½ hours

why this recipe works • Butternut squash puree transforms polenta into a nutritious side dish while enhancing its rustic appeal. How much squash could we add without overpowering polenta's texture and sweet corn flavor? It turned out that for 1 cup of cornmeal, a whole small squash was perfect. Roasting squash halves and scooping out the creamy, fiber-rich flesh kept the process unfussy. For fluffy, creamy polenta, we added a pinch of baking soda, which encouraged the grains to release their starches for a silky consistency with minimal stirring. To round out the flavor, we cooked the polenta with fresh sage and a pinch of nutmeg and then finished with a bit of Parmesan.

- 1 small (1½- to 2-pound) butternut squash, halved lengthwise, seeds removed
- 1 tablespoon extra-virgin olive oil, divided, plus extra for serving
- 1 teaspoon table salt, divided
- ⅛ teaspoon plus ¼ teaspoon pepper, divided
- 1 small onion, chopped fine
- 1½ teaspoons minced fresh sage
- ⅛ teaspoon ground nutmeg
- 5 cups water
- 1 bay leaf
  Pinch baking soda
- 1 cup whole-grain coarse-ground cornmeal
- 1 ounce Parmesan cheese, grated (½ cup), plus extra for serving
- 2 tablespoons pepitas, toasted
  Balsamic vinegar

1 Adjust oven rack to middle position and heat oven to 400 degrees. Line rimmed baking sheet with aluminum foil. Brush cut sides of squash with 1½ teaspoons oil, sprinkle with ¼ teaspoon salt and ⅛ teaspoon pepper, and place cut sides down on prepared baking sheet. Roast until fork inserted into center meets little resistance and sides touching sheet are deep golden brown, 40 to 50 minutes.

2 Remove squash from oven and let cool for 10 minutes. Scoop flesh of squash into medium bowl and set aside; discard skin.

3 Meanwhile, heat remaining 1½ teaspoons oil in large saucepan over medium heat until shimmering. Add onion and remaining ¾ teaspoon salt and cook until softened and lightly browned, 5 to 7 minutes. Add sage and nutmeg and cook until fragrant, about 30 seconds. Stir in water, bay leaf, remaining ¼ teaspoon pepper, and baking soda and bring to boil. Slowly pour cornmeal into water in steady stream while stirring back and forth with wooden spoon or silicone spatula. Bring mixture to boil, stirring constantly, about 1 minute. Reduce heat to lowest setting and cover.

4 After 5 minutes, whisk polenta to smooth out any lumps that may have formed, about 15 seconds. (Make sure to scrape down sides and bottom of saucepan.) Cover and continue to cook, whisking occasionally, until polenta grains are tender but slightly al dente, about 25 minutes longer.

5 Stir in cooked squash, increase heat to medium-low, and cook, stirring occasionally, until squash is well incorporated, about 5 minutes. Off heat, stir in Parmesan and season with salt and pepper to taste. Cover and let sit for 5 minutes. Serve, topping individual portions with extra Parmesan, pepitas, and a drizzle of balsamic vinegar.

| **MAKE IT DAIRY-FREE** • Substitute plant-based Parmesan cheese for the dairy Parmesan cheese or omit.

Warm Rye Berries with Apple and Scallions

serves 4 to 6 • **total time: 1½ hours**

why this recipe works • The earthy, nutty flavor and firm chew of rye berries make them an ideal base for a hearty side. Here we paired the grain with tart Granny Smith apple plus scallions for a pilaf-style dish with an irresistible combination of textures and flavors. We found it easiest (and fastest) to simmer the rye berries in a pot of water until they were tender but still chewy. You can use any whole grain in place of the rye berries; note that cooking times may change (see the chart on page 333).

- 1 cup rye berries, rinsed
- ½ teaspoon table salt, plus salt for cooking rye berries
- 2 tablespoons extra-virgin olive oil
- 3 scallions, white parts sliced thin, green parts sliced thin on bias
- 1 Granny Smith apple, peeled, cored, and cut into ¼-inch pieces
- ¼ teaspoon pepper
- ¼ teaspoon fennel seeds
- 1 teaspoon sherry vinegar

1 Bring 2 quarts water to boil in large saucepan. Stir in rye berries and 2 teaspoons salt. Return to boil, then reduce to simmer and cook until tender, 50 minutes to 1 hour 10 minutes. Drain well. Spread on rimmed baking sheet and let cool for at least 10 minutes.

2 Heat oil in 12-inch skillet over medium heat until shimmering. Add scallion whites, apple, pepper, fennel seeds, and salt and cook, stirring frequently, until apple starts to soften, 2 to 4 minutes. Add rye berries and cook until warmed through, 2 to 5 minutes. Off heat, stir in vinegar and scallion greens. Season with salt and pepper to taste. Serve.

| **MAKE AHEAD** • Cooked rye berries can be refrigerated for up to 2 days.

Spelt Salad with Pickled Fennel, Pea Greens, and Mint

serves 4 to 6 • **total time: 1 hour, plus 30 minutes cooling**

why this recipe works • We love the earthy, nutty flavor and toothsome bite of spelt. We simmered the kernels in a pot of water until they were tender but still retained some of their pleasing chew before letting them cool on a rimmed baking sheet. We combined the spelt with tart and crunchy quick pickled fennel, pea tendrils, and mint and tossed them with a bright dressing for a uniquely delicious salad. You can use any whole grain in place of the spelt; note that cooking times may change (see the chart on page 333). Pea tendrils are also called pea greens or pea shoots. Watercress can be substituted for the pea tendrils.

- 1 cup spelt, rinsed
- ½ teaspoon table salt, divided, plus salt for cooking spelt
- ⅓ cup cider vinegar
- 1 small fennel bulb, 1 tablespoon fronds minced, stalks discarded, bulb halved, cored, and sliced thin
- 3 tablespoons extra-virgin olive oil
- 2 tablespoons lemon juice
- 1 small shallot, minced
- ¼ teaspoon pepper
- 2 ounces pea tendrils, torn into bite-size pieces (2 cups)
- ¼ cup torn fresh mint
- 1 ounce feta cheese, crumbled (¼ cup)

1 Bring 2 quarts water to boil in large saucepan. Add spelt and 2 teaspoons salt and boil gently until grains are tender, 50 minutes to 1 hour 5 minutes. Drain spelt, spread on rimmed baking sheet, and let cool for at least 10 minutes.

2   Meanwhile, bring vinegar and ¼ teaspoon salt to simmer in small saucepan over medium-high heat, stirring occasionally, until sugar dissolves. Off heat, stir in fennel. Cover and let cool completely, about 30 minutes. Drain and discard liquid.

3   Whisk oil, lemon juice, shallot, pepper, and remaining ¼ teaspoon salt together in large bowl. Add cooled spelt, pea tendrils, mint, fennel fronds, and ½ cup pickled fennel (reserve remaining pickled fennel for another use) to dressing and toss to combine. Season with salt and pepper to taste. Sprinkle with feta. Serve.

> **MAKE AHEAD** • Cooked spelt can be refrigerated for up to 2 days.

> **MAKE IT DAIRY-FREE** • Substitute plant-based feta cheese for the dairy feta cheese or omit.

Wheat Berry Salad with Radicchio, Dried Cherries, and Pecans

serves 4 to 6 • total time: 1¾ hours

why this recipe works • Here, wheat berries get paired with a variety of bold mix-ins with a diverse array of textures and flavors. We started by simmering the wheat berries like pasta in a pot of water until they were tender but still chewy. Once cooled, we added them to a bright, red wine vinaigrette along with radicchio, parsley, dried cherries, and pecans. A sprinkling of more pecans and pungent, creamy blue cheese provided the finishing touch. You can use any whole grain in place of the wheat berries; note that cooking times may change (see the chart on page 363).

- 1 cup wheat berries, rinsed
- ½ teaspoon table salt, plus salt for cooking wheat berries
- 3 tablespoons extra-virgin olive oil
- 2 tablespoons red wine vinegar
- 1 small shallot, minced
- ½ teaspoon pepper
- 1 cup chopped radicchio
- 1 cup fresh parsley leaves
- ½ cup pecans, toasted and chopped coarse, divided
- ¼ cup dried cherries
- 1 ounce blue cheese, crumbled (¼ cup)

1   Bring 2 quarts water to boil in large saucepan. Add wheat berries and 2 teaspoons salt and boil gently until grains are tender, 1 hour to 1 hour 20 minutes. Drain wheat berries, spread on rimmed baking sheet, and let cool for at least 10 minutes.

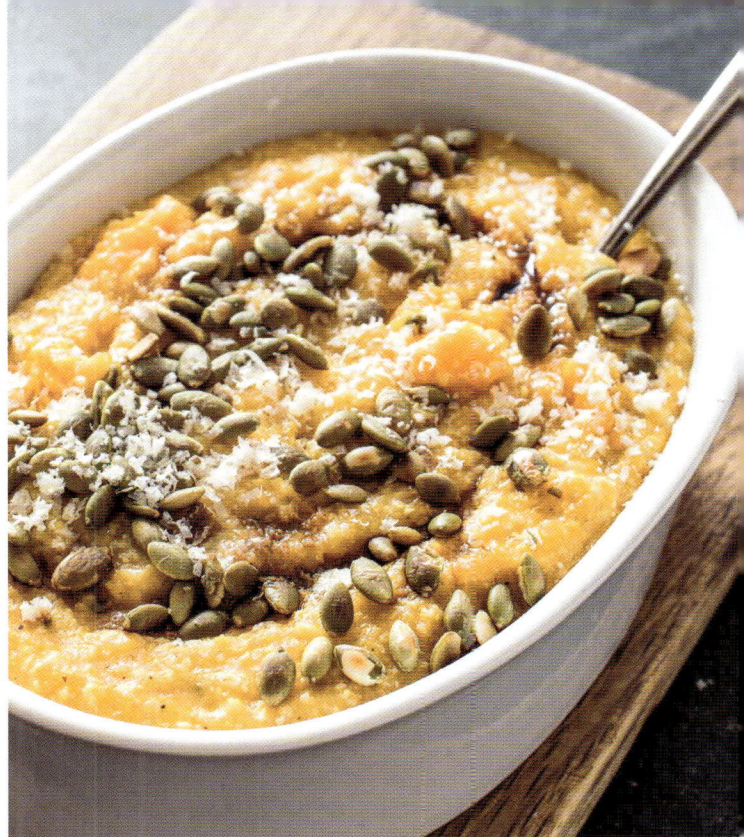

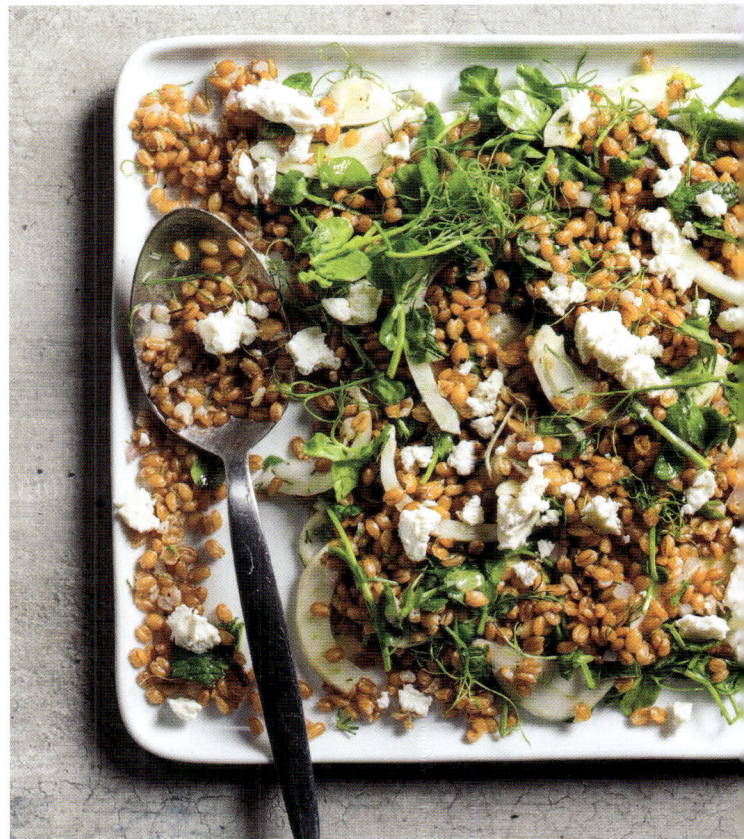

top | *Butternut Squash Polenta*
bottom | *Spelt Salad with Pickled Fennel, Pea Greens, and Mint*

2 Whisk oil, vinegar, shallot, pepper, and salt together in large bowl. Add wheat berries, radicchio, parsley, half of pecans, and cherries and toss to combine. Season with salt and pepper to taste. Sprinkle with blue cheese and remaining pecans. Serve.

> **MAKE AHEAD** • Cooked wheat berries can be refrigerated for up to 2 days.

> **MAKE IT DAIRY-FREE** • Substitute plant-based blue cheese for the dairy blue cheese or omit.

Charred Asparagus with Strawberries

serves 4 • total time: 40 minutes **FAST**

why this recipe works • Strawberries—lightly charred in a cast-iron skillet—add sweetness and a bit of smokiness to balance the delicate vegetal flavor of asparagus. We tossed halved strawberries in olive oil and seared them in a cast-iron skillet before combining them with shallot, red wine vinegar, and a touch of sugar for a bright dressing. We cooked the asparagus next, moving the spears around in the pan until they were deeply browned all over, which brought out their natural nuttiness and more smoky flavor. Chopped pistachios, a finishing sprinkle of mint, and a drizzle of olive oil brought crunch, freshness, and richness. This recipe works best with asparagus spears that are ½ inch thick or larger; thinner asparagus will crowd the pan and overcook.

    8 ounces strawberries, hulled and halved lengthwise (2 cups)
    5 tablespoons extra-virgin olive oil, divided
    ¾ teaspoon table salt, divided
    2 pounds asparagus, trimmed
    ½ teaspoon pepper
    1 shallot, minced
    4 teaspoons red wine vinegar
    ½ teaspoon sugar
    ⅓ cup chopped toasted pistachios
    2 tablespoons torn fresh mint

1 Toss strawberries with 1 tablespoon oil and ¼ teaspoon salt in medium bowl; set aside. Toss asparagus with pepper, 2 tablespoons oil, and remaining ½ teaspoon salt on large plate or baking sheet; set aside.

2 Heat 12-inch cast-iron skillet over medium heat for 3 minutes. Transfer strawberry mixture to skillet and cook, without stirring, until strawberries are charred on bottoms, 5 to 7 minutes, transferring strawberries to now-empty bowl with metal spatula as they finish charring; set aside.

3 Toss asparagus mixture to redistribute oil, then add asparagus to now-empty skillet, using tongs to arrange spears in even layer (some will overlap). Cook over medium heat until spears are char-streaked and tender, 10 to 16 minutes, rotating and turning spears about every 3 minutes. Transfer spears to platter as they finish cooking.

4 Add shallot, vinegar, and sugar to bowl with strawberries and gently stir to combine; season with salt and pepper to taste. Spoon half of berry mixture over asparagus and sprinkle with half of pistachios. Gently turn spears with tongs to distribute berry mixture and nuts. Spoon remaining berry mixture over asparagus. Sprinkle with mint and remaining pistachios. Drizzle with remaining 2 tablespoons oil. Serve warm or at room temperature.

Skillet-Roasted Broccoli with Parmesan and Black Pepper

serves 4 • total time: 35 minutes **FAST**

why this recipe works • Eating your broccoli is easy if it's deeply browned and nutty and cooked evenly from stem to floret. This stovetop method achieves impressive browning quickly. We cut broccoli crowns into wedges to create plenty of flat sides that sat flush with the surface of a generously oiled skillet, and steamed the broccoli initially to soften it. When the water evaporated, the oil filled any gaps between the broccoli and the skillet for optimal heat transfer and browning, yielding crisp wedges with meaty stems and delicate florets. To add flavor without introducing any moisture that would ruin the crisp exterior, we sprinkled the cooked broccoli with a mixture of Parmesan and lemon zest, scattering some of the topping directly on the serving platter in order to season the broccoli from both above and below.

    ½ teaspoon pepper
    ½ teaspoon grated lemon zest
    1 ounce Parmesan cheese, grated (½ cup)
    1¼ pounds broccoli crowns
    5 tablespoons avocado oil
    ¾ teaspoon kosher salt
    2 tablespoons water

1 Using your fingers, mix pepper and lemon zest in small bowl until evenly combined. Add Parmesan and toss with your fingers or fork until lemon zest and pepper are evenly distributed. Sprinkle one-third of topping onto platter.

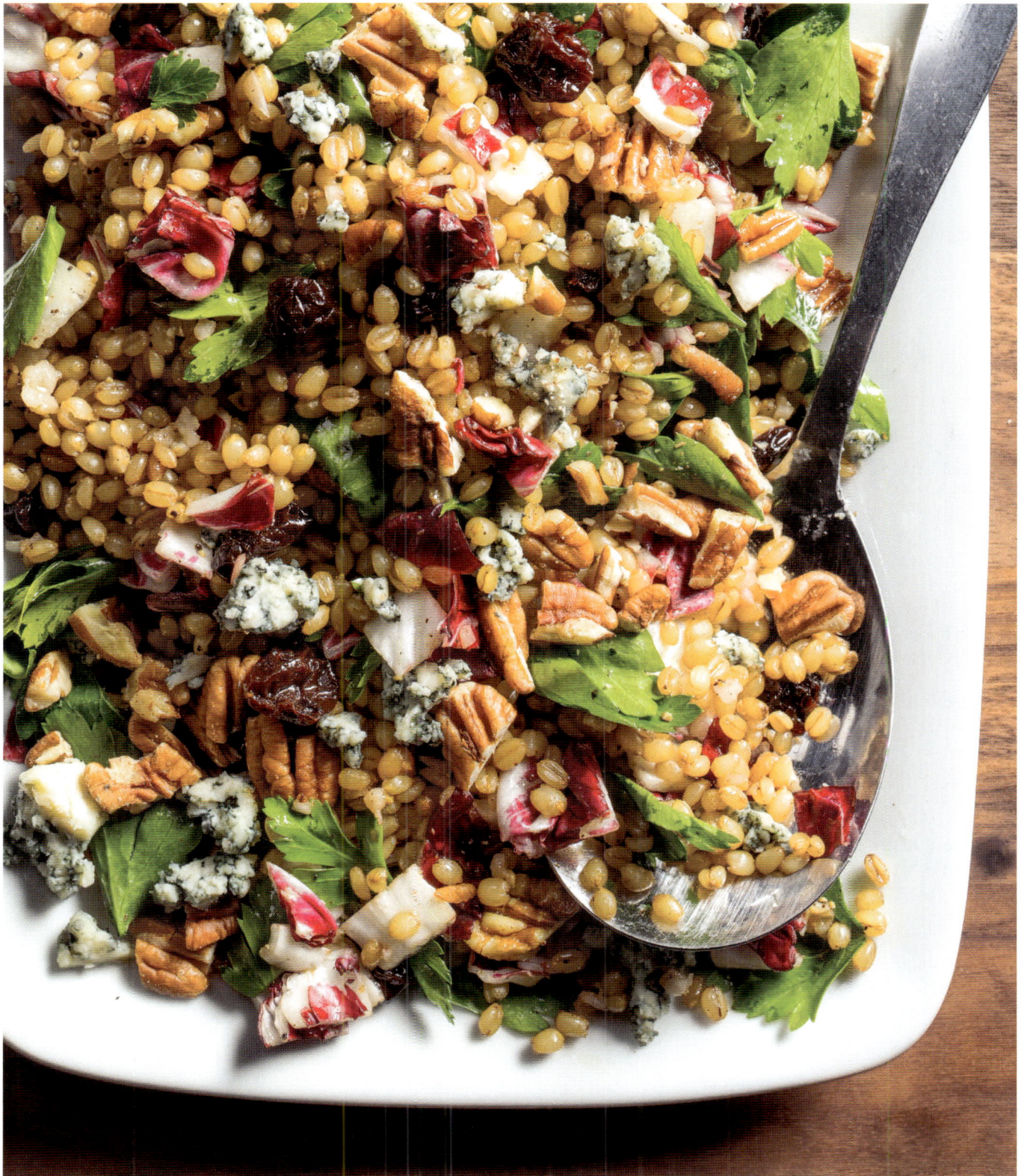

Wheat Berry Salad with Radicchio, Dried Cherries, and Pecans

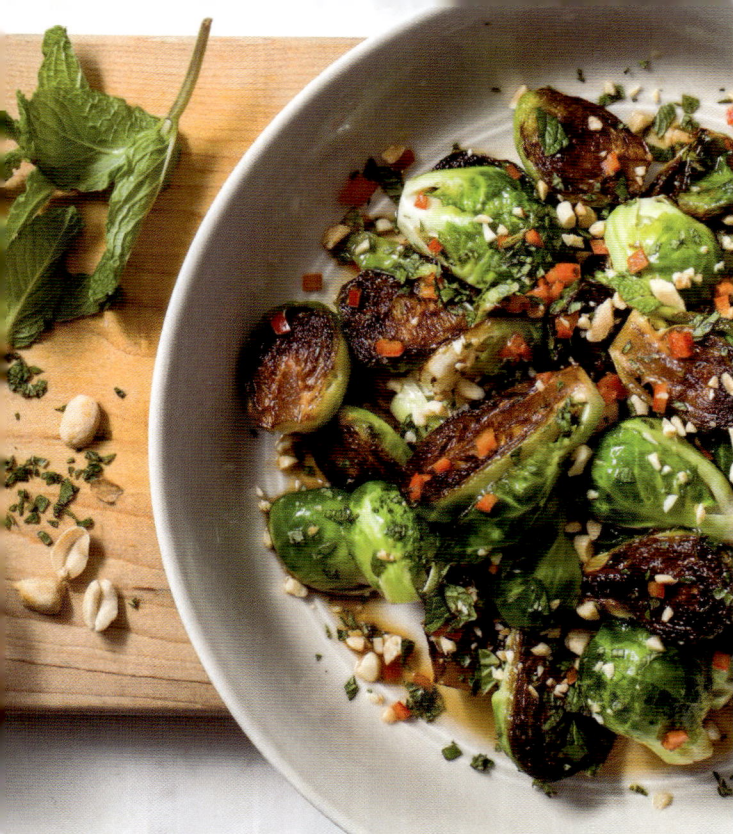

2 Cut broccoli crowns into 4 wedges if 3 to 4 inches in diameter or 6 wedges if 4 to 5 inches in diameter. Add oil to 12-inch non-stick skillet and tilt skillet until oil covers surface. Add broccoli cut side down (pieces will fit snugly; if a few pieces don't fit in bottom layer, place on top). Sprinkle evenly with salt and drizzle with water. Cover and cook over high heat, without moving broccoli, until broccoli is bright green, about 4 minutes.

3 Uncover and press gently on broccoli with back of spatula. Cover and cook until undersides of broccoli are deeply charred and stems are crisp-tender, 4 to 6 minutes. Off heat, uncover and turn broccoli so second cut side is touching skillet. Move any pieces that were on top so they are flush with skillet surface. Continue to cook, uncovered, pressing gently on broccoli with back of spatula, until second cut side is deeply browned, 3 to 5 minutes longer. Transfer to platter, sprinkle with remaining topping, and serve.

MAKE IT DAIRY-FREE • Substitute plant-based Parmesan cheese for the dairy Parmesan cheese or omit.

Skillet-Roasted Brussels Sprouts with Chile, Peanuts, and Mint

serves 4 • total time: 20 minutes   **FAST**

why this recipe works • The best roasted brussels sprouts—well browned but still crisp-tender—need no boost from bacon or cream. We highlight them instead with splashes of lime juice and fish sauce for savory tang, which is accented with sprinklings of mint, chile, and roasted peanuts. To create stovetop brussels sprouts that were deeply browned on the cut sides while still bright green on the uncut sides and crisp-tender within, we started the sprouts in a cold skillet with olive oil and cooked them covered. This gently heated the sprouts and created a steamy environment that cooked them through without adding any extra moisture. We then removed the lid and continued to cook the sprouts cut sides down so that they had time to develop a substantial, caramelized crust. A red jalapeño can be substituted for the Fresno chile. Look for brussels sprouts that are similar in size, with small, tight heads that are no more than 1½ inches in diameter, as they're likely to be sweeter and more tender than larger sprouts.

- 1 pound small (1 to 1½ inches in diameter) brussels sprouts, trimmed and halved
- 5 tablespoons extra-virgin olive oil
- 1 Fresno chile, stemmed, seeded, and minced

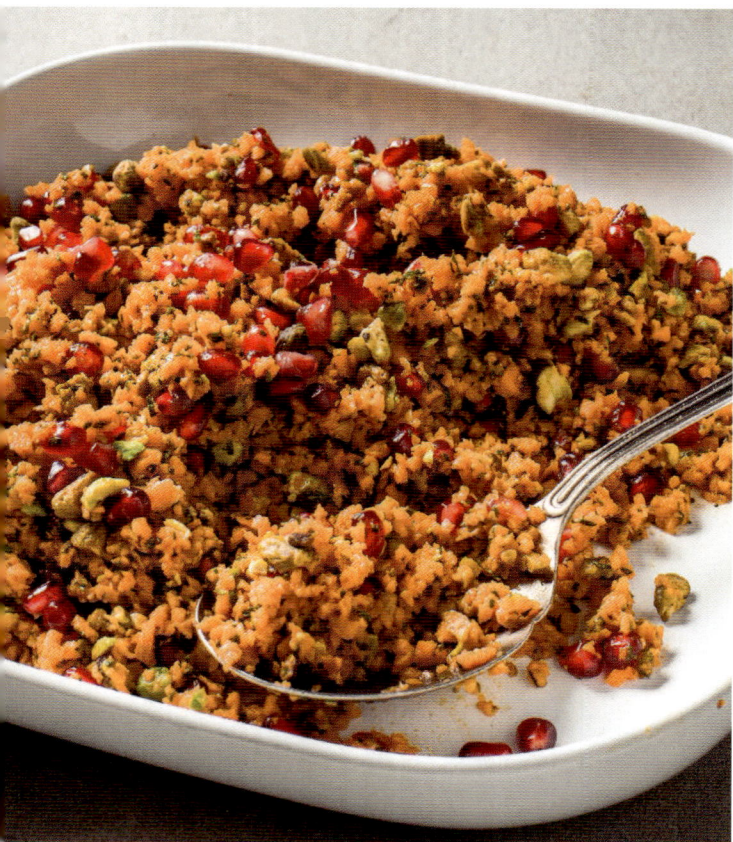

2 teaspoons lime juice

1 teaspoon fish sauce

¼ teaspoon table salt

2 tablespoons finely chopped dry-roasted peanuts

2 tablespoons chopped fresh mint

1   Arrange brussels sprouts in single layer, cut sides down, in 12-inch nonstick skillet. Drizzle oil evenly over sprouts. Cover skillet, place over medium-high heat, and cook until sprouts are bright green and cut sides have started to brown, about 5 minutes.

2   Uncover and continue to cook until cut sides of sprouts are deeply and evenly browned and paring knife slides in with little to no resistance, 2 to 3 minutes longer, adjusting heat and moving sprouts as necessary to prevent them from overbrowning. While brussels sprouts cook, combine Fresno chile, lime juice, fish sauce, and salt in small bowl.

3   Off heat, add chile mixture to skillet and stir to evenly coat brussels sprouts. Season with salt and pepper to taste. Transfer sprouts to large plate, sprinkle with peanuts and mint, and serve.

Roasted Cabbage with Gochujang, Sesame, and Scallion

serves 4 to 6 · total time: 50 minutes

why this recipe works · For roasted cabbage that was well seasoned, attractively caramelized outside, and meltingly tender inside, we started by cutting the head straight through the core to create eight structurally sound wedges. Spreading oil over the cut surfaces and laying those surfaces flush against a baking sheet gave the edge of each leaf its best chance at deep caramelization. We covered the pan tightly with foil for the first 20 minutes of roasting to foster a steamy environment, which cooked the wedges through. We then removed the foil and allowed the exterior to dry out and caramelize. A quick flip halfway through the uncovered roasting period ensured that both sides were equally browned. A sauce of spicy-sweet gochujang, tart rice vinegar, and nutty sesame oil—drizzled over the serving platter and all over the cabbage—turned humble cabbage into a party of flavors. A dense cabbage, one that's heavier than it looks, will hold together best when cut into eight wedges.

1 head green cabbage (2 to 2½ pounds)

3 tablespoons avocado oil, divided

½ teaspoon table salt, divided

¼ teaspoon pepper

2 tablespoons gochujang

1 tablespoon unseasoned rice vinegar

2 teaspoons water

1 teaspoon toasted sesame oil

½ teaspoon sugar

1 tablespoon toasted sesame seeds

2 scallions, green parts only, sliced thin

1   Adjust oven rack to upper-middle position and heat oven to 500 degrees. Quarter cabbage through core and cut each quarter into 2 wedges, leaving core intact. Arrange wedges, 1 flat side down, on rimmed baking sheet. Brush 1½ tablespoons avocado oil on exposed cut sides of wedges and sprinkle with ¼ teaspoon salt. Flip wedges so oiled sides are flush with sheet. Brush second cut sides with remaining 1½ tablespoons avocado oil and sprinkle with pepper and remaining ¼ teaspoon salt. Cover sheet tightly with aluminum foil and roast for 20 minutes.

2   Remove foil (be careful of escaping steam) and continue to cook until cabbage wedges begin to brown on underside, 5 to 10 minutes. Using tongs and thin metal spatula, flip each wedge. Roast until edges are very well browned and some leaves have crisped, 5 to 10 minutes. While cabbage roasts, stir gochujang, vinegar, water, sesame oil, and sugar together in small bowl.

3   Drizzle half of gochujang mixture over serving platter. Transfer cabbage to platter, drizzle with remaining gochujang mixture, sprinkle with sesame seeds and scallions, and serve.

Carrot "Tabbouleh" with Mint, Pistachios, and Pomegranate Seeds

serves 6 · total time: 20 minutes   **FAST**   **SUPERCHARGED**

why this recipe works · We love finding new ways to eat more vegetables; it's a simple yet exciting way to bring variety to your table. We've used beta carotene–loaded carrots to make noodles, and it turns out they can also be transformed into a vibrant tabbouleh-style salad. We took advantage of our food processor, using it first to chop pistachios. After emptying the bowl, we gave our carrots a whir, grinding them to the size of grains. We then tossed them with a simple dressing enlivened with paprika, stirred in the pistachios and some mint, and added antioxidant-rich pomegranate seeds for a pop of color and juicy, tart sweetness. We prefer the convenience and the hint of bitterness that unpeeled carrots lend to this salad; just be sure to scrub the carrots well before using.

¾ cup shelled pistachios, toasted

¼ cup extra-virgin olive oil

3 tablespoons lemon juice

1 teaspoon table salt

½ teaspoon pepper

½ teaspoon smoked paprika

⅛ teaspoon cayenne pepper

1 pound carrots, unpeeled, trimmed and cut into 1-inch pieces

2 cups minced fresh mint leaves

1 cup pomegranate seeds, divided

Pulse pistachios in food processor until coarsely chopped, 10 to 12 pulses. Transfer to bowl. Whisk oil, lemon juice, salt, pepper, paprika, and cayenne in large bowl until combined. Process carrots in now-empty food processor until finely chopped, 10 to 20 seconds, scraping down sides of bowl as needed. Transfer carrots to bowl with dressing; add mint, half of pomegranate seeds, and half of pistachios; and toss to combine. Season with salt to taste. Transfer to serving platter, sprinkle with remaining pomegranate seeds and pistachios, and serve.

VARIATION

Carrot "Tabbouleh" with Fennel, Orange, and Hazelnuts

Omit smoked paprika and cayenne. Substitute toasted, skinned, and chopped hazelnuts for pistachios, 1 halved and cored fennel bulb cut into 1-inch pieces for mint, and orange juice for lemon juice. Add ¼ teaspoon orange zest and 2 tablespoons white wine vinegar to mixture with carrots. Substitute ½ cup minced fresh chives for pomegranate seeds.

Cauliflower Puree

serves 6 · total time: 40 minutes   **FAST**

why this recipe works · The key to silky mashed potatoes is usually loads of butter and cream. To create a creamy, versatile vegetable puree without all the saturated fat, we turned to cauliflower. Not only is cauliflower high in vitamins and fiber, but it's easy to work with and, thanks to its neutral flavor, makes a great stand-in for potatoes. As a bonus, the low starch content meant it pureed like a dream. Steaming the cauliflower before blitzing it in the food processor guaranteed a smooth, velvety texture. To make our puree reminiscent of mashed potatoes, we added thyme and garlic. A dash of white wine vinegar balanced all the flavors.

¼ cup extra-virgin olive oil

2 garlic cloves, minced

2 teaspoons minced fresh thyme or ¾ teaspoon dried

½ teaspoon table salt, plus salt for cooking cauliflower

¼ teaspoon white wine vinegar

1 large head cauliflower (3 pounds), florets cut into 1-inch pieces, core peeled and sliced ¼ inch thick

1   Cook oil and garlic in 8-inch nonstick skillet over low heat, stirring occasionally, until garlic is pale golden, 9 to 12 minutes. Off heat, stir in thyme, salt, and vinegar; transfer to liquid measuring cup and set aside to cool.

2   Meanwhile, bring 2½ cups water and ½ teaspoon salt to boil in Dutch oven over high heat. Add cauliflower, cover, and cook until cauliflower is tender, stirring once halfway through, 14 to 16 minutes.

3   Drain cauliflower and transfer to food processor. Add 2 tablespoons water and process cauliflower until mostly smooth, 3 to 4 minutes, scraping down sides of bowl as needed. With processor running, drizzle in oil-garlic mixture and process until completely smooth, about 30 seconds. (If puree is too thick, add hot water, 1 tablespoon at a time, until desired consistency is reached). Transfer to serving bowl and season with salt and pepper to taste. Serve.

Sautéed Swiss Chard with Currants and Pine Nuts

serves 4 · total time: 30 minutes   **FAST**

why this recipe works · Swiss chard, a sturdy green with a beet-like flavor that mellows when cooked, is a nutritional powerhouse, offering vitamins as well as pigments with anti-inflammatory properties. We sliced the stems on a bias to help them cook evenly and gave the stems a head start, sautéing them with garlic and cumin until lightly caramelized. We added the tender leaves later and in two stages, allowing one batch to begin wilting before adding the rest. Currants and toasted pine nuts brought bursts of chewy sweetness and crunch. We stirred them in off the heat along with some sherry vinegar; the touch of acidity brightened the dish noticeably.

2 tablespoons extra-virgin olive oil

1 garlic clove, minced

¼ teaspoon ground cumin

1½ pounds Swiss chard, stems sliced ¼ inch thick on bias, leaves sliced into ½-inch-wide strips, divided

⅛ teaspoon table salt

2 teaspoons sherry vinegar

3 tablespoons dried currants

3 tablespoons pine nuts, toasted

1 Heat oil in 12-inch nonstick skillet over medium-high heat until shimmering. Add garlic and cumin and cook, stirring constantly, until lightly browned, 30 to 60 seconds. Add chard stems and salt and cook, stirring occasionally, until spotty brown and crisp-tender, about 6 minutes.

2 Add two-thirds of chard leaves and cook, tossing with tongs, until just starting to wilt, 30 to 60 seconds. Add remaining chard leaves and cook, stirring frequently, until leaves are tender, about 3 minutes. Off heat, stir in vinegar, currants, and pine nuts. Season with salt and pepper to taste. Serve.

Sugar Snap Peas with Pine Nuts, Fennel, and Lemon Zest

serves 4 · total time: 25 minutes   **FAST**

why this recipe works · A cross between English peas and snow peas, sugar snap peas have sweet edible pods with small, juicy peas inside. To ensure that the pods and their peas cooked at the same rate, we steamed the peas briefly before quickly sautéing them; the trapped steam transferred heat more efficiently than air, so the peas cooked through faster. Cutting the peas in half reduced the cooking time, so the pods retained more of their snap, and as a bonus, the pockets captured plenty of seasonings. A dukkah-like mix of pine nuts, fennel seeds, lemon zest, salt, and red pepper flakes dressed up the peas with distinct (but not overwhelming) flavor and crunch. Do not substitute ground fennel for the fennel seeds.

- 3 tablespoons pine nuts
- 1 teaspoon fennel seeds
- ½ teaspoon grated lemon zest
- ½ teaspoon kosher salt
- ⅛ teaspoon red pepper flakes
- 2 teaspoons avocado oil
- 12 ounces sugar snap peas, strings removed, halved crosswise on bias
- 2 tablespoons water
- 1 garlic clove, minced
- 3 tablespoons chopped fresh basil

1 Toast pine nuts in 12-inch skillet over medium heat, stirring frequently, until just starting to brown, about 3 minutes. Add fennel seeds and continue to toast, stirring constantly, until pine nuts are lightly browned and fennel is fragrant, about 1 minute. Transfer pine nut mixture to cutting board. Sprinkle lemon zest, salt, and pepper flakes over pine nut mixture. Chop mixture until finely minced and well combined. Transfer to bowl and set aside.

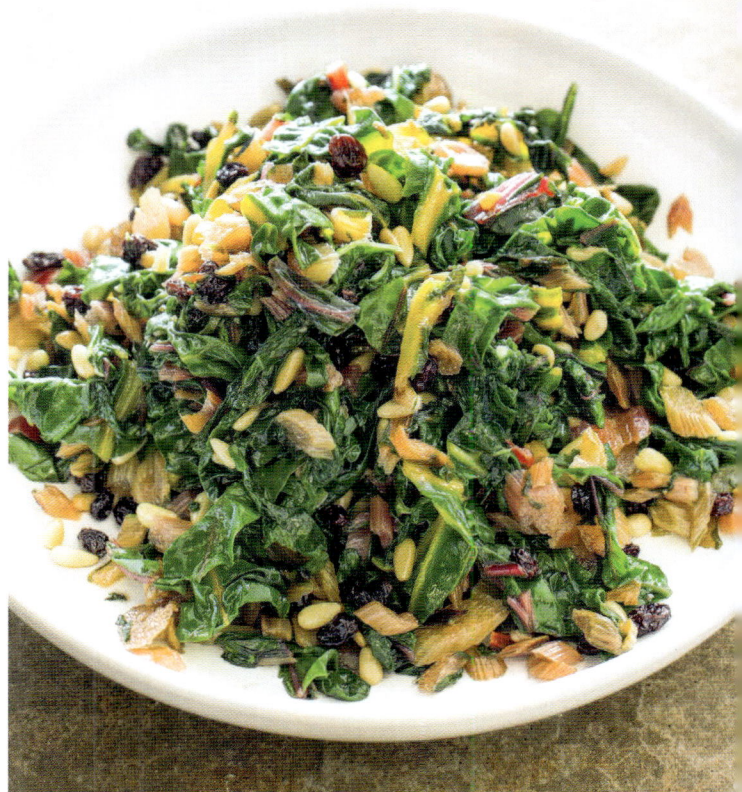

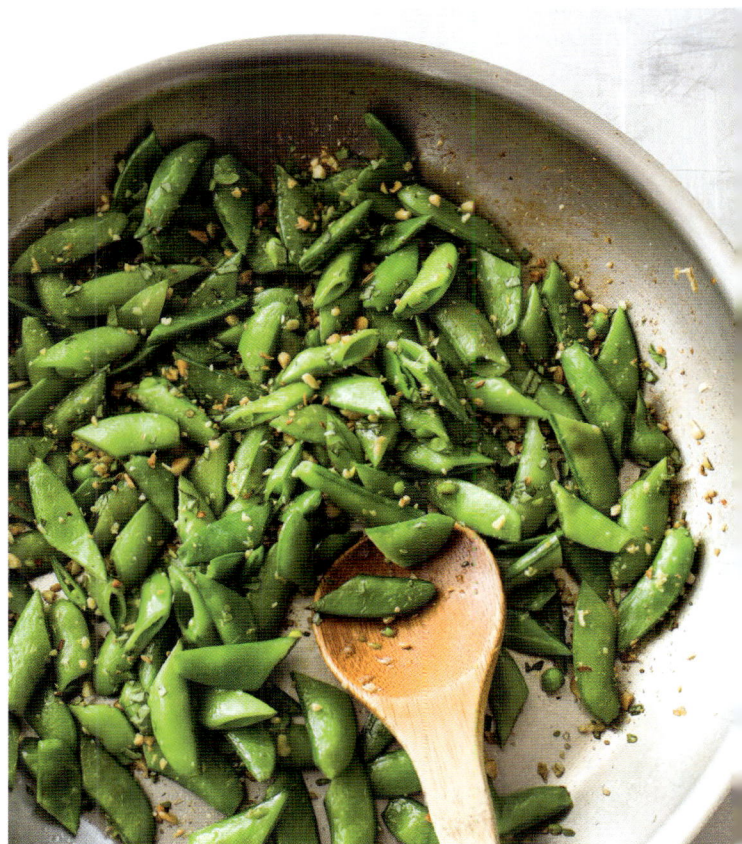

top | Sautéed Swiss Chard with Currants and Pine Nuts
bottom | Sugar Snap Peas with Pine Nuts, Fennel, and Lemon Zest

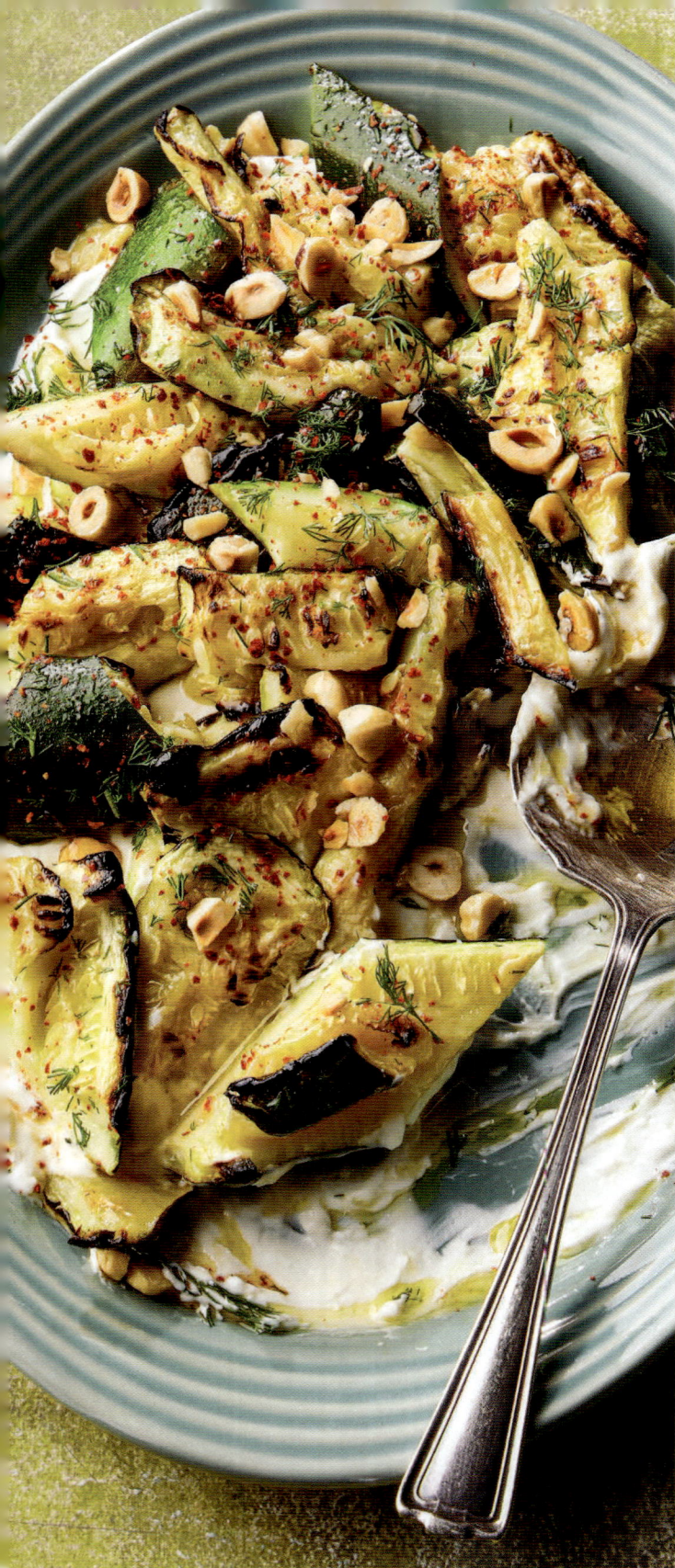

2   Heat oil in now-empty skillet over medium heat until shimmering. Add snap peas and water, immediately cover, and cook for 2 minutes. Uncover, add garlic, and cook, stirring frequently, until moisture has evaporated and snap peas are crisp-tender, about 2 minutes. Remove skillet from heat; stir in three-quarters of pine nut mixture and basil. Transfer snap peas to serving platter, sprinkle with remaining pine nut mixture, and serve.

Cumin and Chili Roasted Sweet Potato Wedges

serves 4 to 6 • total time: 45 minutes   **FAST**

why this recipe works • Roasted sweet potato wedges may taste indulgent, but they're a breeze to prepare and are loaded with beta carotene, making them an easy, healthy addition to your dinner table. Using small potatoes, about 8 ounces each, helped the wedges to fit uniformly on the baking sheet. They should be of similar size so that they cook at the same rate. Be sure to scrub and dry the whole potatoes thoroughly before cutting them into wedges and tossing them with the oil and spices.

   2   pounds small sweet potatoes, unpeeled, cut lengthwise into 1½-inch wedges
   2   tablespoons extra-virgin olive oil
   2   teaspoons ground cumin
   2   teaspoons chili powder
   1   teaspoon garlic powder
   ½   teaspoon table salt
   ½   teaspoon pepper

1   Adjust oven rack to middle position and heat oven to 450 degrees. Line rimmed baking sheet with parchment paper. Toss all ingredients together in bowl.

2   Arrange potatoes, skin side down, in single layer on sheet. Roast until lightly browned and tender, about 30 minutes. Serve.

Roasted Kabocha Squash with Maple and Sage

serves 4 • total time: 1 hour

why this recipe works • Kabocha looks like a small, squat pumpkin with dark green or red skin and a nutty, earthy flavor (the red variety is noticeably sweeter). When roasted, its flesh becomes

Broiled Smashed Zucchini with Garlicky Yogurt

creamy and its skin tender enough to eat, so this recipe gives us more fiber than many other winter squash recipes. Here we used a mix of warm spices (paprika, coriander, and black pepper) to complement the kabocha's sweetness, which we accentuated with a sweet-tart vinaigrette whisked together from a touch of maple syrup, cider vinegar, and sage. The warm squash drank up the dressing to achieve a sweet-savory balance.

- 1 kabocha squash (3 pounds), halved lengthwise and seeded
- ¼ cup extra-virgin olive oil, divided
- 1 garlic clove, minced
- 2 teaspoons paprika
- 1 teaspoon ground coriander
- ½ teaspoon table salt
- ½ teaspoon pepper
- 1 tablespoon cider vinegar
- 1 tablespoon maple syrup
- 2 teaspoons minced fresh sage

1 Adjust oven rack to middle position and heat oven to 475 degrees. Line rimmed baking sheet with parchment paper.

2 Cut each squash half into 2½- to 3-inch pieces. Whisk 2 tablespoons oil, garlic, paprika, coriander, salt, and pepper together in large bowl. Add squash and toss until evenly coated. Arrange squash cut side down in single layer on prepared sheet. Roast until bottoms of most pieces are deep golden brown, 15 to 20 minutes.

3 Remove sheet from oven. Gently flip squash and switch outer pieces with inner pieces on sheet. Continue to roast until squash is tender and most pieces are deep golden brown on second side, 15 to 20 minutes.

4 Whisk vinegar, maple syrup, sage, and remaining 2 tablespoons oil together in small bowl. Transfer squash to serving platter and drizzle with vinaigrette. Serve.

Broiled Smashed Zucchini with Garlicky Yogurt

serves 4 · total time: 50 minutes

why this recipe works · Go ahead, give your zucchini a whack with a meat pounder and then slide the irregular pieces under the broiler. Not only does this create a range of textures, it unlocks a variety of flavors from almost-raw to tender and nutty-sweet to slightly charred. Drizzling the craggy chunks with olive oil and

lemon juice before broiling helped highlight the subtle flavors. We served the zucchini atop a creamy yogurt sauce garnished with crunchy nuts, herbs, pepper flakes, and a drizzle of olive oil. The zucchini do not need to be the same size, though we prefer ones that are 7 to 12 ounces each. We developed this recipe using an electric broiler. If using a gas broiler, adjust the oven rack 4 inches from the broiler element and use tongs to rearrange the zucchini pieces halfway through cooking instead of rotating the pan in step 2.

- 2 pounds zucchini
- 2 tablespoons extra-virgin olive oil, plus extra for drizzling
- 4 teaspoons lemon juice
- 2¼ teaspoons kosher salt, divided
- ½ cup plain Greek yogurt
- 2 tablespoons water
- ½ teaspoon minced garlic
- ¼ cup hazelnuts, toasted, skinned, and chopped
  Chopped fresh dill, basil, parsley, or chives
  Aleppo pepper

1 Adjust oven rack 5 inches from broiler element and heat broiler. Using meat pounder or rolling pin, firmly but gently smash zucchini until flattened and cracked lengthwise. Trim and discard ends. Break each zucchini into 2 to 4 large pieces. Transfer zucchini pieces to large bowl, including any smaller pieces that have been created during smashing and breaking. Add oil and lemon juice and toss until zucchini is evenly coated.

2 Arrange zucchini, skin side down, on aluminum foil–lined rimmed baking sheet. Sprinkle with 2 teaspoons salt, making sure to season thicker pieces more heavily than thinner pieces. Broil until zucchini are lightly charred in spots, 9 to 12 minutes, rotating pan halfway through broiling. Let cool until zucchini are warm to touch, 15 to 20 minutes.

3 Meanwhile, stir yogurt, water, garlic, and remaining ¼ teaspoon salt together in small bowl. Let sit at room temperature to allow flavors to meld, about 10 minutes. Spread yogurt mixture on serving platter. Cut zucchini into bite-size pieces. Arrange zucchini on top of yogurt mixture. Sprinkle with hazelnuts, dill, and Aleppo pepper. Drizzle with oil and serve.

MAKE IT DAIRY-FREE · Substitute plant-based Greek yogurt for the dairy Greek yogurt.

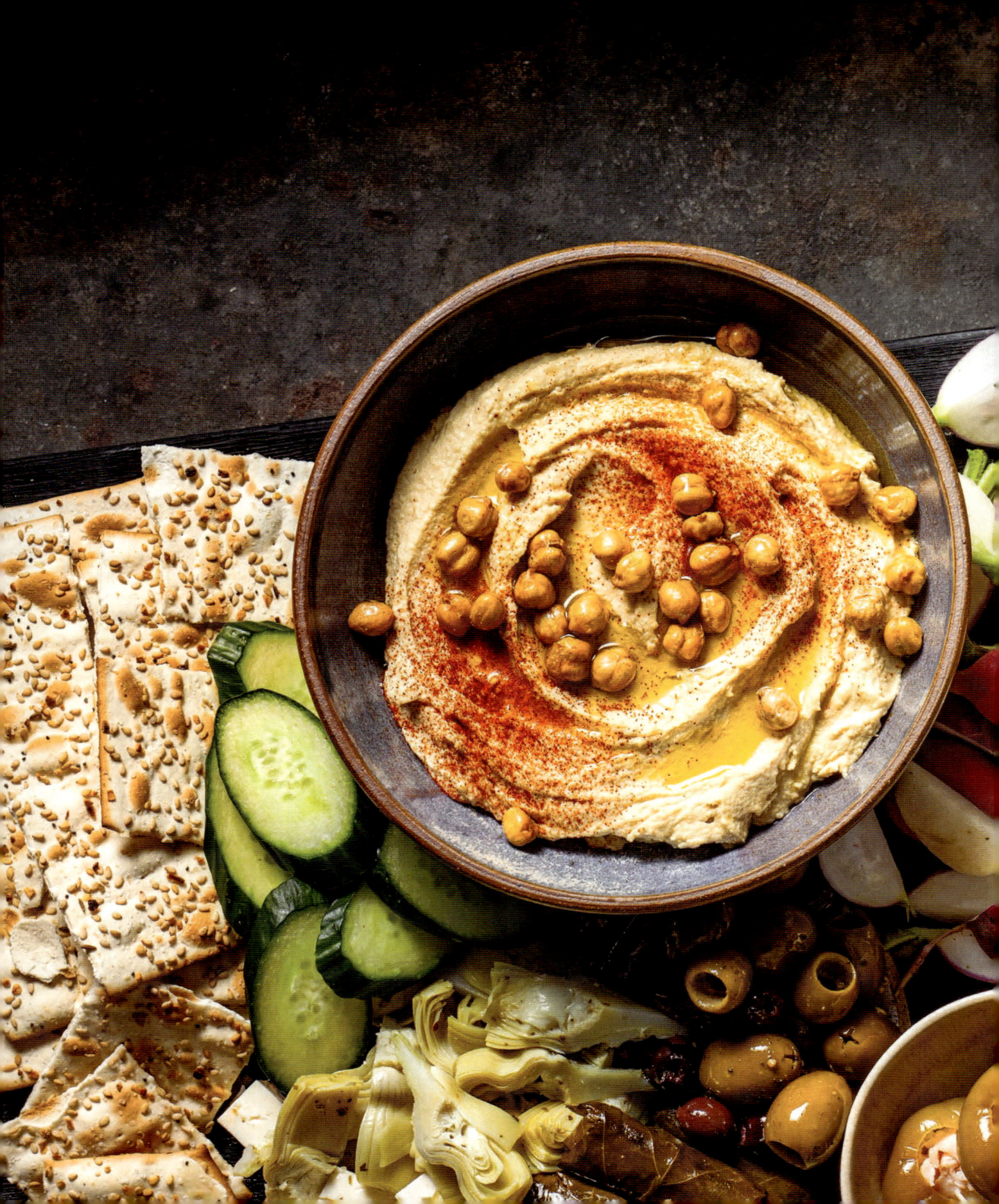

SNACKS

■ FAST   ■ SUPERCHARGED

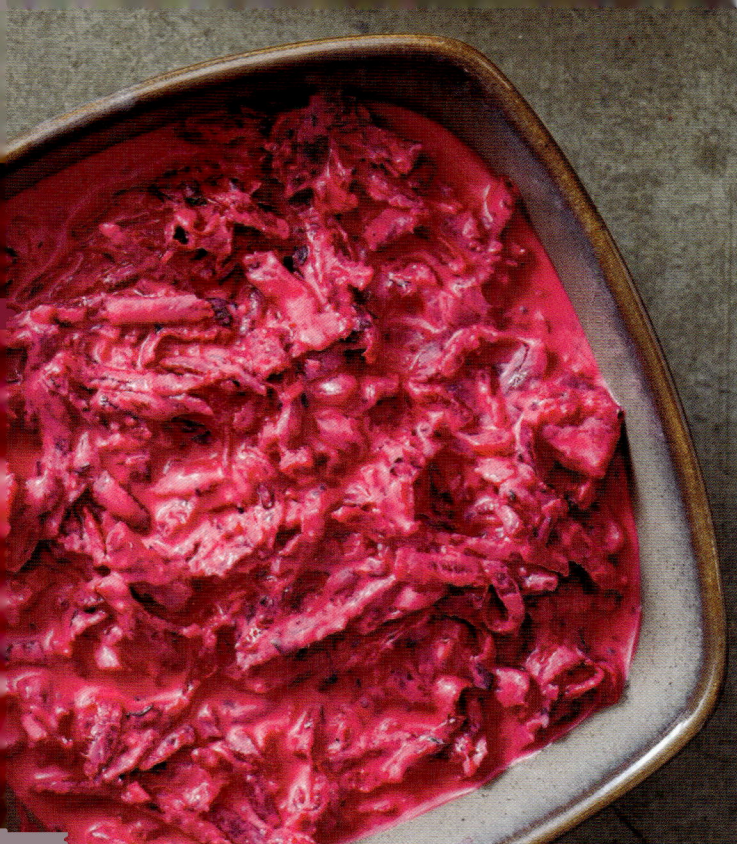

Tzatziki

serves 8 (makes about 2 cups) • **total time: 20 minutes, plus 1 hour chilling**

why this recipe works • Tzatziki is a traditional Greek sauce made from strained yogurt and cucumber; it's equally delicious eaten as a dip with a rainbow of raw, nutrient-dense vegetables as it is dolloped over grilled chicken or lamb. To make our own classic version, we started by shredding a cucumber on a coarse grater, salting it, and letting it drain to keep any excess liquid from watering down the dip. Greek yogurt added a probiotic boost, while the cucumber brought textural interest, crunch, and anti-inflammatory flavonoids. For a vibrantly pink tzatziki with even more anti-inflammatory compounds, we created a variation that includes peeled and grated beets. Using Greek yogurt here is key; do not substitute regular plain yogurt or the sauce will be very watery. Serve with Crudités (page 373), whole-grain tortilla chips, or whole-wheat pita chips.

- 1 (12-ounce) cucumber, peeled, halved lengthwise, seeded, and shredded
- ¼ teaspoon table salt
- 1 cup plain 2 percent Greek yogurt
- 2 tablespoons extra-virgin olive oil
- 2 tablespoons minced fresh mint or dill
- 1 small garlic clove, minced
- ⅛ teaspoon pepper

1 Toss cucumber with salt in colander and let drain for 15 minutes.

2 Whisk yogurt, oil, mint, and garlic together in medium serving bowl, then stir in cucumber. Cover and refrigerate until chilled, at least 1 hour. Stir in pepper before serving.

VARIATION
Beet Tzatziki
Reduce amount of cucumber to 6 ounces and add 6 ounces raw beets, peeled and grated, to cucumber and salt in step 1.

MAKE AHEAD • Tzatziki can be refrigerated for up to 2 days.

MAKE IT DAIRY-FREE • Substitute plant-based Greek yogurt for the dairy yogurt.

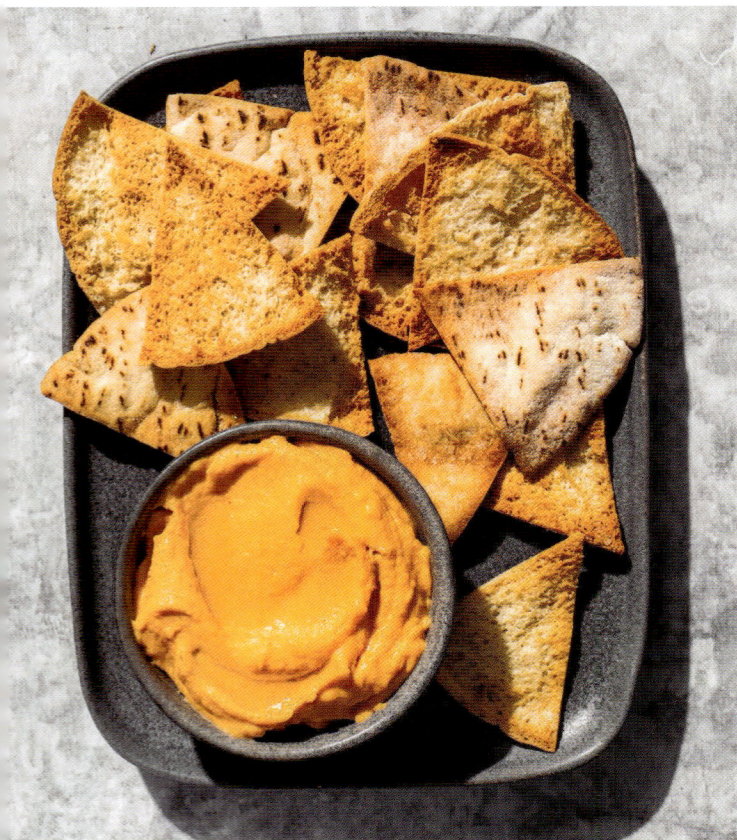

top | *Beet Tzatziki*
bottom | *Sweet Potato Hummus*

Classic Hummus

serves 8 (makes about 2 cups) · total time: 15 minutes, plus 30 minutes resting `FAST`

why this recipe works · With protein and fiber from chickpeas, hummus makes an energizing plant-powered snack, especially if paired with vegetables. Classic hummus is composed of only a few simple ingredients: chickpeas, tahini, olive oil, garlic, and lemon juice. But many traditional recipes are surprisingly complex, and the chickpeas must be soaked overnight and then skinned. We wanted a simple, streamlined recipe for hummus with a light, silky-smooth texture and balanced flavor profile. We used convenient canned chickpeas and brought out the food processor to make quick work of turning them into a smooth puree. But the key to the best texture was to create an emulsion. We started by grinding the chickpeas, then slowly added a mixture of water and lemon juice. We whisked olive oil and a generous amount of tahini together and drizzled the mixture into the chickpeas while processing; this created a lush, light, and flavorful puree. Earthy cumin, garlic, and a pinch of cayenne kept the flavors balanced. If desired, garnish the hummus with 1 tablespoon of minced fresh cilantro or parsley, 2 tablespoons of reserved whole chickpeas, and/or more cayenne. Serve with Crudités (page 373), Whole-Wheat Seeded Crackers (page 375), or whole-wheat pita chips.

- ¼ cup water, plus extra as needed
- 3 tablespoons lemon juice
- 6 tablespoons tahini
- 2 tablespoons extra-virgin olive oil
- 1 (15-ounce) can no-salt-added chickpeas, rinsed
- 1 small garlic clove, minced
- ½ teaspoon table salt
- ¼ teaspoon ground cumin
  Pinch cayenne pepper

1 Combine water and lemon juice in small bowl. In separate bowl, whisk tahini and oil together.

2 Process chickpeas, garlic, salt, cumin, and cayenne in food processor until almost fully ground, about 15 seconds. Scrape down sides of bowl with silicone spatula. With machine running, add lemon juice mixture in steady stream. Scrape down sides of bowl and continue to process for 1 minute. With machine running, add tahini mixture in steady stream and process until hummus is smooth and creamy, about 15 seconds, scraping down sides of bowl as needed.

3 Transfer hummus to serving bowl, cover with plastic wrap, and let sit at room temperature until flavors meld, about 30 minutes. Serve.

VARIATIONS

Roasted Red Pepper Hummus

Omit water and cumin. Add ¼ cup jarred roasted red peppers, rinsed and patted dry, to food processor with chickpeas. Garnish hummus with 2 tablespoons toasted sliced almonds and 2 teaspoons minced fresh parsley.

Artichoke-Lemon Hummus

Omit cumin and increase lemon juice to ¼ cup (2 lemons). Add ¾ cup frozen artichoke hearts, thawed and patted dry, and ¼ teaspoon grated lemon zest to food processor with chickpeas. Garnish hummus with additional ¼ cup thawed frozen artichoke hearts, patted dry and chopped, and 2 teaspoons minced fresh parsley or mint.

❙ **MAKE AHEAD** · Hummus can be refrigerated for up to 5 days.

Sweet Potato Hummus

serves 14 (makes 3½ cups) · total time: 35 minutes, plus 30 minutes resting `SUPERCHARGED`

why this recipe works · This vibrant sweet potato hummus combines creamy chickpeas with earthy sweet potato—for an anthocyanin boost plus a welcome dose of extra fiber. To bring out the tuber's flavor, we tested mixing varying amounts with our classic hummus. We found that one large sweet potato (about 1 pound) offered just the right balance. Microwaving the potato yielded a flavor that was nearly as intense as roasting and a lot faster. As for seasonings, we preferred less tahini than in traditional hummus, so we used just ¼ cup. To complement the sweet potato, we added an antioxidant-rich blend of spices: paprika, coriander, cinnamon, and cumin. Serve with Crudités (page 373), Whole-Wheat Seeded Crackers (page 375), or whole-wheat pita chips.

- 1 large sweet potato (about 1 pound), unpeeled
- ¾ cup water
- ¼ cup lemon juice (2 lemons)
- ¼ cup tahini
- 2 tablespoons extra-virgin olive oil, plus extra for drizzling
- 1 (15-ounce) can no-salt-added chickpeas, rinsed
- 1 small garlic clove, minced
- 1 teaspoon paprika
- 1 teaspoon table salt
- ½ teaspoon ground coriander
- ¼ teaspoon ground cumin
- ⅛ teaspoon ground cinnamon
- ⅛ teaspoon cayenne pepper

1   Prick sweet potato several times with fork, place on plate, and microwave until very soft, about 12 minutes, flipping halfway through microwaving. Slice potato in half lengthwise, let cool, then scrape sweet potato flesh from skin and transfer to food processor; discard skin.

2   Combine water and lemon juice in small bowl. In separate bowl, whisk tahini and oil together.

3   Process sweet potato, chickpeas, garlic, paprika, salt, coriander, cumin, cinnamon, and cayenne in food processor until almost fully ground, about 15 seconds. Scrape down bowl with silicone spatula. With machine running, add lemon juice mixture in steady stream. Scrape down bowl and continue to process for 1 minute. With machine running, add tahini mixture in steady stream and process until hummus is smooth and creamy, about 15 seconds, scraping down bowl as needed.

4   Transfer hummus to serving bowl, cover with plastic wrap, and let sit at room temperature until flavors meld, about 30 minutes. Drizzle with extra oil before serving.

❚ MAKE AHEAD • Hummus can be refrigerated for up to 5 days.

Quick Lemon-Garlic White Bean Dip

serves 8 (makes 2 cups) • total time: 35 minutes   **FAST**

why this recipe works • This bean dip is inspired by the bright flavors of ful medames, a Middle Eastern meze that's made with fava beans and often served alongside hummus and falafel and eaten with pita. The flavors are fresh and simple, with garlic and lemon being the most prominent. We turned to widely available white beans, leaving some whole to add texture to the dip. We topped the dip with a version of tatbeeleh, a common topping for various meze that is made from green chiles, onion, lemon juice, and olive oil. Serve with warm pita, Whole-Wheat Seeded Crackers (page 375), or crudités.

Dip
1   teaspoon extra-virgin olive oil
3   scallions
2   (15-ounce) cans no-salt-added small white beans, 6 tablespoons liquid reserved, beans rinsed
2½ tablespoons lemon juice
2   garlic cloves, minced
1   teaspoon ground cumin
¼   teaspoon table salt

Tatbeeleh Topping
2   jalapeño chiles, stemmed, seeded, and chopped fine
¼   cup finely chopped onion
2   scallions, sliced thin
1   tablespoon lemon juice
¼   cup minced fresh parsley
½   teaspoon table salt
4   teaspoons extra-virgin olive oil, plus extra for drizzling Flake sea salt

1   **For the dip** Heat oil in Dutch oven over medium-high heat until shimmering. Reduce heat to medium, add scallions, and cook until spotty brown, 4 to 6 minutes, flipping halfway through cooking. Add beans, lemon juice, garlic, cumin, and salt and cook over medium-low heat until warmed through, about 10 minutes, stirring occasionally. Discard scallions.

2   Transfer 1½ cups bean mixture to food processor along with reserved bean liquid and process until mostly smooth with some small pieces visible, about 10 seconds. Return processed beans to Dutch oven with remaining whole beans and stir to combine. Season with salt to taste.

3   **For the topping** Combine all ingredients except flake sea salt in bowl. Transfer warm dip to serving bowl and top with tatbeeleh topping. Drizzle with extra oil and sprinkle with sea salt. Serve.

❚ MAKE AHEAD • Dip can be refrigerated for up to 24 hours; reheat gently before topping with tatbeeleh and serving.

Navy Bean and Artichoke Dip

serves 8 (makes about 2 cups) • total time: 35 minutes, plus 30 minutes resting

why this recipe works • Most artichoke dips could justifiably be called mayonnaise-cheese dips, given what goes into them. To create a rendition that didn't go overboard on the saturated fat, we looked to bean dip to provide a creamy base that also contributed protein and fiber. We thought that vegetal artichokes (high in vitamins K and C and various minerals) would partner well with earthy-sweet but mild navy beans, which have a velvety texture. Using canned beans and jarred artichoke hearts kept the recipe streamlined. To increase the creaminess of our dip and add a filling protein boost plus some probiotics, we incorporated Greek yogurt. Finally, a healthy dose of lemon juice, garlic, parsley, and scallion added fresh flavor and brightness. Serve with Crudités (page 373) or Whole-Wheat Seeded Crackers (page 375).

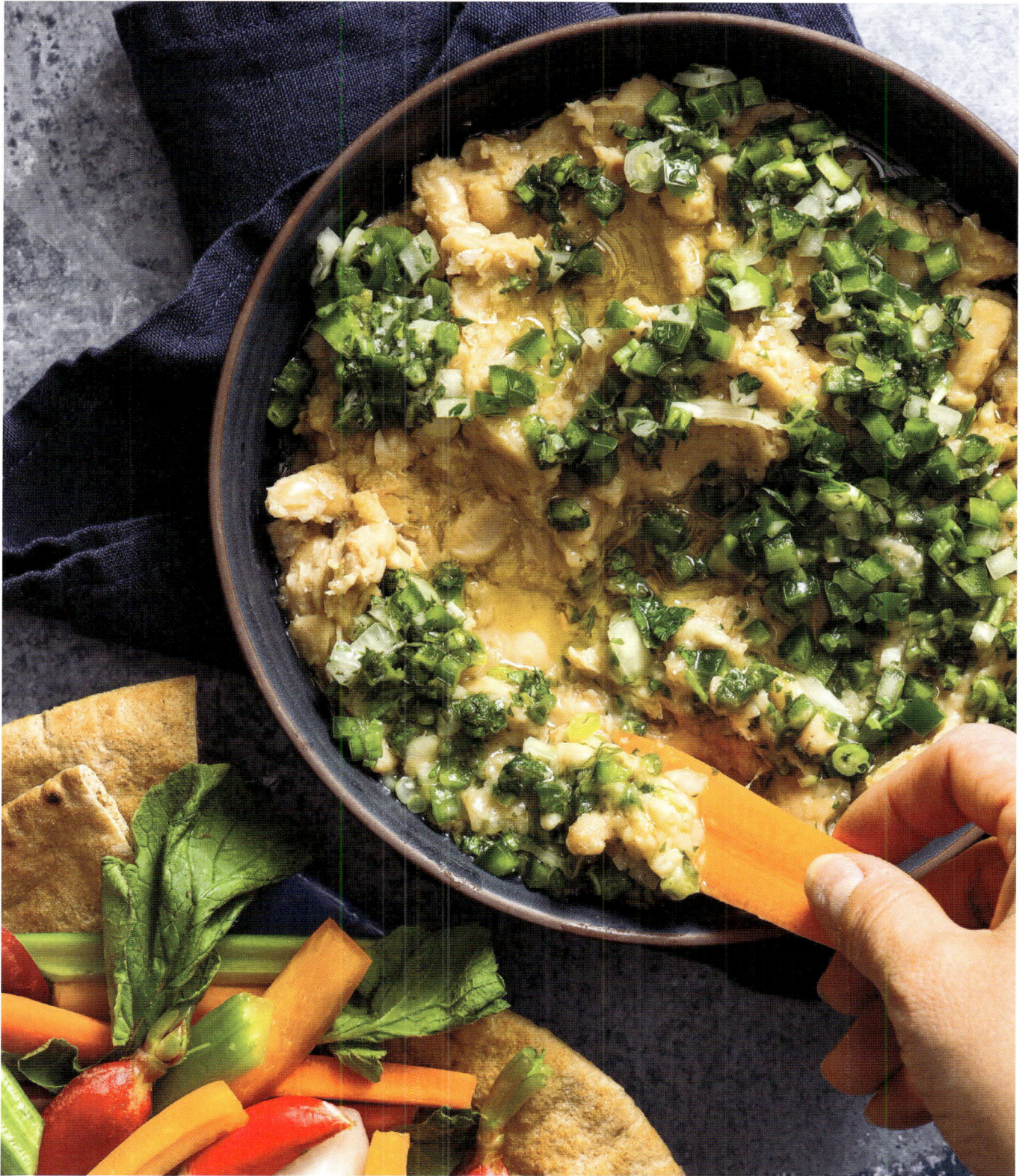

1 teaspoon grated lemon zest plus 2 tablespoons juice

1 small garlic clove, minced

1 (15-ounce) can no-salt-added navy beans, 2 tablespoons liquid reserved, beans rinsed

1 cup jarred whole artichoke hearts packed in water, rinsed and patted dry, 2 tablespoons chopped

¼ cup fresh parsley leaves

1 scallion, white and light green parts cut into ½-inch pieces, dark green part sliced thin on bias

¾ teaspoon table salt

¼ teaspoon ground fennel

Pinch cayenne pepper

¼ cup plain 2 percent Greek yogurt

Extra-virgin olive oil

1 Combine lemon zest and juice and garlic in bowl and let sit for 15 minutes.

2 Pulse garlic–lemon juice mixture, beans, their reserved liquid, whole artichoke hearts, parsley, white and light green scallion pieces, salt, fennel, and cayenne in food processor until finely ground, 5 to 10 pulses, scraping down bowl as needed. Continue to process until uniform paste forms, about 1 minute, scraping down bowl as needed.

3 Add yogurt and continue to process until smooth, about 15 seconds. Transfer to serving bowl, cover, and let stand at room temperature for 30 minutes. Season with salt to taste. Sprinkle with reserved chopped artichokes and dark green scallion parts and drizzle with oil to taste before serving.

MAKE AHEAD • Dip can be refrigerated for up to 24 hours. Sprinkle with artichokes and scallion greens and drizzle with oil before serving.

MAKE IT DAIRY-FREE • Substitute plant-based Greek yogurt for the dairy Greek yogurt.

Beet Dip with Yogurt and Tahini

serves 6 to 8 • total time: 2¼ hours, plus 30 minutes resting **SUPERCHARGED**

why this recipe works • For this bright recipe inspired by beet dips found in Levantine cuisines, we roasted and shredded beets and then mixed them with creamy Greek yogurt, nutty tahini, olive oil, garlic, lemon juice, and seasonings. The tahini added a little bitterness, and the lemon juice added tang to balance the sweetness of the beets. Letting the dip chill for 30 minutes allowed the flavors to meld. A sprinkle of fresh dill gave contrasting color and freshness. To ensure even cooking, look for beets of similar size—roughly 2 to 3 inches in diameter. If you can't find Aleppo pepper, you can substitute ½ teaspoon of paprika plus ⅛ teaspoon of red pepper flakes. Serve with cucumber slices, whole-wheat pita chips, or Whole-Wheat Seeded Crackers (page 375).

1¼ pounds red or golden beets, trimmed

1 cup plain whole-milk Greek yogurt

5 tablespoons extra-virgin olive oil, divided

¼ cup tahini

¼ cup lemon juice (2 lemons)

3 garlic cloves, minced

2 teaspoons dried mint

1½ teaspoons table salt

1 teaspoon ground dried Aleppo pepper, plus extra for seasoning

¼ teaspoon ground cumin

1 tablespoon chopped fresh dill

1 Adjust oven rack to middle position and heat oven to 350 degrees. Wrap beets in aluminum foil packet and place on rimmed baking sheet. Roast until beets offer no resistance when pierced through foil with paring knife, 1¼ to 1½ hours. Carefully open packet and set beets aside to cool completely, about 25 minutes. Rub off skins with paper towels.

2 Meanwhile, whisk yogurt, ¼ cup oil, tahini, lemon juice, garlic, mint, salt, Aleppo pepper, and cumin together in large bowl.

3 Shred cooled beets on large holes of box grater or using shredding disk of food processor. Stir beets into yogurt mixture and refrigerate until flavors meld, about 30 minutes.

4 Stir dip to recombine and season with salt and Aleppo pepper to taste. Transfer to serving bowl, drizzle with remaining 1 tablespoon oil, and sprinkle with dill. Serve chilled or at room temperature.

MAKE AHEAD • Dip can be refrigerated for up to 3 days.

MAKE IT DAIRY-FREE • Substitute plant-based Greek yogurt for the dairy Greek yogurt.

Nutrition Knowledge   This creamy, spiced beet dip is as nutrient-dense as it is visually striking. Beets are rich in betalains, potent antioxidants with anti-inflammatory and detoxifying properties that support liver health and circulation. Tahini, made from ground sesame seeds, brings a dose of healthy fats, plant-based protein, and lignans, which have been shown to reduce inflammatory markers and support hormonal balance. Blended with probiotic-rich Greek yogurt, heart-healthy olive oil, and warming spices such as cumin and Aleppo pepper, the recipe delivers bold flavor and an anti-inflammatory boost. —*Alicia*

NOTES FROM THE TEST KITCHEN

Substituting Precooked Beets

We prefer the balanced flavor that freshly roasted beets bring to this beet dip, but the convenience and nutritional value of precooked beets can't be overlooked. One pound of precooked vacuum-packed beets or one (15-ounce) can of beets can be used in place of the raw beets; skip step 1 and drain any liquid before shredding.

Vacuum-Packed Vacuum-packed beets are often cooked directly in the pouch or steamed without extra water, so they retain their sweetness and flavor, as well as more nutrients. The concentrated flavor will also result in a slightly sweeter dish.

Canned Canned beets are cooked in water, so the colorful juice and much of the beets' soluble sugar leaches out, causing some loss of water-soluble nutrients (though much of the minerals and fiber do remain intact). Canned beets will result in a lighter-colored dip with a slightly more acidic end product. If using canned beets, reduce the salt to 1 teaspoon and season with salt to taste before serving.

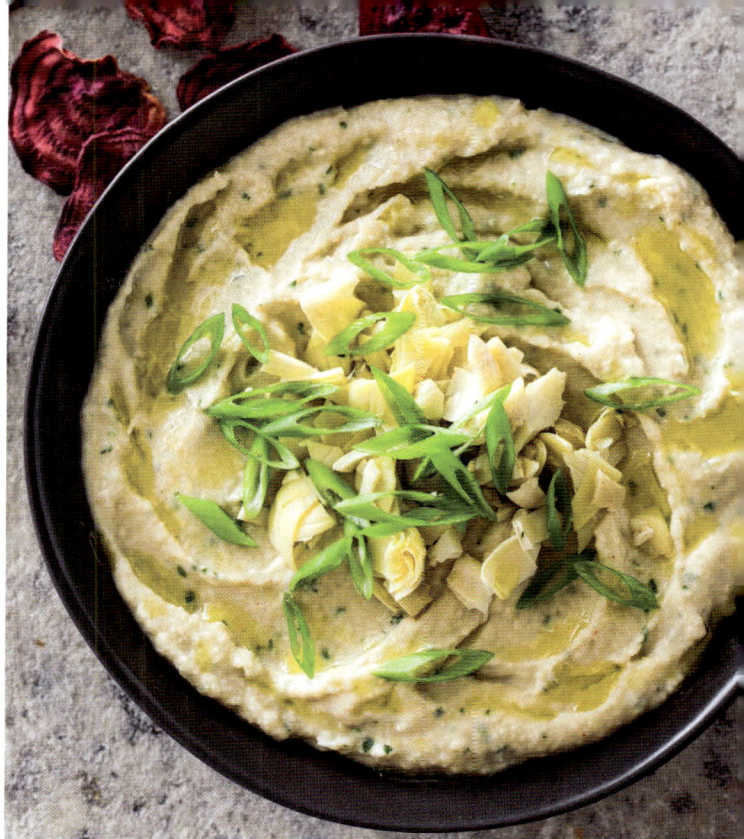

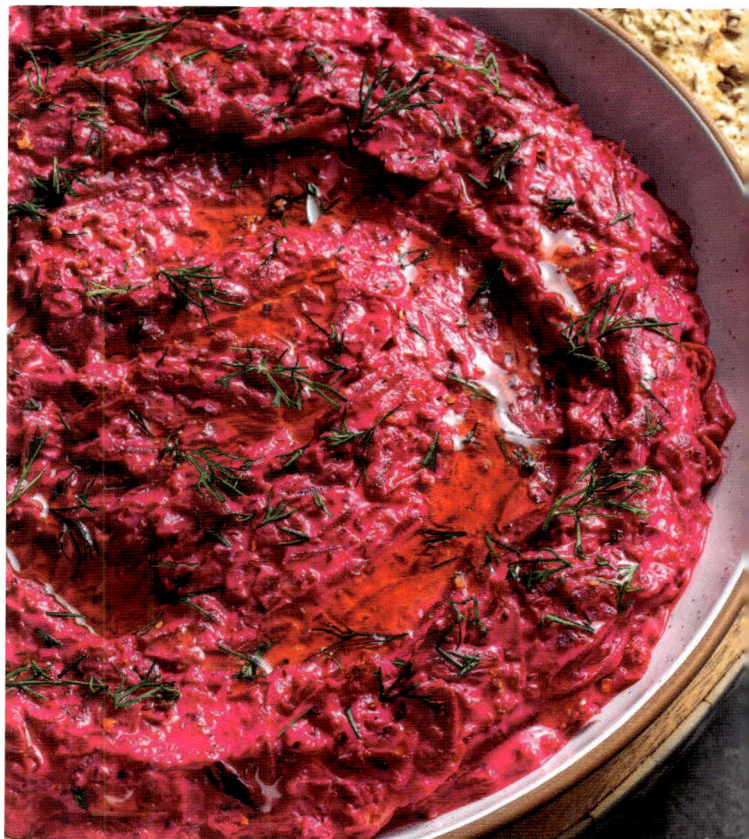

top | *Navy Bean and Artichoke Dip*
bottom | *Beet Dip with Yogurt and Tahini*

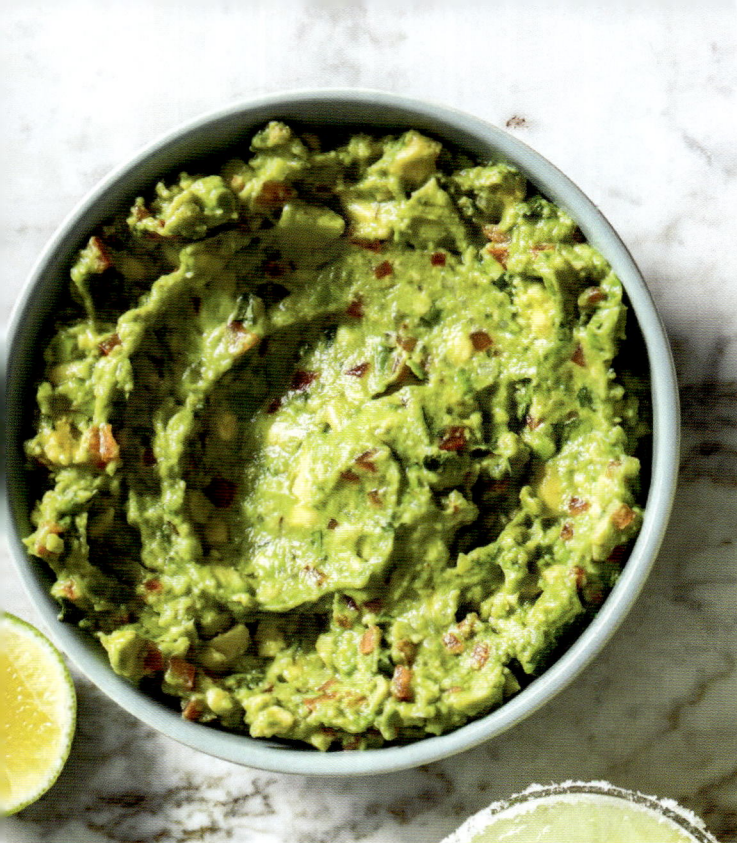

Guacamole

serves 8 (makes about 2 cups) • total time: 15 minutes **FAST**

why this recipe works • Avocados are packed with heart-healthy monounsaturated fats as well as a variety of vitamins and other nutrients that fight inflammation. For the ultimate creamy, big-flavored guacamole, we looked at the traditional methods that typically make a smooth guacamole using the coarse surface of a molcajete, a three-legged Mexican mortar made of volcanic rock. Hoping to make ours without any special equipment, we minced the onion and chile by hand with kosher salt; the coarse crystals broke down the aromatics, releasing their juices and flavors and transforming them into a paste that we combined with the avocado and other ingredients. (The salt will also help the aromatics break down if you do use a mortar and pestle.) Lime zest added further brightness without acidity. We used a whisk to mix and mash the avocado into the paste, creating a creamy but still chunky dip. For a spicier version, mince and add the serrano ribs and seeds to the onion mixture. Be sure to use Hass avocados here; Florida, or "skinny," avocados are too watery for dips. Serve with whole-grain tortilla chips.

- 2 tablespoons finely chopped onion
- 1 serrano chile, stemmed, seeded, and minced
- 1 teaspoon kosher salt
- ¼ teaspoon grated lime zest plus 1½–2 tablespoons juice
- 3 ripe avocados, halved, pitted, and cut into ½-inch pieces
- 1 plum tomato, cored, seeded, and minced
- 2 tablespoons chopped fresh cilantro

Place onion, serrano, salt, and lime zest on cutting board and chop until very finely minced. Transfer onion mixture to medium serving bowl and stir in 1½ tablespoons lime juice. Add avocados and, using sturdy whisk, mash and stir mixture until well combined, with some ¼- to ½-inch chunks of avocado remaining. Stir in tomato and cilantro. Season with up to additional 1½ teaspoons lime juice to taste before serving.

MAKE AHEAD • Guacamole can be refrigerated for up to 24 hours by pressing plastic wrap flush against the surface.

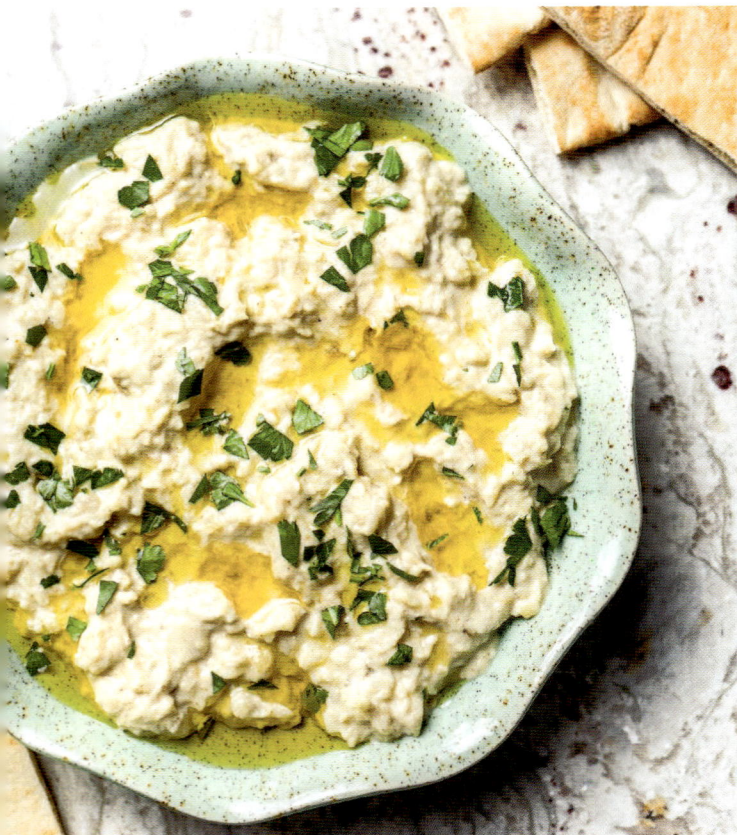

top | *Guacamole*
bottom | *Baba Ghanoush*

Baba Ghanoush

serves 8 (makes 2 cups) · total time: 1 hour, plus 1 hour chilling

why this recipe works · Eggplant turns creamy and soft when roasted, making it the perfect base for the beloved Middle Eastern dip baba ghanoush. Before roasting the eggplants, we pricked their skin to encourage moisture to evaporate and to prevent the skin from splitting open; roasting them whole in a very hot oven resulted in flesh that was meltingly tender. To avoid a watery dip, we scooped the hot pulp into a colander to drain before adding it to the food processor with the other ingredients. We kept the flavorings true to tradition: lemon juice, olive oil, garlic, and tahini. A drizzle of heart-healthy olive oil and a sprinkle of parsley finished our baba ghanoush. In addition to serving as a dip, this makes a great sandwich spread (or filling). Look for eggplants with an even shape for this recipe, as bulbous eggplants won't cook evenly. Serve with warm pita, whole-wheat pita chips, or Whole-Wheat Seeded Crackers (page 375).

- 2 eggplants (1 pound each), pricked all over with fork
- 2 tablespoons tahini
- 2 tablespoons extra-virgin olive oil, plus extra for serving
- 4 teaspoons lemon juice
- 1 small garlic clove, minced
- ¾ teaspoon table salt
- ¼ teaspoon pepper
- 2 teaspoons chopped fresh parsley

1 Adjust oven rack to middle position and heat oven to 500 degrees. Place eggplants on aluminum foil–lined rimmed baking sheet and roast, turning eggplants every 15 minutes, until uniformly soft when pressed with tongs, 40 minutes to 1 hour. Let eggplants cool for 5 minutes on sheet.

2 Set colander over bowl. Trim top and bottom ¼ inch of eggplants, then halve eggplants lengthwise. Using spoon, scoop hot pulp into colander (you should have about 2 cups pulp); discard skins. Let pulp drain for 3 minutes. Discard liquid.

3 Transfer drained eggplant to food processor. Add tahini, oil, lemon juice, garlic, salt, and pepper. Pulse mixture to coarse puree, about 8 pulses. Season with salt and pepper to taste

4 Transfer to serving bowl, cover tightly with plastic wrap, and refrigerate until chilled, about 1 hour. Season with salt and pepper and drizzle with extra oil to taste; sprinkle with parsley before serving.

MAKE AHEAD · Dip can be refrigerated for up to 24 hours.

Carrot-Habanero Dip

serves 10 (makes 2½ cups) · total time: 40 minutes, plus 30 minutes chilling **SUPERCHARGED**

why this recipe works · This flavorful dip is packed with sweet carrot flavor as well as antioxidants. To enliven the earthiness of the beta carotene–rich carrots, we added heat in the form of habaneros, which also brought a dose of capsaicin. To maintain the carrots' brilliant color, we avoided browning them. Instead, we cooked them over an initial blast of heat to break down their cell walls before adding water and simmering them until tender. Processing the mixture produced a smooth dip, which we finished with a drizzle of olive oil and some crunchy pepitas. For a spicier dip, use the higher amount of habanero chiles given, and/or add the seeds from the chiles. Serve with whole-wheat pita chips, Crudités (page 373), or Whole-Wheat Seeded Crackers (page 375).

- 3 tablespoons extra-virgin olive oil, divided, plus extra for serving
- 2 pounds carrots, peeled and sliced ¼ inch thick
- ½ teaspoon table salt
- 1–2 habanero chiles, seeded and minced
- 2 garlic cloves, minced
- ¾ teaspoon ground coriander
- ¾ teaspoon ground cumin
- ¾ teaspoon ground ginger
- ⅛ teaspoon chili powder
- ⅛ teaspoon ground cinnamon
- ⅓ cup water
- 1 tablespoon white wine vinegar
- 1 tablespoon roasted, salted pepitas
- 1 tablespoon minced fresh cilantro

1 Heat 1 tablespoon oil in large saucepan over medium-high heat until shimmering. Add carrots and salt and cook until carrots begin to soften, 5 to 6 minutes. Stir in habanero, garlic, coriander, cumin, ginger, chili powder, and cinnamon and cook until fragrant, about 30 seconds. Add water and bring to simmer. Cover, reduce heat to low, and cook, stirring occasionally, until carrots are tender, 15 to 20 minutes.

2 Transfer carrots to bowl of food processor, add vinegar, and process until smooth, scraping down sides of bowl as needed, 1 to 2 minutes. With processor running, slowly add remaining 2 tablespoons oil until incorporated. Transfer to serving bowl, cover, and refrigerate until chilled, at least 30 minutes. Season with salt and pepper to taste. Sprinkle with pepitas and cilantro and drizzle with extra oil. Serve.

MAKE AHEAD · Dip can be refrigerated for up to 24 hours.

Muhammara

serves 6 (makes 1½ cups) • total time: 15 minutes **FAST**

why this recipe works • In this recipe for muhammara, a spicy-sweet dip of roasted red peppers and walnuts popular in Levantine cuisine, the peppers offer not only smoky depth but also velvety texture. Cracker crumbs absorb extra juice so the dip stays thick. Walnuts add richness, offset by tart pomegranate molasses. We prefer red bell peppers in this dip. Any savory cracker may be used for the crumbs. Crush the crackers in a zipper-lock bag with a rolling pin. We like to use our homemade Roasted Bell Peppers (recipe follows), but you can use store-bought if you prefer. Serve with warm pita, whole-wheat pita chips, or Crudités (page 373), or use as a sandwich spread.

1 cup roasted red bell peppers, chopped coarse
½ cup walnuts, toasted
⅓ cup cracker crumbs
3 scallions, chopped coarse
¼ cup extra-virgin olive oil
4½ teaspoons pomegranate molasses
4 teaspoons lemon juice
1½ teaspoons paprika
1 teaspoon ground cumin
½ teaspoon table salt
⅛ teaspoon cayenne pepper

Process all ingredients in food processor until uniform coarse puree forms, about 15 seconds, scraping down sides of bowl halfway through processing. Transfer to bowl and serve.

MAKE AHEAD • Dip can be refrigerated for up to 3 days.

MAKE IT GLUTEN-FREE • Substitute gluten-free crackers can be substituted for the crackers.

Roasted Bell Peppers

makes 1½ cups • total time: 30 minutes

Cooking times will vary depending on the broiler and the thickness of the bell peppers, so watch them carefully as they cook. Green bell peppers retain some bitterness even when roasted and are best used as a complement to sweeter red, yellow, and orange bell peppers.

3 large bell peppers (1½ pounds)

1 Line rimmed baking sheet with aluminum foil and spray with avocado oil spray. Slice ½ inch from top and bottom of each bell pepper. Gently remove stems from tops. Twist and pull out each core, using knife to loosen at edges if necessary. Cut slit down 1 side of each bell pepper.

2 Turn each bell pepper skin side down and gently press so it opens to create long strip. Slide knife along insides of bell peppers to remove remaining ribs and seeds.

3 Arrange bell pepper strips, tops, and bottoms skin side up on prepared sheet and flatten all pieces with your hand. Adjust oven rack 3 to 4 inches from broiler element and heat broiler. Broil until skin is puffed and most of surface is well charred, 10 to 13 minutes, rotating sheet halfway through broiling.

4 Using tongs, pile bell peppers in center of foil. Gather foil over bell peppers and crimp to form pouch. Let steam for 10 minutes. Open foil packet carefully and spread out bell peppers. When cool enough to handle, peel bell peppers and discard skins.

Fresh Tomato Salsa

serves 8 (makes about 2 cups) • total time: 40 minutes **FAST**

why this recipe works • Salsa is a great option for the appetizer table or daily snacking, but many recipes turn out watery. We found a solution—draining diced tomatoes (skin, seeds, and all) in a colander. This rid them of excess liquid, giving us a chunkier salsa. For supporting ingredients, we chose red onions for punchy flavor, jalapeño chile for vegetal heat, and lime juice for tang. To make this salsa spicier, add the seeds from the chile. Serve with whole-grain tortilla chips or whole-wheat pita chips.

1 pound ripe tomatoes, cored and cut into ½-inch pieces
1 jalapeño chile, stemmed, seeded, and minced
⅓ cup finely chopped red onion
1 small garlic clove, minced
3 tablespoons minced fresh cilantro
1 tablespoon lime juice, plus extra for seasoning
¼ teaspoon table salt

Place tomatoes in colander and let drain for 30 minutes. As tomatoes drain, layer jalapeño, onion, garlic, and cilantro on top. Shake colander to drain excess juice, then transfer salsa to serving bowl. Stir in lime juice and salt. Season with extra lime juice to taste before serving.

MAKE AHEAD • Salsa can be refrigerated for up to 3 days.

crudités

A platter of crudités can be a beautiful, versatile, and very fiberful centerpiece for snacking or entertaining. For perfect crudités, you simply need to prep fresh vegetables properly: Some vegetables must first be blanched and then shocked in ice water; others benefit from being cut in a particular manner. Refrigerate raw vegetables wrapped in damp paper towels in a zipper-lock bag and blanched vegetables in an airtight container for up to 2 days.

Asparagus To remove tough, fibrous ends of asparagus, bend thick end of each stalk until it snaps off. Blanch asparagus for 30 to 60 seconds.

Broccoli and Cauliflower Cut broccoli and cauliflower florets into bite-size pieces by slicing down through stem. Blanch broccoli and cauliflower (separately) for 1 to 1½ minutes.

Carrots and Celery Slice both celery and peeled carrots lengthwise into long, elegant lengths rather than short, stumpy pieces.

Endive Gently pull off leaves one at a time, continuing to trim root end as you work your way toward heart of endive.

Green Beans Line beans up in a row and trim off inedible stem ends with just 1 cut. Blanch beans for 1 minute.

Peppers Slice off top and bottom of pepper and remove seeds and stem. Slice down through side of pepper, unroll it so that it lies flat, then slice into ½-inch-wide strips.

Radishes Choose radishes with green tops still attached so that each half has a leafy handle for grasping and dipping. Slice each radish in half through stem.

Blanching Directions

Bring 6 quarts water and 2 tablespoons table salt to boil in large pot over high heat. Cook vegetables, 1 variety at a time, until slightly softened but still crunchy at core, following times given for individual vegetables above. Transfer blanched vegetables immediately to bowl of ice water until completely cool, then drain and pat dry.

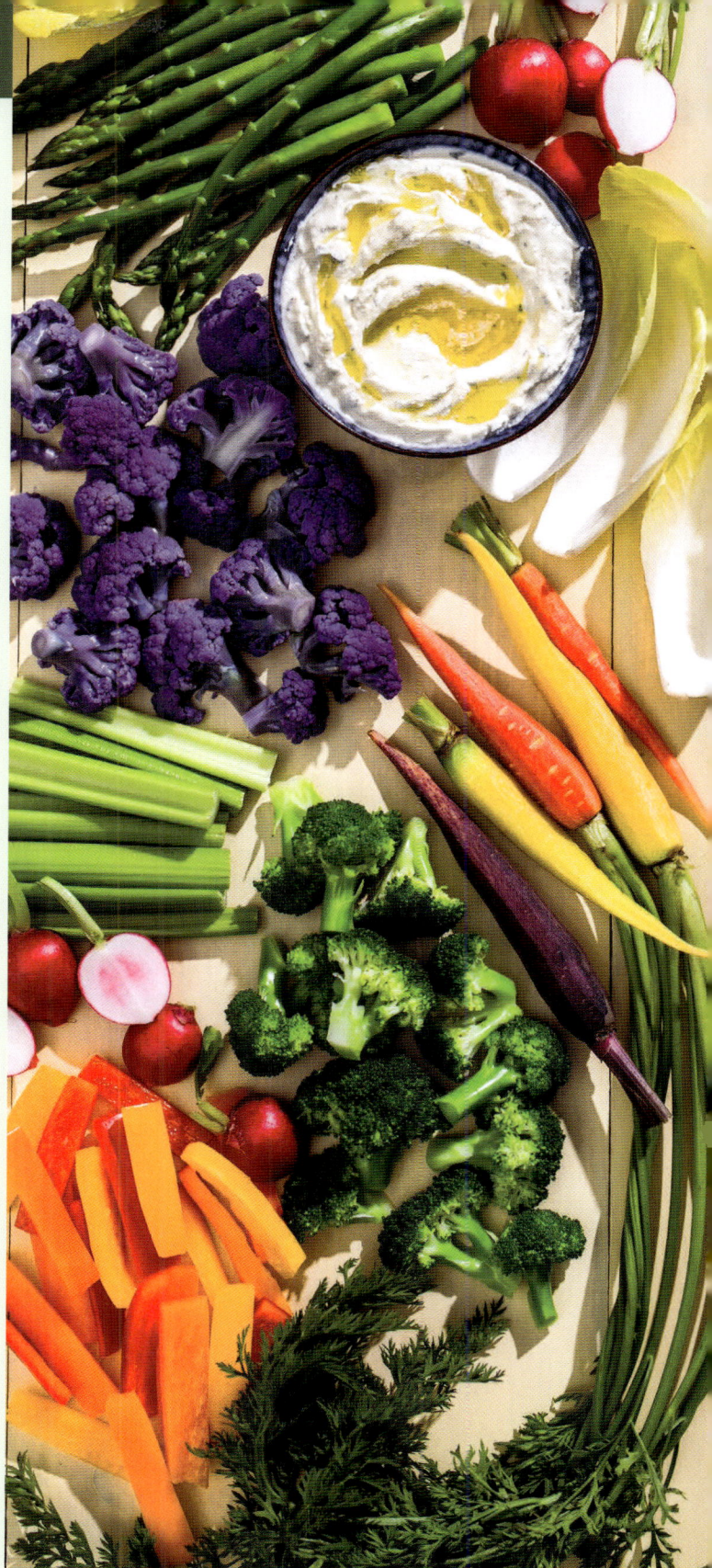

Toasted Corn Salsa

serves 8 (makes about 2 cups) • total time: 25 minutes, plus 1 hour chilling

why this recipe works • Toasted corn kernels and chopped red bell pepper make a summery anti-inflammatory duo. The corn and pepper give this salsa hearty texture, while jalapeño, shallot, and garlic enliven the flavors. Lime juice, cilantro, and cumin round out the mixture. Do not substitute frozen corn for the fresh corn here. Be sure to use a nonstick skillet when toasting the corn. To make this salsa spicier, add the seeds from the chile. Serve with whole-grain tortilla chips or whole-wheat pita chips.

- 4½ teaspoons extra-virgin olive oil, divided
- 2 ears corn, kernels cut from cobs
- 1 red bell pepper, stemmed, seeded, and chopped fine
- ½ jalapeño chile, stemmed, seeded, and minced
- 1 scallion, sliced thin
- 2 garlic cloves, minced
- 2 tablespoons lime juice, plus extra for seasoning
- 2 tablespoons minced fresh cilantro
- ½ teaspoon ground cumin
- ¼ teaspoon table salt
- ⅛ teaspoon pepper

1 Heat 1½ teaspoons oil in 12-inch nonstick skillet over medium-high heat until shimmering. Add corn and cook, stirring occasionally, until golden brown, 6 to 8 minutes.

2 Transfer corn to medium serving bowl and stir in remaining 1 tablespoon oil, bell pepper, jalapeño, scallion, garlic, lime juice, cilantro, cumin, salt, and pepper. Cover and refrigerate until flavors meld, at least 1 hour. Season with extra lime juice to taste before serving.

VARIATION
Toasted Corn and Black Bean Salsa
Reduce amount of corn to 1 ear; use 10-inch skillet when cooking corn in step 1 and reduce cooking time to 4 minutes. Add ¾ cup canned no-salt-added black beans, rinsed, to corn with remaining ingredients.

> **MAKE AHEAD** • Salsa can be refrigerated for up to 2 days.

Orange-Fennel Spiced Almonds

serves 8 (makes 2 cups) • total time: 45 minutes **FAST**

why this recipe works • Making your own spiced nuts is a great way to enjoy them without the added sugar and excess salt that often accompanies store-bought versions. Nuts are a great source of beneficial fats and protein and make an ideal on-the-go anti-inflammatory snack. Watch the nuts carefully during toasting, as they go from golden and fragrant to burnt very quickly.

- 1 tablespoon extra-virgin olive oil
- 1 teaspoon grated orange zest
- 1 teaspoon fennel seeds
- 1 teaspoon table salt
- ¼ teaspoon pepper
- 2 cups raw whole almonds

Adjust oven rack to middle position and heat oven to 350 degrees. Combine oil, orange zest, fennel seeds, salt, and pepper in bowl. Toss almonds with oil mixture until well coated, then spread into single layer on rimmed baking sheet. Bake, stirring often, until fragrant and lightly browned, about 10 minutes. Transfer almonds to serving bowl and let cool completely, about 20 minutes, before serving.

VARIATION
Spicy Chipotle Almonds
Substitute 1 teaspoon ground cumin, ¾ teaspoon chipotle chile powder, and ½ teaspoon garlic powder for orange zest and fennel seeds.

> **MAKE AHEAD** • Almonds can be stored in airtight container for up to 1 week.

Cherry, Chocolate, and Orange Trail Mix

serves 12 (makes about 3 cups) • total time: 35 minutes, plus 20 minutes cooling

why this recipe works • Store-bought trail mix is loaded with sugar and saturated fat; the good news is that it's surprisingly simple to make it yourself. We toasted raw pepitas, almonds, and walnuts—excellent sources of beneficial fats—until fragrant and golden brown. To keep the sugar under control, we used unsweetened dried cherries and just 1 ounce of chopped semisweet chocolate. To pull all the flavors together, we added orange zest for brightness and cinnamon for spice. Watch the nuts carefully during toasting, as they go from golden and fragrant to burnt very quickly.

½ cup raw pepitas
2 tablespoons grated orange zest (2 oranges)
¼ teaspoon ground cinnamon
⅛ teaspoon table salt
¾ cup raw whole almonds
¾ cup raw walnuts, broken into large pieces
½ cup unsweetened dried cherries
1 ounce semisweet chocolate, chopped

1 Adjust oven rack to middle position and heat oven to 350 degrees. Line rimmed baking sheet with parchment paper. Combine pepitas, orange zest, cinnamon, and salt in bowl.

2 Spread almonds and walnuts into single layer on prepared sheet and bake, stirring often, until beginning to turn fragrant, about 6 minutes. Stir in pepita mixture and continue to bake until nuts are fragrant and lightly browned, 3 to 4 minutes. Transfer nut mixture to large bowl and let cool completely, about 20 minutes.

3 Add dried cherries and chocolate to nut mixture and toss to combine. Serve.

VARIATION
Cherry, Coconut, Chili, and Lime Trail Mix
Omit chocolate. Substitute lime zest (3 limes) for orange zest and cayenne pepper for cinnamon. Add ⅓ cup unsweetened flaked coconut to pepita mixture in step 1.

| **MAKE AHEAD** • Trail mix can be stored in airtight container for up to 1 week.

Whole-Wheat Seeded Crackers

serves 12 • total time: 2 hours, plus 2 hours resting and cooling   **SUPERCHARGED**

why this recipe works • These crisp, flavorful crackers take their inspiration from the sturdy Mediterranean lavash cracker, which is typically made with a mix of white, wheat, and semolina flours. For heartiness and nutty flavor, our recipe uses all whole-wheat flour. To give our crackers plenty of texture, not to mention an anti-inflammatory boost, we stirred sesame seeds and flaxseeds into the dough along with a touch of turmeric for its mild warmth—and its curcumin, of course. Letting the dough rest for an hour after mixing made it easier to roll out (between sheets of parchment paper for even greater ease). We pricked the dough all over with a fork to prevent air bubbles, brushed it with egg, and sprinkled it with chia seeds for extra fiber and anti-inflammatory benefits. We

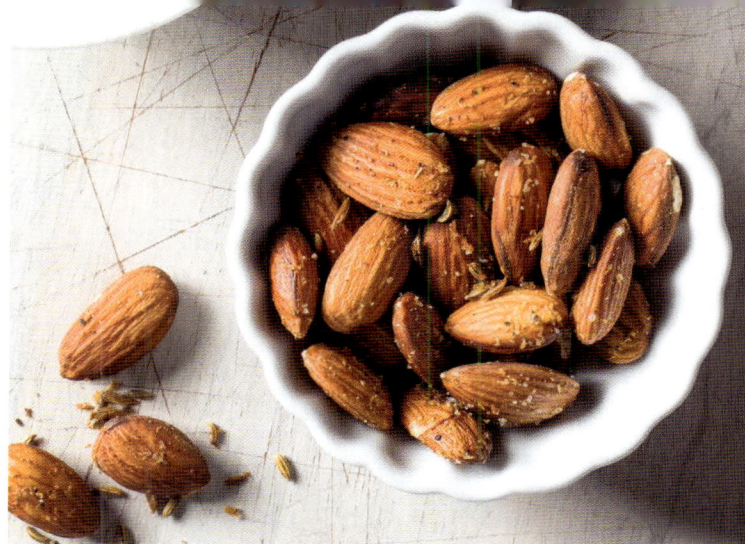
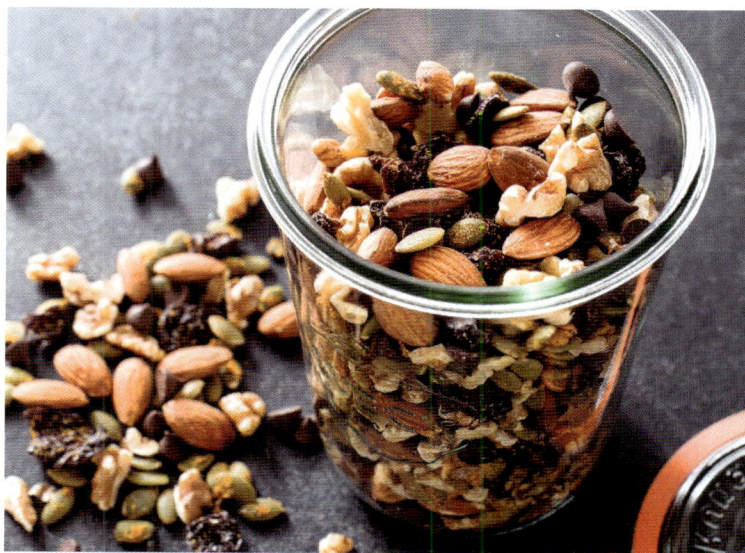
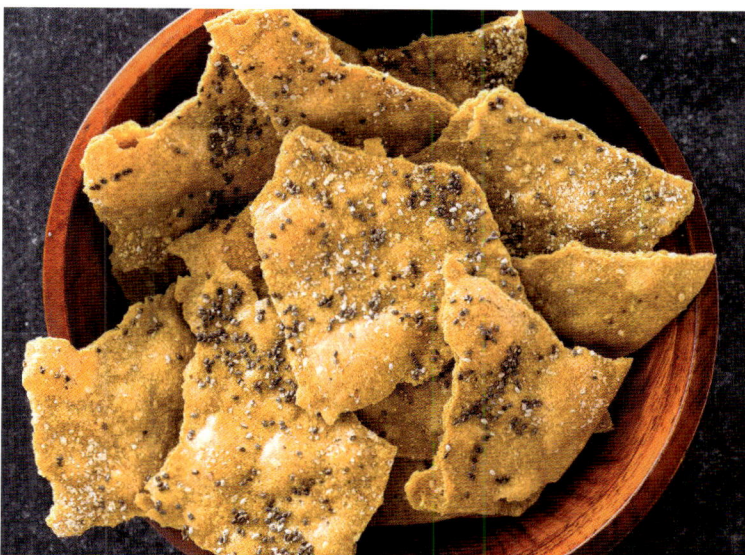

top	Orange-Fennel Spiced Almonds
middle	Cherry, Chocolate, and Orange Trail Mix
bottom	Whole-Wheat Seeded Crackers

baked the giant crackers until deep golden brown and let them cool before breaking them up into rustic pieces. We like golden flaxseeds for their milder flavor, but you can also use brown flaxseeds. We also prefer the larger crystal size of sea salt or kosher salt for sprinkling on the crackers; you can substitute table salt, but reduce the amount by half.

3 cups (16½ ounces) whole-wheat flour
2 tablespoons ground golden flaxseeds
2 tablespoons sesame seeds
1 teaspoon ground turmeric
¾ teaspoon table salt
1 cup (8 ounces) warm water
⅓ cup extra-virgin olive oil, plus extra for brushing
1 large egg, lightly beaten
2 tablespoons chia seeds, divided
2 teaspoons coarse sea salt or kosher salt, divided
½ teaspoon pepper, divided

1 Using stand mixer fitted with dough hook, mix flour, ground flaxseeds, sesame seeds, turmeric, and table salt together on low speed. Gradually add warm water and oil and knead until dough is smooth and elastic, 7 to 9 minutes. Turn dough out onto lightly floured counter and knead by hand to form smooth, round ball. Divide dough into 4 equal pieces, brush with oil, and cover with plastic wrap. Let rest at room temperature for 1 hour.

2 Adjust oven racks to upper-middle and lower-middle positions and heat oven to 400 degrees. Working with 1 piece of dough (keep remaining dough covered with plastic), roll between 2 large sheets of parchment paper into 15 by 11-inch rectangle (about ⅛ inch thick). Remove top sheet of parchment and slide parchment with dough onto baking sheet. Repeat with second piece of dough and second baking sheet.

3 Using fork, poke holes in doughs at 2-inch intervals. Brush doughs with egg, then sprinkle each with 1½ teaspoons chia seeds, ½ teaspoon sea salt, and ⅛ teaspoon pepper. Press gently on seeds and seasonings to help them adhere.

4 Bake crackers until golden brown, 15 to 18 minutes, switching and rotating sheets halfway through baking. Transfer crackers to wire rack and let cool completely, about 30 minutes. Let baking sheets cool completely before rolling out and baking remaining 2 pieces of dough. Break cooled crackers into large pieces and serve.

MAKE AHEAD • Crackers can be stored in airtight container for up to 2 weeks.

NOTES FROM THE TEST KITCHEN

All About Flaxseeds

Flaxseeds are one of the best sources of the beneficial omega-3 fatty acid called alpha-linolenic acid (ALA), which is found only in certain plant foods and oils and must be supplied by our diet. Flaxseeds have a sweet, wheaty flavor, are naturally gluten-free, and are sold both whole and ground in most supermarkets. For our Whole-Wheat Seeded Crackers, we chose ground flaxseeds because grinding improves the release of their nutrients. If you can't find ground flaxseeds, grind whole seeds in a spice grinder or food processor. Flaxseeds, like other nuts and seeds, should be stored in the freezer.

Nutrition Knowledge These seeded whole-wheat crackers are a satisfying way to sneak in serious anti-inflammatory benefits. Whole-wheat flour delivers fiber and polyphenols that support gut health, while flaxseeds and chia seeds are rich in alpha-linolenic acid (ALA). Turmeric gives us a boost of curcumin, a powerful anti-inflammatory compound, and sesame seeds offer healthy fats to support heart health. —*Alicia*

Chickpea Crackers

serves 6 to 8 (makes about 35 crackers) •
total time: 45 minutes, plus 30 minutes cooling

why this recipe works • These crackers are made using chickpea flour, which is rich in protein, fiber, and flavor. Because it is a dense flour, we added olive oil to help create a tender texture, while still keeping the crackers crisp. Warm water was key for hydrating the flour and ensuring that the dough was easy to roll out. The dough will feel dry after mixing in the bowl but should hold together when squeezed. It will come together fully after kneading. Don't be afraid to liberally flour the counter when rolling; it's necessary to roll the dough out to the proper thickness. We prefer 2-inch crackers, but you can use any size round cutter with no change in the baking time. The crackers pair well with cheese and dips but are flavorful enough to be eaten on their own.

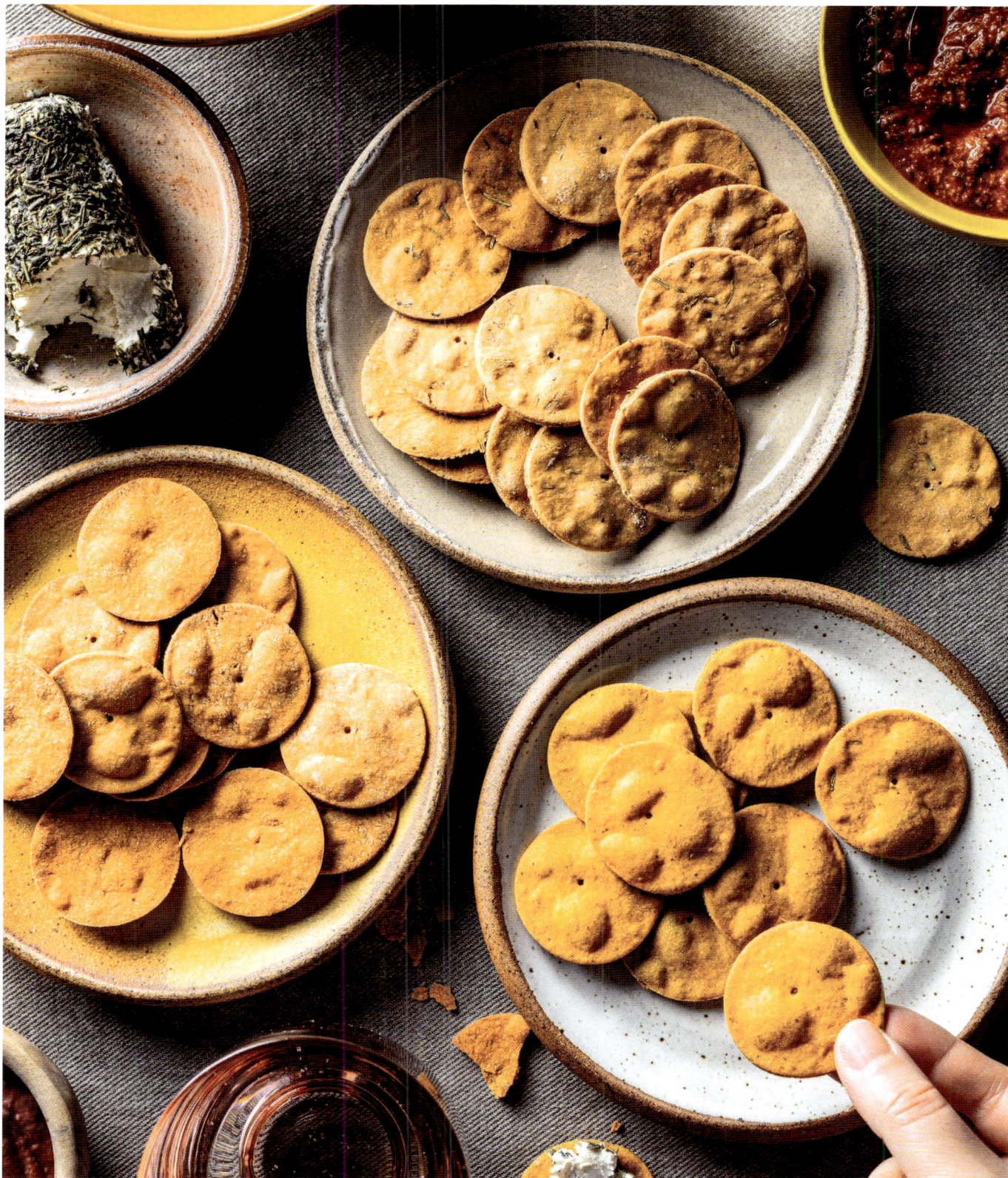

Chickpea Crackers

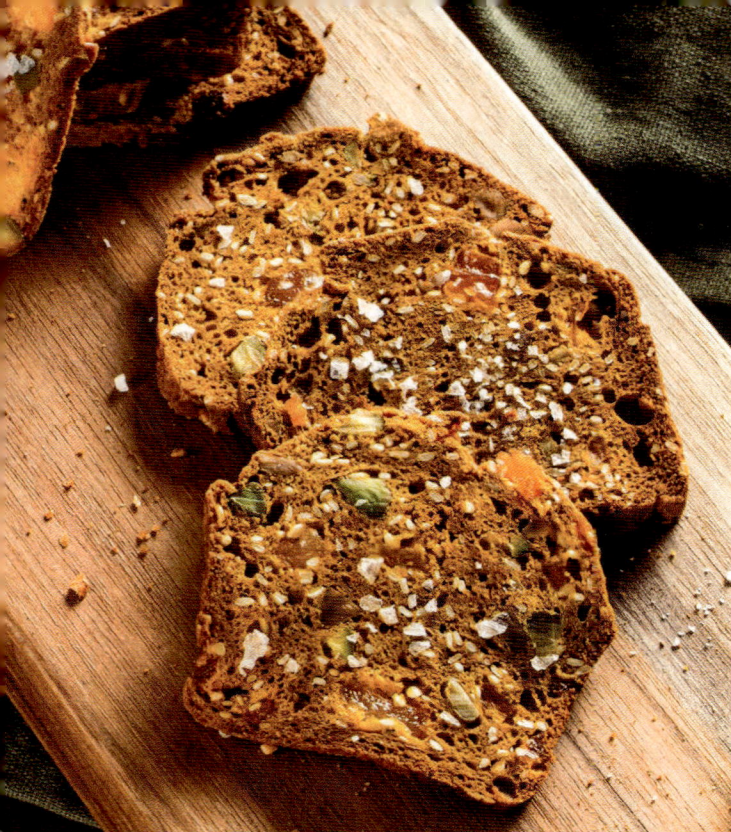

1 cup (4½ ounces) chickpea flour, plus extra for rolling
¼ teaspoon table salt
3 tablespoons plus 1 teaspoon warm water
1 tablespoon extra-virgin olive oil

1 Adjust oven rack to middle position and heat oven to 350 degrees. Line rimmed baking sheet with parchment paper. Whisk flour and salt together in large bowl. Stir in water and oil and mix until shaggy dough forms. Transfer to clean counter and knead dough until no dry flour remains. Shape into 4-inch round, wrap with plastic wrap, and let rest for 10 minutes.

2 On well-floured counter, roll dough into 13-inch round (about ¹⁄₁₆ inch thick), flipping and flouring dough if it begins to stick to counter or resists rolling. Using 2-inch biscuit cutter, cut as many rounds from dough as possible and transfer to prepared sheet.

3 Combine scraps and knead briefly to form cohesive ball. Flatten and reroll dough into 8-inch round (about ¹⁄₁₆ inch thick). Repeat cutting rounds from dough and transferring to sheet. Arrange dough rounds so they are evenly spaced over sheet, then poke each dough round in center with blunt end of toothpick or skewer.

4 Bake crackers until puffed and golden brown, 17 to 19 minutes, rotating sheet halfway through baking. Let crackers cool completely on sheet, about 30 minutes. Serve.

VARIATIONS
Turmeric–Black Pepper Chickpea Crackers
Add 1 teaspoon ground turmeric and ½ teaspoon pepper to flour mixture in step 1.

Herbes de Provence Chickpea Crackers
Add 2 teaspoons herbes de Provence to flour mixture in step 1.

MAKE AHEAD • Crackers can be stored in airtight container for up to 5 days.

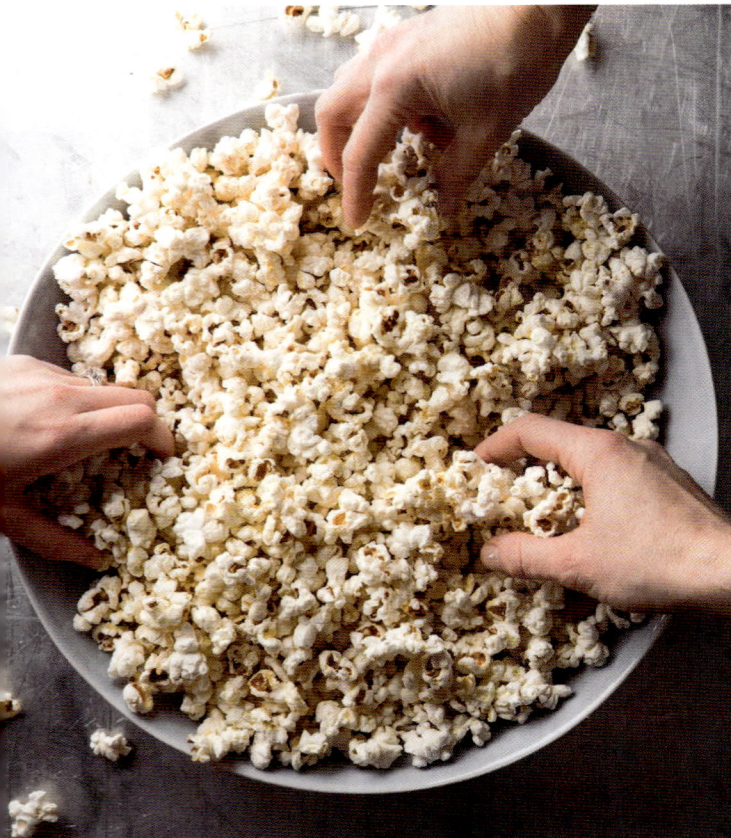

top | *Seeded Pumpkin Crackers*
bottom | *Popcorn with Olive Oil*

Seeded Pumpkin Crackers

serves 8 to 10 (makes 50 crackers) · total time 2 hours, plus 5½ hours chilling and cooling

why this recipe works · For these crackers, we seasoned pumpkin puree with orange zest and baharat, a spice blend of ground red pepper, cardamom, cinnamon, and nutmeg. To the dough we added sesame seeds, pistachios, and dried apricots. Freezing the loaves after the first bake ensured that we could slice the crackers thin for a second bake. This recipe is best made in two 5½ by 3-inch loaf pans. You can use one 8½ by 4½-inch loaf pan instead; bake the loaf for the same amount of time and then slice the frozen loaf down the center before slicing crosswise to achieve the right size crackers. We prefer our homemade Baharat (page 136), but you can use store-bought, if you prefer.

- 1 cup (5 ounces) all-purpose flour
- 1 teaspoon baking powder
- ¼ teaspoon baking soda
- 1 cup canned unsweetened pumpkin puree
- 1 teaspoon baharat
- 1 tablespoon table salt
- ¼ cup (1¾ ounces) sugar
- 2 tablespoons avocado oil
- 2 large eggs
- 1 tablespoon grated orange zest
- ⅓ cup dried apricots, chopped
- ⅓ cup sesame seeds
- ⅓ cup shelled pistachios, toasted and chopped
- 2 tablespoons coarse sea salt

1 Adjust oven rack to middle position and heat oven to 350 degrees. Grease two 5½ by 3-inch loaf pans. Whisk flour, baking powder, and baking soda together in large bowl; set aside. Combine pumpkin puree, baharat, and table salt in 10-inch skillet. Cook over medium heat, stirring occasionally, until reduced to ¾ cup, 6 to 8 minutes; transfer to medium bowl. Stir in sugar and oil and let cool slightly, about 5 minutes.

2 Whisk eggs and orange zest into pumpkin mixture, then fold into reserved flour mixture until combined (some small lumps of flour are OK). Fold in apricots, sesame seeds, and pistachios. Scrape batter into prepared pans, smoothing tops with silicone spatula. Bake until skewer inserted in center comes out clean, 45 to 50 minutes, switching and rotating pans halfway through baking.

3 Let loaves cool in pans on wire rack for 20 minutes. Remove loaves from pans and let cool completely on rack, about 1½ hours. Transfer cooled loaves to zipper-lock bag and freeze until firm, about 3 hours.

4 Heat oven to 300 degrees and line rimmed baking sheet with parchment paper. Using serrated knife, carefully slice each frozen loaf as thin as possible (about ¼ inch thick). Arrange slices in single layer on prepared sheet and sprinkle with sea salt. Bake until dark golden, 25 to 30 minutes, flipping crackers and rotating sheet halfway through baking. Transfer sheet to wire rack and let crackers cool completely, about 30 minutes. Serve.

> **MAKE AHEAD** · Loaves can be prepared through step 3 and frozen for up to 1 month. Cooled crackers can be stored in airtight container for up to 3 days.

Popcorn with Olive Oil

serves 8 to 10 (makes about 14 cups)
total time: 15 minutes **FAST**

why this recipe works · Popcorn can be a nourishing, fiber-rich snack. But add a lot of extra saturated fat in the form of butter and suddenly you've turned this healthy food into a possible source of inflammation. Instead, we seasoned our batch with extra-virgin olive oil for a fruity flavor and some anti-inflammatory benefits. We found that adding a small amount of water to the pot along with the kernels helped them pop more consistently. When cooking the popcorn, be sure to keep the lid on tight and shake the pot vigorously to prevent scorching.

- 1 tablespoon water
- ½ cup popcorn kernels
- 2 tablespoons extra-virgin olive oil
- ½ teaspoon table salt
- ½ teaspoon pepper

Heat Dutch oven over medium-high heat for 2 minutes. Add water and popcorn, cover, and cook, shaking frequently, until first few kernels begin to pop. Continue to cook, shaking vigorously, until popping slows to about 2 seconds between pops. Transfer popcorn to large serving bowl and toss with oil, salt, and pepper. Serve.

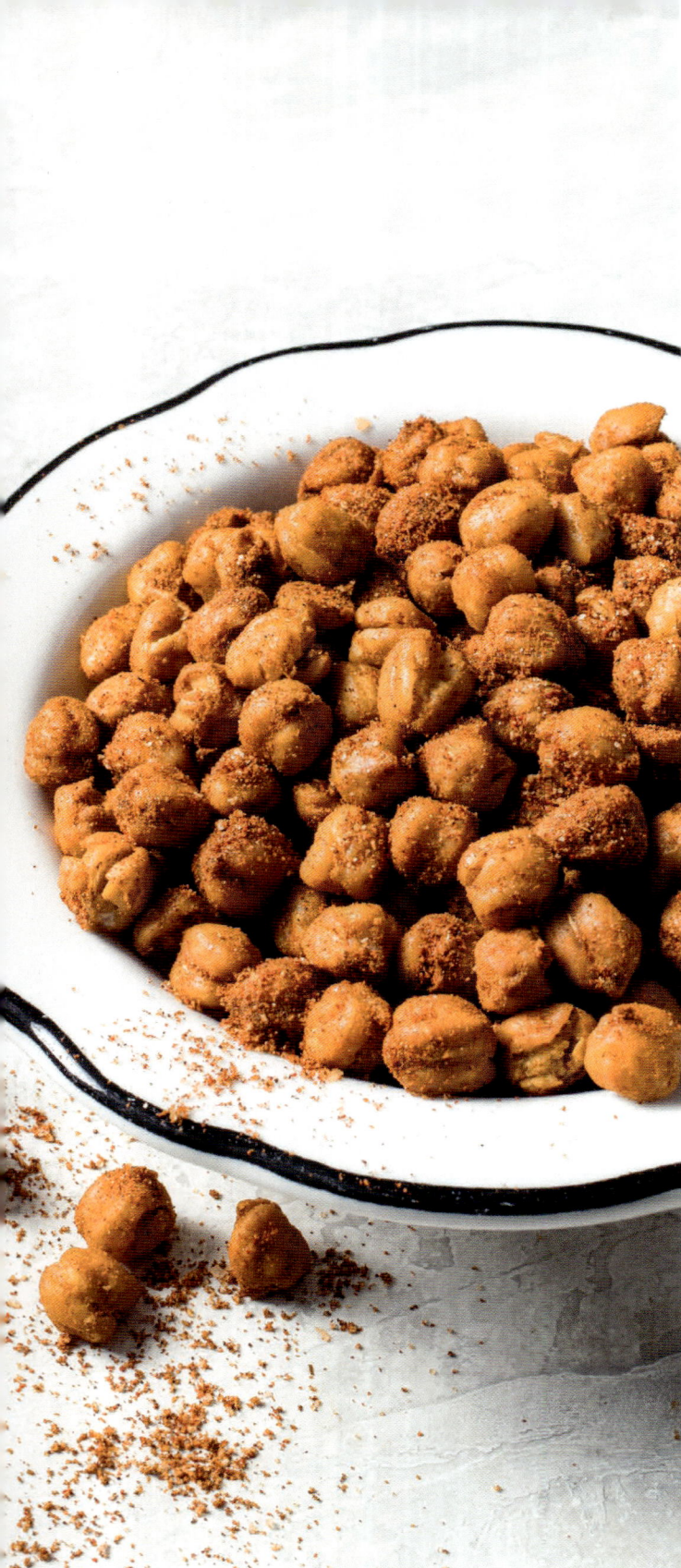

Smoked Paprika–Spiced Roasted Chickpeas

serves 6 (makes 1⅔ cups) · **total time: 1¼ hours, plus 30 minutes cooling**

why this recipe works · You can easily turn a can of chickpeas into a healthy, crunchy snack. Roasted chickpeas have the crunch and saltiness of chips and pretzels but are packed with protein and lighter on oil. We first zapped the chickpeas in the microwave to burst them open at the seams so that they released interior moisture. We coated them with a small amount of olive oil and baked them in a 350-degree oven. To keep them from burning, we crowded them toward the center of the pan for part of the roasting time. We dusted the chickpeas with a mix of smoked paprika, coriander, cumin, salt, and cayenne. There is no need to rinse the chickpeas. This recipe calls for a metal baking pan; using a glass or ceramic baking dish will result in unevenly cooked chickpeas.

- 2 (15-ounce) cans no-salt-added chickpeas
- 3 tablespoons extra-virgin olive oil
- 1 tablespoon smoked paprika
- ½ teaspoon ground coriander
- ¼ teaspoon ground cumin
- ⅛ teaspoon table salt
- ⅛ teaspoon cayenne pepper

1 Adjust oven rack to middle position and heat oven to 350 degrees. Place chickpeas in colander and let drain for 10 minutes. Line large plate with double layer of paper towels. Spread chickpeas over plate in even layer. Microwave until exteriors of chickpeas are dry and many have split slightly at seams, 8 to 12 minutes.

2 Transfer chickpeas to 13 by 9-inch metal baking pan. Add oil and stir until evenly coated. Using spatula, spread chickpeas into single layer. Transfer to oven and roast for 30 minutes. While chickpeas are roasting, combine paprika, coriander, cumin, salt, and cayenne in small bowl.

3 Stir chickpeas and crowd toward center of pan, avoiding edges of pan as much as possible. Continue to roast until chickpeas appear dry, slightly shriveled, and deep golden brown, 20 to 40 minutes longer. (To test for doneness, remove a few paler chickpeas and let cool briefly before tasting; if interiors are soft, return to oven for 5 minutes before testing again.)

4 Transfer chickpeas to large bowl. Toss with spice mixture to coat. Season with salt to taste. Let cool completely before serving, about 30 minutes.

Coriander-Turmeric Roasted Chickpeas

Substitute 2 teaspoons paprika for smoked paprika. Increase ground coriander to 1 teaspoon and ground cumin to ½ teaspoon. Add ½ teaspoon sugar, ½ teaspoon ground turmeric, and ½ teaspoon ground allspice to paprika mixture in step 2.

> **MAKE AHEAD** • Chickpeas can be stored in airtight container for up to 1 week.

Sesame Nori Chips

serves 12 • total time: 35 minutes **FAST**

why this recipe works • Our nori chips are ethereally light and crisp—and full of antioxidants. To create a simple chip with oceanic flavor, we focused on a few elements. A moderately hot oven consistently produced the best chips—pleasantly crisp without being burnt. To highlight the clean nori flavor, we added only sesame seeds, which toasted nicely while the chips baked, and salt. Avocado oil brushed on the chips helped the sesame seeds to adhere while further crisping up the chips. For a sturdier chip, we folded the nori sheets to double their thickness; water brushed between the folded sheets kept them together. You can use either toasted or untoasted nori sheets for this recipe.

10	sheets nori
1¼	teaspoons avocado oil
5	teaspoons sesame seeds

1 Adjust oven racks to upper-middle and lower-middle positions and heat oven to 350 degrees. Line 2 rimmed baking sheets with parchment paper. Working with 1 nori sheet at a time, brush bottom half liberally with water. Fold top half toward you and press firmly until sealed. Brush top of folded nori with ⅛ teaspoon oil, sprinkle with ½ teaspoon sesame seeds, and season with kosher or flake sea salt to taste. Cut nori into 1-inch strips.

2 Arrange nori strips in single layer, spaced evenly apart on prepared sheets. Bake until nori is very crisp and sesame seeds are golden, about 8 minutes, switching and rotating sheets halfway through baking (nori strips should be dark and shriveled slightly). Let cool completely on sheets, 8 to 10 minutes. Serve.

> **MAKE AHEAD** • Chips can be stored in airtight container for up to 1 week.

Walnut-Pomegranate Stuffed Dates

makes 5 dates • total time: 10 minutes **FAST**

why this recipe works • These showstopping stuffed Medjool dates pack a dose of antioxidants. Dates are rich in fiber and flavonoids, so they satiate a sweet tooth without potentially inflammatory refined sugars. Walnuts and shredded coconut add healthy fat, while freeze-dried pomegranate adds textural interest and more antioxidants. You can use walnut pieces in place of the walnut halves; you'll need about 1 teaspoon per date. If you can't find date molasses, you can use pomegranate molasses, though the flavor will be tangier and less caramel-like. This recipe can be easily scaled up to make as many stuffed dates as you'd like.

5	pitted Medjool dates
10	walnut halves
1	teaspoon date molasses
5	teaspoons unsweetened shredded coconut
¾	teaspoon freeze-dried pomegranate seeds

Using paring knife, cut slit down length of each date, without cutting through entirely. Working with 1 date at a time, gently open date at slit and stuff with 2 walnut halves. Place date molasses in small bowl and coconut in second small bowl. Working with one date at a time, dip one end of date in molasses, then dip in coconut, pressing to adhere. Sprinkle freeze-dried pomegranate seeds over walnuts.

VARIATION

Pistachio-Orange Stuffed Dates

Omit walnut halves, date molasses, coconut, and pomegranate seeds. Combine 5 teaspoons chopped pistachios, ¼ teaspoon grated orange zest, and ⅛ teaspoon flake sea salt in bowl. Stuff each date with 1 teaspoon pistachio mixture.

> **MAKE AHEAD** • Dates can be refrigerated for up to 1 month.

Cranberry-Almond No-Bake Energy Bites

makes 12 energy bites • total time: 15 minutes, plus 30 minutes chilling **FAST**

why this recipe works • These energy bites couldn't be simpler to make: Just stir the ingredients together, roll into balls, and chill until firm. In under an hour, you'll have a stash of filling, anti-inflammatory bites ready to eat on the go. You can add 1 tablespoon of chia seeds or ground flaxseed to oat mixture in step 1, if desired.

¾ cup (2¼ ounces) old-fashioned rolled oats
⅓ cup peanut butter, almond butter, or sunflower butter
⅓ cup sliced almonds
⅓ cup dried cranberries
2 tablespoons honey
⅛ teaspoon table salt

1 Add all ingredients to large bowl. Stir with silicone spatula until well combined.

2 Wet your hands. Use your wet hands to roll oat mixture into 12 balls (about 1 tablespoon each). Place balls on plate.

3 Cover plate with plastic wrap and place in refrigerator. Chill balls until firm, at least 30 minutes. Serve.

> **MAKE AHEAD** • Energy bites can be refrigerated for up to 3 days.

Chewy Granola Bars with Hazelnuts, Cherries, and Cacao Nibs

makes 24 bars • total time: 1¼ hours, plus 2 hours cooling

why this recipe works • Most store-bought granola bars contain a lot of added sugar and fillers. For bars that were fiberful, satisfying, and anti-inflammatory, we combined toasted oats, nuts, and seeds with a mixture of pureed apricots and avocado oil. The result was only mildly sweet—and much tastier than store-bought. The nuts, seeds, and fruit can be swapped out according to your preference to make bars that suit a variety of tastes. Be sure to use apricots that are soft and moist, or the bars will not hold together well. Avoid using extra-thick rolled oats here.

1½ cups blanched hazelnuts
2½ cups (7½ ounces) old-fashioned rolled oats
1 cup raw sunflower seeds
1 cup dried apricots
1 cup packed (7 ounces) brown sugar
¾ teaspoon table salt
½ cup avocado oil
3 tablespoons water
1½ cups (1½ ounces) crisped rice cereal
1 cup dried cherries
½ cup cacao nibs

1 Adjust oven rack to middle position and heat oven to 350 degrees. Make foil sling for 13 by 9-inch baking pan by folding 2 long sheets of aluminum foil; first sheet should be 13 inches wide and second sheet should be 9 inches wide. Lay sheets of foil in pan perpendicular to each other, with extra foil hanging over edges of pan. Push foil into corners and up sides of pan, smoothing foil flush to pan. Lightly spray foil with avocado oil spray.

2 Pulse hazelnuts in food processor until finely chopped, 8 to 12 pulses. Spread hazelnuts, oats, and sunflower seeds on rimmed baking sheet and toast until lightly browned and fragrant, 12 to 15 minutes, stirring halfway through toasting. Reduce oven temperature to 300 degrees.

3 While oat mixture is toasting, process apricots, sugar, and salt in food processor until apricots are very finely ground, about 15 seconds. With processor running, add oil and water. Continue to process until homogeneous paste forms, about 1 minute. Transfer paste to large, wide bowl.

4 Add warm oat mixture to bowl and stir with silicone spatula until well coated. Add cereal, cherries, and cacao nibs and stir gently until ingredients are evenly mixed. Transfer mixture to prepared pan and spread into even layer. Place 14-inch sheet of parchment or waxed paper on top of granola and press and smooth very firmly with your hands, especially at edges and corners, until granola is level and compact. Remove parchment and bake granola until fragrant and just beginning to brown around edges, about 25 minutes. Transfer pan to wire rack and let cool for 1 hour. Using foil overhang, lift granola out of pan. Return to wire rack and let cool completely, about 1 hour.

5 Discard foil and transfer granola to cutting board. Using chef's knife, cut granola in half crosswise to create two 6½ by 9-inch rectangles. Cut each rectangle in half to make four 3¼ by 9-inch strips. Cut each strip crosswise into 6 equal pieces. Serve.

VARIATIONS

Chewy Granola Bars with Walnuts and Cranberries
Omit cacao nibs. Substitute walnuts for hazelnuts and pulse until finely chopped, 8 to 10 pulses. Substitute chopped dried cranberries for cherries.

Nut-Free Chewy Granola Bars
Omit hazelnuts, cherries, and cacao nibs. Toast 1 cup raw pepitas, ¼ cup sesame seeds, and ¼ cup chia seeds with oats in step 2. Increase cereal to 2 cups.

> **MAKE AHEAD** • Granola bars can be stored in airtight container for up to 3 weeks.

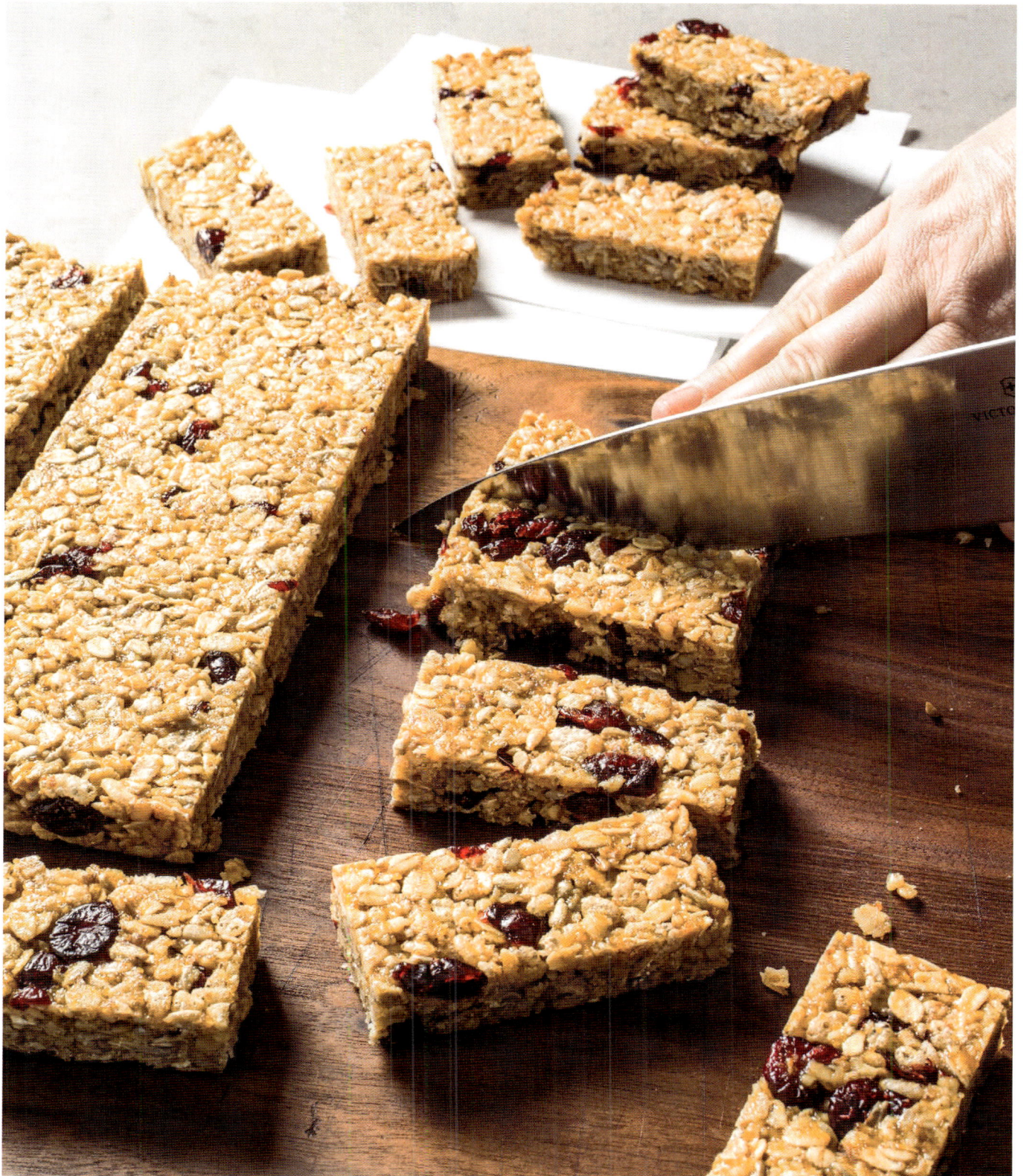

Chewy Granola Bars with Hazelnuts, Cherries, and Cacao Nibs

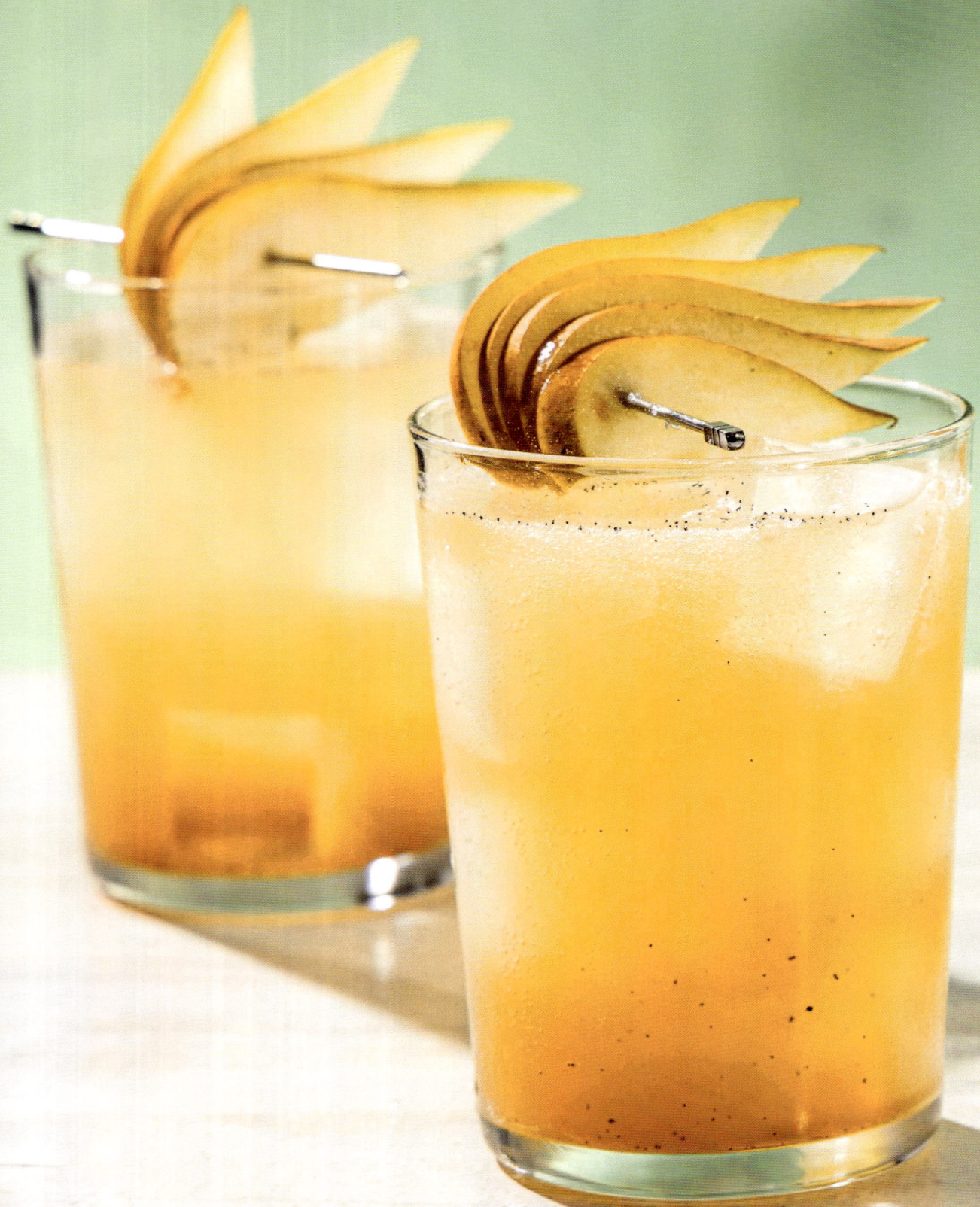

DRINKS

■ FAST   ■ SUPERCHARGED

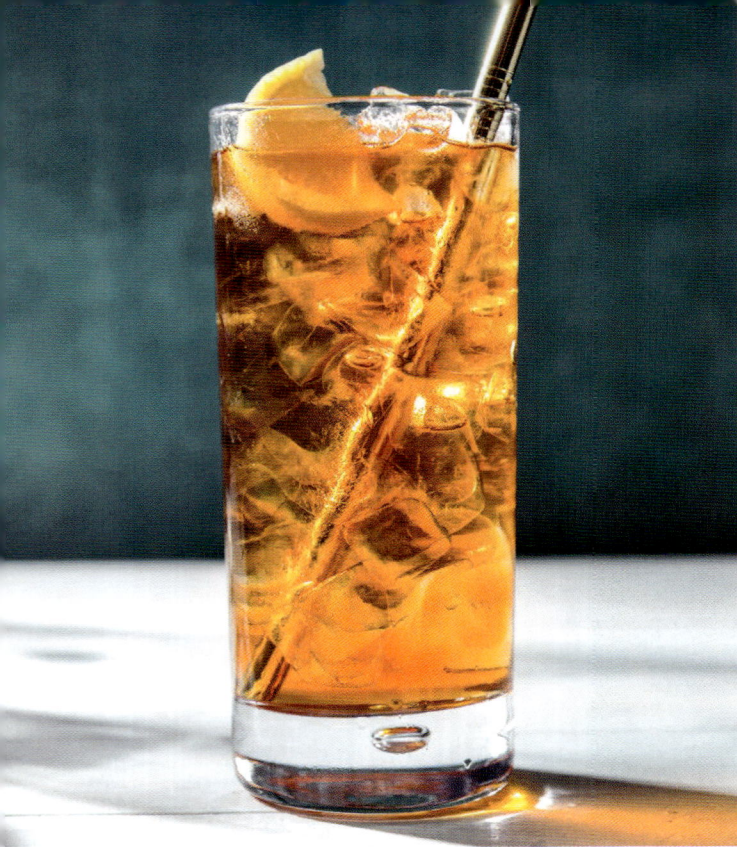

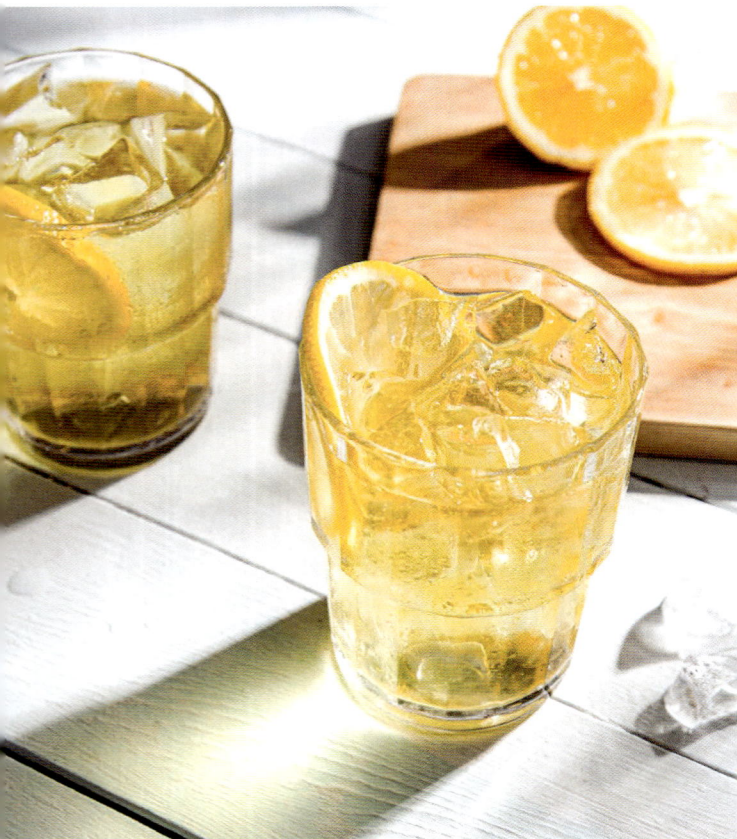

Iced Black Tea

serves 4 · total time: 15 minutes, plus 2 hours steeping and chilling

why this recipe works · Teas, rich in polyphenols and other nutrients, are great to sip for their powerful anti-inflammatory benefits. When you make your own brisk and refreshing iced tea at home, you can control the flavor intensity and sugar amount. When we compared iced teas made from loose-leaf tea versus tea bags, we found the former produced a more flavorful, complex drink. Iced tea can be brewed using cold or boiling water, but we found that a cold-infused tea tasted flat, while boiling water led to bitter results. We devised a technique that produced balanced flavor by combining the two methods. First, we steeped the tea in water that had been brought to a boil, then added ice water and continued to steep for an hour. At this cooler temperature, the aromatic compounds infused the water, while the bitter ones did not. This drink can be served as is, or lightly sweetened with honey, maple syrup, or our Simple Syrup (recipe follows). Both caffeinated and decaffeinated tea work well here. If you don't have loose-leaf black tea, you can substitute 2 black tea bags. For an accurate measurement of boiling water, bring a kettle of water to a boil and then measure out the desired amount. This recipe can easily be doubled.

1½ tablespoons black tea leaves
3 cups boiling water
1 cup ice water
   Lemon wedges

Place tea in medium bowl. Add boiling water and steep for 4 minutes. Add ice water and steep for 1 hour. Strain through fine-mesh strainer into pitcher or large container (or strain into second bowl and transfer to pitcher). Refrigerate until chilled, at least 1 hour or up to 3 days. Serve in ice-filled glasses, garnished with lemon wedges.

VARIATIONS

Raspberry-Basil Iced Black Tea

Omit lemon wedges. Mash 1½ cups thawed frozen raspberries, 3 tablespoons chopped fresh basil, 2 tablespoons sugar (optional), and 2 teaspoons lemon juice in bowl until no whole berries remain. Add mixture to tea with ice water. Garnish each serving with basil sprig.

Ginger-Pomegranate Iced Black Tea

Add ⅔ cup pomegranate juice, 2 tablespoons sugar (optional), and 1½–2 tablespoons grated fresh ginger to tea with ice water. Substitute lime wedges for lemon wedges.

top | *Iced Black Tea*
bottom | *Iced Green Tea*

Apple-Cinnamon Iced Black Tea

Omit lemon wedges. Add ½ cinnamon stick to medium bowl with tea. Add 1 cored and shredded red apple and 1 tablespoon sugar (optional) to tea with ice water.

Simple Syrup

total time: 15 minutes

Because the sugar in simple syrup has already dissolved, it is ideal for sweetening all kinds of drinks (especially cold ones) to your desired sweetness.

Combine equal parts sugar and warm tap water in bowl, then whisk until sugar has dissolved. Let cool completely, about 10 minutes, then transfer to airtight container. Syrup can be refrigerated for up to 1 month. Shake well before using.

Iced Green Tea

serves 4 · total time: 15 minutes, plus 2 hours steeping and chilling

why this recipe works · A beloved drink globally (and especially throughout Asia), green tea is earthy, invigorating, and rich in anti-inflammatory catechins. Sipping it not only fights inflammation but also makes it more enjoyable to stay hydrated. To make it iced, we used the same method as in our Iced Black Tea but adjusted the temperature so as to not over-extract the more sensitive leaves. To achieve a smooth drink, we brewed the tea with 175-degree water, then cooled the extraction. Steeping the tea at this lower temperature slowly drew out more delicate flavor. Chinese green tea will produce a grassy, floral tea, whereas Japanese green tea is more savory. This drink can be served as is, or lightly sweetened with honey, maple syrup, or our Simple Syrup (page 387). Both caffeinated and decaffeinated loose-leaf tea work well here. If you don't have loose-leaf green tea, you can substitute 2 green tea bags. This recipe can easily be doubled.

2 tablespoons green tea leaves
3 cups hot water (175 degrees)
1 cup ice water
  Lemon wedges

Place tea in medium bowl. Add hot water and steep for 4 minutes. Add ice water and steep for 1 hour. Strain through fine-mesh strainer into pitcher or large container (or strain into second bowl and transfer to pitcher). Refrigerate until chilled, at least 1 hour or up to 3 days. Serve in ice-filled glasses, garnished with lemon wedges.

VARIATIONS

Cantaloupe-Mint Iced Green Tea

Omit lemon wedges. Add 1 cup grated cantaloupe pulp, 3 tablespoons chopped fresh mint, 2 tablespoons sugar (optional), and 1 tablespoon lemon juice to tea with ice water. Garnish each serving with mint sprig.

Cucumber-Lime Iced Green Tea

Shred ½ English cucumber on large holes of box grater. Add shredded cucumber, 2 tablespoons sugar (optional), ½ teaspoon grated lime zest, and 1 tablespoon lime juice to tea with ice water. Substitute lime slices for lemon wedges.

Pear-Sage Iced Green Tea

Omit lemon wedges. Add 1 cored and shredded pear, 2 tablespoons sugar (optional), and 1 teaspoon minced fresh sage to tea with ice water.

Hibiscus Iced Tea

serves 4 to 6 · total time: 40 minutes, plus 1 hour cooling
SUPERCHARGED

why this recipe works · Polyphenol-rich hibiscus teas have roots in West Africa, where people use their native plant hibiscus, also called roselle, to make a drink called bissap. This recipe from mixologist Tiffanie Barriere steeps whole dried hibiscus flowers with orange, ginger, and spices for an anti-inflammatory drink. Gently simmer the tea and then strain out the solids. Use whole dried hibiscus flowers, not cut and sifted ones. If you can find only the latter, use the weight listed (1½ ounces), not the volume. You can substitute Simple Syrup (page 387) for the cane syrup, but the flavor will be less complex. This recipe can easily be doubled.

6 cups water
1½ ounces whole dried hibiscus flowers (1½ cups)
6 (3-inch) strips orange zest plus 2 tablespoons juice
6 (2-inch) strips lemon zest plus 2 tablespoons juice
1 (½-inch) piece ginger, peeled and sliced thin
1 cinnamon stick
1 star anise pod
1 whole clove
2–4 tablespoons cane syrup (optional)

1 Bring water, hibiscus flowers, orange zest and juice, lemon zest and juice, ginger, cinnamon stick, star anise, and clove to simmer in large saucepan over medium heat. Reduce heat to low and steep until mixture is fragrant and flavors meld, about 20 minutes.

2 Strain mixture through fine-mesh strainer into large bowl or storage container. Refrigerate until chilled, at least 1 hour or up to 10 days.

3 Transfer strained tea to serving pitcher and stir in cane syrup, if using. Serve in ice-filled glasses.

> **Nutrition Knowledge** Hibiscus flowers contain unique plant compounds such as anthocyanins and polyphenols, which help lower inflammation and protect against cellular damage. Warming spices like cinnamon, clove, and star anise not only add depth of flavor but also deliver potent antimicrobial and anti-inflammatory benefits with compounds such as cinnamaldehyde, eugenol, and anethole. —*Alicia*

Cold Brew Coffee Concentrate

serves 4 (makes about 4 cups) · total time: 25 minutes, plus 24 hours steeping and 1 hour chilling

why this recipe works · If you can't start your day without a cup of joe, here's good news: Coffee is shown to offer protective benefits from the drink's polyphenols, as long as it's consumed in moderation (too much can drive inflammatory stress hormones such as cortisol). Cold brew has mild acidity and bitterness that lets more of the subtle, hidden flavors of coffee come through. Here, we used common household equipment for our steep: a 2-quart Mason jar, strainer, and coffee filter. Using a high ratio of ground beans to water produced a concentrate that was easy to store and could be diluted as desired. Double straining the concentrate ensured that our drink was free of sediment. Our finishing touch was a pinch of kosher salt, which rounded out the cold brew's flavors. If you don't have medium-roast coffee beans, you can substitute light or dark roast. This concentrate needs to be diluted before drinking. We recommend a 1:1 ratio of concentrate to water, but you can dilute it more if you like.

  8 ounces medium-roast coffee beans, ground coarse (3 cups)
  4 cups filtered water, room temperature
    Kosher salt (optional)

1 Stir coffee and water together in 2-quart jar or narrow pitcher. Allow raft of ground coffee to form, about 10 minutes, then stir again to recombine. Cover with plastic wrap and let steep at room temperature for 24 hours.

2 Set fine-mesh strainer over large bowl. Pour concentrate into strainer and, using back of ladle or silicone spatula, gently stir concentrate to help filter through strainer, extracting as much liquid as possible. Discard grounds.

3 Set now-empty strainer over second large bowl and line with large coffee filter. Strain concentrate for a second time through prepared strainer, gently stirring concentrate to help filter through strainer. (This may take up to 10 minutes.) Transfer to airtight container. Refrigerate until chilled, at least 1 hour or up to 1 week.

To make one cup iced coffee Add ½ cup coffee concentrate, ½ cup cold water, and pinch kosher salt, if using, to ice-filled glass. Gently stir to combine, and serve.

VARIATIONS
Pumpkin-Spiced Cold Brew Coffee Concentrate
Add 2 teaspoons toasted and cracked allspice berries, 4 toasted and cracked cinnamon sticks, and 12 toasted whole cloves to coffee and water mixture in step 1.

Star Anise–Orange Cold Brew Coffee Concentrate
Add 1 toasted star anise pod and 1 tablespoon grated orange zest to coffee and water mixture in step 1.

London Fog Tea Latte

serves 1 · total time: 15 minutes **FAST**

why this recipe works · London Fog consists of Earl Grey tea, steamed milk, and sweetened vanilla syrup. We wanted to enjoy it as a hot latte without the sugar concealing the flavor of the Earl Grey. Bergamot is an orange-tasting citrus fruit native to Italy, and it gives Earl Grey its distinctive flavor. The citrus oil provides a floral complexity, so we combined two potent spices to complement that floral nature: vanilla extract and an aromatic cardamom pod. The vanilla provided sweetness without eclipsing the tea, while the cardamom contributed an earthy, spiced note. To turn this drink into a latte, we preferred the simplicity of a saucepan and a whisk to create our steamed milk, but any method will do. If you prefer a more subtle vanilla aroma, use the smaller amount given. For an accurate measurement of boiling water, bring a kettle of water to a boil and then measure out the desired amount.

1½ teaspoons Earl Grey tea leaves
1 green cardamom pod, cracked
½ cup boiling water
½ cup milk
¼–½ teaspoon vanilla extract

1 Add tea and cardamom pod to tea infuser or tea sachet. Steep tea mixture with boiling water in teacup, covered, for 5 minutes.

2 Meanwhile, heat milk and vanilla in small saucepan over medium heat until it registers 140 to 155 degrees, about 5 minutes. Off heat, whisk vigorously to create dense foam on top, about 2 minutes.

3 Remove tea infuser and slowly pour frothed milk over tea, spooning remaining foam over top. Serve immediately.

MAKE IT DAIRY-FREE • Substitute plant-based milk for the dairy milk. (Soy milk will yield less foam, so we recommend using an immersion blender.)

Matcha

serves 1 • total time: 5 minutes **FAST** **SUPERCHARGED**

why this recipe works • Popular in Japan, matcha is a powder made from green tea leaves that are shaded during their growth. This increases the rate of theanine production (an amino acid also found in mushrooms), which gives matcha its characteristic umami taste. Green tea, and hence matcha, is also an excellent source of anti-inflammatory catechins. We found that adding the water in two stages, once to make a paste and then the rest to whisk into a froth, resulted in a beverage that had less undissolved sediment. Using hot rather than boiling water was ideal, as green tea leaves tend to be more delicate than black. Using 1½ teaspoons of matcha per serving resulted in tea with complex—but not bitter—flavor and a rich texture. The matcha was strong and produced a thick layer of foam after whisking. We also created a matcha latte variation, using frothed milk instead of water for a creamier option with subtle sweetness. If you don't have ceremonial-grade matcha, you can substitute premium-grade matcha. Avoid culinary-grade matcha. Matcha is traditionally prepared in a chawan, a Japanese tea bowl, and whisked using a bamboo whisk called a chasen.

1½ teaspoons ceremonial-grade matcha powder
1 cup hot water (175 degrees), divided

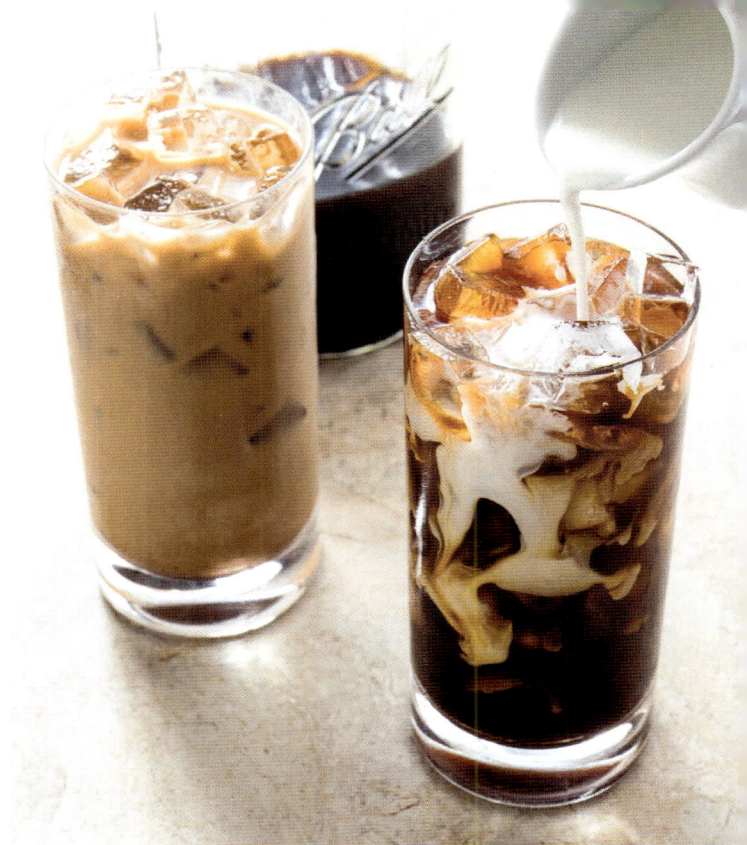

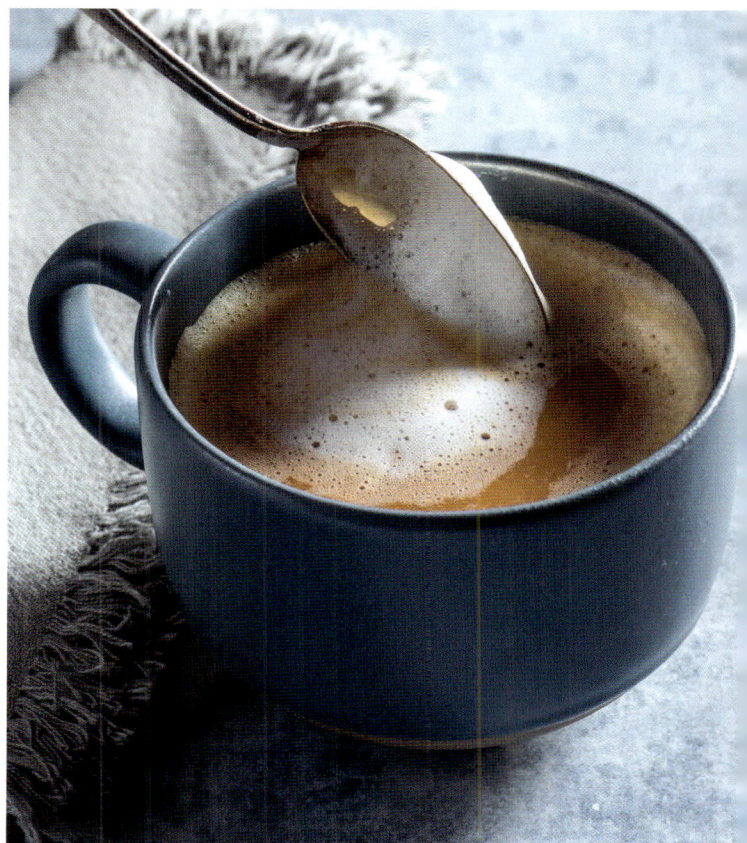

top | *Cold Brew Coffee Concentrate*
bottom | *London Fog Tea Latte*

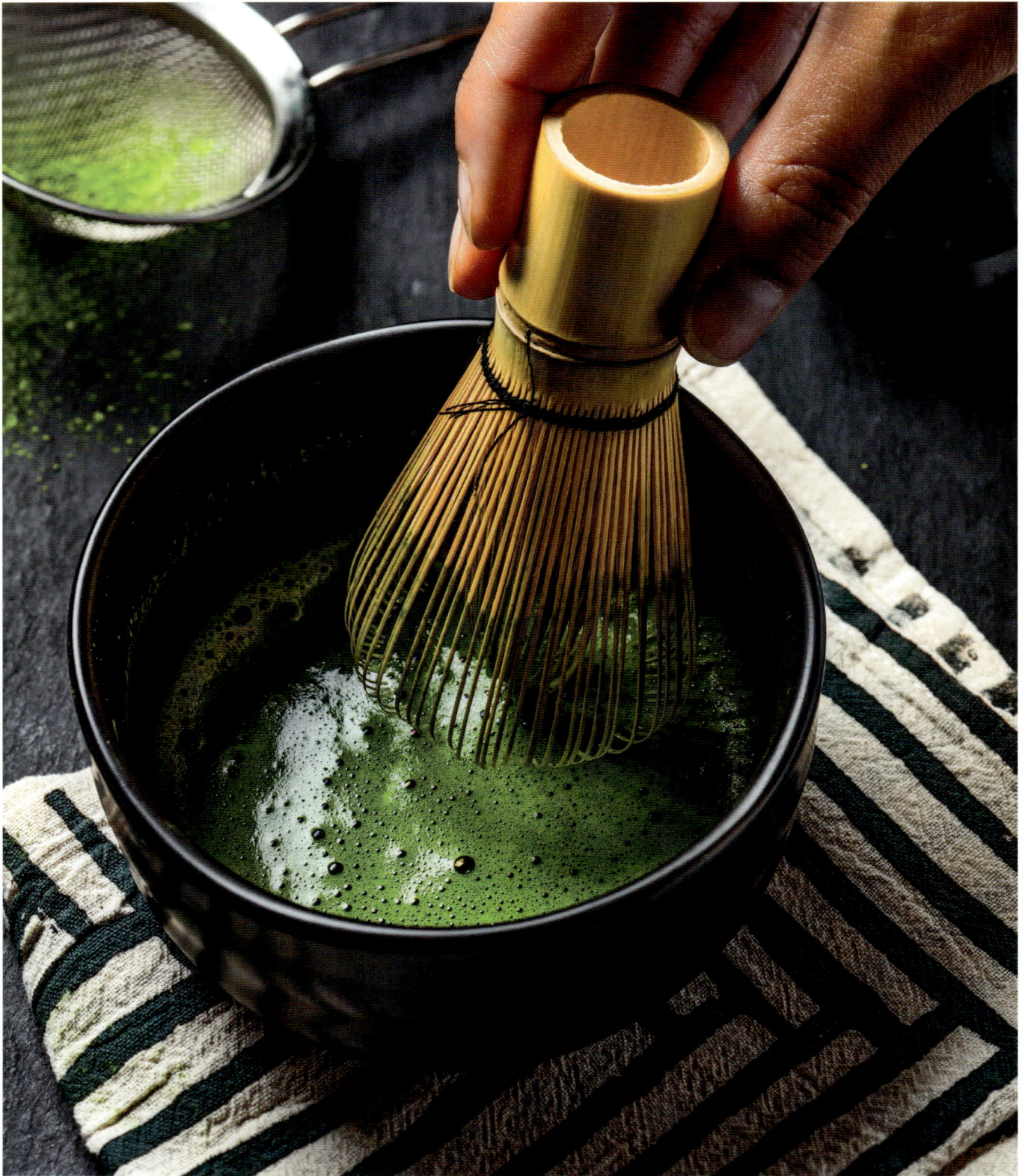

1 Sift matcha powder into chawan or small soup bowl. Using chasen or small whisk, whisk 2 tablespoons hot water into sifted powder until dissolved. Add another 2 tablespoons hot water and quickly whisk using zigzag motion until thick layer of small bubbles form on surface of matcha, about 30 seconds.

2 Stir remaining ¾ cup hot water into matcha. Serve immediately in chawan or teacup.

VARIATION
Matcha Latte

Omit ¾ cup water in step 2. Heat ¾ cup milk in small saucepan over medium heat until it registers 140 to 155 degrees, about 5 minutes. Off heat, whisk vigorously to create dense foam on top, about 2 minutes. Slowly pour frothed milk over prepared matcha, spooning remaining foam over top.

> **MAKE IT DAIRY-FREE** • Substitute plant-based milk for the dairy milk. (Soy milk will yield less foam, so we recommend using an immersion blender.)

Emoliente

serves 4 • total time: 40 minutes   **FAST**   **SUPERCHARGED**

why this recipe works • Often sold in the streets of Lima, Peru, emoliente is a warm, smooth, nourishing drink made with toasted barley, flaxseeds, horsetail, and cat's claw. Cat's claw is a bitter-tasting, woody vine found in the tropical jungles of South and Central America, while horsetail is a grassy-tasting fern; both are known to offer anti-inflammatory protection. Toasted barley is chock-full of nutrients and minerals and produces a nutty flavor when brewed. Flaxseeds thicken the texture and provide omega-3s and antioxidants. To meld these flavors together, we added lemon juice and honey, which brought a hint of acidity and sweetness. Keeping the drink at a simmer for half an hour allowed for proper extraction of the thickening qualities of flaxseeds and for adequate reduction and concentration of flavor. Roasted unhulled barley kernels (sometimes known as toasted barley) is what gives this beverage its distinctive caramel hue and nutty flavor; do not substitute pearl barley. If you don't have stick cat's claw bark, you can substitute 4 teaspoons chipped or shaved cat's claw bark. Dried horsetail and cat's claw bark can be purchased at specialty tea shops, health stores, or online.

1 cup roasted barley
½ cup flaxseeds
¼ cup dried horsetail, crumbled into 1-inch pieces
1 stick (2½ inches long by 1 inch wide) cat's claw bark
2 quarts water
3 tablespoons lemon juice, plus extra for seasoning
2 tablespoons honey, plus extra for seasoning

1 Bring barley, flaxseeds, horsetail, cat's claw, and water to simmer in large saucepan and continue to simmer until liquid is reduced by half, 30 to 35 minutes.

2 Strain mixture through fine-mesh strainer into heatproof bowl. Just before serving, stir in lemon juice and honey. Season with extra lemon juice and honey to taste. (Emoliente can be refrigerated without lemon juice and honey for up to 3 days; mixture will thicken once chilled but loosen again after reheating. To make a single portion, bring 1 cup emoliente to simmer in small saucepan, then stir in 2 teaspoons lemon juice and 1 teaspoon honey.)

VARIATIONS
Emoliente with Chamomile

Add 2 tablespoons dried chamomile to saucepan during last 5 minutes of simmering.

Emoliente with Alfalfa and Anise

Add 2 tablespoons dried alfalfa leaves and 1 teaspoon anise seed to saucepan during last 5 minutes of simmering.

Citrus Burst Black Tea Blend

makes 1 cup dry blend (enough for 24 servings)
total time: 5 minutes   **FAST**

why this recipe works • When you make your own tea blend at home, you can take advantage of tea's anti-inflammatory benefits anytime you want—and stay hydrated throughout the day. Bright, zesty lemon and earthy, tannic black tea are a classic pairing. Lemon verbena added a lemon curd–like richness to our blend because it's both sour and herbal-sweet. To play up the citrus aspect, dried orange peel brought some floral notes, while coriander seeds, which already have a citrusy flavor, added savory depth. We used a spice grinder to break up the lemon verbena into uniform pieces for a well-balanced citrus and black tea flavor. A boldly flavored tea such as Assam is ideal for this recipe; alternatively, use Irish or English breakfast tea. If you don't have coriander seeds you can substitute fennel seeds, and if you don't have dried orange peel you can substitute dried lemon peel. If you have one, a mortar and pestle can be used to crush the spices.

⅔ cup dried lemon verbena
⅓ cup coriander seeds
⅓ cup dried orange peel
⅓ cup black tea leaves

Pulse lemon verbena in spice grinder until coarsely ground and pieces are no larger than ½ inch, about 3 pulses. Add coriander seeds and orange peel and pulse until coarsely ground and pieces of lemon verbena are no larger than ¼ inch, about 4 pulses. Transfer to small bowl and stir in black tea. (Tea blend can be stored in airtight container at room temperature for up to 3 months.)

To make one cup tea Add 2 teaspoons tea blend to tea infuser or tea sachet. Steep tea mixture with 1 cup boiling water in teacup, covered, for 5 minutes. Remove tea infuser and serve immediately.

Cacao, Cardamom, and Rose Herbal Tea Blend

makes 1 cup dry blend (enough for 16 servings)
total time: 5 minutes   **FAST**   **SUPERCHARGED**

why this recipe works • Chocolate and roses don't just make a nice Valentine's Day gift—they also pair nicely in a teacup. We wanted to make a dried tea blend that combined the nutritious benefits and rich flavor of cacao with the fragrance of rose petals. We started with dried rose petals and found our cacao component in flavanol-rich whole nibs, which contributed a milk chocolate flavor. Pulsing them in a spice grinder created extra surface area to extract an even richer chocolate flavor. With the grinder in use, we took the opportunity to grind some whole cardamom pods; their aromatic character mimicked that of roses while giving the chocolate a spiced character. If you have one, a mortar and pestle can be used to crush the spices.

10 green cardamom pods
¾ cup cacao nibs
3 tablespoons food-grade dried rose petals

Pulse cardamom in spice grinder until coarsely ground, about 10 pulses. Add cacao nibs and pulse until cacao nibs are coarsely ground, about 10 pulses. Transfer to small bowl and stir in rose petals. (Tea blend can be stored in airtight container at room temperature for up to 3 months.)

To make one cup tea Add 1 tablespoon tea blend to tea infuser or tea sachet. Steep tea mixture with 1 cup boiling water in teacup, covered, for 10 minutes. Remove tea infuser and serve immediately.

Immunitea Herbal Tea Blend

makes 1 cup dry blend (enough for 16 servings)
total time: 5 minutes   **FAST**   **SUPERCHARGED**

why this recipe works • Regulating immune function goes hand in hand with minimizing inflammation. For this immunity-boosting blend, we picked herbal components with properties known to offer anti-inflammatory protection. Elderberries and rose hips offered a fruity-floral base with a tangy quality, similar to hibiscus but with more depth of flavor from the pairing. Elderberries can be effective in reducing the duration of sickness, while rose hips are incredibly high in antioxidants such as vitamin C, which works to prevent illness in the first place. Echinacea, an herbaceous flower, is also full of antioxidants and thought to be effective at reducing the duration of colds and flus. It lent savory, hay-like notes to the floral blend, and lemon balm provided a light, citrusy flavor with a cooling sensation on the finish to round out the mix. This blend is so flavorful that it'll be easy to stay hydrated all day long. Dried rose hips, lemon balm, and echinacea can be purchased at specialty tea shops, health stores, or online. If you don't have cut and sifted dried echinacea, you can substitute dried echinacea herb or dried echinacea root.

7 tablespoons dried rose hips
¼ cup dried elderberries
3 tablespoons dried lemon balm
3 tablespoons cut and sifted dried echinacea

Combine all ingredients in bowl. (Tea blend can be stored in airtight container at room temperature for up to 3 months.)

To make one cup tea Add 1 tablespoon tea blend to tea infuser or tea sachet. Steep tea mixture with 1 cup boiling water in teacup, covered, for 10 minutes. Remove tea infuser and serve immediately.

Nutrition Knowledge This immunity-boosting blend showcases the healing power of plant botanicals. Rose hips, rich in vitamin C and galactolipids, are known to reduce joint inflammation and support immune health, making them a popular remedy for conditions such as arthritis. Elderberries provide potent antioxidants and antiviral benefits, while lemon balm offers calming properties and gentle anti-inflammatory support. Echinacea, a well-known immune booster, contains alkamides and flavonoids that help regulate inflammation and strengthen the body's natural defenses.   —*Alicia*

Cozy and Calm Herbal Tea Blend

makes 1 cup dry blend (enough for 16 servings)
total time: 5 minutes FAST

why this recipe works • Inspired by relaxing tea blends, we sought to make our own earthy and floral nighttime drink to help us wind down at the end of the day. Passionflower, which is grown in South America, has sedative properties that slow brain activity and promote calmness. Valerian root produces mild sedation, decreasing anxiety and blood pressure. The valerian root can taste bitter, and the passionflower is fairly grassy, but the floral ingredients masked those flavors. Dried chamomile and lavender have been used worldwide for their calming properties, so they perfectly completed our roster of cozy ingredients. Dried passionflower and valerian root can be purchased at specialty tea shops, health stores, or online.

- 6 tablespoons dried chamomile
- 5 tablespoons dried lavender
- 2 tablespoons dried passionflower
- 2 tablespoons dried valerian root

Combine all ingredients in bowl. (Tea blend can be stored in airtight container at room temperature for up to 1 month.)

To make one cup tea Add 1 tablespoon tea blend to tea infuser or tea sachet. Steep tea mixture with 1 cup boiling water in teacup, covered, for 5 minutes. Remove tea infuser and serve immediately.

Tummy Tea Herbal Tea Blend

makes 1 cup dry blend (enough for 16 servings)
total time: 5 minutes FAST SUPERCHARGED

why this recipe works • To aid digestion and calm an irritated tummy, this supercharged blend of soothing ingredients is just what you need. Ginger is a well-known anti-inflammatory that soothes the intestinal tract. We paired it with cooling peppermint, which relaxes muscles in the digestive system, plus fennel seeds, which have antispasmodic properties to lessen stomach cramps. We enhanced the licorice-y fennel by pairing it with actual licorice root. For a fuller-bodied tea with no grit, we used a spice grinder to coarsely grind the fennel, break the licorice root, and increase the surface area of the ginger root. Our final ingredient, lemongrass, is a mild diuretic that can reduce uncomfortable bloating. While this blend's flavor is stimulating to the taste buds, the ingredients are effective at calming and relaxing the digestive tract. If you have one, a mortar and pestle can be used to crush the spices.

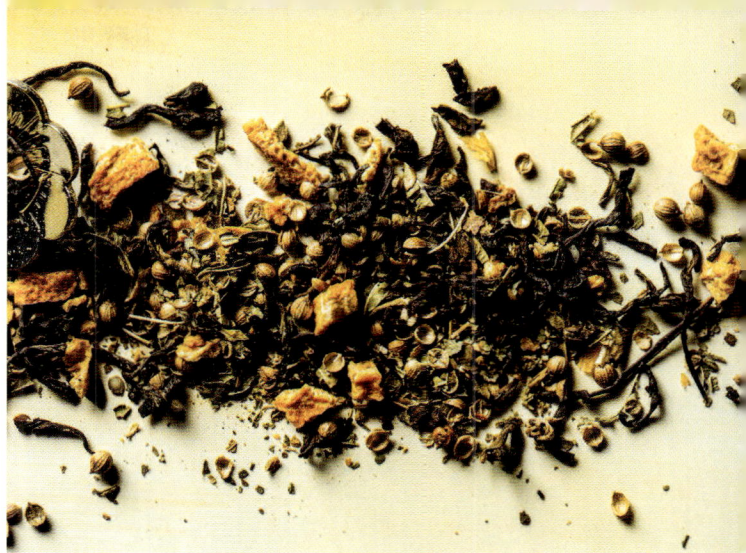
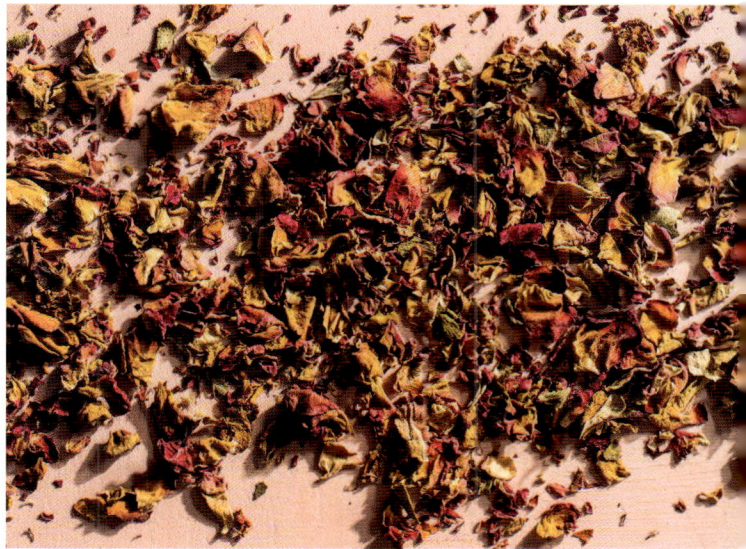
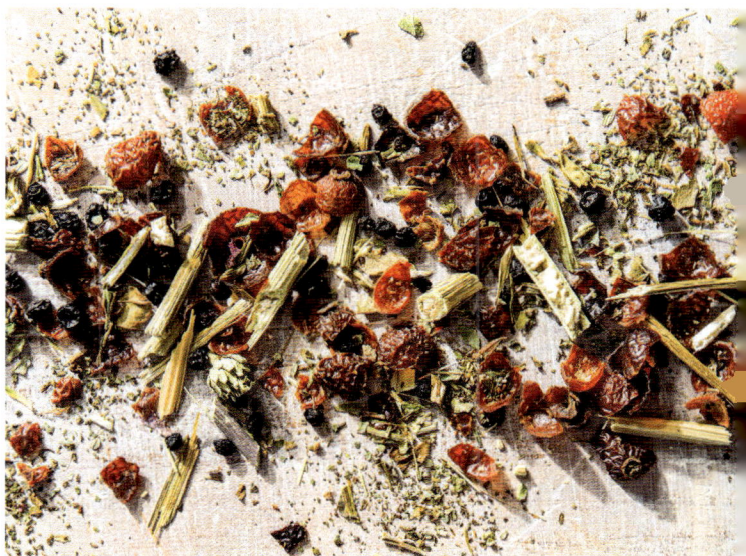

top	*Citrus Burst Black Tea Blend*
middle	*Cacao, Cardamom, and Rose Herbal Tea Blend*
bottom	*Immunitea Herbal Tea Blend*

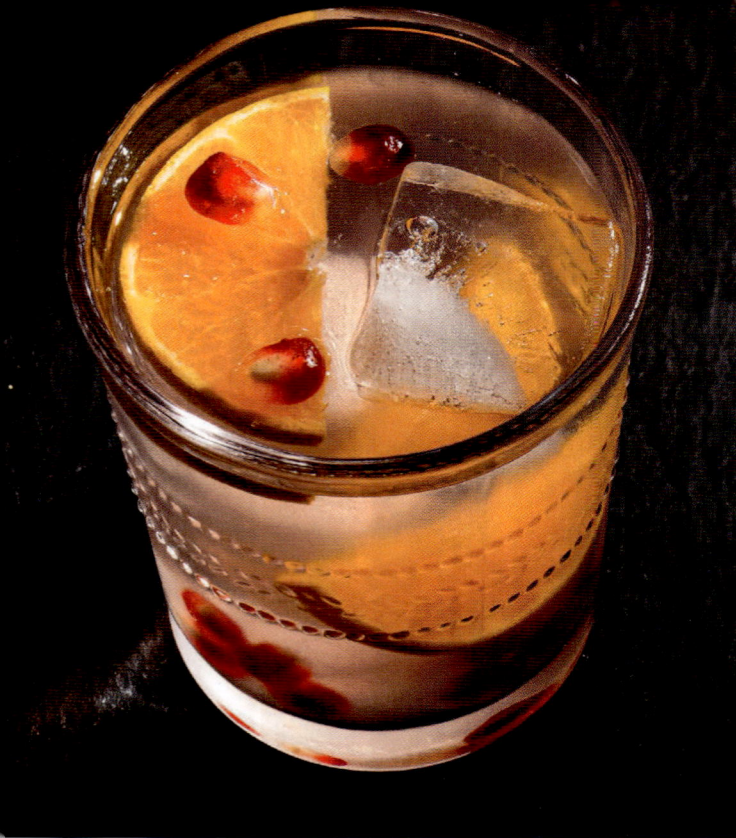

1/3 cup fennel seeds
1/4 cup dried ginger root
1 tablespoon licorice root
3 tablespoons dried lemongrass
3 tablespoons dried peppermint

Pulse fennel seeds, ginger, and licorice in spice grinder until coarsely ground, about 10 pulses. Transfer to small bowl and stir in lemongrass and peppermint. (Tea blend can be stored in airtight container at room temperature for up to 3 months.)

To make one cup tea Add 1 tablespoon tea blend to tea infuser or tea sachet. Steep tea mixture with 1 cup boiling water in teacup, covered, for 10 minutes. Remove tea infuser and serve immediately.

Winter Citrus and Pomegranate Water

serves 6 to 8 · **total time: 10 minutes, plus 30 minutes chilling**
FAST

why this recipe works · Walking around the grocery store during a New England January inspired us to create this winter-friendly fruit water. While berries looked sad and pale in the dead of winter, the citrus stand was a beacon of bright yellows, oranges, and greens that brought to mind a ray of sunshine—and screamed vitamin C, which we could all use to help boost immunity during the colder months. Mandarin oranges had the most inviting color, so they became the base of our drink. What else was in season? Big, beautiful pomegranates. While mandarins have a distinctly juicy, sweet flavor and are lower in acid than other oranges, pomegranates are intensely tart and vibrant (in both acidity and color), not to mention rich with antioxidants. The addition of 1/2 cup of seeds livened up the orange, and the bright flavors melded deliciously to create an appealingly tart berryish combo. If you don't have mandarin orange, you can substitute blood orange.

1 mandarin orange, sliced thin, plus extra for garnish
1/2 cup pomegranate seeds, plus extra for garnish
8 cups water, divided

1 Combine orange, pomegranate seeds, and 1 cup water in 8-cup liquid measuring cup or large bowl. With potato masher or muddler, muddle fruit until broken down and all juice is expressed, about 30 seconds. Stir in 3 cups water. Cover and refrigerate until flavors meld and mixture is chilled, 30 minutes to 1 hour.

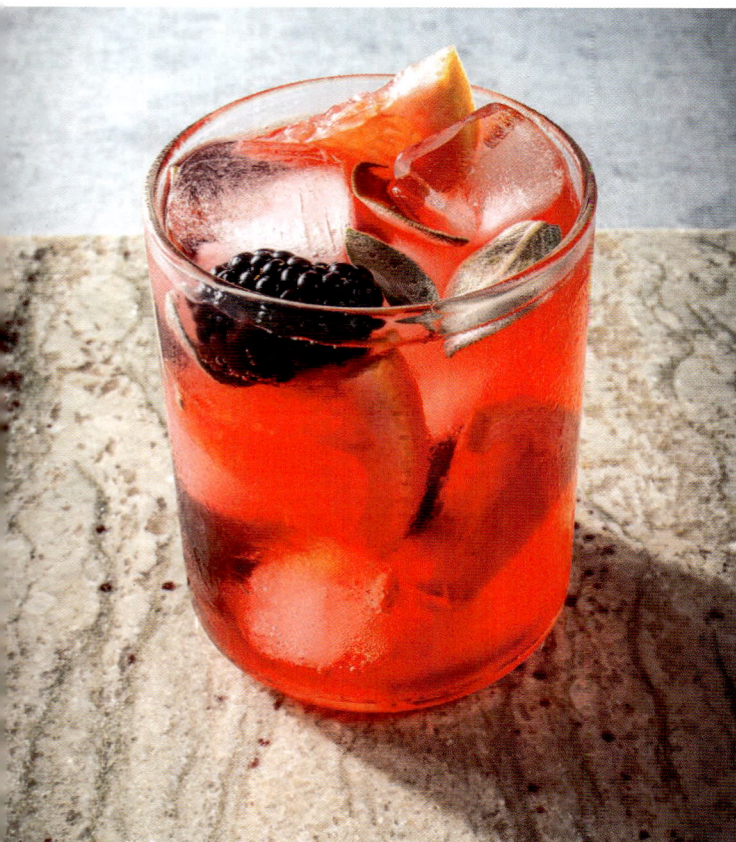

top | *Winter Citrus and Pomegranate Water*
bottom | *Grapefruit, Blackberry, and Sage Water*

2   Strain infused water through fine-mesh strainer into pitcher, pressing on solids to extract as much juice as possible. Discard solids. Stir in remaining 4 cups water and serve in ice-filled glasses garnished with extra orange slices and pomegranate seeds. (Water can be refrigerated for up to 24 hours; garnish with extra orange slices and pomegranate seeds just before serving.)

HOW TO REMOVE POMEGRANATE SEEDS

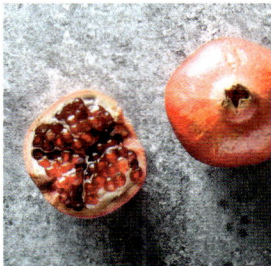

1   Halve pomegranate crosswise.

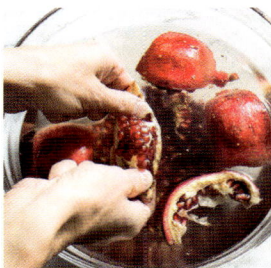

2   Submerge it in bowl of water and gently pull it apart. Seeds will sink, separating from bitter pith and membrane that holds them.

Watermelon-Lime Agua Fresca

serves 6 to 8 · total time: 15 minutes   **FAST**

why this recipe works · Agua fresca, or "fresh water," is a refreshing Mexican fruit drink. The phrase also covers a variety of blended beverages made from fruits, grains, seeds, or flowers along with sugar and water. To make a version with one of summer's favorite fruits—watermelon—we whizzed chunks of the melon with water in a blender and strained out the pulp before accenting the mixture with lime juice for tartness, agave nectar for sweetness, and a pinch of salt to bring out both of these flavors. Agave nectar is extracted as juice from agave plants before being heated to reduce the liquid and concentrate its sweet flavor. While similar to honey, it has a more neutral flavor that blends seamlessly into our subtly sweet watermelon and lime drink. Because watermelons vary in sweetness, we started by tasting our watermelon to determine how much agave nectar to incorporate into the agua fresca. Adjust the amounts of lime juice and sweetener to your taste. If you don't have agave nectar, you can substitute honey.

8   cups 1-inch seedless watermelon pieces
2   cups water
¼   cup lime juice (2 limes)
1–2   tablespoons agave nectar
¼   teaspoon table salt
    Fresh mint leaves

Working in 2 batches, process watermelon and water in blender until smooth, about 30 seconds. Strain mixture through fine-mesh strainer into pitcher; discard solids. Stir in lime juice, agave, and salt until agave and salt have dissolved. Serve in ice-filled glasses, garnished with mint. (Agua fresca can be refrigerated for up to 5 days; stir to recombine before serving.)

Grapefruit, Blackberry, and Sage Water

serves 6 to 8 · total time: 10 minutes, plus 30 minutes chilling
FAST

why this recipe works · For a citrus- and herb-infused water with an unexpected flavor pairing, we turned to grapefruit and sage. Grapefruit gave this water some welcome acidity tinged with bitter notes thanks to oils in the peel, which we left on during muddling. Sage offered a complex herbal quality that is aromatic and grassy. Our final ingredient was blackberries, which provided beautiful color and sweetness to offset the grapefruit. To amp up the herbaceous flavor of this water, we used fresh sage. The ingredients interplayed well, combining their sweet-tart notes and woodsy elements. Be sure to seek out unbruised sage and good-quality, ripe blackberries. If you don't have blackberries, you can substitute raspberries. If you don't have sage, you can substitute 4 thyme or tarragon sprigs. The grapefruit should not be damaged or bruised. Do not infuse for longer than 1 hour, as the grapefruit steadily takes over the other flavors. For ideal flavor, enjoy this infused water on the same day of its preparation.

½   grapefruit, sliced thin, plus extra for garnish
1   cup blackberries, plus extra for garnish
2   tablespoons fresh sage leaves, plus extra for garnish
8   cups water, divided

1   Combine grapefruit, blackberries, sage, and 1 cup water in 8-cup liquid measuring cup or large bowl. With potato masher or muddler, muddle fruit until broken down and all juice is expressed, about 30 seconds. Stir in 3 cups water. Cover and refrigerate until flavors meld and mixture is chilled, 30 minutes to 1 hour.

2   Strain infused water through fine-mesh strainer into pitcher, pressing on solids to extract as much juice as possible. Discard solids. Stir in remaining 4 cups water and serve in ice-filled glasses garnished with extra grapefruit, blackberries, and sage. (Water can be refrigerated for up to 24 hours; garnish with extra grapefruit, blackberries, and sage just before serving.)

Star Fruit, Lime, and Basil Water

serves 6 to 8   •   total time: 10 minutes, plus 30 minutes chilling
FAST

why this recipe works   •   Star fruit is the obvious star (no pun intended) of this lively infused water. Uniquely shaped and aptly named, star fruit is a tropical fruit common in Southeast Asia; it has a sweet-sour honeysuckle flavor that is reminiscent of a kiwi, with similarly textured, juicy flesh. For complementary flavors, we chose lime juice and Thai basil, which are often found in Southeast Asian drinks. When testing, we experimented with differing amounts of muddled lime and discovered that we enjoyed the high levels of brightness and sour acidity that one whole sliced lime brought to the water. Our herbal element of Thai basil gave the drink a refreshing, licorice flavor that combined with the lime and star fruit to taste deliciously invigorating. Star fruit will turn from green to yellow as it ripens; for best results, look for star fruits that are mostly yellow. If you don't have Thai basil, you can substitute Italian basil or tarragon leaves.

1½   star fruits, sliced thin, plus extra for garnish
1   lime, sliced thin, plus extra for garnish
¾   cup fresh Thai basil leaves, plus extra for garnish
8   cups water, divided

1   Combine star fruit, lime, Thai basil, and 1 cup water in 8-cup liquid measuring cup or large bowl. With potato masher or muddler, muddle fruit until broken down and all juices are expressed, about 30 seconds. Stir in 3 cups water. Cover and refrigerate until flavors meld and mixture is chilled, 30 minutes to 1 hour.

2   Strain infused water through fine-mesh strainer into pitcher, pressing on solids to extract as much juice as possible. Discard solids. Stir in remaining 4 cups water and serve in ice-filled glasses garnished with extra star fruit, lime, and basil. (Water can be refrigerated for up to 24 hours; garnish with extra star fruit, lime, and basil just before serving.)

Green Apple, Lemon, and Dill Water

serves 6 to 8   •   total time: 10 minutes, plus 30 minutes chilling
FAST

why this recipe works   •   For a naturally flavored apple water, we experimented with infusing different varieties to achieve the most exciting flavor. We tried Braeburn, Honeycrisp, Fuji, and Golden Delicious apples only to discover that although they all worked just fine, they were similar—tasty, but generic. When we tested Granny Smiths, however, they stood out as distinctly green and bright in both color and flavor. Granny Smiths are pleasantly tart, but this quality was lessened once infused, so we emphasized it with a little fresh lemon. Adding dill gave the water an herbal flavor that stood up to the tart apples and lemon while enhancing the fresh taste of this infused water. If you don't have a Granny Smith apple, you can substitute a Fuji, Gala, or Honeycrisp apple.

1   Granny Smith apple, cored and shredded, plus extra for garnish
½   lemon, sliced thin, plus extra for garnish
¼   cup fresh dill, plus extra for garnish
8   cups water, divided

1   Combine apple, lemon, dill, and 1 cup water in 8-cup liquid measuring cup or large bowl. With potato masher or muddler, muddle fruit until broken down and all juice is expressed, about 30 seconds. Stir in 3 cups water. Cover and refrigerate until flavors meld and mixture is chilled, 30 minutes to 1 hour.

2   Strain infused water through fine-mesh strainer into pitcher, pressing on solids to extract as much juice as possible. Discard solids. Stir in remaining 4 cups water and serve in ice-filled glasses garnished with extra apple, lemon, and dill. (Water can be refrigerated for up to 24 hours; garnish with extra apple, lemon, and dill just before serving.)

Honeydew-Lemon Agua Fresca

serves 6 to 8   •   total time: 15 minutes   **FAST**

why this recipe works   •   This honeydew melon and lemon agua fresca is a great way to switch up your hydration game or provide your brunch guests with a unique alcohol-free beverage. To keep this drink mildly sweet, we derived sweetness mostly from the melon itself and added just a bit of agave nectar. Honeydew has a mild flavor, so we enlivened it with punchy lemon juice for brightness and citrus vitamins. Using only ¼ cup allowed the citrus to mellow into the background and not turn the drink sour. Because honeydew melons vary in sweetness, we started by tasting our honeydew to determine how much agave nectar to incorporate into the agua fresca. Adjust the amounts of lemon juice and agave to your taste. If you don't have honeydew, you can substitute cantaloupe, and if you don't have agave nectar, you can substitute honey.

    8   cups 1-inch honeydew pieces
    2   cups water
    ¼   cup lemon juice (2 lemons)
    1–2 tablespoons agave nectar
    ¼   teaspoon table salt
        Fresh basil leaves (optional)

Working in 2 batches, process honeydew and water in blender until smooth, about 30 seconds. Strain mixture through fine-mesh strainer into pitcher; discard solids. Stir in lemon juice, agave, and salt until agave and salt have dissolved. Serve in ice-filled glasses garnished with basil, if using. (Agua fresca can be refrigerated for up to 5 days; stir to recombine before serving.)

Cantaloupe and Fresno Chile Spritzer

serves 4 · total time: 10 minutes   **FAST**

why this recipe works · We love the delicately sweet taste of cantaloupe and wanted to kick it up a notch for a stimulating spritzer. Spice and fruit are a proven twosome, so we paired our melon with the subtle heat and fresh spiciness of Fresno chiles. When processed, the cantaloupe created a frothy and colorful puree, and the chile deepened the color to a rich orange. When trying different levels of spice, we landed on half a seeded chile for a result that was pleasantly spicy and not painfully so. Straining the blend before stirring it into seltzer filtered out the bits of pepper skin for a smooth drink. If you don't have cantaloupe, you can substitute honeydew, and if you don't have a Fresno chile, you can substitute a jalapeño.

    2   cups 1-inch cantaloupe pieces
    ½   Fresno chile, stemmed, seeded, and chopped
    3   cups seltzer, chilled

1   Process cantaloupe and Fresno chile in food processor until smooth, scraping down sides of bowl as needed, about 1 minute. Strain mixture through fine-mesh strainer into pitcher. (Puree can also be stored in airtight container in refrigerator for up to 2 days; transfer puree to pitcher before proceeding.)

2   Just before serving, gently stir seltzer into puree until combined. Pour into ice-filled glasses. (You can also make a single portion by combining ¼ cup puree and ¾ cup seltzer in glass before adding ice.)

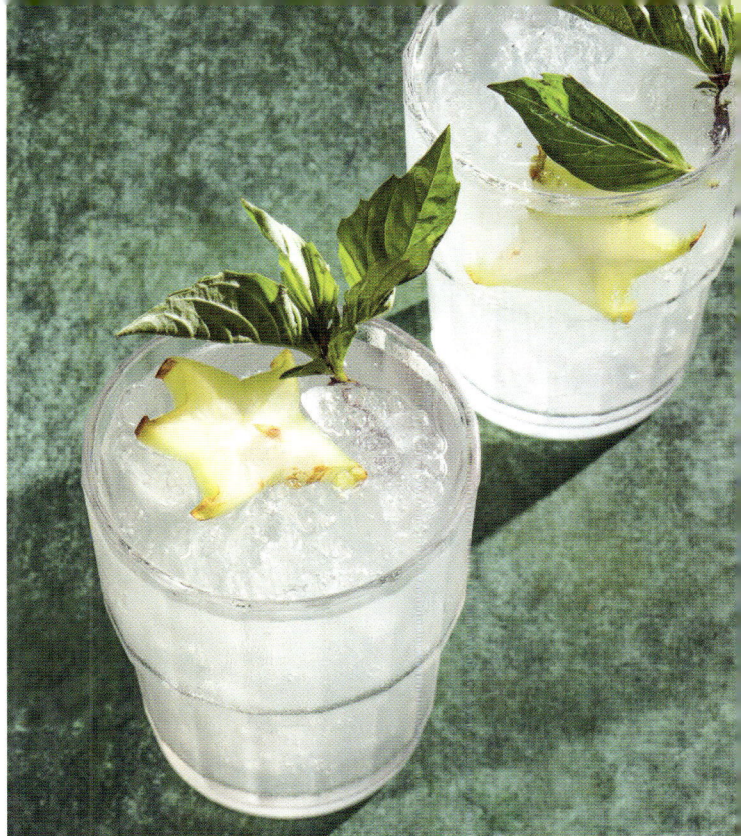

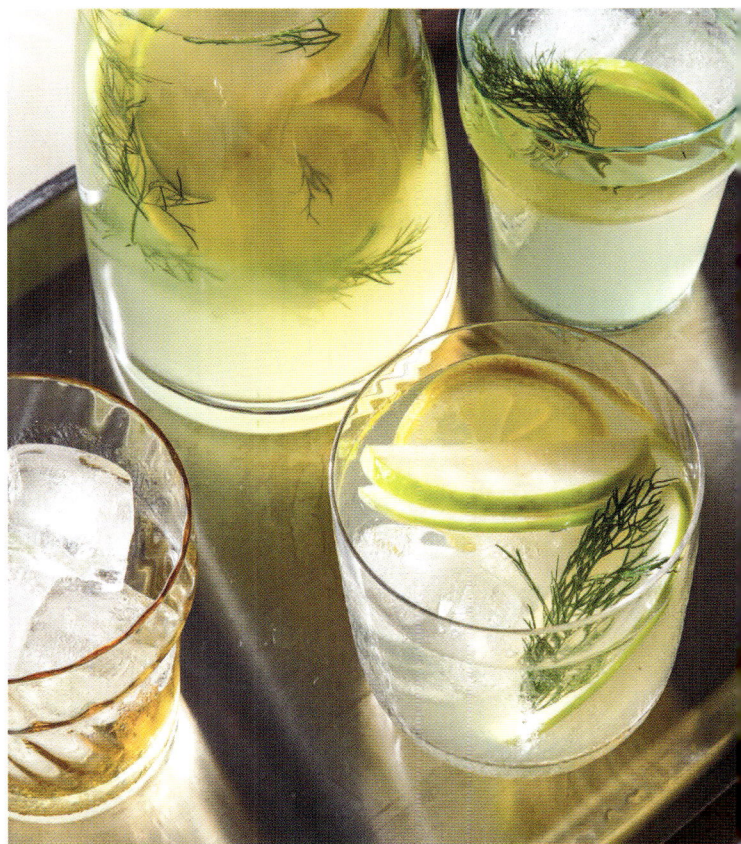

top | Star Fruit, Lime, and Basil Water
bottom | Green Apple, Lemon, and Dill Water

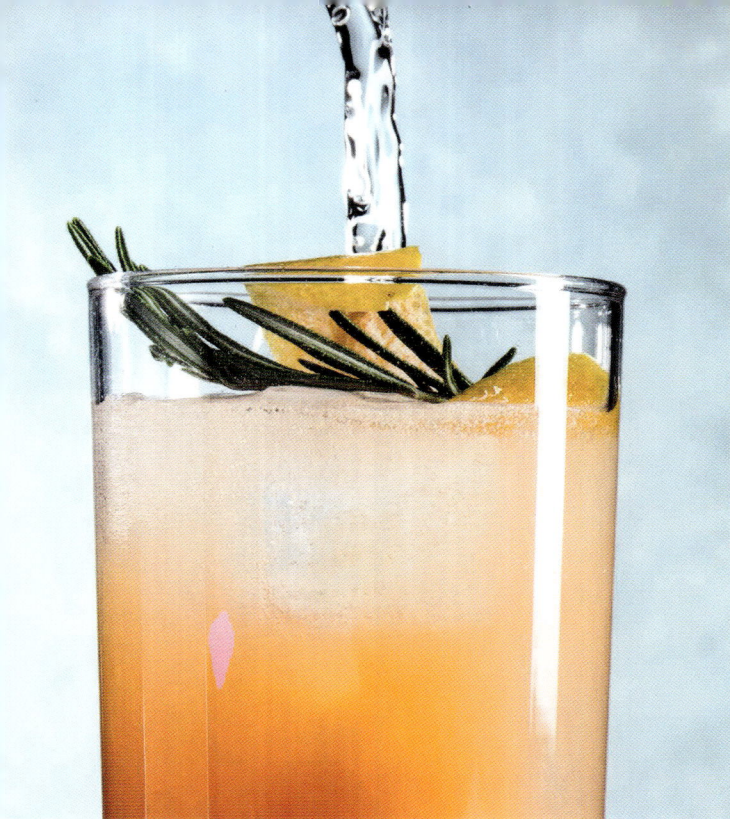

Grapefruit-Rosemary Spritzer

serves 1 · **total time: 5 minutes** `FAST`

why this recipe works · With its citrus and herbal flavors, this simple but sophisticated drink is perfect for brightening up any gathering. Fresh grapefruit juice, seltzer, and rosemary syrup add up to far more than the sum of their parts. Our preferred method for infusing a drink with herbal flavors is via a flavored syrup because it disperses so evenly. Just a tablespoon of the syrup's piney flavor tempered the grapefruit's tartness and offered intriguing savory notes. We like to use fresh juice for this spritzer (you can use yellow, pink, or red grapefruit), but you can also substitute unsweetened store-bought juice. You can substitute herb syrup with thyme or sage for the herb syrup with rosemary.

- ½ cup grapefruit juice plus 1 strip zest, for garnish
- 1 tablespoon Herb Syrup with rosemary (recipe follows)
- ½ cup seltzer, chilled
- Rosemary sprig (optional)

Fill chilled glass halfway with ice. Add grapefruit juice and rosemary syrup and stir to combine. Add seltzer and, using spoon, gently lift juice mixture from bottom of glass to top to combine. Top with additional ice and garnish with grapefruit zest and rosemary sprig, if using. Serve.

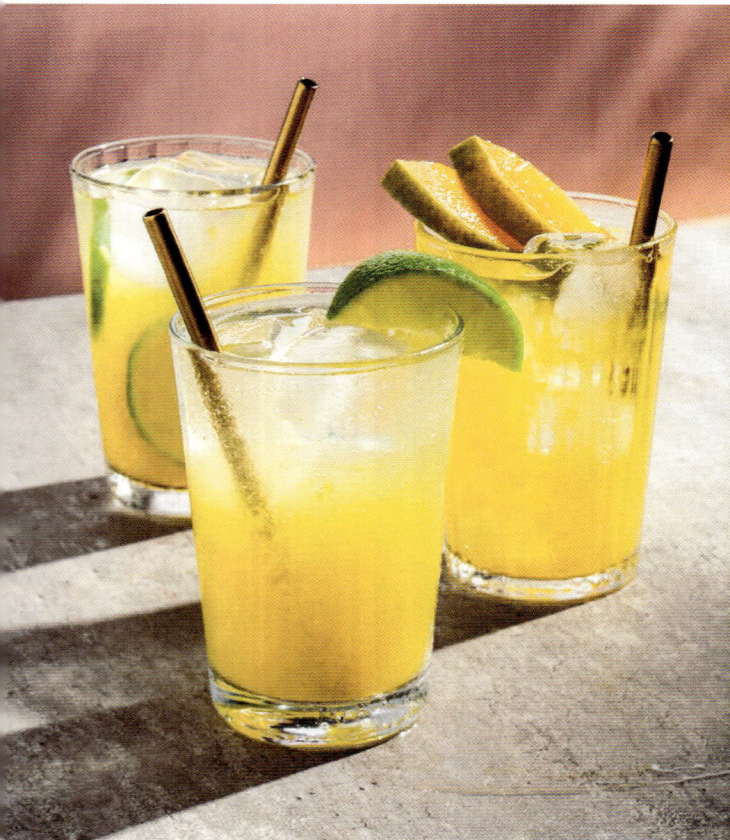

Citrus Syrup

Makes 1 cup (enough for 16 sodas)

- ¾ cup sugar
- ⅔ cup water
- 2 teaspoons grated grapefruit, lemon, lime, or orange zest

Heat sugar, water, and zest in small saucepan over medium heat, whisking often, until sugar has dissolved, about 5 minutes; do not boil. Let cool completely, about 30 minutes. Strain syrup through fine-mesh strainer into airtight container; discard solids. (Syrup can be refrigerated for up to 1 month.)

To make Herb Syrup Substitute ½ cup fresh herb leaves (basil, dill, mint, sage, or tarragon), 12 fresh thyme sprigs, or 1 fresh rosemary sprig for citrus zest, adding herb after simple syrup is removed from heat.

---

top | *Grapefruit-Rosemary Spritzer*
bottom | *Mango and Lime Spritzer*

Pear and Vanilla Spritzer

serves 4 · total time: 10 minutes **FAST**

why this recipe works · For a sugar-free drink inspired by cream soda, we processed half a vanilla bean with ripened pears and combined the mixture with bubbly seltzer. We opted to use vanilla bean instead of vanilla extract because, while the latter worked in this recipe and is traditionally beneficial in baking, it tasted slightly of alcohol. The pears contributed enhanced body and complexity that complemented the vanilla flavor; the fruit tasted vaguely of warm spices and became velvety in the food processor, which added a nice texture to our final drink. Adding pear also brought in a dose of gut-supporting fiber. Be sure the pears are perfectly ripe. The puree will hold well in the fridge for up to 2 days. It may get slightly darker as the day progresses. If you don't have a vanilla bean you can substitute ¼ teaspoon vanilla extract, and if you don't have Bosc pears you can substitute Anjou or Bartlett pears.

> ### NOTES FROM THE TEST KITCHEN
>
> #### Pear Primer
>
> There are all kinds of pears to use when cooking, baking, or making drinks. Here are some of our favorites for giving a dish a sweet fiber boost.
>
> **Asian Pear** Also known as "pear-apples," Asian pears are rounder and squatter than other varieties. They are crunchy and do not soften as they ripen. They add crisp texture to salads or slaws.
>
> **Anjou Pear** Available with red or green skin, Anjou pears are squat and plump, with wider necks than other varieties. Their flesh is creamy, tender, and incredibly juicy when ripe.
>
> **Bartlett Pear** Green when underripe, these pears turn yellowish when ripe. They have a floral sweetness and thin, delicate skin. (Bartletts are the variety typically used for canned pears.)
>
> **Bosc Pear** Easy to recognize by their brownish skin and elongated necks, Bosc pears are sweet and fragrant when ripe and are our favorite pears for baking. They're naturally firmer than other varieties, so they don't turn as mushy when cooked.

½ vanilla bean
2 Bosc pears, peeled, halved, and cored
3 cups seltzer, chilled

1 Cut vanilla bean in half lengthwise. Using tip of paring knife, scrape out seeds; discard empty pod (or save for another use). Process pears and vanilla seeds in food processor until smooth, scraping down sides of bowl as needed, about 90 seconds. Strain mixture through fine-mesh strainer into pitcher. (Puree can also be stored in airtight container in refrigerator for up to 2 days; transfer puree to pitcher before proceeding.)

2 Just before serving, gently stir seltzer into puree until combined. Pour into ice-filled glasses. (You can also make a single portion by combining ¼ cup puree and ¾ cup seltzer in glass before adding ice.)

Mango and Lime Spritzer

serves 4 · total time: 15 minutes **FAST**

why this recipe works · Fresh mango was essential to this spritzer because it is one of only two add-ins. We found that without other flavors to meld with or stand behind, frozen mango was not assertive enough; this beverage needed the fresh and juicy flesh of ripe mango. For a tropical pairing, we processed the fresh mango with lime juice and some zest for a bold citrus aroma and much-needed acidity to balance out the sweet fruit (plus a vitamin C boost). When the mango was broken down in the food processor, it created a beautifully thick puree. Straining this blend was essential to filter out the pulp and lime zest, which imparted nice flavor but can taste bitter. If you don't have a lime, you can substitute lemon or orange, and if you don't have seltzer, you can substitute coconut water.

2 mangos, peeled, pitted, and coarsely chopped
½ teaspoon grated lime zest plus 1 tablespoon juice
3 cups seltzer, chilled

1 Process mangos and lime zest and juice in food processor until smooth, scraping down sides of bowl as needed, about 1 minute. Strain mixture through fine-mesh strainer into pitcher. (Puree can also be stored in airtight container in refrigerator for up to 2 days; transfer puree to pitcher before proceeding.)

2 Just before serving, gently stir seltzer into puree until combined. Pour into ice-filled glasses. (You can also make a single portion by combining ¼ cup puree and ¾ cup seltzer in glass before adding ice.)

fermenting 101

Fermented drinks are known to have probiotic benefits that can help improve digestive health, which is key for fighting inflammation. Fermenting drinks at home may sound intimidating, but we've worked hard to make it simpler and less prone to failure. We developed recipes for tepache, kefir, and kombucha that are easy to follow and offer big rewards. Fermenting is inherently wild, so you can never truly control the process; we standardized our recipes to make the results as predictable as possible, but outcomes still do vary depending on a number of factors.

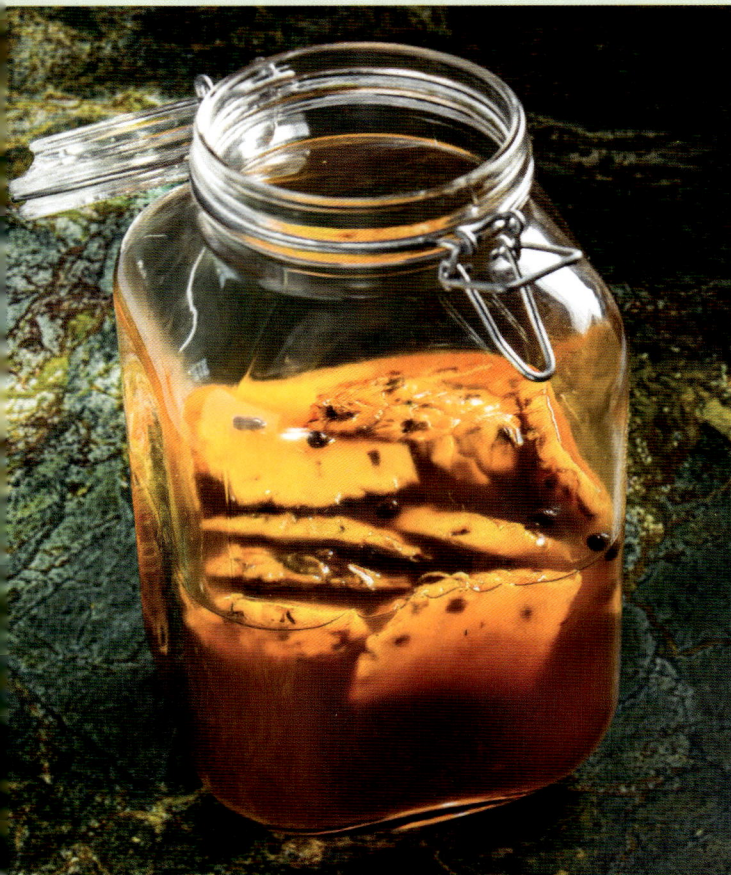

Sanitation Matters

Cleanliness is important for any drink you make at home, but it's especially so for fermented ones. The ideal environment for fermentation is also ideal for unwanted bacteria, so sanitation is essential. Wash, sanitize, and air-dry all utensils, jars, and bottles that will come in contact with your homemade beverage. In the test kitchen we use a dye-free, fragrance-free detergent for washing and an iodophor sanitizer, a disinfectant containing iodine (prepared to the manufacturer's instructions), when necessary. If your dishwasher has a sterilization setting, you can use that instead. Always use clean parchment and zipper-lock bags.

Many factors can affect fermentation. It is largely impacted by temperature and the amount of cultures present, so fermentation rates may vary.

Where to Ferment

You need a consistent temperature range for your beverage (the recommended temperature will vary, but it's typically somewhere between 70 and 80 degrees), and less fluctuation is better. The cooler the space, the longer the fermentation may take—sometimes never succeeding at all. If it's too warm and the process occurs too quickly, there will be less nuanced flavor and you're more likely to overferment and miss the optimal stopping point. Plus, it can lead to a greater production of alcohol.

Why Your Water Matters

During our fermentation experimentation, we tested with tap, distilled, spring, and filtered water. They all worked, but we ended up choosing filtered water or spring water to ensure the best quality outcome. Distilled water lacks minerals, which yeast needs to grow effectively. Additionally, some tap water is highly chlorinated, which is harmful to the microbes, and other tap water may have pathogens. So filtered or spring water was deemed best for safety and optimal brewing conditions.

Drink Responsibly

The creation of alcohol occurs naturally as a by-product of the fermentation process. The fermented beverages in this chapter can contain between 0.5 and 3 percent alcohol by volume depending on duration of fermentation time and ingredients used. Kefir is at the lower end of the range, and tepache and kombucha are at the higher end. If a drink overferments, it can lead to agreater percentage of alcohol by volume.

| top | Tepache |
| right | Milk Kefir |

Eat Your Mistakes

The best way to tell if you have overfermented your beverage is by taste. If it is too tart and vinegar-forward to enjoy as a drink, you have overfermented, but you can still use the results.

Kombucha Kombucha will essentially turn into vinegar, so use it however you would a standard vinegar. Or simmer leftover kombucha in a saucepan until reduced to a sweet syrup. Use in alcohol-free cocktails and flavored waters.

Kefir This tangy drink can replace buttermilk in dressings or enrich smoothies. Or, strain through cheesecloth to make yogurt.

Tepache It's hardly a mistake if your tepache overferments (it's often fermented longer so that it becomes more alcoholic. Enjoy it as is, though be aware the alcohol content will be higher.

The Ins and Outs of Kefir

Troubleshooting Kefir Fermentation

Visual cues are key here. Once properly fermented and ready to strain, the milk kefir will have thickened and gelled (easy to see if you gently tilt the jar).

Underfermented The milk and grains have not thickened and the mixture has not achieved kefir's pleasantly sour smell within the prescribed time. Increasing the room temperature a few degrees or doubling the grains in step 2 will speed up the fermentation.

Overfermented The whey separates noticeably from the milk curd in step 2. Decreasing the ambient room temperature or having the amount of grains will slow down the fermentation cycle.

Sharing and Storing Activated Kefir Grains

You will end up with more grains than you need after activation, plus, the fermentation process produces excess grains over time. After activation, unused grains can be refrigerated or frozen.

Refrigerate Store grains in an airtight jar with enough milk to submerge the grains (about 1 cup of milk for every 1 tablespoon of grains) for up to 2 weeks. To make kefir with refrigerated grains, skip reactivation and continue with step 2 of the recipe.

Freeze Rinse the grains with filtered water, pat dry, toss with dry milk powder (1 tablespoon for every 1 tablespoon of grains), and store in a freezer bag with the air pressed out for up to 6 months. To make kefir with frozen grains, start recipe with one 36-hour reactivation period before proceeding to step 2.

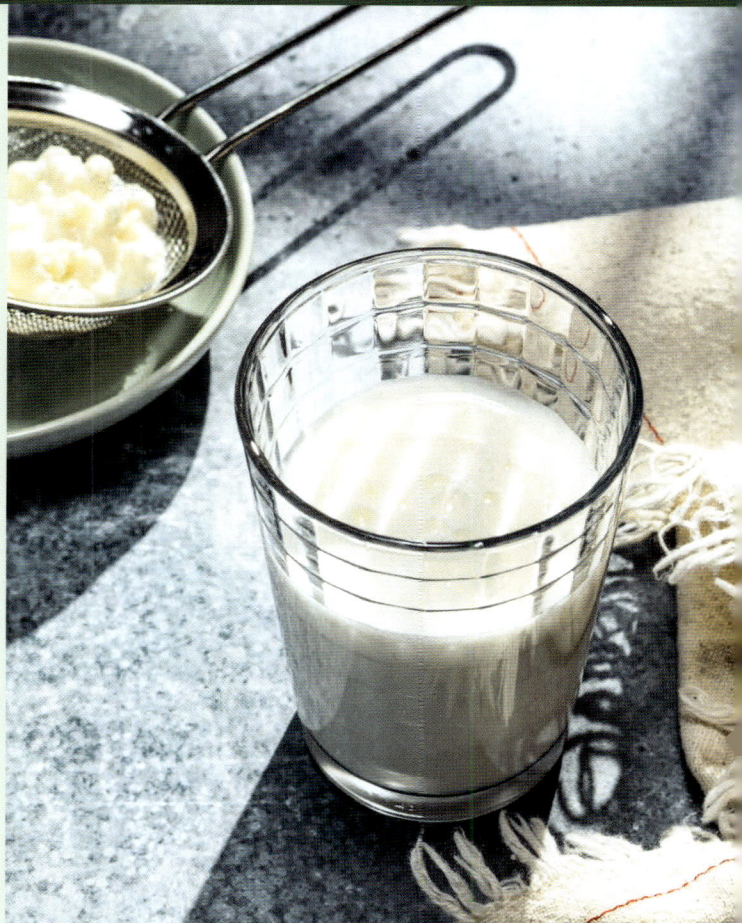

NOTES FROM THE TEST KITCHEN

Sharing Your Pellicle

The pellicle, or SCOBY (symbiotic culture of bacteria and yeast), refers to the jellyfish-like membrane or skin that forms on the surface of the fermenting kombucha. This can be split and shared with others to make more kombucha, as the pellicle forms a new layer every time it's disturbed. Using gloved (or very clean) hands, you can pull apart the individual layers. Store the pellicle in 1 cup of kombucha at room temperature to guarantee you have at least ¾ cup of mature kombucha to start your next batch. Store the pellicle and mature kombucha for up to 2 weeks at room temperature.

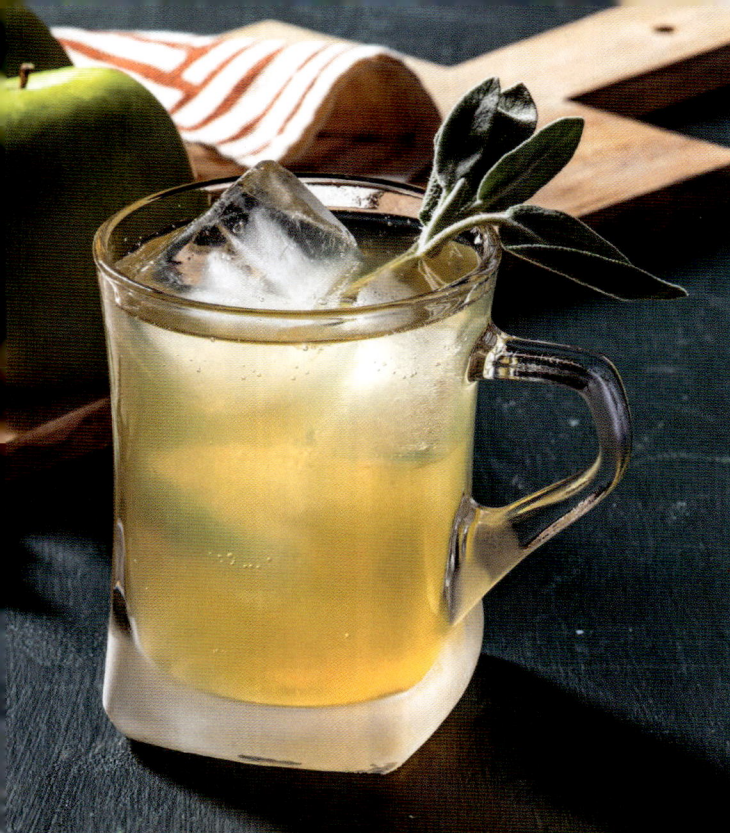

Bubbly Sage Cider

serves 1 · total time: 5 minutes FAST

why this recipe works · Whether baked, roasted, or sipped, apples and sage are an autumnal match made in heaven. The sweetly aromatic juice of apples is tempered by the herbaceous, slightly bitter greenness of sage, so we wanted to turn this winning combo into a drink. We found the best expression of apple as a liquid to come in the form of apple cider. However, apple cider is so concentrated that we needed only ¼ cup (to ¾ cup of seltzer) for its flavor to shine through the bubbles. We used our lightly sweetened herb syrup to infuse the drink with sage flavor without the need for muddling. To balance the sweetness of this drink, we decided to forgo our normal citrus route and instead turned to apple cider vinegar. Not only did this naturally fermented condiment offer acidity, it also added complexity through secondary notes of apples. You can substitute Herb Syrup with thyme or rosemary (page 398) for the herb syrup with sage.

- ¼ cup apple cider
- 1 tablespoon Herb Syrup with sage (page 398)
- ½ teaspoon apple cider vinegar
- ¾ cup seltzer, chilled
   Apple slices (optional)
   Fresh sage leaves (optional)

Fill chilled glass halfway with ice. Add apple cider, sage syrup, and vinegar and stir to combine. Add seltzer and, using spoon, gently lift cider mixture from bottom of glass to top to combine. Top with additional ice and garnish with apple slices and sage leaves, if using. Serve.

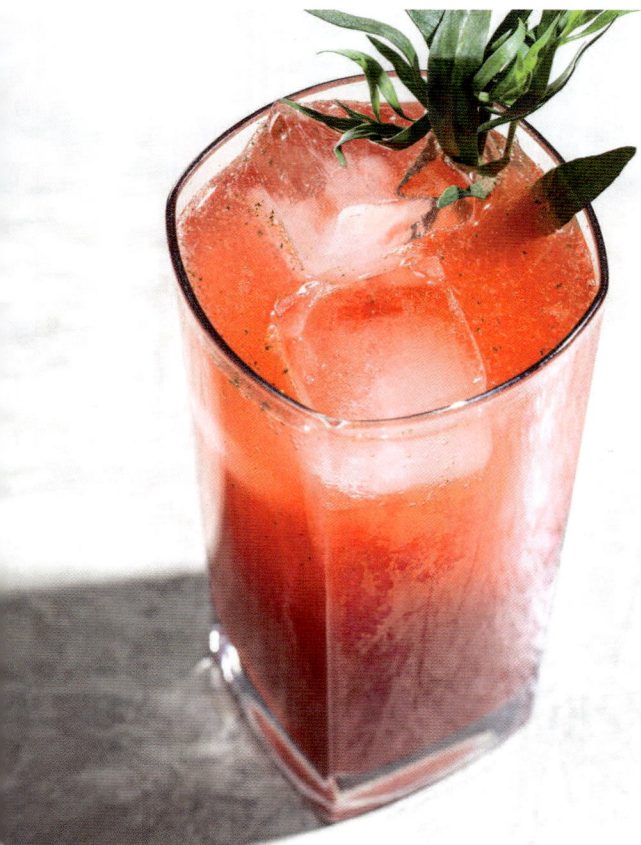

Sicilian Sunrise

serves 1 · total time: 10 minutes FAST

why this recipe works · Blood oranges are a beautiful winter standout and feature prominently in Sicilian cuisine. When juiced, these oranges make for a striking dark-magenta drink with raspberry notes and a whisper of bitterness. To help them shine in a refreshing, alcohol-free mixed drink, we turned to fresh tarragon, whose anise-licorice notes combine with citrus in many Mediterranean dishes. A tablespoon of herb syrup gave us plenty of tarragon flavor, and lemon juice balanced the acidity of the freshly squeezed orange juice. Poured over ice and topped with chilled seltzer, our beverage was rich in citrus flavor, with a unique herbal back note. If you don't have blood oranges, you can substitute navel oranges. You can substitute Simple Syrup (page 387) or Herb Syrup with basil (page 398) for the Herb Syrup with tarragon.

½ cup blood orange juice (3 oranges)
1½ teaspoons lemon juice
1 tablespoon Herb Syrup with tarragon (page 398)
½ cup seltzer, chilled
Tarragon sprig (optional)

Fill chilled glass halfway with ice. Add orange juice, lemon juice, and tarragon syrup and stir to combine. Add seltzer and, using spoon, gently lift juice mixture from bottom of glass to top to combine. Top with additional ice and garnish with tarragon sprig, if using. Serve.

Tepache

serves 4 to 6 • total time: 25 minutes, plus 3 days fermenting and 1 hour chilling

why this recipe works • Tepache is a spiced and fruity fermented Mexican beverage. It's great for the gut and easy to make at home, as it does not require the addition of cultures. We decided to make our version as simple as possible by using pineapple peels, cinnamon, and the iconic piloncillo. Piloncillo, also known as panela or panocha, is an unrefined cane sugar used throughout Central and South America. It is traditionally used in tepache and adds rich, caramel-like sweetness. Technique and temperature are of utmost importance to ensure proper and safe fermentation of this recipe. We submerged all ingredients in filtered water with the assistance of parchment paper and a makeshift weight made from a water-filled zipper-lock bag. Maintaining a temperature range from 72 to 75 degrees was also crucial, as any less and the tepache will not ferment. We recommend using a serrated knife to break the piloncillo into smaller pieces for accurate measurement. You will need a 1-gallon wide-mouth glass jar for this recipe. If you don't have piloncillo, you can substitute turbinado (such as Sugar in the Raw) or demerara sugar. You will need spring or filtered tap water for this recipe.

1 pineapple, rinsed
4½ ounces piloncillo, broken into small pieces (½ cup packed)
1 cinnamon stick
½ teaspoon allspice berries (optional)

1 Discard pineapple crown and peel pineapple. Cut peels into rough 3-inch pieces and set aside; enjoy pineapple flesh separately. Cut out parchment paper round to match diameter of 1-gallon wide-mouth jar.

2 Heat piloncillo, 1 cup spring or filtered tap water, cinnamon stick, and allspice berries, if using, in large saucepan over medium-high heat until piloncillo has dissolved, about 5 minutes. Add

pineapple peels, piloncillo syrup, and 4 cups room-temperature spring or filtered tap water to 1-gallon wide-mouth jar and stir to combine. Press parchment round flush against surface of peels. Fill 1-quart zipper-lock bag with 1 cup water, squeeze out air, and seal well. Place bag of water on top of parchment and gently press down to submerge pineapple. Cover jar with large coffee filter or triple layer of cheesecloth and secure with rubber band. Place jar in 72- to 75-degree location away from direct sunlight and let ferment for 3 to 5 days.

3 After 3 days, taste tepache daily until it has reached desired flavor. Beverage should be fruit-forward with caramel and spice undertones and have mild fermented flavor, with slight effervescence.

4 When tepache has reached desired flavor, strain liquid through fine-mesh strainer into storage container; discard solids. Chill tepache for at least 1 hour or up to 1 week. Serve over ice.

Milk Kefir

serves 1 • total time: 30 minutes, plus 4½ days fermenting

why this recipe works • Milk kefir, made from fermented dairy and kefir grains, is a tart, creamy probiotic drink that is great for gut health. Milk kefir grains contain bacteria and yeast and, as a result, have higher amounts of probiotics than yogurt. These grains culture dairy milk in only 24 hours, so we made a recipe that produces 1 cup of kefir a day. During shipping, the bacteria balances can be thrown off, so it is important to activate them upon arrival. The kefir grains need time to acclimate to their new environment and build up to their full potential for a balanced beverage—a bit yeasty with a yogurt-like flavor. Any dairy milk will produce delicious kefir, but we preferred the richness of whole milk. Package sizes for kefir grains can vary by manufacturer. We call for the minimum amount necessary for success; however, you should include the entire amount of kefir grains in step 1 if a greater amount is provided. You will need a 2-cup glass jar with a lid for this recipe. Your kefir jar should be covered well but loosely. We find inverting the lid of a Mason jar before sealing it with the screw top is an easy way to create a covered but breathable environment for the kefir. This recipe can easily be doubled. For information on storing kefir grains, see pages 400-401.

4-5 cups whole milk, divided, plus extra as needed
1 (¼-ounce) package live kefir culture

1   To activate kefir Combine 1 cup milk and kefir grains with their packing liquid in 2-cup glass jar. Cover loosely with lid, place in 68- to 72-degree location away from direct sunlight, and let ferment for 36 hours.

2   Strain mixture through fine-mesh strainer; reserve grains and discard milk. Clean jar. Combine reserved grains and 1 cup fresh milk in now-empty jar, place in 68- to 72-degree location away from direct sunlight, and let ferment for 24 hours. Repeat straining and refreshing grain and milk mixture until milk lightly sours and thickens to buttermilk consistency within 24-hour period, 1 to 2 more times. Strain mixture, reserving activated kefir grains and discarding milk.

3   To make kefir Combine ⅛ teaspoon activated kefir grains and 1 cup fresh milk in clean jar. Cover loosely with lid, place in 68- to 72-degree location away from direct sunlight, and let ferment until milk lightly sours and thickens to buttermilk consistency, about 24 hours. Store remaining activated kefir grains for later use. Kefir should not show signs of separation within fermentation cycle; if it does, it has overfermented.

4   Strain kefir through fine-mesh strainer into serving glass or storage container, gently stirring mixture to help separate grains from kefir; reserve grains to make another batch or store with remaining activated kefir grains. Serve, or refrigerate kefir for up to 3 days.

5   To make future batches of kefir Repeat recipe from step 3, using reserved kefir grains. The grains will increase in volume over multiple batches of kefir; we recommend discarding excess grains once they measure over ⅛ teaspoon.

VARIATION

Milk Kefir with Vanilla

Stir ½ teaspoon vanilla extract into strained kefir in step 4 until fully combined.

Kombucha

serves 4 to 6 (makes 1½ quarts) · **total time: 20 minutes, plus 6 days fermenting and 1 hour chilling**

why this recipe works · It is surprisingly easy and economical to make kombucha at home: Just add sweetened, cooled tea to mature kombucha and allow it to ferment in a warm environment and you'll have an effervescent, gut-friendly drink. You can consume your kombucha either as a still beverage or let it undergo a secondary fermentation in the bottle to become a sparkling one. Once you have mature kombucha and some simple equipment, you'll have all you need to make a consistently satisfying drink. If you don't have loose-leaf tea, you can substitute 4 tea bags. You will need a 1-gallon wide-mouth glass jar and three 16-ounce glass bottles with caps for this recipe. Look for a mature starter online. For information on storing the pellicle, see pages 400-401.

- 8 cups spring or filtered tap water, room temperature, divided
- 2 tablespoons loose-leaf black or green tea
- ½ cup (3½ ounces) sugar
- ¾ cup mature kombucha plus 1 ounce kombucha pellicle
- 3 tablespoons Simple Syrup (page 387) (optional)

1   Bring 2 cups water to boil in small saucepan over high heat; remove from heat. (If steeping green tea, allow boiled water to cool to 175 degrees.) Using reusable tea infuser or disposable tea bag, steep tea in water for 5 minutes (if using black tea) or 3 minutes (if using green tea). Discard tea. Whisk in sugar until dissolved.

2   Add sweetened tea and remaining 6 cups water to 1-gallon wide-mouth jar and stir to combine (mixture should be less than 100 degrees; let cool, if necessary, before proceeding). Stir in mature kombucha and pellicle. Cover jar with large coffee filter and secure with rubber band. Place jar in 73- to 83-degree location away from direct sunlight and let ferment for 6 days. After 6 days, taste kombucha daily until it has reached desired sweet-tart balance.

3   When kombucha has reached desired flavor, transfer pellicle to bowl, using tongs or slotted spoon, along with 1 cup mature kombucha; set aside at room temperature for up to 2 weeks. Stir remaining kombucha to recombine.

4a   For still kombucha Using funnel and ladle, divide kombucha evenly among three 16-ounce bottles, filling each bottle to within 1 inch of top. (Enjoy excess kombucha immediately or refrigerate in separate small container.) Secure bottle caps and refrigerate until chilled, at least 1 hour or up to 1 month. Serve.

4b   For sparkling kombucha Using funnel and ladle, fill three 16-ounce bottles halfway with kombucha, add 1 tablespoon simple syrup, and top with remaining kombucha to within 1 inch of top. (Enjoy excess kombucha immediately or refrigerate in separate small container.) Secure bottle caps and gently shake to combine ingredients. Store bottles in 73- to 83-degree location away from direct sunlight for 7 days to carbonate. Refrigerate carbonated kombucha until chilled, at least 1 hour or up to 1 month. Serve, opening bottles slowly to prevent foaming.

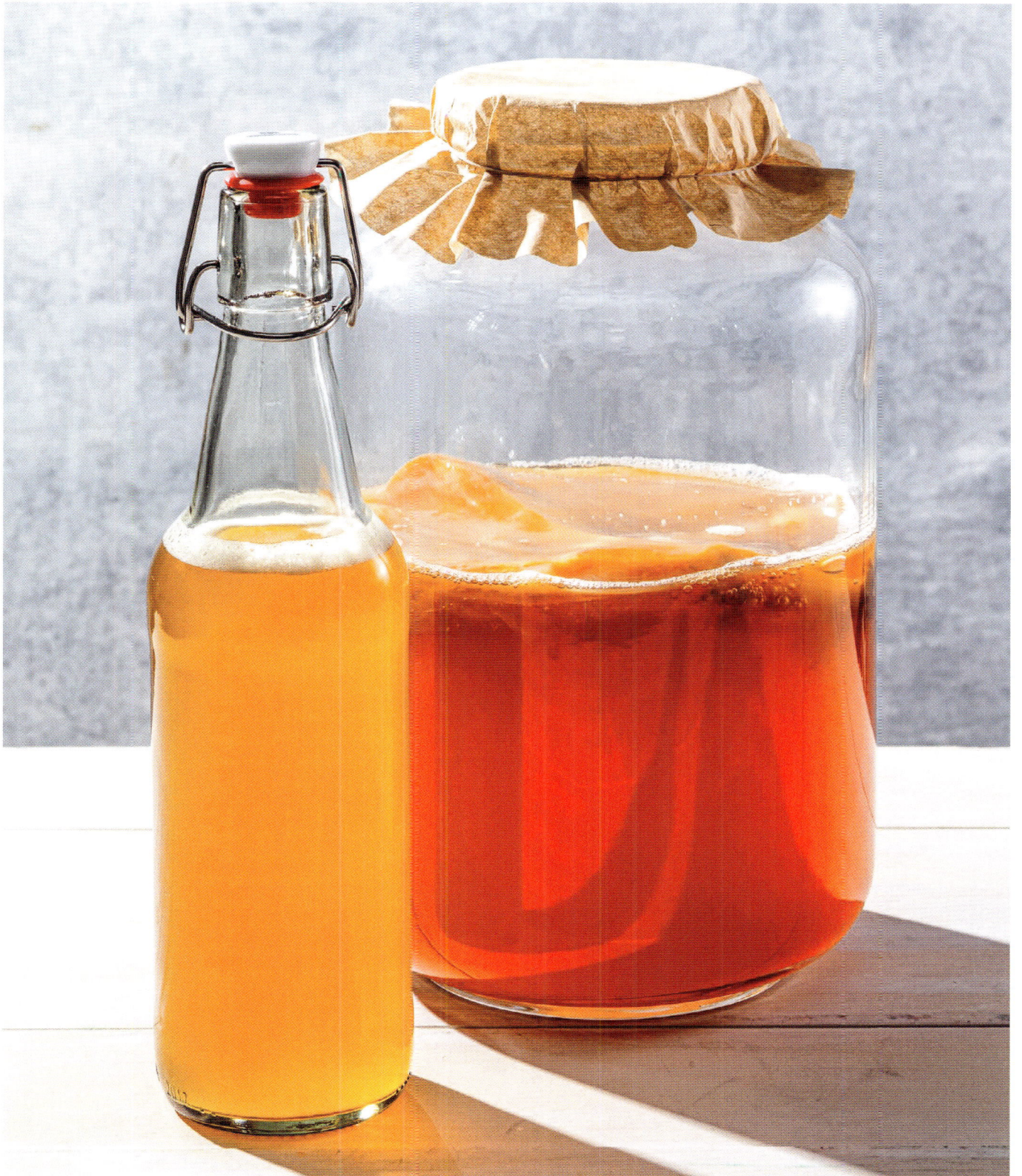

5 To make future batches of kombucha Repeat recipe, using reserved pellicle and mature kombucha in step 2. The pellicle will continue to increase in size over multiple batches of kombucha; we recommend sharing or discarding excess pellicle once it weighs over 5 ounces.

VARIATIONS

Sparkling Blue Ginger-Lime Kombucha

Add 1 teaspoon (¼-inch) dried ginger pieces, 1 teaspoon blue or green spirulina (optional), and ¼ teaspoon grated lime zest to each bottle with simple syrup in step 4b. Reduce carbonating time to 5 days.

Sparkling Spicy Pineapple Kombucha

Process 8 ounces thawed frozen organic pineapple chunks and 1 tablespoon minced, seeded Fresno chile in blender until smooth, about 1 minute. Strain mixture through fine-mesh strainer into small bowl, pressing on solids to extract as much juice as possible; discard solids. Substitute ¼ cup pineapple puree for simple syrup in each bottle in step 4b. Reduce carbonating time to 5 days.

Sparkling Mixed Berry Kombucha

Process 8 ounces thawed frozen organic mixed berries in blender until smooth, about 1 minute. Strain mixture through fine-mesh strainer into small bowl, pressing on solids to extract as much juice as possible; discard solids and stir in ½ teaspoon vanilla extract (optional). Substitute ¼ cup berry puree for simple syrup in each bottle in step 4b. Reduce carbonating time to 5 days.

Raw Hot Chocolate

serves 2 • total time: 15 minutes   **FAST**

why this recipe works • Inspired by hot cacao beverages enjoyed by ancient Mayan society, we wanted to make a decadent-tasting hot chocolate that used no added processed sugar at all. We infused our beverage with deep chocolaty flavor by blooming cacao nibs in milk alongside vanilla beans, whose floral and aromatic notes nicely complemented the complexity of the cacao. To give our drink some unrefined sweetness, we added pitted dates to our simmered mixture, which allowed the dates to soften enough for blending while imparting a honeyed and fruity flavor. After simmering, we blended the still-warm mixture and strained it to remove distracting particulates for smooth sipping. We took care to strain the mixture gently and avoided pressing on the solids, as this resulted in a slightly bitter drink. Our hot chocolate was delectably rich without being overwhelmingly sweet.

½ vanilla bean
2½ cups milk
3 pitted dates
½ cup cacao nibs

1 Cut vanilla bean in half lengthwise. Using tip of paring knife, scrape out seeds. Bring vanilla seeds and bean, milk, dates, and cacao nibs to simmer in medium saucepan over medium-high heat and cook, stirring occasionally, until dates soften and flavors meld, about 5 minutes.

2 Carefully transfer cacao mixture to blender and process until smooth, about 1 minute. Strain mixture through fine-mesh strainer into serving mugs, discarding solids. Serve.

MAKE IT DAIRY-FREE • Substitute plant-based milk for the dairy milk (we especially like oat milk here).

Haldhicha Dudh

serves 2 • total time: 10 minutes   **FAST**

why this recipe works • Haldhicha dudh (in the Marathi language of Western India) is a traditional beverage that is used to soothe a cold or cough. Translated as "turmeric milk," haldhicha dudh combines turmeric with heated and lightly sweetened milk. When developing the proportions for our recipe, we relied on the advice of our colleague Kaumudi Marathé, who grew up with the drink. Because fresh turmeric is seasonal, this drink is made with ground turmeric so that it can be enjoyed year-round. Turmeric is a spice that's sensitive to temperature, so we whisked it into the milk off heat to allow it to bloom without overcooking and tasting bitter. We found that 2 teaspoons was ideal—any more and the drink became gritty and tannic (like oversteeped tea), and any less resulted in a drink that was too dairy-forward. Instead of sugar, we sweetened our milk with honey because it balanced the earthy turmeric. We enjoyed trying out additional ingredients that paired nicely with the turmeric and found black pepper and ginger to be exciting add-ins thanks to their invigorating flavors and antioxidant load. Once we added additional aromatics, a short steep time was necessary to draw out their flavors.

2 cups whole milk
2 teaspoons ground turmeric
2 teaspoons honey

Bring milk to simmer in small saucepan over medium-high heat. Off heat, whisk in turmeric and honey until fully combined. Strain into serving mugs, discarding solids. Serve.

VARIATIONS

Haldhicha Dudh with Black Pepper
Add 1 teaspoon cracked black peppercorns with turmeric and honey. Let steep, covered, for 5 minutes before straining and serving.

Haldhicha Dudh with Ginger
Add 1 teaspoon grated fresh ginger with turmeric and honey. Let steep, covered, for 5 minutes before straining and serving.

Switchel

serves 6 to 8 • total time: 15 minutes, plus 7 hours cooling and chilling

why this recipe works • You could consider switchel to be the original energy drink or health tonic, since both cider vinegar and maple syrup contain potassium, an electrolyte, and ginger contains gingerol, an anti-inflammatory compound. Traditionally served to farmers working in the fields during haying season, it is sometimes referred to as "haymaker's punch" and is still served in some Amish communities. We liked the balance of ¾ cup cider vinegar to ½ cup maple syrup. Two tablespoons of grated fresh ginger contributed the spicy warmth we were looking for without overpowering the delicate maple flavor. Last but not least, some rolled oats provided hearty body. The longer you let the switchel chill before straining, the stronger the ginger flavor will be. Feel free to adjust the tartness with water to suit your taste.

    6   cups water
    ¾   cup cider vinegar
    ½   cup pure maple syrup
    ¼   cup old-fashioned rolled oats
    2   tablespoons grated fresh ginger
    1   teaspoon grated lemon zest, plus lemon slices for garnish
    ¼   teaspoon table salt

1 Bring all ingredients to brief simmer in large saucepan over medium-high heat. Let cool to room temperature, about 1 hour. Transfer switchel to bowl, cover, and refrigerate until flavors meld, at least 6 or up to 24 hours.

2 Strain mixture through fine-mesh strainer set over serving pitcher or large container, pressing on solids to extract as much liquid as possible; discard solids. Serve in chilled old-fashioned glasses or Mason jars filled with ice, garnishing individual portions with lemon slices.

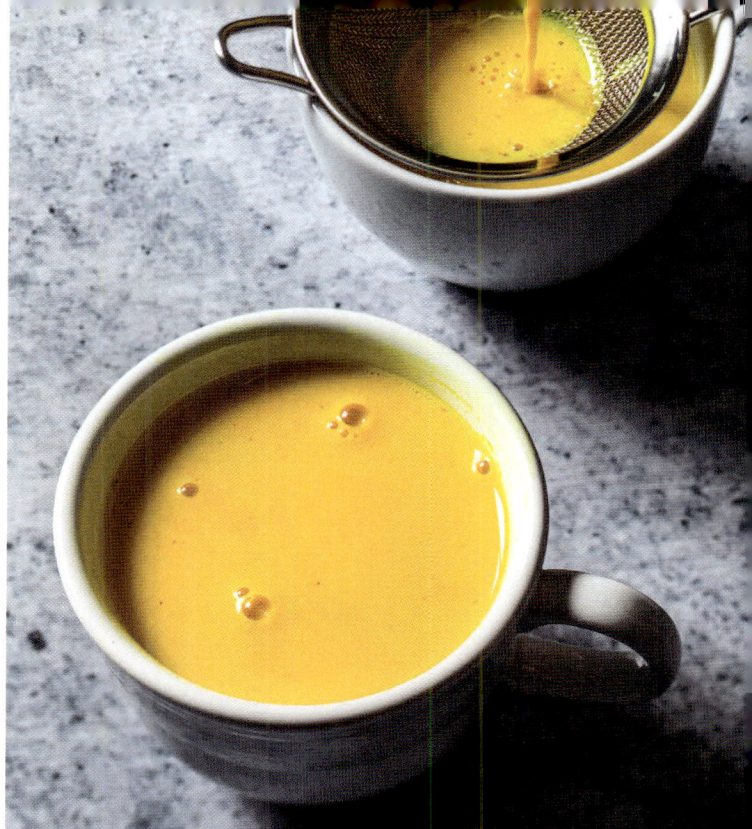

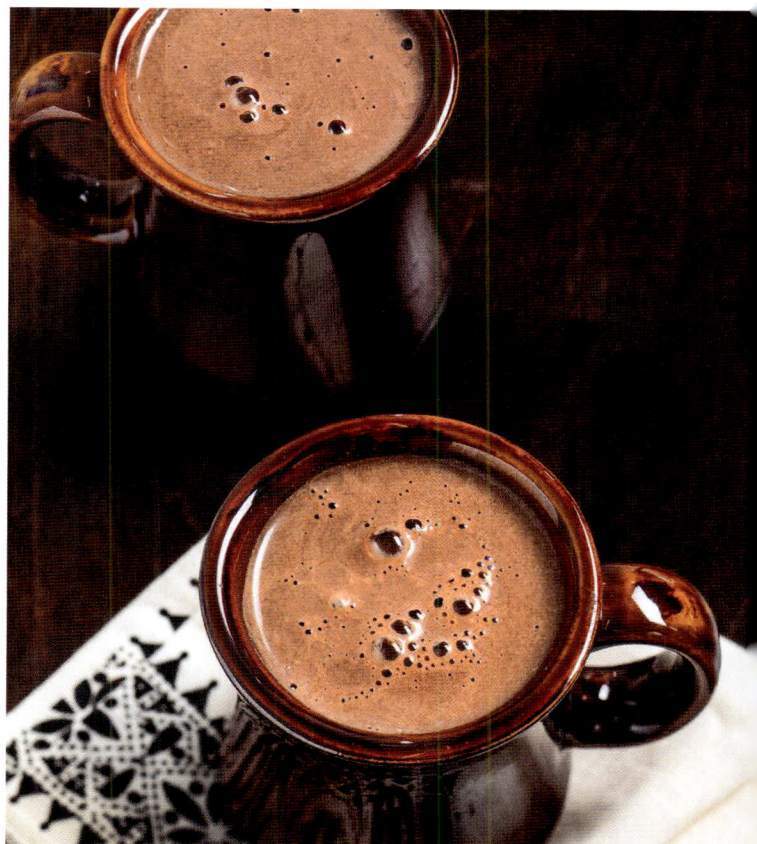

top	*Haldhicha Dudh*
bottom	*Raw Hot Chocolate*

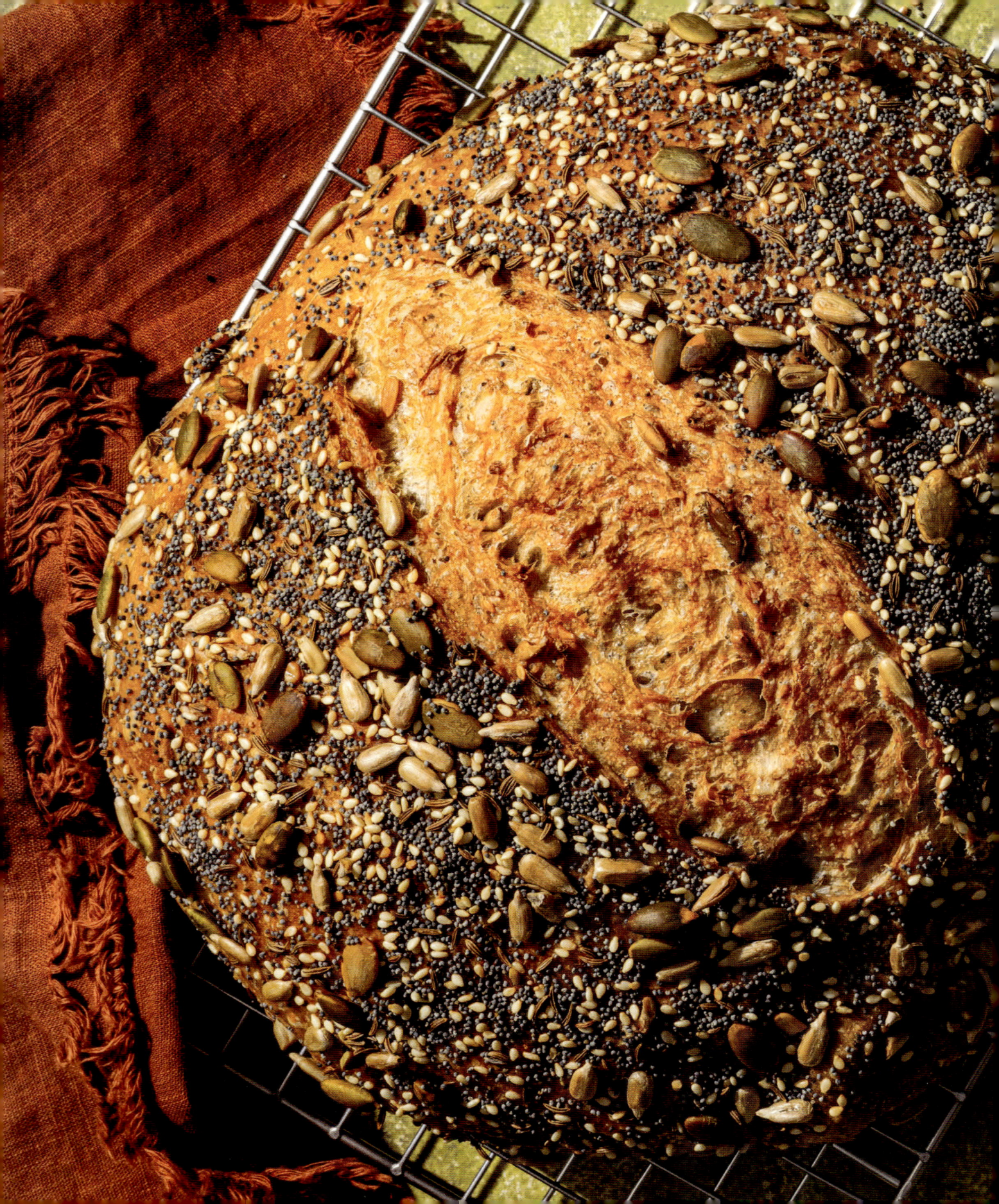

BREADS

Nutrition Knowledge   Thanks to an extended fermentation process, our no-knead loaves are easier to digest and may be gentler on the gut than kneaded breads. The slow rise breaks down gluten and phytic acid, helping your body absorb more nutrients and supporting more stable energy. Plus, they're totally hands-off—just time doing the work for you.   *—Alicia*

■ FAST   ■ SUPERCHARGED

Flourless Nut and Seed Loaf

makes 1 loaf • total time: 1½ hours, plus 4 hours resting and cooling **SUPERCHARGED**

why this recipe works • Flourless nut and seed loaves have gained popularity for a reason: They're high in protein and all-around nutritious, with hearty bite. A slice, toasted and slathered with a nut or seed butter rich in beneficial fats, or some fruit preserves, makes a quick and easy anti-inflammatory breakfast. To start, we toasted the nuts and seeds—a heart-healthy combination of sunflower seeds, sliced almonds, and pepitas—to amplify their flavor. To bind them, we combined oats with flaxseeds and powdered psyllium husk, which, when hydrated, created a gel with strong binding properties. Maple syrup added subtle sweetness. To ensure that the bread stayed together, we let the dough hydrate for a couple hours in the pan before baking. Fully baking this bread in the pan resulted in a wet loaf; to fix this, we baked the loaf for 20 minutes to let the outside set and then turned it out to finish baking free-form. The test kitchen's preferred loaf pan measures 8½ by 4½ inches; if you use a 9 by 5-inch loaf pan, start checking for doneness 5 minutes earlier than advised in the recipe.

    1 cup raw sunflower seeds
    1 cup sliced almonds
    ½ cup raw unsalted pepitas
 1¾ cups (5¼ ounces) old-fashioned rolled oats
    ¼ cup whole flaxseeds
    3 tablespoons powdered psyllium husk
 1½ cups (12 ounces) water
    3 tablespoons extra-virgin olive oil
    2 tablespoons maple syrup
    ¾ teaspoon table salt

1 Adjust oven rack to middle position and heat oven to 350 degrees. Line bottom of 8½ by 4½-inch loaf pan with parchment paper and spray with avocado oil spray. Combine sunflower seeds, almonds, and pepitas on rimmed baking sheet and bake, stirring occasionally, until lightly browned, 10 to 12 minutes. Transfer to bowl and let cool slightly, about 5 minutes.

2 Stir oats, flaxseeds, and psyllium into bowl with toasted seed-nut mixture. Whisk water, oil, maple syrup, and salt in second bowl until well combined. Using silicone spatula, stir water mixture into nut-seed mixture, then transfer to prepared pan. Using your wet hands, press dough into corners of pan and smooth top.

3 Cover loosely with plastic wrap and let sit at room temperature until mixture is fully hydrated and cohesive, about 2 hours.

4 Adjust oven rack to middle position and heat oven to 350 degrees. Remove plastic and bake loaf for 20 minutes. Invert loaf onto wire rack set in rimmed baking sheet. Remove loaf pan and discard parchment. Bake loaf (still inverted) until deep golden brown and loaf sounds hollow when tapped, 35 to 45 minutes. Let loaf cool completely on wire rack, about 2 hours. Slice and serve.

Soda Bread with Nuts and Cacao Nibs

makes 1 loaf • total time: 1¼ hours, plus 1 hour cooling

why this recipe works • What you usually find in the United States as "Irish soda bread" is a fairly sweet white bread made with butter, eggs, raisins, and caraway seeds. While delicious, it's not actually Irish. Traditional Irish soda bread, made with whole-wheat flour and without raisins, butter, or eggs, is the simple, savory counterpart to its sweeter Americanized cousin. It's craggy, hearty, and nutty, perfect for enjoying alongside soup or a cup of tea. Our rendition is true to this whole-wheat, not-sweet Irish ethos. Adding both wheat bran and wheat germ to the flour mixture created complex flavor and a rustic, coarse texture—not to mention a more fiber-rich end result. We did still take some decidedly nontraditional liberties with the mix-ins, studding the bread with toasted walnuts and cacao nibs for a dose of beneficial fats. The cacao nibs provided the intense flavor of chocolate without any sweetness. The dough came together in just one bowl and required a bare minimum of shaping.

    2 cups (11 ounces) whole-wheat flour
    1 cup (5 ounces) all-purpose flour
    1 cup wheat bran
    ¼ cup wheat germ
    2 teaspoons sugar
 1½ teaspoons baking powder
 1½ teaspoons baking soda
    1 teaspoon table salt
    2 cups (16 ounces) buttermilk
    1 cup walnuts, toasted and chopped
    6 tablespoons cacao nibs

1 Adjust oven rack to middle position and heat oven to 375 degrees. Lightly grease 8-inch round cake pan.

2 Whisk whole-wheat flour, all-purpose flour, wheat bran, wheat germ, sugar, baking powder, baking soda, and salt together in large bowl. Stir in buttermilk, walnuts, and cacao nibs until all flour is moistened and dough forms soft, ragged mass.

3 Transfer dough to counter and gently shape into 6-inch round (surface will be craggy). Using serrated knife, cut ½-inch-deep cross about 5 inches long on top of loaf. Transfer to prepared pan.

4 Bake until loaf is lightly browned and center registers 185 degrees, 50 minutes to 1 hour, rotating pan halfway through baking. Remove bread from pan and let cool on wire rack for at least 1 hour. Slice and serve.

Oatmeal Dinner Rolls

makes 12 rolls · total time: 1½ hours, plus 2 hours rising and cooling

why this recipe works · These delightfully homey rolls avoid the dense texture that both whole-wheat flour and oats can create. We started by soaking old-fashioned oats in boiling water. During a short rest the oats absorbed most of the water (and turned to meal), effectively hiding extra moisture in this dough, which turned to steam in the oven. The resulting rolls turned out unexpectedly fluffy and plush. For this strategy, we drew inspiration from the tangzhong method—a Chinese technique that involves cooking a portion of flour and liquid into a thick paste before adding it to the rest of the dough—but let the oats, rather than flour, do the absorbing. As a bonus, the high hydration of the dough and moisture-holding capabilities of whole grains also extended the rolls' shelf life, so they can be enjoyed for a few days. We supplemented the whole-wheat flour in the dough with white bread flour for structure, and also added molasses, which lent complexity and sweetness to the rolls. Nestling the dough balls close together in a round cake pan ensured that they supported each other in an upward, rather than outward, expansion. For an accurate measurement of boiling water, bring a kettle of water to a boil and then measure out the desired amount. Avoid blackstrap molasses here, as it's too bitter.

- ¾ cup (2¼ ounces) plus 4 teaspoons old-fashioned rolled oats, divided
- ⅔ cup (5⅓ ounces) boiling water plus ½ cup (4 ounces) cold water
- 2 tablespoons unsalted butter, cut into 4 pieces
- 1½ cups (8¼ ounces) bread flour
- ¾ cup (4⅛ ounces) whole-wheat flour
- ¼ cup molasses
- 1½ teaspoons instant or rapid-rise yeast
- 1 teaspoon table salt
- 1 large egg lightly beaten with 1 tablespoon water and pinch table salt

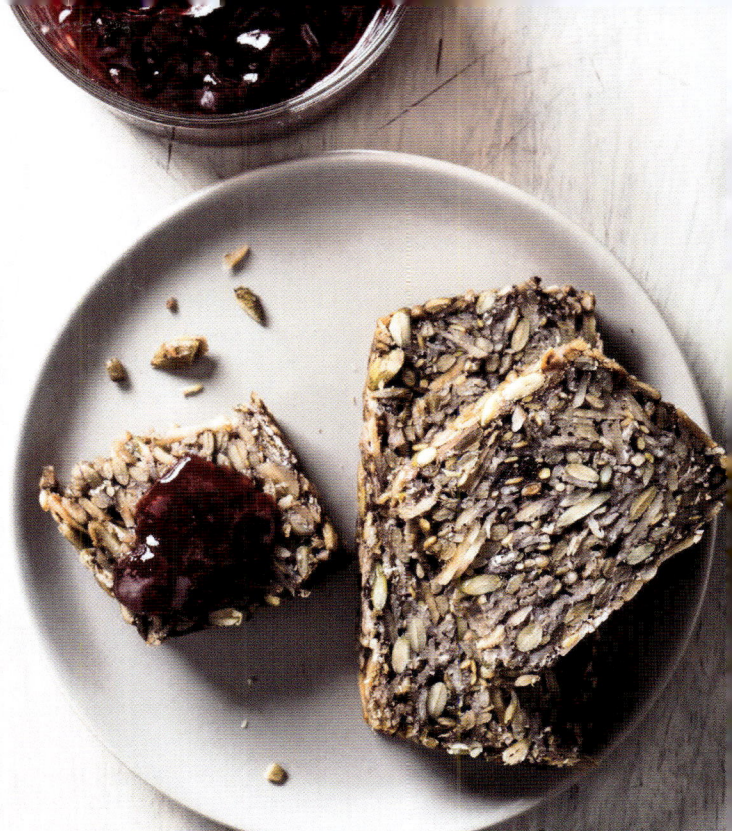

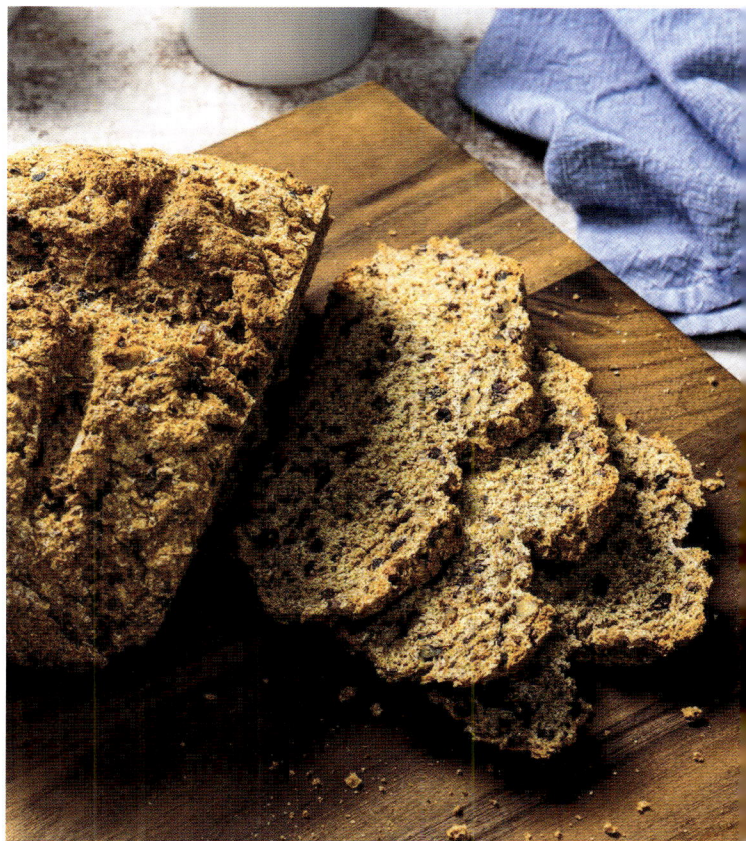

1 Stir ¾ cup oats, boiling water, and butter together in bowl of stand mixer and let sit until butter is melted and most of water has been absorbed, about 10 minutes.

2 Add bread flour, whole-wheat flour, cold water, molasses, yeast, and salt. Using dough hook on low speed, mix until flour is moistened, about 2 minutes (dough may look dry). Increase speed to medium-low and mix until dough clears sides of bowl (it will still stick to bottom), about 8 minutes, scraping down dough hook halfway through mixing (dough will be sticky). Transfer dough to clean counter and knead by hand to form smooth, round ball, about 30 seconds.

3 **First rise** Place dough seam side down in lightly greased large bowl or container, cover with plastic wrap, and let rise unti doubled in volume, 1 to 1½ hours.

4 Grease 9-inch round cake pan. Press down on dough to deflate. Transfer dough to lightly floured counter and pat dough gently into 8-inch square. Cut dough into 12 equal pieces and cover loosely with plastic. Working with 1 piece of dough at a time (keep remaining pieces covered), form each piece into rough ball by stretching dough around your thumb and pinching edges together so that top is smooth. Place ball seam side down on clean counter and, using your cupped hand, drag in small circles until dough feels taut and round. Arrange dough balls seam side down in prepared pan, placing 9 dough balls around edge of pan and remaining 3 dough balls in center.

5 **Second rise** Cover with plastic and let rise until doubled in size, no gaps are visible between rolls, and dough springs back minimally when poked gently with your finger, 45 minutes to 1 hour.

6 Adjust oven rack to lower-middle position and heat oven to 375 degrees. Gently brush rolls with egg wash and sprinkle with remaining 4 teaspoons oats. Bake until rolls are deep brown and register at least 195 degrees, 25 to 30 minutes. Let rolls cool in pan on wire rack for 3 minutes; invert rolls onto rack, then reinvert. Let rolls cool for 20 minutes. Serve warm or at room temperature.

NOTES FROM THE TEST KITCHEN

What is Tangzhong?

Tangzhong, the technique that inspired our Oatmeal Dinner Rolls, is a method traditionally used for Japanese milk bread. We frequently employ it in the test kitchen to create wetter doughs that remain easy to handle and aren't overly sticky. The tangzhong method involves briefly cooking a portion of the bread's flour and water to make a thick, pudding-like paste, which is then combined with the rest of the ingredients. This paste allows you to add even more liquid to the dough without making it sticky, since flour can absorb about twice as much hot water as it can cold. The technique is especially handy for rolled or braided creations that need workability, and for incredibly fluffy, tender dinner rolls. The extra water also converts to steam in the oven, contributing to rise and creating a lighter crumb. The added hydration also increases gluten development, giving the bread the structure it needs to trap steam effectively rather than letting it escape. The end result is exceptionally soft, moist bread—something particularly helpful when working with whole-wheat flours.

Whole-Wheat Oatmeal Loaf

makes 1 loaf · total time: 1¾ hours, plus 5 hours rising and cooling

why this recipe works · Our Oatmeal Dinner Rolls (page 411) are a favorite for us. We decided to take that dough and bake it in a loaf pan: With a soft crumb, a sweet wheat-and-oat flavor, and a pretty exterior, it's ideal for dressing up sandwiches (and getting in whole grains at lunch to boot). The sandwich bread is just as plush and delicious as the rolls—and available by the slice. For an accurate measurement of boiling water, bring a kettle of water to a boil and then measure out the desired amount. We strongly recommend measuring the flour by weight. Avoid blackstrap molasses here, as it's too bitter. The test kitchen's preferred loaf pan measures 8½ by 4½ inches; if you use a 9 by 5-inch loaf pan, increase the shaped rising time and start checking for doneness 10 minutes earlier than advised in the recipe.

¾ cup (2¼ ounces) plus 4 teaspoons old-fashioned rolled oats, divided

⅔ cup (5⅓ ounces) boiling water plus ½ cup (4 ounces) water, room temperature

2 tablespoons unsalted butter, cut into 4 pieces

1½ cups (8¼ ounces) bread flour

¾ cup (4⅛ ounces) whole-wheat flour

¼ cup molasses

1½ teaspoons instant or rapid-rise yeast

1 teaspoon table salt

1 Stir ¾ cup oats, boiling water, and butter together in bowl of stand mixer and let sit until butter is melted and most of water has been absorbed, about 10 minutes.

2 Add bread flour, whole-wheat flour, room temperature water, molasses, yeast, and salt. Using dough hook on low speed, mix until cohesive dough starts to form and no dry flour remains, about 2 minutes, scraping down sides of bowl as needed (dough may look dry). Increase speed to medium-low and mix until dough clears sides of bowl (it will still stick to bottom), about 8 minutes, scraping down dough hook halfway through mixing (dough will be sticky). Transfer dough to lightly floured counter and knead to form smooth, round ball, about 30 seconds.

3 **First rise** Place dough seam side down in lightly greased large bowl or container, cover tightly with plastic wrap, and let rise until doubled in volume, 1 to 1½ hours.

4 Grease 8½ by 4½-inch loaf pan. Press down on dough to deflate. Transfer dough to lightly floured counter (side of dough that was against bowl should now be facing up). Press and stretch dough into 8 by 6-inch rectangle, with long side parallel to counter edge. Roll dough away from you into firm cylinder, keeping roll taut by tucking it under itself as you go. Pinch seam closed and place loaf seam side down in prepared pan, tucking ends as needed to match size of pan and pressing dough gently into corners.

5 **Second rise** Cover loosely with greased plastic and let rise until loaf reaches ½ inch above lip of pan at lowest point and dough springs back minimally when poked gently with your finger, about 1 hour.

6 Adjust oven rack to lower-middle position and heat oven to 350 degrees. Mist loaf with water and sprinkle with remaining 4 teaspoons oats. Bake until loaf is deep golden brown and registers at least 205 degrees, 35 to 40 minutes, rotating pan halfway through baking. Let loaf cool in pan for 15 minutes. Remove loaf from pan and let cool completely on wire rack, about 3 hours, before slicing and serving.

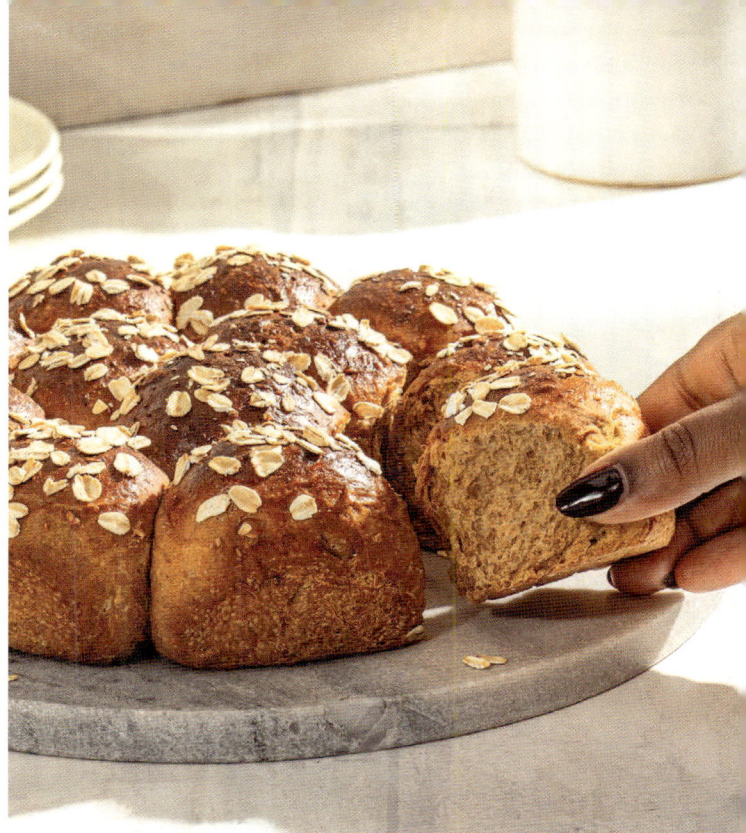

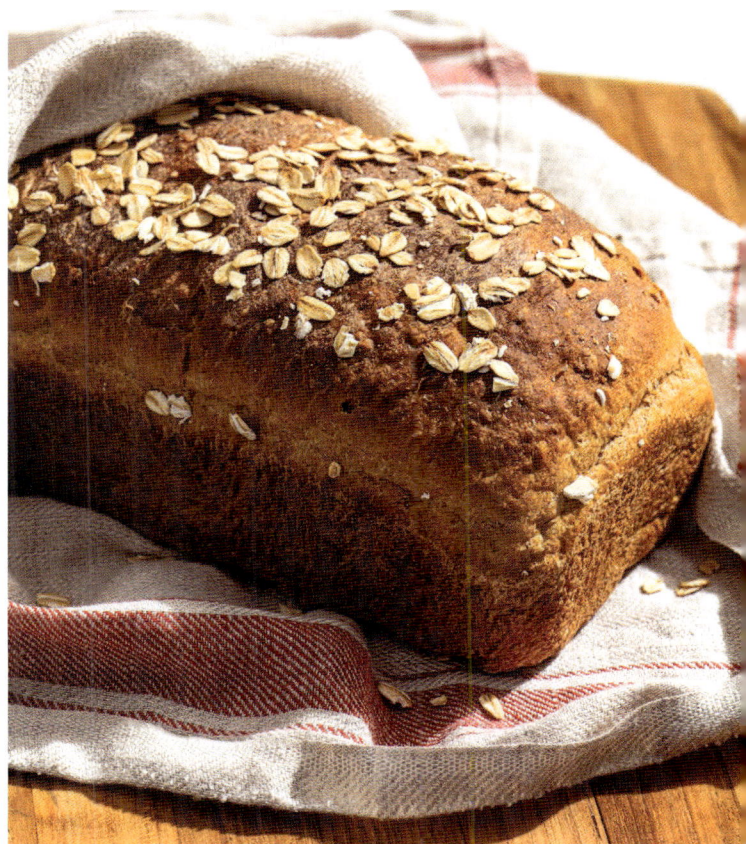

top | *Oatmeal Dinner Rolls*

bottom | *Whole-Wheat Oatmeal Loaf*

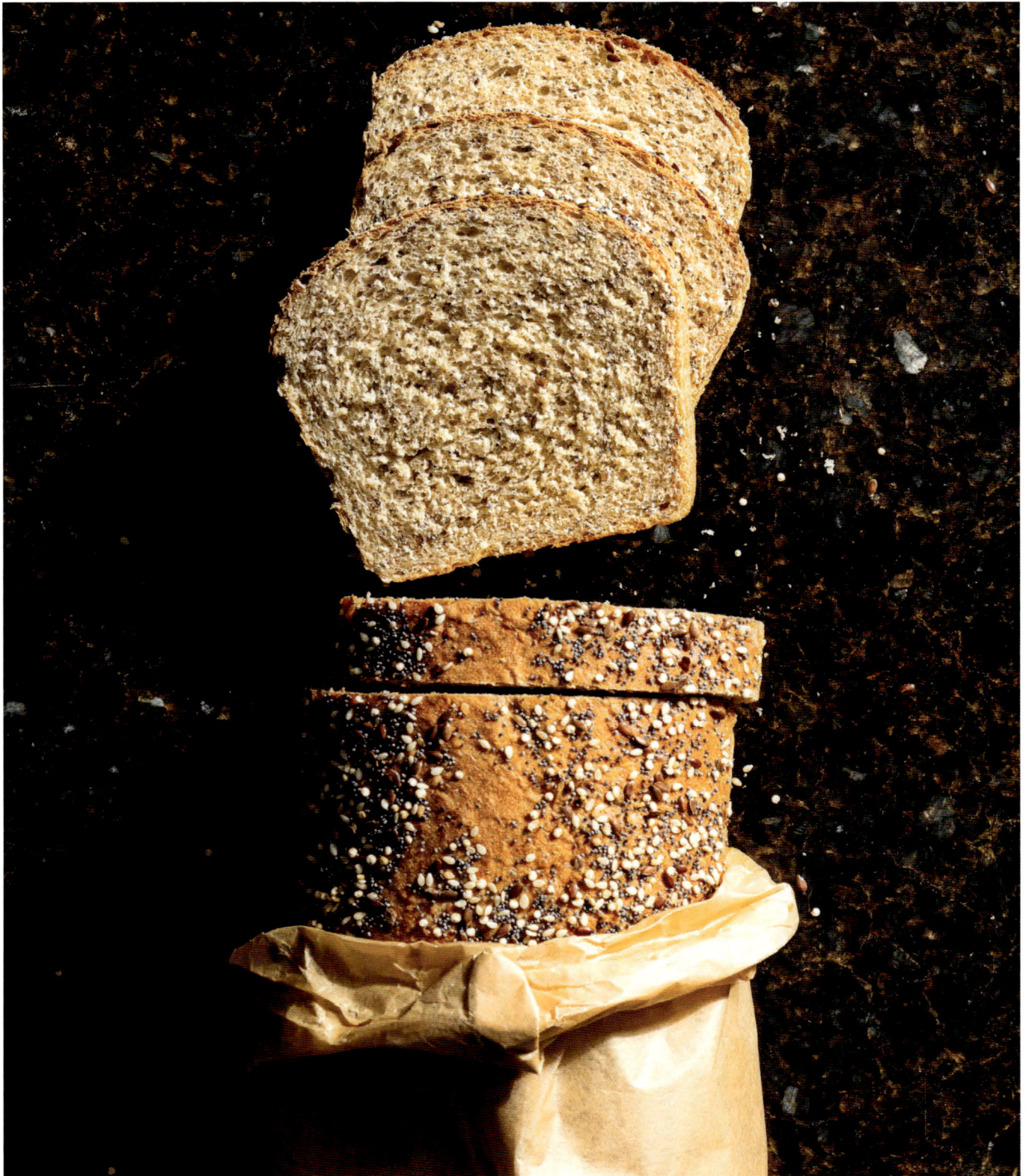

Quinoa Whole-Wheat Bread

Quinoa Whole-Wheat Bread

makes 1 loaf · total time: 2 hours, plus 5½ hours rising and cooling

why this recipe works · This hearty sandwich bread made with quinoa, whole-wheat flour, and flax, poppy, and sesame seeds will jump-start your day with fiber and protein. Cooking the quinoa in the microwave before adding it to the dough prevented it from sucking up moisture from the loaf, giving us a pleasantly chewy yet tender bread. A quarter-cup of seeds stirred into the dough added fun crunch that kept this loaf from being stodgy. We like the convenience of prewashed quinoa; rinsing removes the quinoa's bitter protective coating (called saponin). If you buy unwashed quinoa, rinse it and then spread it out on a clean dish towel to dry for 15 minutes. The test kitchen's preferred loaf pan measures 8½ by 4½ inches; if you use a 9 by 5-inch loaf pan, increase the shaped rising time and start checking for doneness 10 minutes earlier than advised in the recipe.

    1   cup (8 ounces) water, room temperature, divided
    ⅓   cup (1¾ ounces) plus 1 teaspoon prewashed white quinoa, divided
    1⅔ cups (9⅛ ounces) bread flour
    1   cup (5½ ounces) whole-wheat flour
    2   tablespoons plus 1 teaspoon flaxseeds, divided
    1   tablespoon plus 1 teaspoon poppy seeds, divided
    1   tablespoon plus 1 teaspoon sesame seeds, divided
    2   teaspoons instant or rapid-rise yeast
    1½ teaspoons table salt
    ¾   cup (6 ounces) whole milk, room temperature
    2   tablespoons honey
    1   tablespoon avocado oil
    1   large egg lightly beaten with 1 tablespoon water and pinch table salt

1 Microwave ¾ cup water and ⅓ cup quinoa in covered bowl at 50 percent power until water is almost completely absorbed, 8 to 12 minutes, stirring halfway through microwaving. Uncover quinoa and let sit until cooled slightly and water is completely absorbed, about 10 minutes.

2 Whisk bread flour, whole-wheat flour, 2 tablespoons flaxseeds, 1 tablespoon poppy seeds, 1 tablespoon sesame seeds, yeast, and salt together in bowl of stand mixer. Whisk milk, honey, oil, and remaining ¼ cup water in 4-cup liquid measuring cup until honey has dissolved, then whisk in cooked quinoa. Using dough hook on low speed, slowly add milk-quinoa mixture to flour mixture and mix until cohesive dough starts to form and no dry flour remains, about 2 minutes, scraping down bowl as needed. Increase speed

to medium-low and knead until dough is elastic but still sticky, about 8 minutes. Transfer dough to lightly floured counter and knead by hand to form smooth, round ball, about 30 seconds.

3 First rise Place dough seam side down in lightly greased large bowl or container, cover bowl with plastic wrap, and let rise until doubled in volume, 1½ to 2 hours.

4 Grease 8½ by 4½-inch loaf pan. Press down on dough to deflate. Transfer dough to lightly floured counter (side of dough that was against bowl should now be facing up) and press into 8 by 6-inch rectangle, with long side parallel to counter edge. Roll dough away from you into firm cylinder, keeping roll taut by tucking it under itself as you go. Pinch seam closed, then place loaf seam side down in prepared pan, tucking ends as needed to match size of pan and pressing dough gently into corners.

5 Second rise Cover dough loosely with greased plastic and let rise until loaf reaches 1 inch above lip of pan at lowest point and dough springs back minimally when poked gently with your finger, 1 to 1½ hours.

6 Adjust oven rack to lower-middle position and heat oven to 350 degrees. Combine remaining 1 teaspoon quinoa, 1 teaspoon flaxseeds, 1 teaspoon poppy seeds, and 1 teaspoon sesame seeds in bowl. Brush loaf gently with egg wash and sprinkle with quinoa mixture. Bake until loaf is golden brown and registers at least 205 degrees, 45 to 50 minutes, rotating pan halfway through baking. Let loaf cool in pan for 15 minutes. Remove loaf from pan and let cool completely on wire rack, about 3 hours, before slicing and serving.

No-Knead Whole-Wheat Rustic Loaf

makes 1 loaf · total time: 1¾ hours, plus 12 hours rising and cooling

why this recipe works · The nutty complexity of whole-wheat flour in a rustic loaf produces a textural delight. But whole-wheat flour can be challenging to work with because it results in lower gluten development. Our solution was to replace only a third of the flour in one of our no-knead loaves with whole-wheat flour and increase the hydration; this produced a light, moist bread with a chewy crust. We prefer King Arthur brand bread flour in this recipe; the dough will be slightly stickier if you use a lower-protein bread flour. While we prefer the flavor that beer adds, you can substitute an equal amount of water. You will need a bowl that is at least 9 inches wide and 4 inches deep to cover the dough in step 6.

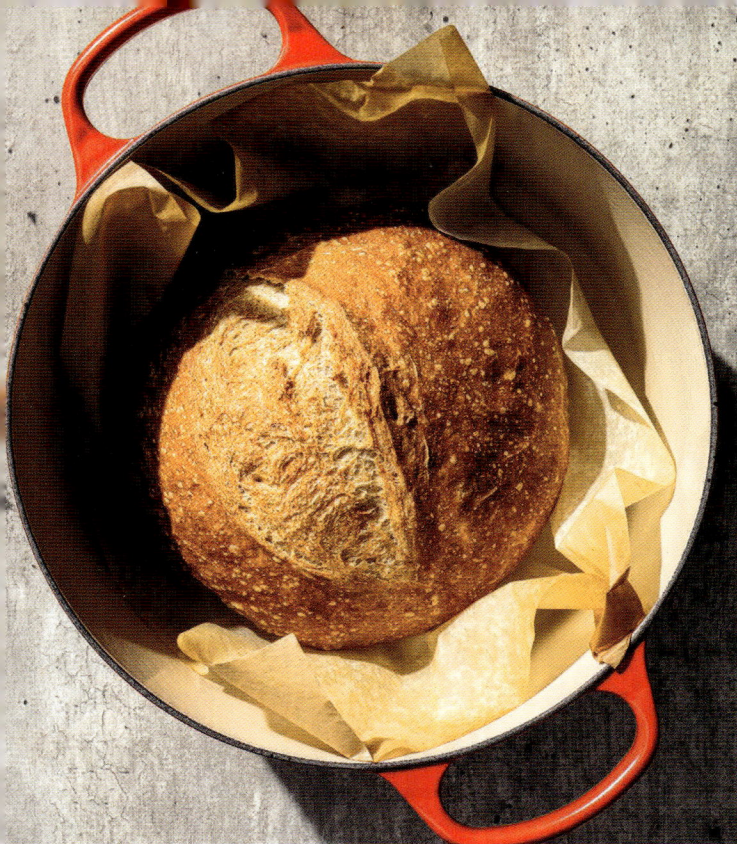

2 cups (11 ounces) bread flour
1 cup (5½ ounces) whole-wheat flour
1½ teaspoons table salt
¼ teaspoon instant or rapid-rise yeast
1 cup (8 ounces) water, room temperature
½ cup (4 ounces) mild lager, room temperature
1 tablespoon distilled white vinegar

1 Whisk bread flour, whole-wheat flour, salt, and yeast together in large bowl. Using silicone spatula, fold water, beer, and vinegar into flour mixture, scraping up dry flour from bottom of bowl and pressing dough until cohesive and shaggy and all flour is incorporated.

2 **First rise** Cover bowl tightly with plastic wrap and let sit at room temperature for at least 8 hours or up to 18 hours.

3 Using greased bowl scraper or your wet fingertips, fold dough over itself by lifting and folding edge of dough toward middle and pressing to seal. Turn bowl 90 degrees and fold dough again; repeat turning bowl and folding dough 6 more times (for a total of 8 folds). Flip dough seam side down in bowl, cover with plastic, and let rest for 15 minutes.

4 Lay 18 by 12-inch sheet of parchment paper on counter and spray lightly with avocado oil spray. Transfer dough seam side up onto lightly floured counter and pat into rough 9-inch circle using your lightly floured hands. Using bowl scraper or your floured fingertips, lift and fold edge of dough toward center, pressing to seal. Repeat 5 more times (for a total of 6 folds), evenly spacing folds around circumference of dough. Press down on dough to seal, then use bench scraper to gently flip dough seam side down.

5 Using both hands, cup side of dough furthest away from you and pull dough toward you, keeping pinky fingers and side of palm in contact with counter and applying slight pressure to dough as it drags to create tension. (If dough slides across surface of counter without rolling, remove excess flour. If dough sticks to counter or your hands, lightly sprinkle counter or hands with flour.) Rotate dough ball 90 degrees, reposition dough ball at top of counter, and repeat pulling dough until taut round ball forms, at least 4 more times. Using your floured hands or bench scraper, transfer dough seam side down to center of prepared parchment.

6 **Second rise** Cover dough with inverted large bowl. Let rise until dough has doubled in size and dough springs back minimally when poked gently with your finger, 1 to 2 hours.

7 Thirty minutes before baking, adjust oven rack to middle position, place Dutch oven with lid on rack and heat oven to

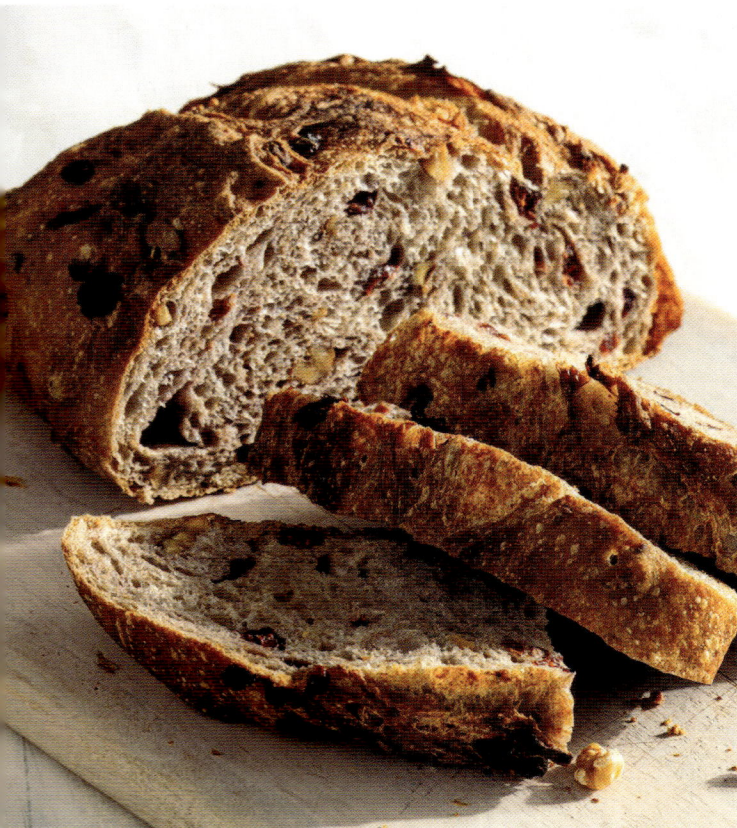

475 degrees. Using sharp knife or single-edge razor blade, make one 6-inch-long, ½-inch-deep slash with swift, fluid motion along top of loaf. Carefully remove hot pot from oven and, using parchment as sling, gently transfer dough to hot pot. Working quickly and reinforcing score in top of loaf if needed, cover pot and return to oven.

8 Reduce oven temperature to 425 degrees and bake loaf in covered pot for 30 minutes. Remove lid and continue to bake until loaf is deep golden brown and registers at least 205 degrees, 10 to 15 minutes. Using parchment sling, carefully remove loaf from hot pot and transfer to wire rack; discard parchment. Let cool completely, about 3 hours, before slicing and serving.

No-Knead Cranberry-Walnut Bread

makes 1 loaf · total time: 1¾ hours, plus 12 hours rising and cooling

why this recipe works · Tart dried cranberries and rich walnuts stud this hearty, chewy loaf that tastes equally delicious toasted and slathered with nut butter for breakfast or sandwiched with meat and cheese for a hearty lunch. For the best distribution of cranberries and walnuts, we added them at the mixing stage, toasting the walnuts first to bring out their nuttiness. Using a combination of bread flour and whole-wheat flour created the chewy yet hearty texture we wanted, and incorporating a bit more water than in our regular whole-wheat loaf kept the crumb moist and tender even when adding a generous amount of thirsty dried fruit. We prefer King Arthur brand bread flour in this recipe; the dough will be slightly stickier if you use a lower-protein bread flour. You will need a bowl that is at least 9 inches wide and 4 inches deep to cover the dough in step 6.

- 2 cups (11 ounces) bread flour
- 1 cup (5½ ounces) whole-wheat flour
- ½ cup dried cranberries
- ½ cup walnuts, toasted and chopped
- 1½ teaspoons table salt
- ¼ teaspoon instant or rapid-rise yeast
- 1½ cups plus 2 tablespoons (13 ounces) water, room temperature
- 1 tablespoon distilled white vinegar

1 Whisk bread flour, whole-wheat flour, cranberries, walnuts, salt, and yeast together in large bowl. Using silicone spatula, fold water and vinegar into flour mixture, scraping up dry flour from bottom of bowl and pressing dough until cohesive and shaggy and all flour is incorporated.

2 **First rise** Cover bowl tightly with plastic wrap and let sit at room temperature for at least 8 hours or up to 18 hours.

3 Using greased bowl scraper or your wet fingertips, fold dough over itself by lifting and folding edge of dough toward middle and pressing to seal. Turn bowl 90 degrees and fold dough again; repeat turning bowl and folding dough 6 more times (for a total of 8 folds). Flip dough seam side down in bowl, cover with plastic, and let rest for 15 minutes.

4 Lay 18 by 12-inch sheet of parchment paper on counter and spray lightly with avocado oil spray. Transfer dough seam side up onto lightly floured counter and pat into rough 9-inch circle using your lightly floured hands. Using bowl scraper or your floured fingertips, lift and fold edge of dough toward center, pressing to seal. Repeat 5 more times (for a total of 6 folds), evenly spacing folds around circumference of dough. Press down on dough to seal, then use bench scraper to gently flip dough seam side down.

5 Using both hands, cup side of dough furthest away from you and pull dough toward you, keeping pinky fingers and side of palm in contact with counter and applying slight pressure to dough as it drags to create tension. (If dough slides across surface of counter without rolling, remove excess flour. If dough sticks to counter or your hands, lightly sprinkle counter or hands with flour.) Rotate dough ball 90 degrees, reposition dough ball at top of counter, and repeat pulling dough until taut round ball forms, at least 4 more times. Using your floured hands or bench scraper, transfer dough seam side down to center of prepared parchment.

6 **Second rise** Cover dough with inverted large bowl. Let rise until dough has doubled in size and dough springs back minimally when poked gently with your finger, 1 to 2 hours.

7 Thirty minutes before baking, adjust oven rack to middle position, place Dutch oven with lid on rack, and heat oven to 475 degrees. Using sharp knife or single-edge razor blade, make one 6-inch-long, ½-inch-deep slash with swift, fluid motion along top of loaf. Carefully remove hot pot from oven and, using parchment as sling, gently transfer dough to hot pot. Working quickly and reinforcing score in top of loaf if needed, cover pot and return to oven.

8 Reduce oven temperature to 425 degrees and bake loaf in covered pot for 30 minutes. Remove lid and continue to bake until loaf is deep golden brown and registers at least 205 degrees, 10 to 15 minutes. Using parchment sling, carefully remove loaf from hot pot and transfer to wire rack; discard parchment. Let cool completely, about 3 hours, before slicing and serving.

No-Knead Seeded Oat Bread

makes 1 loaf · total time: 2¼ hours, plus 12 hours rising and cooling **SUPERCHARGED**

why this recipe works · We love this superlatively nourishing loaf that delivers plenty of anti-inflammatory ingredients in every bite. We packed in three star players: oats, a medley of seeds, and whole-wheat flour. But so many water-hungry components can lead to an overly dense loaf; to avoid this, we hydrated old-fashioned rolled oats with boiling water and upped the overall hydration of the loaf. For the best distribution of seeds, we incorporated toasted seeds during mixing and then covered the loaf with more seeds for nutty crunch. This is a hearty bread you can really sink your teeth into, yet it still maintains the moist texture and springy crumb of a proper rustic loaf. We prefer King Arthur brand bread flour in this recipe; the dough will be slightly stickier if you use a lower-protein bread flour. While we prefer the flavor that beer adds, you can substitute an equal amount of water. You will need a bowl that is at least 9 inches wide and 4 inches deep to cover the dough in step 7. For an accurate measurement of boiling water, bring a kettle of water to a boil and then measure out the desired amount.

- 3 tablespoons raw pepitas
- 3 tablespoons raw sunflower seeds
- 4 teaspoons sesame seeds
- 4 teaspoons poppy seeds
- 2 teaspoons caraway seeds
- ⅔ cup (2 ounces) old-fashioned rolled oats
- ½ cup (4 ounces) boiling water plus ¾ cup (6 ounces) water, room temperature
- ½ cup (4 ounces) mild lager, room temperature
- 1 tablespoon distilled white vinegar
- 2 cups (11 ounces) bread flour
- ⅔ cup (3⅔ ounces) whole-wheat flour
- 1½ teaspoons table salt
- ¼ teaspoon instant or rapid-rise yeast

1 Adjust oven rack to middle position and heat oven to 325 degrees. Combine pepitas, sunflower seeds, sesame seeds, poppy seeds, and caraway seeds in bowl. Measure out 6 tablespoons seed mixture, spread into even layer on rimmed baking sheet, and roast until seeds are lightly golden and fragrant, about 10 minutes. Transfer to wire rack and set aside to cool for 15 minutes. Reserve remaining untoasted seed mixture.

2 Meanwhile, combine oats and boiling water in medium bowl; let sit until water is absorbed and oats have cooled to room temperature, about 15 minutes. Stir in room-temperature water, beer, and vinegar. Whisk bread flour, whole-wheat flour, salt, yeast, and cooled toasted seed mixture together in large bowl. Using silicone spatula, fold oat mixture into flour mixture, scraping up dry flour from bottom of bowl and pressing dough until cohesive and shaggy and all flour is incorporated.

3 First rise Cover bowl tightly with plastic wrap and let sit at room temperature for at least 8 hours or up to 18 hours.

4 Using greased bowl scraper or your wet fingertips, fold dough over itself by lifting and folding edge of dough toward middle and pressing to seal. Turn bowl 90 degrees and fold dough again; repeat turning bowl and folding dough 6 more times (for a total of 8 folds). Flip dough seam side down in bowl, cover with plastic, and let rest for 15 minutes.

5 Lay 18 by 12-inch sheet of parchment paper on counter and spray lightly with avocado oil spray. Transfer dough seam side up onto lightly floured counter and pat into rough 9-inch circle using your lightly floured hands. Using bowl scraper or your floured fingertips, lift and fold edge of dough toward center, pressing to seal. Repeat 5 more times (for a total of 6 folds), evenly spacing folds around circumference of dough. Press down on dough to seal, then use bench scraper to gently flip dough seam side down.

6 Using both hands, cup side of dough furthest away from you and pull dough toward you, keeping pinky fingers and side of palm in contact with counter and applying slight pressure to dough as it drags to create tension. (If dough slides across surface of counter without rolling, remove excess flour. If dough sticks to counter or your hands, lightly sprinkle counter or hands with flour.) Rotate dough ball 90 degrees, reposition dough ball at top of counter, and repeat pulling dough until taut round ball forms, at least 4 more times. Using your floured hands or bench scraper, transfer dough seam side down to center of prepared parchment, then spray or gently brush top of loaf with water. Sprinkle reserved untoasted seed mixture over top and use your hands to gently press seeds onto sides of loaf.

7 Second rise Cover dough with inverted large bowl. Let rise until dough has doubled in size and dough springs back minimally when poked gently with your finger, 1 to 2 hours.

8 Thirty minutes before baking, adjust oven rack to middle position, place Dutch oven with lid on rack, and heat oven to 475 degrees. Using sharp knife or single-edge razor blade, make one 6-inch-long, ½-inch-deep slash with swift, fluid motion along top of loaf. Carefully remove hot pot from oven and, using parchment as sling, gently transfer dough to hot pot. Working quickly and reinforcing score in top of loaf if needed, cover pot and return to oven.

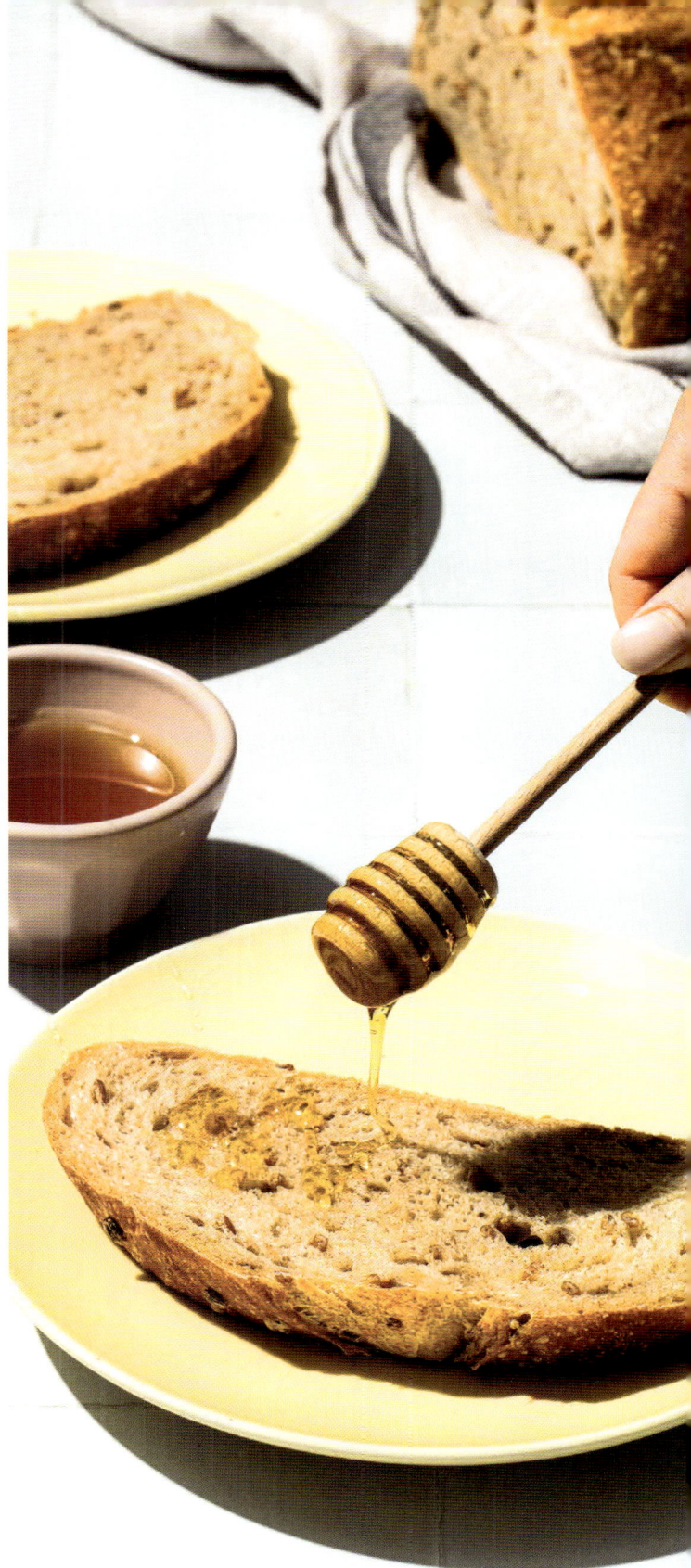

9 Reduce oven temperature to 425 degrees and bake loaf in covered pot for 30 minutes. Remove lid and continue to bake until loaf is deep golden brown and registers at least 205 degrees, 10 to 15 minutes. Using parchment sling, carefully remove loaf from hot pot and transfer to wire rack; discard parchment. Let cool completely, about 3 hours, before slicing and serving.

No-Knead Sprouted Wheat Berry Bread

makes 1 loaf · total time: 1¾ hours, plus 44 hours sprouting, rising, and cooling

why this recipe works · Sprouted grains have nutritional benefits beyond common whole-grain flour, plus a wholesome flavor and texture. When grains begin to sprout, or germinate, their digestibility increases dramatically. In our quest for the ideal sprouted grain to use in our bread, we tried quinoa, millet, lentils, buckwheat, and wheat berries. We chose wheat berries for their exceptionally nutty flavor and pleasant chew. We also employed sprouted wheat flour: Apart from adding nutrition, sprouted grain flours have a longer shelf life and initiate higher enzymatic activity, breaking down more starches in the dough into fermentable sugars for the yeast to feed on. What that meant for our loaf was increased volume and a more open and soft crumb. A touch of honey balanced the earthy flavors of the whole grains. If you can't find sprouted wheat flour, you can use traditional whole-wheat flour. We prefer King Arthur brand bread flour in this recipe; the dough will be slightly stickier if you use a lower-protein bread flour. While we prefer the flavor that beer adds, you can substitute an equal amount of water. You will need a bowl that is at least 9 inches wide and 4 inches deep to cover the dough in step 7. You will need filtered water for soaking and rinsing the grains in this recipe.

¼ cup (1¾ ounces) wheat berries, rinsed

2 cups (16 ounces) water, room temperature, divided

2 cups (11 ounces) bread flour

1 cup (5½ ounces) sprouted wheat flour

1½ teaspoons table salt

¼ teaspoon instant or rapid-rise yeast

½ cup (4 ounces) mild lager, room temperature

1 tablespoon distilled white vinegar

1 tablespoon honey

1   Combine wheat berries and 1 cup filtered water in medium bowl, cover tightly with plastic wrap, and let sit at room temperature until wheat berries are softened, at least 8 hours or up to 16 hours. Drain wheat berries in fine-mesh strainer, return to bowl, and cover with plastic. Puncture plastic with paring knife 8 to 10 times. Let grains sit at room temperature, rinsing with filtered water and draining grains every 8 hours, until grains begin to sprout, 24 to 36 hours.

2   Whisk bread flour, sprouted wheat flour, salt, and yeast together in large bowl. Whisk remaining 1 cup water, beer, vinegar, and honey in 2-cup liquid measuring cup until honey is dissolved. Using silicone spatula, fold sprouted wheat berries and water mixture into flour mixture, scraping up dry flour from bottom of bowl and pressing dough until cohesive and shaggy and all flour is incorporated.

3   **First rise** Cover bowl tightly with plastic and let sit at room temperature for at least 8 hours or up to 18 hours.

4   Using greased bowl scraper or your wet fingertips, fold dough over itself by lifting and folding edge of dough toward middle and pressing to seal. Turn bowl 90 degrees and fold dough again; repeat turning bowl and folding dough 6 more times (for a total of 8 folds). Flip dough seam side down in bowl, cover with plastic, and let rest for 15 minutes.

5   Lay 18 by 12-inch sheet of parchment paper on counter and spray lightly with avocado oil spray. Transfer dough seam side up onto lightly floured counter and pat into rough 9-inch circle using your lightly floured hands. Using bowl scraper or your floured fingertips, lift and fold edge of dough toward center, pressing to seal. Repeat 5 more times (for a total of 6 folds), evenly spacing folds around circumference of dough. Press down on dough to seal, then use bench scraper to gently flip dough seam side down.

6   Using both hands, cup side of dough furthest away from you and pull dough toward you, keeping pinky fingers and side of palm in contact with counter and applying slight pressure to dough as it drags to create tension. (If dough slides across surface of counter without rolling, remove excess flour. If dough sticks to counter or your hands, lightly sprinkle counter or hands with flour.) Rotate dough ball 90 degrees, reposition dough ball at top of counter, and repeat pulling dough until taut round ball forms, at least 4 more times. Using your floured hands or bench scraper, transfer dough seam side down to center of prepared parchment.

7   **Second rise** Cover dough with inverted large bowl. Let rise until dough has doubled in size and dough springs back minimally when poked gently with your finger, 1 to 2 hours.

8   Thirty minutes before baking, adjust oven rack to middle position, place Dutch oven with lid on rack and heat oven to 475 degrees. Using sharp knife or single-edge razor blade, make one 6-inch-long, ½-inch-deep slash with swift, fluid motion along top of loaf. Carefully remove hot pot from oven and, using parchment as sling, gently transfer dough to hot pot. Working quickly and reinforcing score in top of loaf if needed, cover pot and return to oven.

9   Reduce oven temperature to 425 degrees and bake loaf in covered pot for 30 minutes. Remove lid and continue to bake until loaf is deep golden brown and registers at least 205 degrees, 10 to 15 minutes. Using parchment sling, remove loaf from pot and transfer to wire rack; discard parchment. Let cool completely, about 3 hours, before slicing and serving.

NOTES FROM THE TEST KITCHEN

Sprouted Grains

Grains that have been sprouted are said to have an improved texture and flavor, and their vitamins, minerals, and protein become easier to absorb. Sprouting activates enzymes that are dormant in dried seeds and grains. These enzymes increase digestibility and taste sweeter because enzymes break starches down into simple sugars. Not only are sprouted grains brimming with health benefits, but their delicately chewy texture and sweet, nutty flavor are also a welcome change from cooked grains. Since sprouted grains are consumed raw, the treatment of them during sprouting is crucial: Use only filtered water for soaking and rinsing and be sure to use the grains within four days of starting the sprouting process.

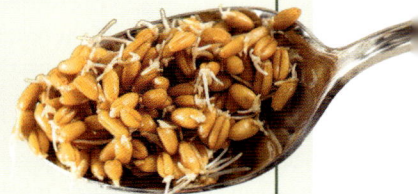

No-Knead Spelt Bread

makes 1 loaf · total time: 1¾ hours, plus 12 hours rising and cooling

why this recipe works · Spelt is an ancient grain that's seen a surge in popularity in the West in recent years. There are a lot of reasons to like spelt flour: It's full of fiber, protein, and vitamins, and, because of its high water solubility, its nutrients are quickly absorbed by the body. We're also delighted by the grain's rich, sweet, nutty flavors, so we used it to make a rustic bread that puts these flavors on display. Combining spelt flour with bread flour, as we usually do with whole-grain flours, gave us a sturdy loaf with wheaty flavor and the appropriate chew. While we prefer the flavor that beer adds, you can substitute an equal amount of water. You will need a bowl that is at least 9 inches wide and 4 inches deep to cover the dough in step 6.

- 2 cups (11 ounces) bread flour
- 1 cup (5½ ounces) spelt flour
- 1½ teaspoons table salt
- ¼ teaspoon instant or rapid-rise yeast
- 1 cup (8 ounces) water, room temperature
- ½ cup (4 ounces) mild lager, room temperature
- 1 tablespoon distilled white vinegar

1 Whisk bread flour, spelt flour, salt, and yeast together in large bowl. Using silicone spatula, fold water, beer, and vinegar into flour mixture, scraping up dry flour from bottom of bowl and pressing dough until cohesive and shaggy and all flour is incorporated.

2 **First rise** Cover bowl tightly with plastic wrap and let sit at room temperature for at least 8 hours or up to 18 hours.

3 Using greased bowl scraper or your wet fingertips, fold dough over itself by lifting and folding edge of dough toward middle and pressing to seal. Turn bowl 90 degrees and fold dough again; repeat turning bowl and folding dough 6 more times (for a total of 8 folds). Flip dough seam side down in bowl, cover with plastic, and let rest for 15 minutes.

4 Lay 18 by 12-inch sheet of parchment paper on counter and spray lightly with avocado oil spray. Transfer dough seam side up onto lightly floured counter and pat into rough 9-inch circle using your lightly floured hands. Using bowl scraper or your floured fingertips, lift and fold edge of dough toward center, pressing to seal. Repeat 5 more times (for a total of 6 folds), evenly spacing folds around circumference of dough. Press down on dough to seal, then use bench scraper to gently flip dough seam side down.

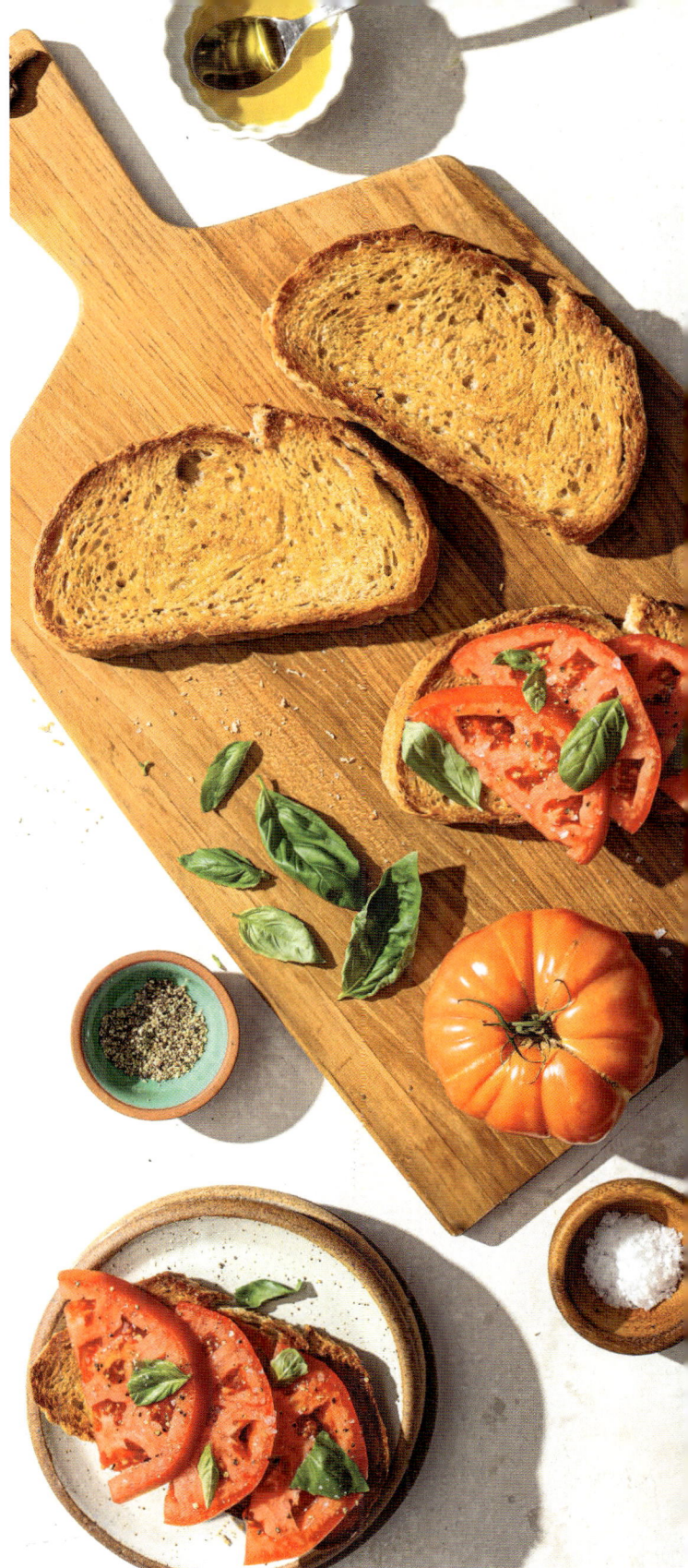

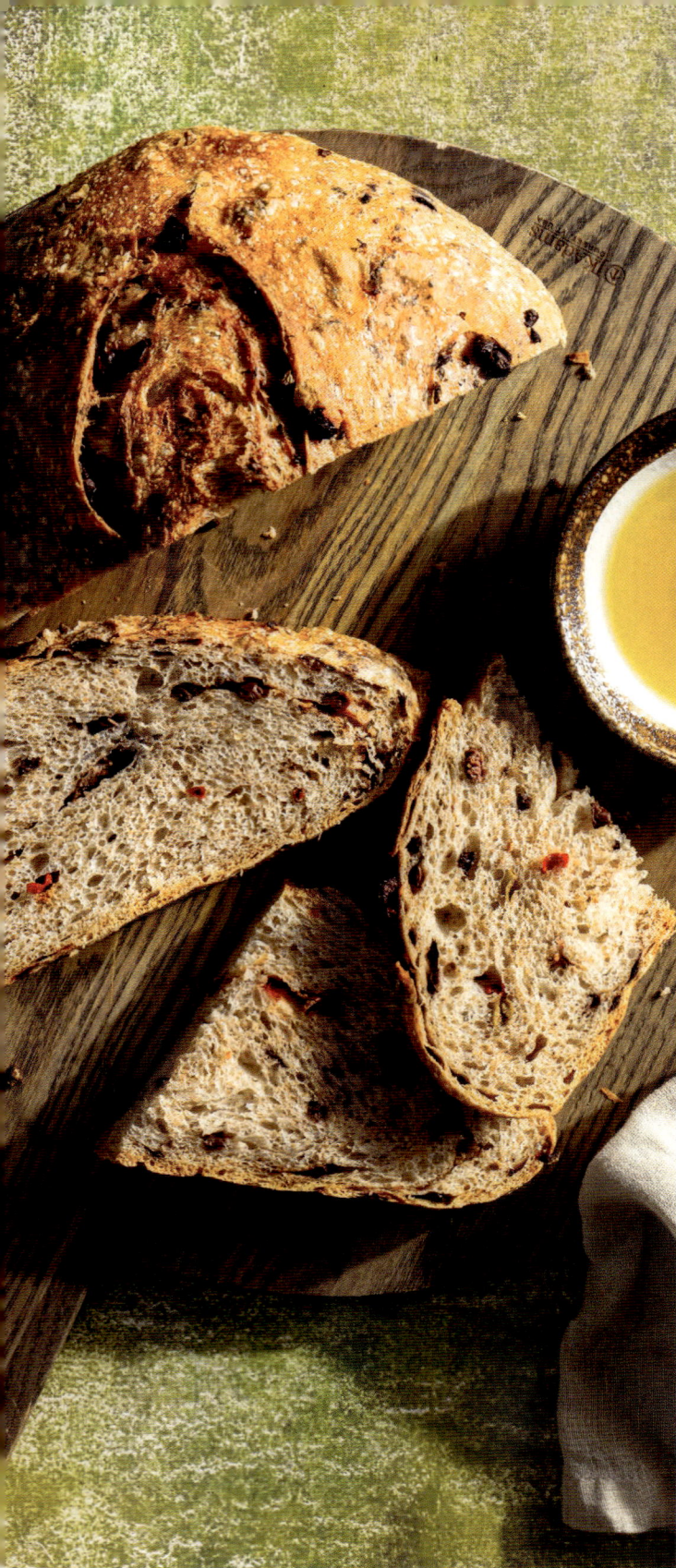

5 Using both hands, cup side of dough furthest away from you and pull dough toward you, keeping pinky fingers and side of palm in contact with counter and applying slight pressure to dough as it drags to create tension. (If dough slides across surface of counter without rolling, remove excess flour. If dough sticks to counter or your hands, lightly sprinkle counter or hands with flour.) Rotate dough ball 90 degrees, reposition dough ball at top of counter, and repeat pulling dough until taut round ball forms, at least 4 more times. Using your floured hands or bench scraper, transfer dough seam side down to center of prepared parchment.

6 **Second rise** Cover dough with inverted large bowl. Let rise until dough has doubled in size and dough springs back minimally when poked gently with your finger, 1 to 2 hours.

7 Thirty minutes before baking, adjust oven rack to middle position, place Dutch oven with lid on rack, and heat oven to 475 degrees. Using sharp knife or single-edge razor blade, make one 6-inch-long, ½-inch-deep slash with swift, fluid motion along top of loaf. Carefully remove hot pot from oven and, using parchment as sling, gently transfer dough to hot pot. Working quickly and reinforcing score in top of loaf if needed, cover pot and return to oven.

8 Reduce oven temperature to 425 degrees and bake loaf in covered pot for 30 minutes. Remove lid and continue to bake until loaf is deep golden brown and registers at least 205 degrees, 10 to 15 minutes. Using parchment sling, carefully remove loaf from hot pot and transfer to wire rack; discard parchment. Let cool completely, about 3 hours, before slicing and serving.

No-Knead Spicy Olive Spelt Bread

makes 1 loaf · **total time: 1¾ hours, plus 12 hours rising and cooling**

why this recipe works · Olives bring enlivening briny bites to hearty breads; we wanted to elevate them further by adding some heat to an olive loaf—for spicy character as well as a dose of capsaicin. We landed on vibrantly hot Calabrian chiles (jarred, as any fresh chile was too harsh). As for the olives, patting them dry before chopping and folding them in prevented their moisture from altering the hydration, which would have made the dough sticky and unworkable. Adding the olives in two batches ensured an equal distribution of add-ins. We enjoyed the contrast between these pockets of flavor and the deep, nutty taste of spelt flour. We like cutting generous slices of this bread for sandwiches and boards, or for serving with soups and stews. We prefer King Arthur brand bread flour in this recipe; the dough will be slightly stickier if you use a lower-protein bread flour. While we prefer the flavor that beer adds, you can substitute an equal amount of water. If you can't find Calabrian chiles, you can use 1½ teaspoons red pepper flakes. Avoid oil-cured olives in this recipe as their flavor will be too intense. You will need a bowl that is at least 9 inches wide and 4 inches deep to cover dough in step 6.

2 cups (11 ounces) bread flour
1 cup (5½ ounces) spelt flour
1½ teaspoons table salt
¼ teaspoon instant or rapid-rise yeast
1 cup (8 ounces) water, room temperature
½ cup (4 ounces) mild lager, room temperature
1 tablespoon distilled white vinegar
¾ cup pitted olives, rinsed, patted dry, and chopped
2 tablespoons minced fresh oregano
1 tablespoon minced, stemmed oil-packed Calabrian chiles

1 Whisk bread flour, spelt flour, salt, and yeast together in large bowl. Using silicone spatula, fold water, beer, and vinegar into flour mixture, scraping up dry flour from bottom of bowl and pressing dough until cohesive and shaggy and all flour is incorporated.

2 First rise Cover bowl tightly with plastic wrap and let sit at room temperature for at least 8 hours or up to 18 hours.

3 Mix olives, oregano, and chiles together in small bowl. Sprinkle half of olive mixture evenly over dough. Using greased bowl scraper or your wet fingertips, fold dough over itself by lifting and folding edge of dough toward middle and pressing to seal. Turn bowl 90 degrees and fold dough again; repeat turning bowl and folding dough 2 more times. Sprinkle remaining olive mixture over dough and repeat folding dough 4 more times (for a total of 8 folds). Flip dough seam side down in bowl, cover with plastic, and let rest for 15 minutes.

4 Lay 18 by 12-inch sheet of parchment paper on counter and spray lightly with avocado oil spray. Transfer dough seam side up onto lightly floured counter and pat into rough 9-inch circle using your lightly floured hands. Using bowl scraper or your floured fingertips, lift and fold edge of dough toward center, pressing to seal. Repeat 5 more times (for a total of 6 folds), evenly spacing folds around circumference of dough. Press down on dough to seal, then use bench scraper to gently flip dough seam side down.

5 Using both hands, cup side of dough furthest away from you and pull dough toward you, keeping pinky fingers and side of palm in contact with counter and applying slight pressure to dough as it drags to create tension. (If dough slides across surface

of counter without rolling, remove excess flour. If dough sticks to counter or your hands, lightly sprinkle counter or hands with flour.) Rotate dough ball 90 degrees, reposition dough ball at top of counter, and repeat pulling dough until taut round ball forms, at least 4 more times. Using your floured hands or bench scraper, transfer dough seam side down to center of prepared parchment.

6 Second rise Cover dough with inverted large bowl and let rise until dough has doubled in size and dough springs back minimally when poked gently with your finger, 1 to 2 hours.

7 Thirty minutes before baking, adjust oven rack to middle position, place Dutch oven with lid on rack and heat oven to 475 degrees. Using sharp knife or single-edge razor blade, make one 6-inch-long, ½-inch-deep slash with swift, fluid motion along top of loaf. Carefully remove hot pot from oven and, using parchment as sling, gently transfer dough to hot pot. Working quickly and reinforcing score in top of loaf if needed, cover pot and return to oven.

8 Reduce oven temperature to 425 degrees and bake loaf in covered pot for 30 minutes. Remove lid and continue to bake until loaf is deep golden brown and registers at least 205 degrees, 10 to 15 minutes. Using parchment sling, carefully remove loaf from hot pot and transfer to wire rack; discard parchment. Let cool completely, about 3 hours, before slicing and serving.

ADDING OLIVES TO BREAD DOUGH

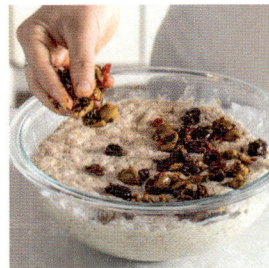

1 Sprinkle olive mixture over dough

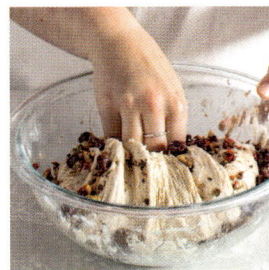

2 Fold dough over itself toward middle, pressing to seal.

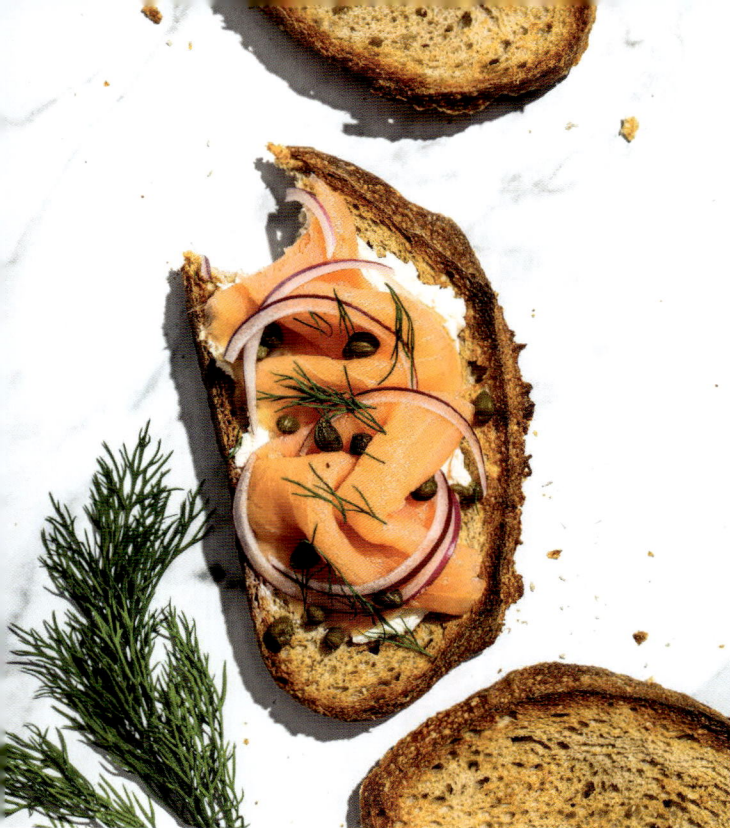

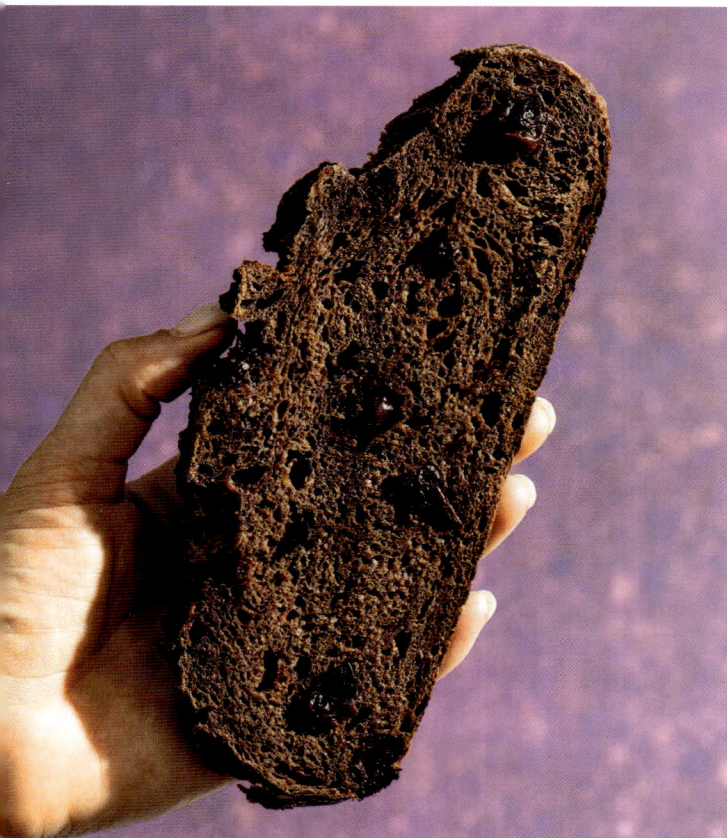

No-Knead Rye Bread

makes 1 loaf · total time: 1¾ hours, plus 12 hours rising and cooling

why this recipe works · To maintain a moist, sliceable texture, recipes for rye breads incorporate a minimal amount rye flour (you might mistake its flavor for that of the caraway seeds that are sometimes in the dough). We wanted the nuttiness of a really rye-forward loaf, not with the closed crumb of a deli bread but with the chewy, open texture of a hearty rustic loaf. To pack in more rye flour without making the loaf dry or crumbly, we added more water than most recipes call for. For the fermented tang of this bread, beer tasted out of place with the rye flour, so we replaced it with an equal amount of extra water with great results. We prefer King Arthur brand bread flour in this recipe; the dough will be slightly stickier if you use a lower-protein bread flour. You will need a bowl that is at least 9 inches wide and 4 inches deep to cover dough in step 6.

  2 cups (11 ounces) bread flour
  1 cup (5½ ounces) medium rye flour
1½ teaspoons table salt
  ¼ teaspoon instant or rapid-rise yeast
1¼ cups plus 2 tablespoons (11 ounces) water, room temperature
  1 tablespoon distilled white vinegar

1 Whisk bread flour, rye flour, salt, and yeast together in large bowl. Using silicone spatula, fold water and vinegar into flour mixture, scraping up dry flour from bottom of bowl and pressing dough until cohesive and shaggy and all flour is incorporated.

2 First rise Cover bowl tightly with plastic wrap and let sit at room temperature for at least 8 hours or up to 18 hours.

3 Using greased bowl scraper or your wet fingertips, fold dough over itself by lifting and folding edge of dough toward middle and pressing to seal. Turn bowl 90 degrees and fold dough again; repeat turning bowl and folding dough 6 more times (for a total of 8 folds). Flip dough seam side down in bowl, cover with plastic, and let rest for 15 minutes.

4 Lay 18 by 12-inch sheet of parchment paper on counter and spray lightly with avocado oil spray. Transfer dough seam side up to lightly floured counter and pat into rough 9-inch circle using your lightly floured hands. Using bowl scraper or your floured fingertips, lift and fold edge of dough toward center, pressing to seal. Repeat 5 more times (for a total of 6 folds), evenly spacing folds around circumference of dough. Press down on dough to seal, then use bench scraper to gently flip dough seam side down.

5 Using both hands, cup side of dough furthest away from you and pull dough toward you, keeping pinky fingers and side of palm in contact with counter and applying slight pressure to dough as it drags to create tension. (If dough slides across surface of counter without rolling, remove excess flour. If dough sticks to counter or your hands, lightly sprinkle counter or hands with flour.) Rotate dough ball 90 degrees, reposition dough ball at top of counter, and repeat pulling dough until taut round ball forms, at least 4 more times. Using your floured hands or bench scraper, transfer dough seam side down to center of prepared parchment.

6 Second rise Cover dough with inverted large bowl. Let rise until dough has doubled in size and dough springs back minimally when poked gently with your finger, 1 to 2 hours.

7 Thirty minutes before baking, adjust oven rack to middle position, place Dutch oven with lid on rack, and heat oven to 475 degrees. Using sharp knife or single-edge razor blade, make one 6-inch-long, ½-inch-deep slash with swift, fluid motion along top of loaf. Carefully remove hot pot from oven and, using parchment as sling, gently transfer dough to hot pot. Working quickly and reinforcing score in top of loaf if needed, cover pot and return to oven.

8 Reduce oven temperature to 425 degrees and bake loaf in covered pot for 30 minutes. Remove lid and continue to bake until loaf is deep golden brown and registers at least 205 degrees, 10 to 15 minutes. Using parchment sling, carefully remove loaf from hot pot and transfer to wire rack; discard parchment. Let cool completely, about 3 hours, before slicing and serving.

No-Knead Cocoa-Cherry Rye Bread

makes 1 loaf · total time: 1¾ hours, plus 12 hours rising and cooling

why this recipe works · Chocolate and rye have become a popular pairing in everything from cookies to coffee cake for a reason: The bitter notes of chocolate with the earthy, nutty rye flour taste complex and sophisticated. For our chocolate-rye bread, we simply added cocoa powder (and a little extra water) to our rye bread recipe. We found that Dutch-processed cocoa powder created a taller, more open-crumbed loaf than one made with more acidic natural cocoa. To balance the dark, earthy backdrop, we added a couple tablespoons of brown sugar and a handful of tart dried cherries. We prefer King Arthur brand bread flour in this recipe; the dough will be slightly stickier if you use a lower-protein bread flour. You will need a bowl that is at least 9 inches wide and 4 inches deep to cover dough in step 6.

    2 cups (11 ounces) bread flour
    1 cup (5½ ounces) medium rye flour
    ⅓ cup (1 ounce) Dutch-processed cocoa powder
    2 tablespoons packed brown sugar
   1½ teaspoons table salt
    ¼ teaspoon instant or rapid-rise yeast
   1½ cups plus 2 tablespoons (13 ounces) water,
        room temperature
    1 tablespoon distilled white vinegar
    ¾ cup dried cherries, divided

1 Whisk bread flour, rye flour, cocoa, sugar, salt, and yeast together in large bowl. Using silicone spatula, fold water and vinegar into flour mixture, scraping up dry flour from bottom of bowl and pressing dough until cohesive and shaggy and all flour is incorporated.

2 First rise Cover bowl tightly with plastic wrap and let sit at room temperature for at least 8 hours or up to 18 hours.

3 Sprinkle half of dried cherries over dough. Using greased bowl scraper or your wet fingertips, fold dough over itself by lifting and folding edge of dough toward middle and pressing to seal. Turn bowl 90 degrees and fold dough again; repeat turning bowl and folding dough 2 more times. Sprinkle remaining dried cherries over dough, and fold dough 4 more times (for a total of 8 folds). Flip dough seam side down in bowl, cover with plastic, and let rest for 15 minutes.

4   Lay 18 by 12-inch sheet of parchment paper on counter and spray lightly with avocado oil spray. Transfer dough seam side up to lightly floured counter and pat into rough 9-inch circle using your lightly floured hands. Using bowl scraper or your floured fingertips, lift and fold edge of dough toward center, pressing to seal. Repeat 5 more times (for a total of 6 folds), evenly spacing folds around circumference of dough. Press down on dough to seal, then use bench scraper to gently flip dough seam side down.

5   Using both hands, cup side of dough furthest away from you and pull dough toward you, keeping pinky fingers and side of palm in contact with counter and applying slight pressure to dough as it drags to create tension. (If dough slides across surface of counter without rolling, remove excess flour. If dough sticks to counter or your hands, lightly sprinkle counter or hands with flour.) Rotate dough ball 90 degrees, reposition dough ball at top of counter, and repeat pulling dough until taut round ball forms, at least 4 more times. Using your floured hands or bench scraper, transfer dough seam side down to center of prepared parchment.

6   Second rise   Cover dough with inverted large bowl. Let rise until dough has doubled in size and dough springs back minimally when poked gently with your finger, 1 to 2 hours.

7   Thirty minutes before baking, adjust oven rack to middle position, place Dutch oven with lid on rack, and heat oven to 475 degrees. Using sharp knife or single-edge razor blade, make one 6-inch-long, ½-inch-deep slash with swift, fluid motion along top of loaf. Carefully remove hot pot from oven and, using parchment as sling, gently transfer dough to hot pot. Working quickly and reinforcing score in top of loaf if needed, cover pot and return to oven.

8   Reduce oven temperature to 425 degrees and bake loaf in covered pot for 30 minutes. Remove lid and continue to bake until loaf registers at least 205 degrees, 10 to 15 minutes. Using parchment sling, carefully remove loaf from hot pot and transfer to wire rack; discard parchment. Let cool completely, about 3 hours, before slicing and serving.

Whole-Wheat Pita Breads

serves 8 • total time: 1¾ hours, plus 16 hours rising

why this recipe works • Adding significant whole-wheat flavor to pita bread turned out to be surprisingly simple. We used a 50/50 combination of bread flour and whole-wheat flour for the perfect amount of nuttiness without compromising the pita's pocket. This blend struck a balance between hearty flavor and enough gluten development to create steam-driven puffing in the oven. Adding oil to the recipe ensured that the pitas were moist. We prefer King Arthur brand bread flour in this recipe; the dough will be slightly stickier if you use a lower-protein bread flour. The pitas are best eaten within 24 hours of baking. Reheat leftover pitas by wrapping them in aluminum foil, placing them in a cold oven, setting the temperature to 300 degrees, and baking for 15 to 20 minutes.

1⅓ cups (7⅓ ounces) whole-wheat flour
1⅓ cups (7⅓ ounces) bread flour
2¼ teaspoons instant or rapid-rise yeast
  1 cup plus 2 tablespoons (9 ounces) ice water
  ¼ cup extra-virgin olive oil
  4 teaspoons honey
1¼ teaspoons table salt
      Avocado oil spray

1   Sift whole-wheat flour through fine-mesh strainer into bowl of stand mixer; discard bran remaining in strainer. Whisk bread flour and yeast into whole-wheat flour. Add ice water, oil, and honey on top of flour mixture. Fit stand mixer with dough hook and mix on low speed until all flour is moistened, 1 to 2 minutes. Let dough rest for 10 minutes.

2   Add salt to dough and mix on medium speed until dough forms satiny, sticky ball that clears sides of bowl, 6 to 8 minutes. Transfer dough to lightly oiled counter and knead until smooth, about 1 minute.

3   Divide dough into 8 equal pieces and cover with plastic wrap. Working with 1 piece of dough at a time (keep remaining pieces covered), form into rough ball by stretching dough around your thumbs and pinching edges together so that top is smooth. Place ball seam side down on clean counter and, using your cupped hand, drag in small circles until dough feels taut and round.

4   Rise   Spray tops of balls lightly with oil spray, then cover tightly with plastic and refrigerate for at least 16 hours or up to 24 hours.

5 One hour before baking, adjust oven rack to lowest position, set baking stone on rack, and heat oven to 425 degrees. Remove dough from refrigerator. Coat 1 dough ball generously on both sides with flour and place on well-floured counter, seam side down. Use heel of your hand to press dough ball into 5-inch circle. Using rolling pin, gently roll into 7-inch circle, adding flour as necessary to prevent sticking. Roll slowly and gently to prevent any creasing. Repeat with second dough ball. Brush both sides of each dough round with pastry brush to remove any excess flour. Transfer dough rounds to unfloured peel, making sure side that was facing up when you began rolling is face up again.

6 Slide both dough rounds carefully onto stone and bake until evenly inflated and lightly browned on undersides, 1 to 3 minutes. Using peel, slide pitas off stone and, using your hands or spatula, gently invert. (If pitas do not puff after 3 minutes, flip immediately to prevent overcooking.) Return pitas to stone and bake until lightly browned in center of second side, about 1 minute. Transfer pitas to wire rack to cool, covering loosely with clean dish towel. Repeat shaping and baking with remaining 6 pitas in 3 batches. Let pitas cool for 10 minutes before serving.

Socca with Sautéed Onions and Rosemary

Serves 6 to 8 · total time: 40 minutes **FAST**

why this recipe works · These thin, crisp, nutty-tasting chickpea pancakes, known as socca, will transport you right to the French Riviera, where the dish is a popular snacking choice as street food or alongside a glass of chilled rosé at an outdoor café. Traditionally, the socca batter is baked in a large cast-iron skillet in a very hot wood-burning oven. Once the large pancake is infused with smoky flavor and blistered on top, it is cut into wedges for serving. To make socca at home, we cooked supereasy smaller versions entirely on the stovetop, using a preheated non-stick skillet and flipping them to get a great crust on both sides. These smaller socca were easier to flip than one large pancake, and the direct heat of the stovetop ensured a crispy exterior on both sides, giving the socca a higher ratio of crunchy crust to tender interior. A topping of golden caramelized onions, enhanced with rosemary, complemented the savory flatbreads.

Batter

- 1½ cups (12 ounces) water
- 1⅓ cups (6 ounces) chickpea flour
- ¼ cup extra-virgin olive oil, divided, plus extra for drizzling
- 1 teaspoon table salt
- ¼ teaspoon ground cumin

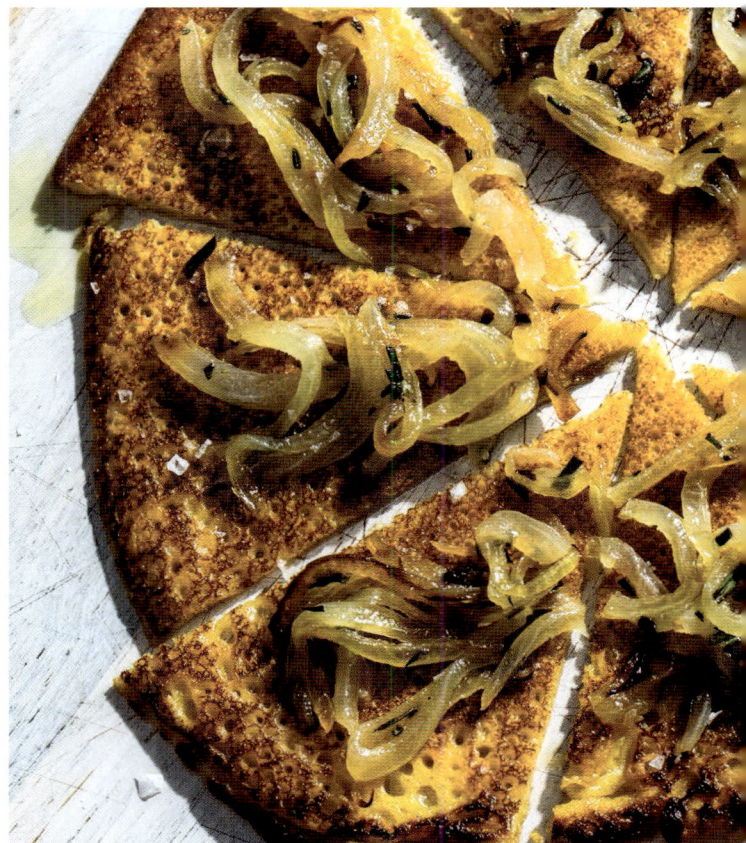

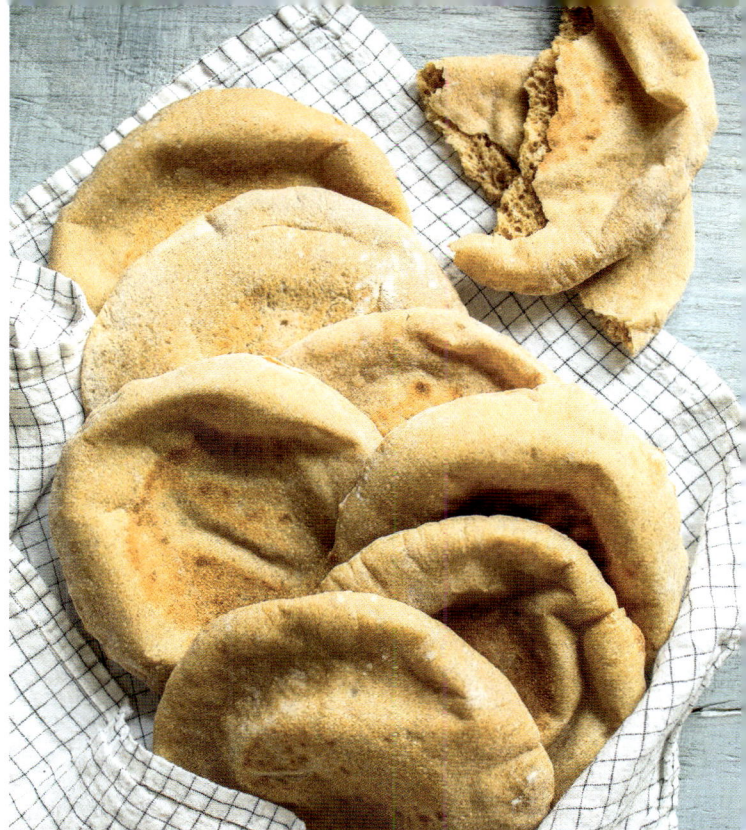

| top | Whole-Wheat Pita Breads |
| bottom | Socca with Sautéed Onions and Rosemary |

Topping
2 tablespoons extra-virgin olive oil
2 cups thinly sliced onions
½ teaspoon table salt
1 teaspoon chopped fresh rosemary
Coarse sea salt

1 For the batter Adjust oven rack to middle position and heat oven to 200 degrees. Set wire rack in rimmed baking sheet and place in oven. Whisk water, flour, 4 teaspoons oil, salt, and cumin in bowl until no lumps remain. Let batter rest while preparing topping, at least 10 minutes.

2 For the topping Heat oil in 10-inch nonstick skillet over medium-high heat until just smoking. Add onions and table salt and cook until onions start to brown around edges but still have some texture, 7 to 10 minutes. Add rosemary and cook until fragrant, about 1 minute. Transfer onion mixture to bowl; set aside. Wipe skillet clean with paper towels.

3 Heat 2 teaspoons oil in now-empty skillet over medium-high heat until just smoking. Lift skillet off heat and pour ½ cup batter into far side of skillet; swirl gently in clockwise direction until batter evenly covers bottom of skillet. Return skillet to heat and cook socca, without moving it, until well browned and crisp around bottom edge, 3 to 4 minutes (you can peek at underside of socca by loosening it from side of skillet with silicone spatula). Flip socca with silicone spatula and cook until second side is just cooked, about 1 minute. Transfer socca, browned side up, to prepared wire rack in oven.

4 Repeat 3 more times, using 2 teaspoons oil and ½ cup batter per batch. Transfer socca to cutting board and cut each into wedges. Serve, topped with sautéed onions, drizzled with extra oil, and sprinkled with sea salt.

Chapatis

Serves 4 · total time: 45 minutes, plus 30 minutes resting

why this recipe works · Chapatis are wheaty, unleavened Indian flatbreads often used in place of utensils for scooping up a number of sumptuous dishes. They're traditionally made from a finely ground hard wheat flour known as atta. We found that a combination of whole-wheat and all-purpose flours yielded a more tender and elastic chapati than one made with only (comparatively coarse) American whole-wheat flour. To simulate the results

achieved by cooking chapatis on the griddle known as a tava, we turned to a well-seasoned cast-iron skillet. This recipe can easily be doubled.

¾ cup (4⅛ ounces) whole-wheat flour
¾ cup (3¾ ounces) all-purpose flour
1 teaspoon table salt
½ cup (4 ounces) warm water
3 tablespoons plus 2 teaspoons avocado oil, divided

1 Whisk whole-wheat flour, all-purpose flour, and salt together in bowl. Stir in water and 3 tablespoons oil until cohesive dough forms. Transfer dough to lightly floured counter and knead by hand to form smooth ball, 1 minute.

2 Divide dough into 4 pieces and cover with plastic wrap. Working with 1 piece of dough at a time (keep remaining pieces covered), form into rough ball by stretching dough around your thumb and pinching edges together so that top is smooth. Place ball seam side down on clean counter and, using your cupped hand, drag in small circles until dough feels taut and round. Repeat with remaining dough pieces. Place on plate seam side down.

3 Cover dough with plastic and let sit for 30 minutes. (Dough can be refrigerated for up to 3 days.)

4 Line rimmed baking sheet with parchment paper. Roll 1 dough ball into 9-inch circle on lightly floured counter (keep remaining pieces covered). Transfer to prepared sheet and top with additional sheet of parchment. Repeat with remaining dough balls.

5 Heat 12-inch cast-iron or nonstick skillet over medium heat for 3 minutes. Add ½ teaspoon oil to skillet, then use paper towels to carefully wipe out skillet, leaving thin film of oil on bottom; skillet should be just smoking. (If using 12-inch nonstick skillet, heat ½ teaspoon oil over medium heat in skillet until shimmering, then wipe out skillet.) Place 1 dough round in hot skillet and cook until dough is bubbly and bottom is browned in spots, about 2 minutes. Flip dough and cook until puffed and second side is spotty brown, 1 to 2 minutes. Transfer to clean plate and cover with dish towel to keep warm. Repeat with remaining oil and dough rounds. Serve. (Cooked chapatis can be refrigerated for up to 3 days or frozen for up to 3 months. To freeze, layer flatbreads between parchment and store in zipper-lock bag. To serve, stack flatbreads on plate, cover with damp dish towel, and microwave until warm, 60 to 90 seconds.)

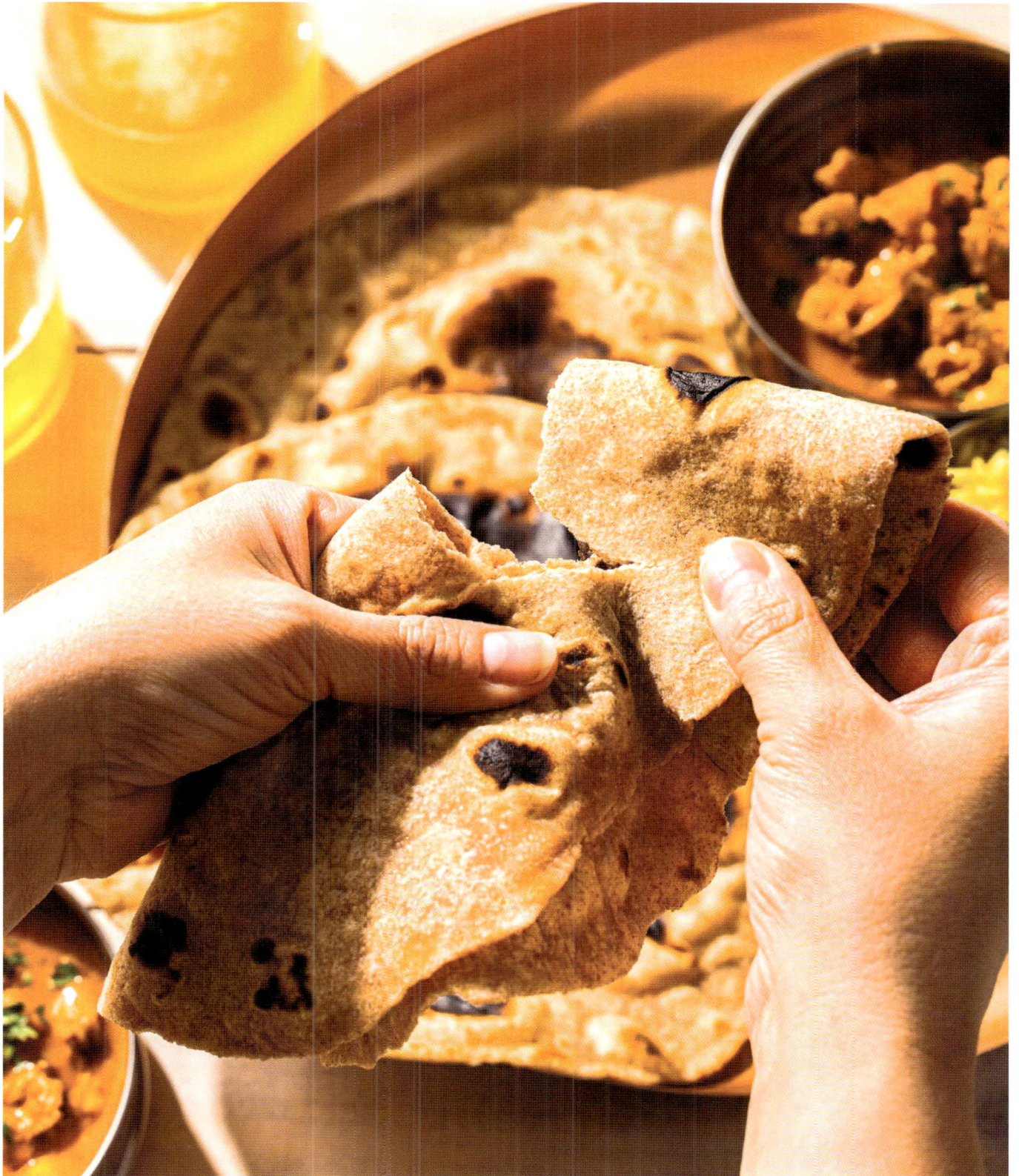

Nutritional Information For Our Recipes

We calculate the nutritional values of our recipes per serving; if there is a range in the serving size, we used the highest number of servings to calculate the nutritional values. We entered all the ingredients, using weights for important ingredients such as meat, cheese, and most vegetables. We also used our preferred brands in these analyses. We did not include additional salt or pepper for food that's "seasoned to taste."

	Cal	Total Fat (g)	Sat Fat (g)	Chol (mg)	Sodium (mg)	Carbs (g)	Fiber (g)	Total Sugar (g)	Added Sugar (g)	Protein (g)
FRONT MATTER										
Chicken Broth (per 1 cup)	20	0	0	0	276	0	0	0	0	4
Vegetable Broth (per 1 cup)	20	0	0	0	310	0	1	2	0	1
Oat Milk	80	2.5	0	0	80	13	2	0	0	2
Almond Milk	260	23	2	0	80	8	4	2	0	9
Soy Milk	100	4.5	0.5	0	75	7	2	2	0	8
BREAKFAST										
Avocado and Bean Toast	260	14	2	0	480	28	9	3	0	9
Quick Pickled Red Onions (per 1 tbsp)	5	0	0	0	0	1	0	0	0	0
Sautéed Grape and Almond Butter Toast	420	25	3	0	250	42	7	25	3	12
Fried Egg Sandwiches with Hummus and Sprouts	450	18	4.5	200	840	53	9	10	0	20
Kale and Black Bean Breakfast Burritos	320	13	2.5	185	560	37	8	2	0	16
Smoked Trout Hash	340	15	3	210	400	32	7	4	0	22
Brussels Sprout Hash	280	15	2	0	800	35	8	7	0	7
Fried Eggs	180	14	3.5	370	140	1	0	0	0	13
Scrambled Eggs	180	14	3.5	370	290	1	0	0	0	13
Poached Eggs	70	5	1.5	185	105	0	0	0	0	6
Easy-Peel Hard-Cooked Eggs	70	5	1.5	185	70	0	0	0	0	6
Easy-Peel Soft-Cooked Eggs	70	5	1.5	185	70	0	0	0	0	6
Frittata Bites with Broccoli and Sun-Dried Tomatoes	430	18	5	380	640	42	7	7	0	24
Scrambled Eggs with Asparagus, Smoked Salmon, and Chives	270	21	5	375	380	3	1	1	0	17
Scrambled Eggs with Pinto Beans and Cotija Cheese	320	23	6	380	500	12	3	1	0	18
Stir-Fried Breakfast Grain Bowls with Gochujang Sauce	480	24	2.5	0	350	55	12	6	0	15
Green Shakshuka	440	32	6	370	960	19	7	3	0	20
Microwave-Fried Garlic Chips (per 1 tbsp)	30	2	0	0	0	3	0	0	0	1
Blueberry and Almond Oatmeal	330	16	2	0	170	41	7	7	3	9
Savory Oatmeal with Tex-Mex Flavors	350	15	5	20	630	44	6	3	0	12
Baked Oatmeal with Apple and Pecans	500	28	3	0	300	60	10	25	0	8
with Banana and Cacao	378	17	5	0	384	29	11	9	0	5
Chia Pudding Parfaits with Pineapple and Kiwi	400	16	3.5	15	220	56	14	34	0	12

	Cal	Total Fat (g)	Sat Fat (g)	Chol (mg)	Sodium (mg)	Carbs (g)	Fiber (g)	Total Sugar (g)	Added Sugar (g)	Protein (g)
BREAKFAST CONTINUED										
Pepita, Almond, and Goji Berry Muesli	350	14	3.5	10	65	45	7	19	0	14
Green Granola	240	12	2	0	50	25	3	5	5	8
100 Percent Whole-Wheat Pancakes	140	6	1	25	250	19	2	4	2	5
Pear-Blackberry Topping (per ¼ cup)	35	0	0	0	15	9	2	6	1	0
Apple-Cranberry Topping (per ¼ cup)	45	0	0	0	15	11	1	9	1	1
Plum-Apricot Topping (per ¼ cup)	45	0	0	0	15	12	1	9	1	0
Raspberry-Chia Compote (per ¼ cup)	60	1.5	0	0	50	11	4	6	4	1
Sweet Yogurt Sauce (per ¼ cup)	60	1.5	1	5	25	9	0	9	6	2
Orange-Honey Yogurt (per ¼ cup)	60	1	0.5	0	15	9	0	9	6	4
Blueberry-Oat Pancakes	350	12	2	65	390	48	5	14	6	12
Berry-Oat Smoothie	170	4.5	1.5	10	30	32	6	13	0	6
Super Greens Smoothie	160	8	1	0	55	23	6	15	0	4
Passionate Dragon Smoothie	110	1.5	0	0	15	15	2	12	0	5
Matcha Fauxba	120	1.5	0	0	35	21	6	14	0	6
Green Apple Pie Smoothie	280	18	4	15	95	24	4	17	0	9
Ruby Red Smoothie	140	2	1.5	10	120	30	8	18	0	4
SOUPS AND STEWS										
Silkie Chicken Soup with Goji Berries and Jujubes	270	15	4	105	960	11	3	6	0	20
Gingery Turmeric Chicken Soup	440	22	4.5	75	940	29	5	3	0	35
Tortilla Soup with Black Beans and Spinach	280	11	1	55	560	28	4	3	0	18
Carrot Ribbon, Chicken, and Coconut Curry Soup	420	29	14	75	850	23	4	11	3	23
Chorba Frik	290	13	2.5	40	610	29	7	4	0	15
Italian Wedding Soup with Kale and Farro	310	7	2.5	25	680	38	6	7	0	26
Provençal Fish Soup	170	4.5	0.5	30	700	5	2	2	0	21
Miso Dashi Soup with Soba and Halibut	340	6	0.5	30	680	53	3	5	0	20
Spring Vegetable Soup with Charred Croutons	400	25	3.5	0	650	38	7	9	0	8
Shiitake, Tofu, and Mustard Greens Soup	210	8	1	0	760	21	5	6	0	14
Spiced Eggplant and Kale Soup	310	26	6	5	630	15	6	7	0	6
Creamy Hawaij Cauliflower Soup with Zhoug	270	24	3.5	0	740	12	4	4	0	4
Hawaij (per 1 tbsp)	15	0.5	0	0	0	3	1	0	0	1
Pink Pickled Turnips (per ½ cup)	10	0	0	0	95	2	1	2	0	0
Garlicky Wild Rice Soup with Artichokes	420	12	1.5	5	640	63	8	8	0	16
Beet and Wheat Berry Soup with Dill Cream	260	11	3	15	720	36	8	12	0	7
Turkish Bulgur and Lentil Soup	340	9	1.5	0	630	53	10	4	0	16
Lentil and Escarole Soup	270	10	1.5	0	540	34	10	5	0	11

	Cal	Total Fat (g)	Sat Fat (g)	Chol (mg)	Sodium (mg)	Carbs (g)	Fiber (g)	Total Sugar (g)	Added Sugar (g)	Protein (g)
SOUPS AND STEWS CONTINUED										
Creamy White Bean Soup with Pickled Celery	190	11	1.5	0	500	18	6	2	0	5
Aash Reshteh	400	19	2	0	850	44	10	6	0	17
Almost Beefless Beef Stew	350	11	2	45	600	36	5	10	0	20
Squash, Pork, and Tamarind Curry	310	13	4.5	40	770	37	6	10	0	14
Kimchi Jjigae	230	13	2	20	1190	10	1	4	1	19
Mapo Tofu	310	20	4	25	760	9	1	2	0	18
Maeuntang	210	6	0.5	40	580	8	1	3	0	30
Green Gumbo	220	15	1	0	710	19	5	3	0	5
Palak Dal	280	9	4.5	20	620	36	9	3	0	16
Vegetable Tagine with Chickpeas and Olives	520	18	2	0	970	76	13	25	0	13
Garam Masala (per 1 tsp)	5	0	0	0	0	1	0	0	0	0
Chickpea Bouillabaisse	770	32	4.5	30	800	89	10	10	2	22
Roasted Poblano and White Bean Chili	280	10	0.5	0	680	41	10	9	0	11
White Chicken Chili	290	9	1	85	740	22	4	5	0	30
Simple Beef Chili with Kidney Beans	480	23	5	75	570	40	15	14	0	31
SALADS AND BOWLS										
Chicken and Arugula Salad with Figs and Warm Spices	490	23	3	60	380	39	9	19	0	32
Perfect Poached Chicken (per ½ cup)	200	4.5	1	125	220	0	0	0	0	38
Dijon Chicken Salad with Raspberries and Avocado	550	34	4	95	640	11	7	2	0	42
Super Cobb Salad	330	18	4.5	145	630	21	8	7	0	25
Sichuan-Style Chicken Salad	260	15	2	85	360	5	2	1	0	27
Beet and Carrot Noodle Salad with Chicken	510	23	4	125	980	31	8	16	1	47
Salmon and Watercress Salad with Grapefruit and Avocado	330	19	2.5	45	520	23	11	11	0	21
Mediterranean Tuna Salad	190	4.5	0.5	30	750	16	5	3	0	21
Carrot and Endive Salad with Smoked Salmon	210	11	1.5	10	440	20	7	10	0	9
Fennel and Apple Salad with Smoked Trout	320	19	3	45	420	20	5	14	0	18
Edamame and Shrimp Salad	410	24	2.5	105	870	20	8	10	4	29
Napa Cabbage Salad with Tofu and Creamy Miso Dressing	340	18	2	0	520	31	5	12	0	17
Chopped Winter Salad with Butternut Squash and Apple	400	28	5	15	460	35	7	13	0	8
Roasted Cauliflower and Grape Salad with Chermoula	340	28	4	0	510	22	6	11	0	6
Roasted Carrot and Beet Salad with Harissa	320	20	3.5	140	540	33	9	17	0	11
Harissa (per 1 tbsp)	110	11	1.5	0	150	3	1	0	0	1
Roasted Pattypan Squash Salad with Dandelion Green Pesto	410	29	3.5	0	470	35	6	15	3	9
Turmeric Rice and Chicken Salad with Herbs	430	16	2.5	70	670	45	4	5	0	27
Harvest Salad with Wild Rice and Sweet Potatoes	320	14	4.5	15	540	41	6	14	0	8
Bulgur Salad with Curry Roasted Sweet Potatoes and Chickpeas	520	28	5	5	720	57	10	11	0	12
Pesto Farro Salad with Cherry Tomatoes and Artichokes	470	28	4.5	5	490	46	7	5	0	13
Quinoa, Black Bean, and Mango Salad with Lime Dressing	450	27	3.5	0	600	45	8	3	0	10

	Cal	Total Fat (g)	Sat Fat (g)	Chol (mg)	Sodium (mg)	Carbs (g)	Fiber (g)	Total Sugar (g)	Added Sugar (g)	Protein (g)
SALADS AND BOWLS CONTINUED										
Lentil and Brown Rice Salad with Fennel, Mushrooms, and Walnuts	610	29	3.5	0	770	66	11	7	0	16
Chilled Soba Noodle Salad with Spring Vegetables	340	9	1	0	810	55	2	8	0	11
California Chicken Salad Bowls	460	24	4	120	590	24	8	13	0	50
Quinoa Bowls with Turkey Meatballs, Green Beans, and Roasted Garlic Dressing	520	31	6	85	900	35	5	11	1	27
Roasted Garlic (per 1 tsp)	15	0.5	0	0	20	2	0	0	0	0
Black Rice Bowls with Roasted Salmon and Miso Dressing	540	18	2.5	60	360	64	9	7	0	31
Beet Poke Bowls	670	28	4	0	930	94	14	13	0	22
Shrimp Saganaki Zoodle Bowls	340	23	4.5	120	920	18	4	8	0	19
Fattoush Salad Bowls	300	18	2	0	490	29	9	5	0	9
Tofu Sushi Bowls	430	24	3	0	790	40	7	6	0	14
Spicy Peanut Noodle Bowls	490	23	3	0	630	61	8	8	0	12
VEGETARIAN MAINS										
Jackfruit Tinga Tacos	330	15	2	0	590	47	8	7	0	5
Spiced Cauliflower Burgers	430	20	4.5	100	950	52	5	18	0	15
Ras el Hanout (per 1 tbsp)	25	1	0	0	25	5	2	0	0	1
Pinto Bean–Beet Burgers	430	20	2.5	0	770	55	5	7	0	11
Shawarma-Spiced Tofu Wraps	580	34	5	0	970	49	3	13	8	24
Sumac Onions (per ¼ cup)	25	2	0	0	75	2	0	1	0	0
Stir-Fried Portobellos with Soy-Maple Glaze	290	14	1.5	0	450	34	4	23	9	8
Stir Fried Tempeh with Orange Sauce	310	13	1.5	0	600	33	3	7	0	16
Stir-Fried Tofu, Shiitakes, and Green Beans	340	19	2	0	450	31	5	9	3	15
Baharat Cauliflower and Eggplant with Chickpeas	560	27	3	0	870	68	12	12	1	19
Baharat (per 1 tbsp)	20	1	0	0	0	5	2	0	0	1
Overstuffed Sweet Potatoes with Tofu and Thai Curry	560	34	4	0	790	51	7	13	0	15
Loaded Sweet Potato Wedges with Tempeh	430	20	3	0	770	54	9	14	0	12
Avocado-Yogurt Sauce (per ¼ cup)	70	6	1	0	65	4	3	1	0	1
Mushroom Bourguignon	340	16	2	0	480	26	6	12	0	11
Saag Tofu	430	26	5	10	640	31	8	12	1	20
Misir Wot	290	12	1.5	0	600	37	10	5	0	12
Chana Masala	340	12	1	0	710	41	10	5	0	14
Vindaloo-Style Potatoes	340	8	1	0	980	60	10	14	0	8
Mexican-Style Spaghetti Squash Casserole	420	24	4.5	10	890	46	13	9	0	13
Big-Batch Meatless Meat Sauce with Chickpeas and Mushrooms (per ½ cup)	130	7	1	0	310	12	3	4	0	4
Fava Bean Pesto Pasta	470	24	4.5	5	550	51	10	3	0	15
Whole-Wheat Spaghetti with Greens, Beans, and Tomatoes	460	13	1.5	0	610	69	15	6	0	17
Farfalle and Summer Squash with Tomatoes, Basil, and Pine Nuts	470	18	2.5	0	210	66	2	9	0	13

	Cal	Total Fat (g)	Sat Fat (g)	Chol (mg)	Sodium (mg)	Carbs (g)	Fiber (g)	Total Sugar (g)	Added Sugar (g)	Protein (g)
VEGETARIAN MAINS CONTINUED										
Orecchiette with Broccoli Rabe and White Beans	440	15	2.5	5	410	60	13	3	0	19
Spaghetti with Spring Vegetables	430	18	2.5	5	480	56	11	5	0	15
Baked Ziti with Creamy Leeks, Kale, and Sun-Dried Tomatoes	480	12	1.5	0	560	79	12	8	0	13
Thai Curry Rice Noodles with Crispy Tofu and Broccoli	510	22	8	0	890	63	2	5	1	16
Sweet Potato Noodles with Shiitakes and Spinach	330	17	2	0	610	41	6	17	9	5
Vegetable Lo Mein	450	17	2	35	950	63	8	39	0	11
Udon Noodles and Mustard Greens with Shiitake-Ginger Sauce	230	5	0.5	0	630	55	6	8	0	12
Soba Noodles with Roasted Eggplant and Sesame	630	27	3.5	0	520	87	9	14	0	13
Curry Roasted Cabbage Wedges with Tomatoes and Chickpeas	520	26	3	0	700	57	15	12	2	15
Lentils and Roasted Broccoli with Lemony Bread Crumbs	420	16	1.5	0	440	55	12	11	0	16
Koshari	580	17	2	0	580	92	16	15	0	21
Crispy Onions (per ¼ cup)	100	5	0.5	0	780	13	0	6	0	1
Mujaddara	460	14	2.5	5	420	70	9	9	1	14
Red Lentil Kibbeh	270	9	1.5	5	500	39	7	4	0	11
Burst Cherry Tomato Puttanesca with Roman Beans	420	14	2	0	1060	60	16	7	0	17
Anchovy Substitute (per 1 tsp)	10	0	0	0	160	2	0	1	0	1
Spicy Braised Chickpeas and Turnips with Couscous	430	9	1	0	490	69	14	11	0	16
Stuffed Delicata Squash	550	34	6	10	960	59	11	8	0	12
Vegetable Fried Rice with Gai Lan and Shiitake Mushrooms	450	21	2	0	640	65	8	8	0	8
Saffron Cauliflower Rice	500	20	4	10	790	70	6	11	0	11
Herb-Yogurt Sauce (per ¼ cup)	40	2	1.5	0	30	3	0	3	2	2
Beet Barley Risotto	330	7	1.5	5	500	51	11	7	0	10
Barley with Lentils, Mushrooms, and Tahini-Yogurt Sauce	440	15	2.5	0	600	63	15	3	0	16
Tahini-Yogurt Sauce (per ¼ cup)	40	3	1	0	115	2	0	0	0	1
Farro and Broccoli Rabe Gratin	410	12	2	5	460	63	11	5	0	17
Wild Mushroom Ragout with Farro	380	3	0	0	440	76	12	15	0	16
Teff-Stuffed Acorn Squash with Lime Crema and Roasted Pepitas	460	14	5	20	700	75	12	11	0	11
Joloff-Inspired Fonio	270	14	2	0	410	33	2	4	1	3
Curried Fonio with Roasted Vegetables and Hibiscus Vinaigrette	540	30	4.5	0	910	67	7	8	2	7
POULTRY										
Perfect Poached Chicken with Warm Tomato-Ginger Vinaigrette	300	12	2	125	420	5	1	2	0	39
Cold-Start Pan-Seared Chicken Breasts with Sun-Dried Tomato Relish	350	19	2.5	125	450	2	1	0	0	39
with Chimichurri	400	26	3.5	125	520	2	0	0	0	39
Chicken Breasts and Asparagus Mimosa	440	24	4	215	950	7	3	3	0	46
Seared Chicken Breasts with Chickpea Salad	630	27	4	125	710	39	9	4	1	50
Sautéed Chicken with Cherry Tomatoes, Olives, and Feta	340	17	3.5	130	620	5	1	3	0	40

POULTRY CONTINUED

	Cal	Total Fat (g)	Sat Fat (g)	Chol (mg)	Sodium (mg)	Carbs (g)	Fiber (g)	Total Sugar (g)	Added Sugar (g)	Protein (g)
Chicken Baked in Foil with Fennel and Sun-Dried Tomatoes	480	24	3.5	125	600	26	4	3	0	42
with Potatoes and Carrots	450	22	3	125	540	22	2	3	0	41
with Sweet Potato and Radish	440	22	3.5	125	580	19	4	6	0	40
Lemon-Thyme Chicken with Garlicky Greens and White Beans	440	20	3	130	910	19	6	2	0	46
Chicken and Couscous with Fennel, Apricots, and Orange	730	34	5	125	720	58	9	21	0	47
Penne with Chicken, Roasted Cherry Tomatoes, and Spinach	610	23	3	85	880	63	12	6	0	40
Parmesan Chicken with Warm Arugula, Radicchio, and Fennel Salad	410	25	5	160	560	17	4	5	0	29
Za'atar Chicken Cutlets with Sweet Potato Wedges and Cabbage Salad	550	22	3	110	850	56	11	15	0	28
Za'atar (per 1 tbsp)	20	1	0	0	120	2	1	2	0	1
Sheet-Pan Chicken Souvlaki	510	25.5	5.5	90	1080	34	6	5	0	36
Smoked Paprika Chicken and Corn Salad with Lime	550	25	3.5	125	970	33	6	7	0	47
Cajun-Spiced Chicken and Okra Tacos	350	18	2	45	560	34	3	3	0	17
Bulgur Bowls with Chicken Meatballs and Sumac Kale	510	27	4.5	65	710	51	9	10	0	24
Tahini-Garlic Sauce (per ¼ cup)	35	2.5	0	0	75	2	0	1	0	1
One Big Cast-Iron Chicken and Chard Enchilada	390	19	6	80	1070	35	7	7	0	25
Golden Chicken Korma	410	25	4.5	75	950	14	3	6	0	31
Skillet-Roasted Chicken Breasts with Garlic-Ginger Broccoli	400	16	4	140	890	10	4	3	0	54
Skillet-Roasted Chicken Breasts with Harissa-Mint Carrots	400	13	3.5	140	840	18	5	9	0	51
Skillet-Roasted Chicken Breasts with Garlicky Green Beans	410	16	5	145	900	10	4	4	0	56
One-Pan Chicken with Butternut Squash and Kale	690	30	5	170	820	49	8	18	0	58
One-Pan Roasted Chicken Breasts with Sweet Potatoes, Poblanos, and Tomatillo Salsa	610	22	5	140	960	45	8	10	0	55
One-Pan Ratatouille with Chicken	640	27	7	145	960	25	6	10	0	51
Spiced Ginger Chicken with Potatoes, Cauliflower, and Pickled Onions	610	27	4.5	100	950	52	10	9	0	44
Green Mole with Chayote and Chicken	420	22	3	105	920	25	9	10	0	34
Chicken Mole with Cilantro-Lime Rice and Beans	560	16	2.5	105	500	77	11	7	0	34
Pulled Jackfruit and Chicken Sandwiches	410	12	2	80	890	52	6	18	4	24
Easy Barbecue Sauce (per 2 tbsps)	122	4	0	0	564	23	1	19	3	1
Cardamom-Spiced Chicken Curry with Tomatoes	330	15	3.5	165	920	10	3	5	0	36
Harissa-Rubbed Chicken Thighs with Charred Cucumber and Carrot Salad	320	20	3	105	630	10	3	5	0	24
Braised Chicken with Mushrooms and Tomatoes	340	10	2.5	180	790	10	2	4	0	39
Chicken and Spiced Freekeh with Cilantro and Preserved Lemon	330	11	1.5	55	680	39	9	2	0	21
Quick Preserved Lemon (per 1 tsp)	5	0	0	0	190	1	0	0	0	0
Crispy Brown Rice with Soy Chicken and Shiitake Mushrooms	380	14	2	70	900	41	3	2	0	21
Arroz con Pollo	330	6	1	70	840	46	2	3	0	21
Sarza Criolla (per 1 tbsp)	5	0	0	0	75	1	0	0	0	0

	Cal	Total Fat (g)	Sat Fat (g)	Chol (mg)	Sodium (mg)	Carbs (g)	Fiber (g)	Total Sugar (g)	Added Sugar (g)	Protein (g)
POULTRY CONTINUED										
Gochujang Turkey Meatballs with Edamame and Sugar Snap Peas	310	16	3	85	780	17	3	3	0	24
Turkey Meatballs with Lemony Brown Rice and Sun-Dried Tomatoes	460	13	3.5	90	580	48	3	3	0	39
Turkey Zucchini Burgers with Cranberry Relish	350	7	3	45	810	41	5	19	13	33
Turkey Shepherd's Pie	370	14	4	90	940	29	9	12	0	39
Turkey Cutlets with Barley and Swiss Chard	610	15	2.5	75	830	64	14	2	0	56
SEAFOOD										
Poached Salmon with Dijon-Herb Vinaigrette	310	14	2	95	460	3	1	1	0	34
Salmon with Sweet Potatoes, Asparagus, and Yogurt	480	19	3.5	100	760	37	8	13	0	41
Salmon Peperonata	430	25	3.5	95	920	14	3	6	0	36
Coriander Salmon with Beets, Oranges, and Avocados	590	36	5	95	990	30	11	16	0	38
Roasted Salmon and Broccoli Rabe with Pistachio Gremolata	400	24	3.5	95	550	6	4	1	0	39
Salmon Cakes with Sautéed Beet Greens and Lemon-Parsley Sauce	350	19	3	65	680	17	6	2	0	28
Saumon aux Lentilles	450	18	2.5	95	810	25	6	5	0	44
Glazed Salmon with Black-Eyed Peas, Walnuts, and Pomegranate	600	31	4	95	550	38	7	14	0	44
Roasted Salmon with White Beans, Fennel, and Tomatoes	550	21	3	105	980	40	14	12	0	49
Sautéed Tilapia with Grapefruit-Basil Relish	260	11	2	55	350	17	6	10	0	24
Sautéed Tilapia with Blistered Green Beans and Pepper Relish	330	21	2.5	55	960	11	4	6	0	27
Sheet Pan Mexican Rice with Tilapia	400	14	4	50	860	48	2	4	0	21
Pan-Seared Trout with Brussels Sprouts	480	29	4	100	700	17	4	3	0	39
Moroccan Fish and Couscous Packets	510	18	2.5	55	950	55	9	5	1	33
Thai Curry Rice with Mahi-Mahi	490	8	3.5	125	890	63	2	3	0	40
Seared Tilapia with Olive Vinaigrette and Warm Chickpea Salad	530	32	4.5	55	910	27	7	3	0	31
Roasted Snapper and Vegetables with Mustard Sauce	530	26	4	65	960	29	5	7	4	41
Pan-Roasted Cod with Cilantro Chimichurri	310	19	2.5	75	680	2	1	0	0	31
Nut-Crusted Cod Fillets with Broiled Broccoli Rabe	370	20	3	120	810	10	4	2	0	36
Lemon-Poached Halibut with Roasted Fingerling Potatoes	480	15	2	40	810	64	9	4	0	23
Pan-Roasted Sea Bass with Wild Mushrooms	350	18	2.5	70	570	11	2	6	0	36
Cod Baked in Foil with Leeks and Carrots	330	15	2	75	710	12	2	4	0	32
Cod with Cilantro Rice	600	34	4	75	610	36	2	0	0	34
Baked Halibut with Cherry Tomatoes and Chickpeas	500	21	3	85	750	32	8	5	0	41
Tabil Couscous with Sardines	460	15	2.5	55	640	61	12	8	0	22
Tabil (per 1 tbsp)	20	1	0	0	0	3	2	0	0	1
Seared Tuna Steaks with Cucumber-Mint Farro Salad	530	21	4	45	820	50	6	3	0	38
Pan-Seared Shrimp with Tangy Soy-Citrus Sauce	170	8	1	180	890	3	0	0	0	20
Salmon Tacos with Super Slaw	550	24	3	95	700	44	9	2	0	39
Tilapia Tacos with Quick Corn Relish	420	16	5	75	870	40	3	6	3	28
Spicy Shrimp Lettuce Wraps	190	12	2	105	960	9	2	2	0	13

	Cal	Total Fat (g)	Sat Fat (g)	Chol (mg)	Sodium (mg)	Carbs (g)	Fiber (g)	Total Sugar (g)	Added Sugar (g)	Protein (g)
SEAFOOD CONTINUED										
Nopales and Shrimp Tacos	370	17	3.5	115	690	39	10	6	0	18
Avocado Crema (per 1 tbsp)	45	4	1.5	5	105	2	1	0	0	1
Braised Halibut with Carrots and Coriander	380	17	2	85	560	17	4	8	0	33
Swordfish en Cocotte with Shallots, Cucumber, and Mint	440	29	5	110	510	8	3	3	0	35
Chraime	290	12	2	90	820	14	4	6	0	31
Halibut Puttanesca	350	18	2.5	90	900	9	3	3	0	35
Fish Tagine	390	23	2.5	75	600	13	4	6	0	32
Baked Shrimp with Fennel, Potatoes, and Olives	310	13	4	160	930	26	5	5	0	21
Seared Shrimp with Tomato, Avocado, and Lime Quinoa	510	20	3	180	510	53	10	5	0	31
Farrotto Primavera with Shrimp	550	23	3	105	960	64	11	5	0	27
Shrimp and White Bean Salad	350	20	2.5	105	610	26	7	4	0	19
Warm White Bean Salad with Sautéed Squid and Pepperoncini	430	24	3.5	265	670	27	7	3	0	25
Shaved Salad with Seared Scallops	450	25	4	35	1000	35	8	19	4	21
Seared Scallops with Watermelon, Cucumber, and Jicama Salad	460	31	4.5	35	1080	28	6	14	3	21
LEAN PORK AND BEEF										
Perfect Pan-Seared Pork Tenderloin Steaks with Orange, Jicama, and Pepita Relish	540	29	4.5	140	910	18	6	7	1	49
Pan-Seared Pork Cutlets with Tomato Chutney	230	7	1.5	105	530	6	1	5	3	34
Seared Pork Chops with Couscous and Celery Salad	630	21	4	110	890	60	10	12	0	48
Greek-Spiced Pork Chops with Warm Zucchini Salad	320	16	4.5	85	690	11	3	5	0	35
Sesame Pork Cutlets with Wilted Napa Cabbage Salad	660	31	3.5	235	820	27	9	6	0	60
Pork Chops with Sweet Potatoes and Rosemary-Maple Sauce	600	18	4.5	125	880	53	8	14	3	54
Pork Chops with Spicy Tomato-Braised Escarole	420	16	4.5	130	990	16	9	6	0	56
Fennel-Crusted Pork Chops with Apples, Shallots, and Prunes	760	21	5	125	910	85	7	20	0	58
One-Pan Roasted Pork Chops and Vegetables with Parsley Vinaigrette	500	19	4.5	95	800	39	7	8	0	42
Fried Brown Rice with Pork and Shrimp	410	13	2.5	175	640	53	6	2	0	24
Chorizo and Potato Tacos	380	20	4.5	25	1060	40	6	1	0	11
Orecchiette with Broccoli Rabe, Fennel, and Spiced Pork	480	17	5	35	610	61	9	0	0	24
Pork Tenderloin with Black Bean, Orange, and Quinoa Salad	550	23	3.6	100	740	44	9	7	0	41
Miso-Glazed Pork with Squash and Brussels Sprouts	520	23	3.5	140	950	30	5	14	6	50
Pork Tenderloin with White Beans and Mustard Greens	620	17	5	150	840	49	17	3	0	66
Spice-Rubbed Pork Tenderloin with Fennel, Tomatoes, Artichokes, and Olives	490	21	4	145	890	22	11	8	0	52
One-Pan Pork Tenderloin and Panzanella Salad	470	23	3.5	100	830	25	2	5	0	36
Chao Nian Gao	350	9	1	25	510	50	3	2	0	14
Maple-Ginger Roasted Pork Tenderloin with Swiss Chard and Carrots	480	18	3	145	750	26	6	15	9	53
Caraway-Crusted Pork Tenderloin with Sauerkraut and Apples	420	12	2.5	140	920	28	6	19	7	46

	Cal	Total Fat (g)	Sat Fat (g)	Chol (mg)	Sodium (mg)	Carbs (g)	Fiber (g)	Total Sugar (g)	Added Sugar (g)	Protein (g)
LEAN PORK AND BEEF CONTINUED										
Greek-Style Braised Pork with Leeks	330	13	3	60	700	22	3	8	0	21
Mexican Pork and Rice	440	13	3.5	75	560	56	11	8	0	35
Steak Tacos with Jicama Slaw	310	13	3	50	340	28	3	1	0	19
Orange-Sesame Beef and Vegetable Stir-Fry	310	18	4	50	520	18	4	7	0	22
Stir-Fried Beef with Gai Lan and Oyster Sauce	350	21	4	70	640	13	5	4	3	31
Flank Steak with Farro and Mango Salsa	650	21	4.5	65	850	85	9	7	0	35
Steak Fajitas	330	11	3	65	890	31	3	4	1	26
Flank Steak with Parsnips and Baby Kale	420	20	5	70	760	35	9	9	0	26
Steak Tips with Spiced Millet and Spinach	470	12	2	50	650	56	9	9	0	31
Sirloin Steak Tips with Charro Beans	630	22	4	105	1010	51	16	5	0	55
Coffee-Rubbed Steak with Sweet Potatoes and Apples	570	25	6	55	790	63	11	28	2	23
Braised Steaks with Root Vegetables	460	18	6	115	560	31	6	8	0	41
Spiced Meatballs, Carrots, and Radishes with Couscous and Dried Cherries	560	16	5	85	810	74	11	19	0	29
Tamale Pie	330	17	5	50	550	25	6	3	0	19
PRESSURE COOKER										
Pressure-Cooker Chicken Noodle Soup with Shells, Tomatoes, and Zucchini	480	12	2.5	210	1000	21	3	6	0	69
Pressure-Cooker Chicken Harira	340	14	2	65	1100	24	6	4	0	30
Pressure-Cooker White Chicken Chili with Zucchini	320	8	1	90	880	29	15	4	0	33
Pressure-Cooker Spiced Chicken Soup with Squash and Chickpeas	290	8	1.5	80	800	23	5	4	0	29
Pressure-Cooker Smoky Turkey Meatball Soup with Kale and Manchego	310	12	4.5	50	1030	14	3	5	0	38
Pressure-Cooker Double Vegetable Beef Stew with Lemon Zest	360	11	3	75	800	30	5	8	0	31
Pressure-Cooker Pork Pozole Rojo	400	17	3	85	920	35	1	2	0	27
Pressure-Cooker Swordfish Stew with Tomatoes, Capers, and Pine Nuts	320	16	3	75	720	16	2	10	0	25
Pressure-Cooker Chicken and Braised Radishes with Dukkah	410	20	3.5	130	760	14	4	5	0	45
Pressure-Cooker Chicken and Black Rice Bowl with Peanut-Sesame Sauce	600	30	3	135	800	63	8	6	1	47
Peanut-Sesame Sauce (per 1 tbsp)	50	3.5	0.5	0	115	4	1	2	2	2
Pressure-Cooker Shredded Chicken Tacos with Mango Salsa	560	18	4	150	710	60	3	19	0	44
Pressure-Cooker Chipotle Chicken and Black Beans with Pickled Cabbage	440	24	6	120	770	32	1	4	1	29
Pressure-Cooker Javaher Polo with Chicken	760	29	5	90	890	87	4	29	0	39
Pressure-Cooker Chicken with Spring Vegetables	470	24	6	120	840	34	7	8	0	30
Pressure-Cooker Chicken and Couscous with Prunes and Olives	610	27	6	120	810	62	9	18	0	28
Pressure-Cooker Shredded Beef Tacos with Jicama Slaw	400	13	3	75	500	40	5	7	1	30
Pressure-Cooker Pork and Bulgur Bowls with Parsley-Pepita Sauce	550	25	5	85	750	50	9	6	3	33
Quick-Pickled Vegetables (per ¼ cup)	15	0	0	0	20	3	0	2	1	0

	Cal	Total Fat (g)	Sat Fat (g)	Chol (mg)	Sodium (mg)	Carbs (g)	Fiber (g)	Total Sugar (g)	Added Sugar (g)	Protein (g)
PRESSURE COOKER CONTINUED										
Pressure-Cooker Haddock with Tomatoes, Escarole, and Crispy Garlic	310	12	1.5	90	830	9	4	3	0	30
Pressure-Cooker Swordfish with Braised Green Beans, Tomatoes, and Feta	470	17	4.5	120	740	38	3	9	0	41
Pressure-Cooker Braised Striped Bass with Zucchini and Tomatoes	320	12	2	135	600	15	4	8	0	34
Pressure-Cooker Halibut with Couscous and Ras el Hanout	540	22	3.5	85	750	43	8	7	0	42
Pressure-Cooker Southwestern Shrimp and Oat Berry Bowls	610	25	4	110	660	71	13	6	0	27
Chipotle-Yogurt Sauce (per 1 tbsp)	10	0.5	0	0	5	1	0	1	0	1
Pressure-Cooker Shrimp and White Beans with Butternut Squash and Sage	370	10	1.5	105	800	45	10	7	0	23
Pressure-Cooker Bulgur with Chickpeas, Spinach, and Za'atar	310	12	1.5	0	360	44	9	2	0	10
Pressure-Cooker Bean and Sweet Potato Chili	400	8	1	0	810	67	6	13	0	16
Pressure-Cooker Farro Salad with Asparagus, Snap Peas, and Tomatoes	420	16	3.5	15	490	62	8	8	0	13
Pressure-Cooker Black Beans and Brown Rice	330	5	0	0	820	65	5	6	0	12
Pressure-Cooker Spaghetti and Turkey Meatballs	460	10	3	65	900	61	11	8	0	34
Pressure-Cooker Parmesan Penne with Chicken and Asparagus	440	11	2.5	50	870	53	10	4	0	28
Pressure-Cooker Rigatoni with Mushroom Ragu	410	10	1	0	840	63	9	10	0	14
Pressure-Cooker Fideos with Chickpeas, Fennel, and Spinach	420	13	1.5	0	850	61	15	8	0	15
GRAIN, BEAN, AND VEGETABLE SIDES										
Quinoa Pilaf with Herbs and Lemon	210	7	1	0	300	29	3	2	0	6
Basic Beans	110	0	0	0	85	20	8	3	0	6
Baked Brown Rice	200	4	0.5	0	125	37	2	1	0	4
Rice and Bean Pilaf	220	4	0	0	160	39	3	1	0	6
Southwestern Black Bean Salad	260	16	2	0	230	26	8	4	0	7
Cuban-Style Black Beans and Rice	250	4	0.5	0	480	46	1	4	0	9
Succotash Salad with Butter Beans and Basil	230	15	2	0	790	22	4	5	0	6
Black-Eyed Pea Salad with Peaches and Pecans	170	9	1	0	330	19	5	5	0	6
Stewed Chickpeas and Spinach with Dill and Lemon	180	6	0.5	0	170	22	6	1	0	8
Chickpeas with Garlic and Parsley	190	10	1.5	0	140	18	4	2	0	6
Edamame Salad with Arugula and Radishes	230	14	1.5	0	300	14	1	7	3	13
Sautéed Fava Beans, Asparagus, and Leeks	220	6	1	0	240	36	15	18	0	16
Lentil Salad with Olives, Mint, and Feta	350	21	3.5	5	200	31	8	2	0	12
with Hazelnuts and Goat Cheese	390	24	4	5	170	31	8	2	0	13
with Carrots and Cilantro	330	19	2.5	0	105	33	8	3	0	11
Lentilles du Puy with Spinach and Crème Fraîche	160	6	2.5	15	370	15	3	3	0	8
Turkish Pinto Bean Salad with Tomatoes, Eggs, and Parsley	270	18	3	70	160	20	6	3	0	9
Cannellini Beans with Roasted Red Peppers and Kale	230	12	2	5	340	20	5	4	0	8
Sicilian White Beans and Escarole	140	4.5	0.5	0	370	20	8	4	0	7

	Cal	Total Fat (g)	Sat Fat (g)	Chol (mg)	Sodium (mg)	Carbs (g)	Fiber (g)	Total Sugar (g)	Added Sugar (g)	Protein (g)
GRAIN, BEAN, AND VEGETABLE SIDES CONTINUED										
White Bean Salad with Oranges and Celery	250	14	2	0	105	25	7	6	0	7
Wild Rice Pilaf with Pecans and Cranberries	370	11	1	0	330	63	3	13	0	8
with Scallions, Cilantro, and Almonds	310	8	1	0	320	51	3	2	0	9
Barley Salad with Celery and Miso Dressing	190	4.5	0.5	0	350	34	7	2	0	4
Barley Salad with Pomegranate, Pistachios, and Feta	280	10	2.5	10	410	41	7	9	2	7
Buckwheat Tabbouleh	280	15	2	0	350	31	3	4	0	6
Bulgur with Chickpeas, Spinach, and Za'atar	310	12	1.5	0	360	44	9	2	0	10
Farro Salad with Asparagus, Snap Peas, and Tomatoes	280	11	2.5	10	230	41	6	5	0	9
Warm Farro with Mushrooms and Thyme	250	9	1	0	125	39	4	4	0	7
Warm Kamut with Carrots and Pomegranate	190	8	1	0	160	27	5	5	0	6
Oat Berry, Chickpea, and Arugula Salad	270	11	2.5	10	280	31	6	4	1	9
Butternut Squash Polenta	130	4.5	1	5	380	21	4	2	0	4
Warm Rye Berries with Apple and Scallions	160	5	0.5	0	220	27	6	3	0	3
Spelt Salad with Pickled Fennel, Pea Greens, and Mint	200	9	1.5	5	280	26	4	4	0	6
Wheat Berry Salad with Radicchio, Dried Cherries, and Pecans	200	11	2	5	190	22	4	3	0	5
Charred Asparagus with Strawberries	270	23	3	0	440	14	5	7	1	5
Skillet-Roasted Broccoli with Parmesan and Black Pepper	220	20	3.5	5	370	7	3	2	0	7
Skillet-Roasted Brussels Sprouts with Chile, Peanuts, and Mint	240	20	3	0	230	13	5	3	0	5
Roasted Cabbage with Gochujang, Sesame, and Scallion	140	9	1.5	0	240	12	4	6	0	3
Carrot "Tabbouleh" with Mint, Pistachios, and Pomegranate Seeds	230	17	2.5	0	440	18	5	8	0	5
with Fennel, Orange, and Hazelnuts	220	18	2	0	450	12	4	6	0	3
Cauliflower Puree	140	10	1.5	0	290	12	5	4	0	4
Sautéed Swiss Chard with Currants and Pine Nuts	160	12	1.5	0	440	12	3	7	0	4
Sugar Snap Peas with Pine Nuts, Fennel, and Lemon Zest	100	7	0.5	0	140	8	3	3	0	3
Cumin and Chili Roasted Sweet Potato Wedges	170	5	0.5	0	300	28	5	8	0	3
Roasted Kabocha Squash with Maple and Sage	240	14	2	0	290	28	4	13	3	4
Broiled Smashed Zucchini with Garlicky Yogurt	190	15	4	5	660	9	3	6	0	6
SNACKS										
Tzatziki	60	4	1	0	85	2	0	2	0	3
Beet Tzatziki	60	4	1	0	100	4	1	3	0	3
Classic Hummus	140	10	1.5	0	160	9	2	0	0	4
Roasted Red Pepper Hummus	150	10	1.5	0	180	9	2	1	0	4
Artichoke-Lemon Hummus	140	10	1.5	0	170	10	3	1	0	4
Sweet Potato Hummus	90	4.5	0.5	0	190	11	2	2	0	2

	Cal	Total Fat (g)	Sat Fat (g)	Chol (mg)	Sodium (mg)	Carbs (g)	Fiber (g)	Total Sugar (g)	Added Sugar (g)	Protein (g)
SNACKS CONTINUED										
Quick Lemon-Garlic White Bean Dip	100	3.5	0	0	250	13	4	1	0	4
Navy Bean and Artichoke Dip	60	0	0	0	420	10	3	1	0	4
Beet Dip with Yogurt and Tahini	190	16	4.5	5	490	8	2	4	0	5
Guacamole	120	11	1.5	0	150	7	5	1	0	2
Baba Ghanoush	80	6	1	0	220	8	3	4	0	2
Carrot-Habanero Dip	80	5	0.5	0	180	8	2	4	0	1
Muhammara	180	16	2	0	330	9	1	4	0	2
Roasted Bell Peppers	20	0	0	0	0	4	1	2	0	1
Fresh Tomato Salsa	15	0	0	0	75	3	1	2	0	1
Toasted Corn Salsa	50	3.5	0	0	75	6	1	2	0	1
Toasted Corn and Black Bean Salsa	60	3	0	0	75	7	2	1	0	2
Orange-Fennel Spiced Almonds	220	20	1.5	0	290	8	5	2	0	8
Spicy Chipotle Almonds	230	20	1.5	0	290	8	5	2	0	8
Cherry, Chocolate, and Orange Trail Mix	150	12	1.5	0	30	9	2	4	1	5
Cherry, Coconut, Chili, and Lime Trail Mix	150	12	2.5	0	30	7	2	3	0	5
Whole-Wheat Seeded Crackers	220	9	1.5	15	340	30	5	0	0	7
Chickpea Crackers	80	3	0	0	85	9	2	2	0	4
Turmeric-Black Pepper Chickpea Crackers	80	3	0	0	85	10	2	2	0	4
Herbes de Provence Chickpea Crackers	80	3	0	0	85	9	2	2	0	4
Seeded Pumpkin Crackers	180	8	1	35	870	23	1	9	5	5
Popcorn with Olive Oil	60	3	0	0	115	7	1	0	0	1
Smoked Paprika–Spiced Roasted Chickpeas	160	8	1	0	70	16	4	1	0	5
Coriander-Turmeric Roasted Chickpeas	160	8	1	0	70	16	4	1	0	5
Sesame Nori Chips	20	1	0	0	40	1	1	0	0	1
Walnut-Pomegranate Stuffed Dates	110	4	1	0	0	20	2	17	0	1
Pistachio-Orange Stuffed Dates	80	1	0	0	45	19	2	16	0	1
Cranberry-Almond No Bake Energy Bites	100	5	1	0	55	12	1	7	3	3
Chewy Granola Bars with Hazelnuts, Cherries, and Cacao Nibs	260	14	2	0	90	31	3	19	8	4
Chewy Granola Bars with Walnuts and Craberries	240	12	1.5	0	90	31	3	20	8	3
Nut-Free Chewy Granola Bars	230	12	2	0	90	27	4	16	8	6

	Cal	Total Fat (g)	Sat Fat (g)	Chol (mg)	Sodium (mg)	Carbs (g)	Fiber (g)	Total Sugar (g)	Added Sugar (g)	Protein (g)
DRINKS										
Iced Black Tea	0	0	0	0	0	0	0	0	0	0
Raspberry-Basil	30	0	0	0	0	6	3	2	0	1
Ginger-Pomegranate	25	0	0	0	0	0	0	5	0	0
Apple-Cinnamon	0	0	0	0	0	0	1	5	0	0
Simple Syrup (per 1 tbsp)	35	0	0	0	0	9	0	9	9	0
Iced Green Tea	0	0	0	0	0	0	0	0	0	0
Cantaloupe-Mint	15	0	0	0	5	3	0	3	0	0
Cucumber-Lime Iced Green Tea	5	0	0	0	0	1	0	1	0	0
Pear-Sage Iced Green Tea	30	0	0	0	0	8	2	5	0	0
Hibiscus Iced Tea	5	0	0	0	0	1	0	1	0	0
Cold Brew Coffee Concentrate	0	0	0	0	0	0	0	0	0	0
Pumpkin-Spiced	0	0	0	0	0	0	0	0	0	0
Star Anise–Orange	0	0	0	0	0	0	0	0	0	0
London Fog Tea Latte	70	4	2.5	10	50	6	0	6	0	4
Matcha	0	0	0	0	0	0	0	0	0	0
Matcha Latte	110	6	3.5	20	80	9	0	9	0	6
Emoliente	35	0	0	0	0	0	0	8	8	0
with Chamomile	35	0	0	0	0	0	0	8	8	0
with Alfalfa and Anise	35	0	0	0	0	0	0	8	8	0
Citrus Burst Black Tea Blend *(per 2 tsp)*	0	0	0	0	0	0	0	0	0	0
Cacao, Cardamom, and Rose Herbal Tea Blend *(per tbsp)*	0	0	0	0	0	0	0	0	0	0
Immunitea Herbal Tea Blend *(per tbsp)*	0	0	0	0	0	0	0	0	0	0
Cozy and Calm Herbal Tea Blend *(per tbsp)*	0	0	0	0	0	0	0	0	0	0
Tummy Tea Herbal Tea Blend *(per tbsp)*	0	0	0	0	0	0	0	0	0	0
Winter Citrus and Pomegranate Water	5	0	0	0	0	1	0	1	0	0
Watermelon-Lime Agua Fresca	60	0	0	0	75	14	0	11	2	1
Grapefruit, Blackberry, and Sage Water	0	0	0	0	0	0	0	0	0	0
Star Fruit, Lime, and Basil Water	0	0	0	0	0	0	0	0	0	0
Green Apple, Lemon, and Dill Water	0	0	0	0	0	0	0	0	0	0
Honeydew-Lemon Agua Fresca	70	0	0	0	105	18	0	16	2	1
Cantaloupe and Fresno Chile Spritzer	20	0	0	0	10	5	0	4	0	1
Grapefruit-Rosemary Spritzer	90	0	0	0	0	23	0	12	12	1
Citrus Syrup (per 1 tbsp)	35	0	0	0	0	9	0	9	9	0
Pear and Vanilla Spritzer	60	0	0	0	0	16	0	10	0	0
Mango and Lime Spritzer	100	0.5	0	0	0	25	0	23	0	1
Bubbly Sage Cider	80	0	0	0	5	19	0	18	12	0

	Cal	Total Fat (g)	Sat Fat (g)	Chol (mg)	Sodium (mg)	Carbs (g)	Fiber (g)	Total Sugar (g)	Added Sugar (g)	Protein (g)
DRINKS CONTINUED										
Sicilian Sunrise	100	0	0	0	0	25	0	22	12	1
Tepache*	35	0	0	0	0	8	0	8	8	0
Milk Kefir*	25	0	0	5	15	2	0	2	2	0
with Vanilla	25	0	0	5	15	2	0	2	2	0
Kombucha*	35	0	0	0	0	8	0	8	8	0
Sparkling Blue Ginger-Lime	35	0	0	0	0	8	0	8	8	0
Sparkling Spicy Pineapple	45	0	0	0	0	11	0	10	8	0
Sparkling Mixed Berry	35	0	0	0	0	9	0	9	8	0
Raw Hot Chocolate	200	10	6	30	130	18	0	17	0	10
Haldhicha Dudh	170	8	4.5	25	105	17	0	17	5	8
with Black Pepper	170	8	4.5	25	105	17	0	17	5	8
with Ginger	170	8	4.5	25	105	17	0	17	5	8
Switchel	60	0	0	0	75	14	0	12	12	0
BREADS										
Flourless Nut and Seed Loaf	380	26	7	0	115	31	10	9	3	11
Soda Bread with Nuts and Cacao Nibs	400	15	3.5	5	670	56	11	5	1	13
Oatmeal Dinner Rolls	240	4	2	10	330	44	2	8	8	7
Whole-Wheat Oatmeal Loaf	260	4.5	2	10	300	47	5	8	7	9
Quinoa Whole-Wheat Bread	290	6	1	25	460	46	5	3	1	11
No-Knead Whole-Wheat Rustic Loaf	220	0	0	0	440	43	3	0	0	8
No-Knead Cranberry-Walnut Bread	290	5	0	0	440	51	4	7	0	9
No-Knead Seeded Oat Bread	280	5	1	0	440	45	5	0	0	10
No-Knead Sprouted Wheat Berry Bread	240	0	0	0	440	50	4	2	2	9
No-Knead Spelt Bread	220	0.5	0	0	440	43	4	0	0	8
No-Knead Spicy Olive Spelt Bread	260	4	0	0	720	44	3	0	0	8
No-Knead Rye Bread	210	0	0	0	440	44	4	0	0	7
No-Knead Cocoa-Cherry Rye Bread	280	0.5	0	0	440	60	5	12	3	8
Whole-Wheat Pita Breads	260	8	1	0	370	41	4	3	3	7
Socca with Sautéed Onions and Rosemary	190	12	1.5	0	990	15	3	3	0	5
Chapatis	310	14	1.5	0	580	41	4	0	0	7

*Values are an estimate and will vary based on fermention conditions.

Conversions & Equivalents

Some say cooking is a science and an art. We would say that geography has a hand in it too. Flours and sugars manufactured in the United Kingdom and elsewhere will feel and taste different from those manufactured in the United States. So we cannot promise that the loaf of bread you bake in Canada or England will taste the same as a loaf baked in the States, but we can offer guidelines for converting weights and measures. We also recommend that you rely on your instincts when making our recipes. Refer to the visual cues provided.

The recipes in this book were developed using standard U.S. measures following U.S. government guidelines. The charts below offer equivalents for U.S. and metric measures. All conversions are approximate and have been rounded up or down to the nearest whole number.

1 teaspoon	=	4.9292 milliliters, rounded up to 5 milliliters
1 ounce	=	28.3495 grams, rounded down to 28 grams

Volume Conversions

U.S.	Metric
1 teaspoon	5 milliliters
2 teaspoons	10 milliliters
1 tablespoon	15 milliliters
2 tablespoons	30 milliliters
¼ cup	59 milliliters
⅓ cup	79 milliliters
½ cup	118 milliliters
¾ cup	177 milliliters
1 cup	237 milliliters
1¼ cups	296 milliliters
1½ cups	355 milliliters
2 cups (1 pint)	473 milliliters
2½ cups	591 milliliters
3 cups	710 milliliters
4 cups (1 quart)	0.946 liter
1.06 quarts	1 liter
4 quarts (1 gallon)	3.8 liters

NOTES FROM THE TEST KITCHEN

CONVERTING FAHRENHEIT TO CELSIUS

We include temperatures in some of the recipes in this book, and we recommend an instant-read thermometer for the job. To convert Fahrenheit degrees to Celsius, use this simple formula:

Subtract 32 degrees from the Fahrenheit reading, then divide the result by 1.8 to find the Celsius reading. For example, to convert 160°F to Celsius:

160°F − 32 = 128°
128° ÷ 1.8 = 71.11°C   →   rounded down to 71°C

Weight Conversions

Because measuring by weight is far more accurate than measuring by volume, and thus more likely to achieve reliable results, we often provide ounce measures for many ingredients.

Ounces	Grams
½	14
¾	21
1	28
1½	43
2	57
2½	71
3	85
3½	99
4	113
4½	128
5	142
6	170
7	198
8	227
9	255
10	283
12	340
16 (1 pound)	454

Index

Note: Page references in *italics* indicate photographs.

A

Aash Reshteh, *74,* 74–75
Agua Fresca
　　Honeydew-Lemon, 396–97
　　Watermelon-Lime, 395
Alfalfa and Anise, Emoliente with, 391
Allergies and food sensitivities, 18
Almond Butter and Sautéed Grape Toast, *24,* 25–26
Almond(s)
　　and Blueberry Oatmeal, 37–38, *39*
　　Cherry, Chocolate, and Orange Trail Mix, 374–75, *375*
　　Cherry, Coconut, Chili, and Lime Trail Mix, 375
　　Chicken and Arugula Salad with Figs and Warm Spices, 92, *93*
　　-Cranberry No-Bake Energy Bars, 381–82
　　Flourless Nut and Seed Loaf, 410, *411*
　　Milk, 19
　　Orange-Fennel Spiced, 374, *375*
　　Pepita, and Goji Berry Muesli, 41
　　Pressure-Cooker Javaher Polo with Chicken, *310,* 310–11
　　Roasted Carrot and Beet Salad with Harissa, *90,* 106
　　Sautéed Grape and Almond Butter Toast, *24,* 25–26
　　Scallions, and Cilantro, Wild Rice Pilaf with, 346
　　Spicy Chipotle, 374
Anchovy(ies)
　　Halibut Puttanesca, *254,* 254–55
　　Substitute, 162
Anise and Alfalfa, Emoliente with, 391
Anthocyanins, 5
Anti-inflammatory diet
　　best cooking methods, 17
　　best foods for, 4–7
　　FAQs, 18
　　favorite recipe makeovers, 20–21

Anti-inflammatory diet (cont.)
　　guide to, 8–12
　　smart shopping for, 13–14
Antioxidants, 4
Apple(s)
　　and Butternut Squash, Chopped Winter Salad with, 104, *105*
　　-Cinnamon Iced Black Tea, 387
　　-Cranberry Topping, 44, *44*
　　and Fennel Salad with Smoked Trout, 100–101, *101*
　　Green, Lemon, and Dill Water, 396, *397*
　　Harvest Salad with Wild Rice and Sweet Potatoes, 109
　　and Pecans, Baked Oatmeal with, 39, *39*
　　Pie Smoothie, Green, 50, *51*
　　and Sauerkraut, Caraway-Crusted Pork Tenderloin with, 282, *283*
　　and Scallions, Warm Rye Berries with, 352–53, *353*
　　Shallots, and Prunes, Fennel-Crusted Pork Chops with, *270,* 270–271
　　and Sweet Potatoes, Coffee-Rubbed Steak with, 292, *293*
Apricot(s)
　　Chewy Granola Bars with Hazelnuts, Cherries, and Cacao Nibs, 382, *383*
　　Chewy Granola Bars with Walnuts and Cranberries, 382
　　dried, about, 41
　　Fennel, and Orange, Chicken and Couscous with, 182–84, *183*
　　Nut-Free Chewy Granola Bars, 382
　　-Plum Topping, 44, *45*
　　Seeded Pumpkin Crackers, *378,* 378–79
Arroz con Pollo, 211–12, *212*
Artichoke(s)
　　and Cherry Tomatoes, Pesto Farro Salad with, 112, *112*
　　Fennel, Tomatoes, and Olives, Spice-Rubbed Pork Tenderloin with, *277,* 277–78
　　Garlicky Wild Rice Soup with, 68–69, *69*
　　-Lemon Hummus, 365
　　and Navy Bean Dip, 366–68, *369*
　　Shrimp Saganaki Zoodle Bowls, 119–20
Arugula
　　and Chicken Salad with Figs and Warm Spices, 92, *93*
　　Edamame and Shrimp Salad, *102,* 102–3

Arugula (cont.)
　　Fennel and Apple Salad with Smoked Trout, 100–101, *101*
　　Oat Berry, and Chickpea Salad, *350,* 351
　　Radicchio, and Fennel Salad, Warm, Parmesan Chicken with, *184,* 185–86
　　and Radishes, Edamame Salad with, 339–40
　　Roasted Butternut Squash Salad with Creamy Tahini Dressing, 358, *359*
　　Seared Tuna Steaks with Cucumber-Mint Farro Salad, *244,* 245
　　Shrimp and White Bean Salad, *258,* 259
　　Three-Bean Salad with, *359,* 359–60
Asparagus
　　and Chicken, Pressure-Cooker Parmesan Penne with, 326, *327*
　　Crudités, *373,* 373
　　Farrotto Primavera with Shrimp, *257,* 257–58
　　Fava Bean, and Leek, Sautéed, 340, *341*
　　Garlicky Wild Rice Soup with Artichokes, 68–69, *69*
　　Mimosa and Chicken Breasts, *178,* 179
　　Pressure-Cooker Chicken with Spring Vegetables, *310,* 311
　　Smoked Salmon, and Chives, Scrambled Eggs with, *32,* 33
　　Snap Peas, and Tomatoes, Farro Salad with, 349, *349*
　　Snap Peas, and Tomatoes, Pressure-Cooker Farro Salad with, 323–24, *324*
　　Spaghetti with Spring Vegetables, *148,* 149–50
　　Spring Vegetable Soup with Charred Croutons, *63,* 63–64
　　Sweet Potatoes, and Yogurt, Salmon with, 220–22, *221*
　　trimming ends of, 33
Avocado oil, 13
Avocado(s)
　　and Bean Toast, 24, *24*
　　Beet Poke Bowls, 118–19, *119*
　　Beets, and Oranges, Coriander Salmon with, 224, *224*
　　Black Rice Bowls with Roasted Salmon and Miso Dressing, *116,* 117–18
　　buying, 24
　　Chorizo and Potato Tacos, 272–73, *273*
　　Crema, 250

Granola, Green, 42, *43*

Granola Bars

Chewy, with Hazelnuts, Cherries, and Cacao Nibs, 382, *383*

Chewy, with Walnuts and Cranberries, 382

Nut-Free Chewy, 382

Grapefruit

and Avocado, Salmon and Watercress Salad with, 98, *99*

-Basil Relish, 229

Blackberry, and Sage Water, *394,* 395–96

-Rosemary Spritzer, 398, *398*

Ruby Red Smoothie, 51, *51*

Grape(s)

California Chicken Salad Bowls, 115, *115*

Roasted, and Cauliflower Salad with Chermoula, *105,* 105–6

Sautéed, and Almond Butter Toast, *24,* 25–26

Greek-Spiced Pork Chops with Warm Zucchini Salad, *266,* 266–67

Greek-Style Braised Pork with Leeks, 282–83, *283*

Green Beans

Blistered, and Pepper Relish, Sautéed Tilapia with, 231

Braised, Tomatoes, and Feta, Pressure-Cooker Swordfish with, *316,* 317

Crudités, 373, *373*

Garlicky, Skillet-Roasted Chicken Breasts with, 197, *197*

Green Gumbo, *80,* 81

Pressure-Cooker Double Vegetable Beef Stew with Lemon Zest, 302–4, *303*

Three-Bean Salad with Arugula, *359,* 359–60

Tofu, and Shiitakes, Stir-Fried, *133,* 133–35

Turkey Meatballs, and Roasted Garlic Dressing, Quinoa Bowls with, *116,* 116–17

Greens

dark leafy, health benefits, 6

see also specific greens

Guacamole, 370, *370*

Gumbo, Green, *80,* 81

Gut-friendly foods, 7

Gut health, 18

H

Haddock

Chraime, 252–54, *253*

Pressure-Cooker, with Tomatoes, Escarole, and Crispy Garlic, 315–16, *316*

Hake

Provençal Fish Soup, *60,* 61

Haldhicha Dudh, 406–7, *407*

with Black Pepper, 407

with Ginger, 407

Halibut

Baked, with Cherry Tomatoes and Chickpeas, 242, *243*

Braised, with Carrots and Coriander, 250–51, *251*

Lemon-Poached, with Roasted Fingerling Potatoes, *240,* 240–41

Pressure-Cooker, with Couscous and Ras el Hanout, 318

Puttanesca, *254,* 254–55

and Soba, Miso Dashi Soup with, *60,* 61–62

Harira, Chicken, Pressure-Cooker, *299,* 299–300

Harissa, 106

-Mint Carrots, Skillet-Roasted Chicken Breasts with, 196, *197*

Roasted Carrot and Beet Salad with, *90,* 106

-Rubbed Chicken Thighs with Charred Cucumber and Carrot Salad, *206,* 206–7

Hash

Brussels Sprout, *28,* 29

Smoked Trout, *28,* 28–29

Hawaij, 68

Hawaij Cauliflower Soup, Creamy, with Zhoug, *66,* 67–68

Hazelnuts

Cherries, and Cacao Nibs, Chewy Granola Bars with, 382, *383*

Chopped Winter Salad with Butternut Squash and Apple, 104, *105*

and Goat Cheese, Lentil Salad with, 341

Orange, and Hazelnuts, Carrot "Tabbouleh" with, 361

Hemp hearts

Green Granola, 42, *43*

Herb(s)

fresh, storing, 75

Herbes de Provence Chickpea Crackers, 378

and Lemon, Quinoa Pilaf with, 332, *332*

-Yogurt Sauce, 166

see also specific herbs

Hibiscus

Iced Tea, 387–88

Vinaigrette and Roasted Vegetables, Curried Fonio with, 172–73, *173*

Hominy

Pressure-Cooker Pork Pozole Rojo, *304,* 304–5

White Chicken Chili, 87–88

Honey

Haldhicha Dudh, 406–7, *407*

Haldhicha Dudh with Black Pepper, 407

Haldhicha Dudh with Ginger, 407

-Orange Yogurt, 45

Honeydew-Lemon Agua Fresca, 396–97

Horsetail

Emoliente, 391

Emoliente with Alfalfa and Anise, 391

Emoliente with Chamomile, 391

Hummus

Artichoke-Lemon, 365

Classic, *362,* 365

Roasted Red Pepper, 365

and Sprouts, Fried Egg Sandwiches with, 26, *27*

Sweet Potato, *364,* 365–66

Hydration, 3

I

Immunitea Herbal Tea Blend, 392, *393*

Inflammation, 2, 18

see also Chronic inflammation

Insoluble fiber, 7

Italian Wedding Soup with Kale and Farro, *60,* 60–61